D1265896

INJURY AND VIOLENCE PREVENTION

INJURY AND VIOLENCE PREVENTION

Behavioral Science Theories, Methods, and Applications

Andrea Carlson Gielen
David A. Sleet
Ralph J. DiClemente
Editors

Forewords by Martin Fishbein
and David C. Grossman

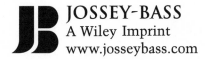

JOSSEY-BASS
A Wiley Imprint
www.josseybass.com

Published by Jossey-Bass
A Wiley Imprint
989 Market Street, San Francisco, CA 94103-1741   www.josseybass.com

Library of Congress Cataloging-in-Publication Data

Injury and violence prevention : behavioral science theories, methods, and
    applications / edited by Andrea Carlson Gielen, David A. Sleet, and Ralph
    J. DiClemente.
      p. cm.
    Includes bibliographical references and index.
    ISBN-13: 978-0-7879-7764-1 (alk. paper)
    ISBN-10: 0-7879-7764-0 (alk. paper)
    1. Accidents—United States—Prevention.   2. Wounds and injuries—
United States—Prevention.   3. Violence—United States—Prevention.
I. Gielen, A. C. (Andrea Carlson)   II. Sleet, David A.   III. DiClemente, Ralph J.
    [DNLM: 1. Accident Prevention—United States.   2. Behavior Therapy
  —United States.   3. Wounds and Injuries—prevention & control—United
States.   4. Violence—prevention & control—United States.   WA 250
I555   2006]
    HV676.A2I65 2006
    363.1—dc22   2005024318

Printed in the United States of America
FIRST EDITION
HB Printing   10 9 8 7 6 5 4 3 2 1

CONTENTS

FOREWORD

Every three minutes, someone in the United States dies from an injury due to such causes as fires and burns, poisons, falls, homicide, suicide, and motor vehicle crashes (Centers for Disease Control and Prevention, 2005). Unintentional injuries and violence are the leading cause of death for Americans from ages one to forty-four. But deaths due to injury are only part of the picture. Millions of Americans sustain nonfatal injuries each year. According to the Centers for Disease Control and Prevention (2005), there were almost 30 million nonfatal injuries requiring emergency care in 2004. In addition to being costly, nonfatal injuries often result in lifelong disability, chronic pain, and dramatic changes in an individual's lifestyle, including his or her ability to be gainfully employed.

But how does one prevent, or lessen the impact of, an injury? At least until recently, injury prevention science has primarily focused on product development and environmental engineering. As this book testifies, this focus has led to a significant decrease in injuries. Clearly the introduction of such products as seat belts, child car safety seats, bicycle helmets, fire-resistant clothing, and smoke alarms has significantly reduced both morbidity and mortality due to injury. In addition to introducing new products, injury prevention scientists have been involved in environmental redesign, making playgrounds and workplaces safer, for example, and in the promotion of safety legislation and other regulations. Thus, even more than most behavioral scientists, injury prevention scientists have taken an ecological perspective that has led them to pay important attention to the interaction between people and their environment.

But as this book recognizes, designing new products, redesigning environments, or passing legislation is only part of the battle. In order to reduce the public health burden of injury, people have to be aware of and appropriately use these products and environments and comply with the laws and regulations. There are literally dozens of behaviors that, if performed, would prevent or significantly reduce the impact of an injury. As the chapter authors so eloquently argue, most injuries have a behavioral component and are therefore preventable. Indeed, as is the case with many of our most pressing health problems, what one does is a critical determinant of whether one will or will not be injured. One immediate implication is the need for behavioral scientists to play a greater role in developing the science of injury prevention.

Fortunately, the social and behavioral sciences have come a long way in identifying the determinants of any given behavior. Indeed, as this book makes clear, a number of empirically supported theories of behavior and behavior change (among them, the health belief model, social cognitive theory, the theories of reasoned action and planned behavior, and protection motivation theory) are relevant to injury prevention. To a certain extent, by identifying a critical set of variables that are assumed to underlie any behavior, these theories provide the diagnostic tools necessary for behavioral understanding. Clearly, the more one knows about the determinants of a given behavior, the more likely is one to be able to develop effective interventions to reinforce or change that behavior.

Although this book provides excellent examples of the use of some of these theories in injury prevention, it recognizes that much more can be done. Indeed, following in the footsteps of such champions of prevention as Mayhew Derryberry in health education and William Haddon in injury control, this book challenges researchers in human behavior to test some of their theories in the area of injury prevention. But even more important than testing the applicability of theory for predicting and understanding injury-related behaviors, this book suggests that the real challenge is to demonstrate the usefulness of theory in designing, developing, and evaluating the effectiveness of injury prevention behavior change interventions.

Although I personally believe that behavior change should be at the heart of most injury prevention interventions, behavioral and social science researchers must not lose sight of the importance of legislation, product development, and environmental engineering. For example, increasing the likelihood that one will use seat belts, bicycle helmets, or smoke alarms is possible only if these products are available. And if application of behavioral theory indicates that the failure to use a particular safety product is related to one's beliefs that the product is uncomfortable, unaesthetic, or too difficult to use, a successful intervention should address product redesign. Injury prevention science is multidisciplinary, and effective injury prevention interventions are most likely to result when behavioral and social scientists work with a variety of other disciplines such as engineering, epidemiology, and law.

For behavioral and social scientists unfamiliar with, or interested in, injury prevention science, this book is required reading. It not only points to the critical role of behavior and behavior change in this domain, but raises important theoretical and methodological questions about technology transfer, behavioral maintenance, and appropriate designs for evaluating intervention effectiveness. Given the enormous public health burden associated with injury, it seems clear that those of us who are studying behavior and behavior change have an obligation to try to prevent both unintentional injuries and violence. I hope that this book, by suggesting new lines of research and multidisciplinary collaborations, will serve as a stimulus to behavioral and social scientists to participate more fully in this challenging and exciting field of injury prevention.

Martin Fishbein
Annenberg School for Communications
University of Pennsylvania

Reference

Centers for Disease Control and Prevention. (2005, July 6). *Web-based Injury Statistics Query and Reporting System (WISQARS)*. Retrieved Oct. 30, 2005, from www.cd.gov/ncipc/wisqars.

FOREWORD

When I was in medical school in the early 1980s, I learned that changing a patient's behavior was one of the most difficult challenges a doctor faced in medical practice. Lifestyle modification, medication adherence, and addictions were just a few of the thorny recurrent issues faced by primary care physicians, issues that might attract a Sisyphus into medicine. But I do not remember learning any of the principles, and certainly none of the art, of behavioral interventions. Not until my residency training did I began to learn about behavioral theory and behavior modification and how to practice the latter. I learned it from a psychologist who worked with medical doctors in the community.

A decade later, when I was receiving training in public health, I heard the same message about behavior and the challenge for public health researchers and practitioners interested in the same list of problems. Researchers could describe the boundaries of a public health problem, its associated risk and protective factors, and even its costs and prognosis, but few could speak with confidence about changing the behaviors that lay at the foundation of that problem. Soon, however, there would be many in public health with training as behavioral scientists who brought that skill to the problems of chronic disease prevention and health promotion. Only more recently have these skills been directed toward injury control.

Entering the field of injury control, I learned about William Haddon, a preventive medicine physician and visionary in automotive medicine who moved the long-standing discourse on motor vehicle injury prevention away from driver be-havior and toward vehicle safety and crashworthiness. During the 1960s, design changes to cars and highways were recognized to have a substantial impact on safety. Seat belts, collapsible steering wheels, breakaway light poles, and divided highways required technological advances and changes in vehicle and road de-sign standards to improve safety. Haddon's vision about the importance of vehi-cle and road environment change to prevent injury had a far-reaching impact on the design and manufacture of vehicles and roads, but little impact on the be-havioral side of the equation. Some of the major causes of crash deaths, such as behaviors of seat belt use, drunk driving, and speeding, still seemed out of reach during Haddon's time.

It was not long before the topic of human factors in the injury field resur-faced. In the mid-1980s, controversy erupted over the issue of whether automak-ers should be required to install air bags in cars (the passive solution) or whether seat belt use should be mandated (the active solution). In the eye of this intense debate lay some basic uncertainties about the likelihood for behavior change in injury control and the role of human factors, a prospect that made many injury control advocates uneasy.

As the field of injury control has matured as a recognizable discipline in pub-lic health, our paradigms require reexamination. Few purely passive solutions to injury control problems remain untapped. Even formerly "pure" solutions, such as air bags, have devolved into mixed solutions; for example, air bag on-off switches and the need to place children in the rear seat away from the air bag clearly demonstrate the need for behavioral change expertise. Numerous other in-jury problems requiring effective intervention share a similar need to address both engineering and behavioral solutions. Moreover, the complexity of human be-havior demands a paradigm that expands the well-rehearsed 3E model of pre-vention (education, enforcement, and engineering) into one that includes efforts to better explicate and positively influence the behavioral components of injury problems.

Our field is catching up. When the U.S. Institute of Medicine's (IOM) panel on Injury in America convened and issued its landmark report in 1987, only a sin-gle page in the entire 150-page document was devoted to the role of behavior change, and the tone was laden with skepticism. Biomechanics was heralded as the key basic science of injury control. When a new panel reconsidered the IOM report in 1997, much more extensive mention was made of the need for research in the behavioral sciences, such as risk perception and risk-taking research and more extensive study of social and behavioral antecedents and consequences of injury. Cross-disciplinary research was openly encouraged among public health, medicine, and social and behavioral scientists.

Many in our field now recognize that behavior is at the foundation for many injuries and that behavior change, in addition to the other approaches we use, is needed to prevent injuries. Preventing injuries and violence will require greater efforts to understand behaviors, attitudes, and community norms that lead to injury and also identify effective behavioral change interventions. Ultimately the best solutions will combine innovative approaches to modifying individual and community behavior, along with technical and environmental factors that enable and reinforce behavior change.

Gielen, Sleet, and DiClemente have crossed the divide, bringing together contributors who are both behavioral scientists and injury prevention professionals. This fine book is part of the evolutionary change taking place in our field and represents a review of the best thinking on the subject of behavior change theory and applications in injury control. It will be of great interest to researchers who are looking for new intervention paradigms and practitioners who want to apply the fundamentals. The chapters address state-of-the-art theoretical frameworks, as well as examples of practical applications of these theories in intervention design and evaluation. These are the principles and applications most of us missed out on in our training, and few are getting even today. After reading this book, I would argue that behavior change theory has become one of the basic sciences for many of us in injury control, public health, and preventive medicine. Our successes in the future will partly hinge on how well we adapt and integrate these models into the interventions of tomorrow.

David C. Grossman
Center for Health Studies
Group Health Cooperative
Seattle, Washington

PREFACE

Injuries and violence exact a substantial toll on the public's health and are the leading cause of death of children and young adults in the United States. Injury prevention draws on the full breadth and depth of other scientific disciplines, practices, and knowledge, and behavioral science is among its most important underpinnings. Human behavior contributes in many ways as a causal factor in injuries and an essential element for their prevention. According to the Centers for Disease Control and Prevention, the National Academy of Science's Institute of Medicine, and the American Psychological Association, behavioral science is one of the core disciplines in the field of injury prevention and control.

Much is being done to facilitate behavioral science research in the injury and violence prevention field. For example, federal support for funding theory-based approaches to injury prevention and behavioral safety is on the increase, and many behavioral scientists have joined federal agencies focusing on injury prevention and academic institutions supporting research in injury control. Over the past several years, national and international conferences on injury prevention and control, health education, and psychology have all included sessions featuring the work of behavioral scientists. Special issues of several scholarly journals have been devoted to behavioral and health promotion aspects of injury and violence prevention, and systematic reviews of injury prevention strategies have highlighted the need for more effective educational approaches and behavior change applications to injury and violence prevention. There is now a substantial body of published research demonstrating the contributions of behavioral science to injury and violence prevention.

The purpose of this book is to introduce the discipline of behavioral science and provide examples of its application to injury and violence prevention policies, programs, and research. In particular, the book emphasizes the specific theories, methods, and applications that make behavioral science approaches relevant and central to reducing injury-related harm. The growing appreciation for the role of behavioral science in addressing public health problems in general, and injuries in particular, makes this book especially timely. No current book brings together the behavior change theories and methods as they have been (or could be) applied to the problems of injuries and violence. With the scholarly and thoughtful contributions of each of our widely respected chapter authors, we are pleased to offer this first such text.

The book is divided into four parts. The chapters in Part One focus on some of the most frequently used behavior change theories and models and how they have been applied (or could be applied) to injury problems. The chapter authors describe specific theories and models and provide examples of how they can be used to understand and influence safety-related behaviors. Because risk communication is such a central element of much of the work in injury prevention, one chapter focuses on this topic. We also address theories that are appropriate at individual and community levels, as well as integrative models that are particularly useful for intervention planning, implementation, and evaluation.

The chapters in Part Two introduce the most commonly used research methods for understanding and influencing behavior change. One chapter explores basic descriptive correlational research that is particularly useful for conducting needs assessments of safety knowledge, attitudes, beliefs, and practices. Another chapter addresses intervention research and program evaluation, which are essential for planning, implementing, and evaluating behavior change interventions. The Appendix includes a listing of databases that will be useful for injury prevention research and program development.

Behavior change issues for specific injury topic areas are covered by the chapters in Part Three. Here we focus on both unintentional injuries (motor vehicle safety, including the role of alcohol; sports and recreational injuries; home injuries, including fires; and occupational injuries) and intentional injuries (intimate partner violence, self-directed violence, and youth violence). Each chapter provides information about the epidemiology of the injuries being addressed, behavioral risk and protective factors, and a discussion of the role of behavioral theory and behavior change experiences and options.

The chapters in Part Four are devoted to cross-cutting issues that have the potential to influence many injury risk behaviors simultaneously or are relevant to many injury outcomes, such as child supervision, posttraumatic stress, and the role of legislation and engineering in changing behavior and, more broadly, promoting injury prevention.

We hope this book will be a useful tool for interventionists. The field of injury and violence prevention is increasingly moving more toward intervention development, implementation, and dissemination, activities that cannot ignore the powerful influence of human behavior. For example, we know a great deal about how to prevent injuries; the effectiveness of bike helmets, smoke alarms, seat belts, and car safety seats has been demonstrated. A primary challenge in injury prevention is how to implement these interventions broadly in communities and among those particularly high-risk and vulnerable populations. Because this often requires an ecological approach, this challenge can be met by understanding the theories and methods of behavior change at multiple levels. Conceptual frameworks and methods from behavioral science are particularly critical for researchers interested in intervention trials and practitioners interested in program design, implementation, evaluation, and dissemination.

Most researchers in public health know and use contemporary behavior change theories and methods to combat infectious and chronic disease, but they rarely are trained in injury control. Paradoxically, injury professionals, usually trained in epidemiology and occupational and environmental health, are cognizant of the concepts related to injury content but lack specific training in behavior change theory or methods. We prepared this book to address this gap. We hope it will serve as a bridge to link the field of behavioral science with injury control.

Behavioral and social scientists have had a long-standing interest and involvement in public health research, but the careful use of behavioral science theories, methods, and applications to injury prevention is fairly recent. Even more recent is the integration of behavioral science research in injury prevention funding portfolios and curricula. It is our hope that the body of work in this book will encourage public health students, researchers, and practitioners to look carefully and creatively at ways to incorporate behavioral strategies into their injury and violence prevention work.

Acknowledgments

We acknowledge the many authors in this book who shared their research and knowledge of behavioral science and injury to make this book possible. They are among a small but growing number of researchers and practitioners who apply behavioral science principles to injury and violence prevention. Their commitment, enthusiasm, and persistence in documenting the impact of behavioral research on injury prevention will surely benefit the future health of communities, families, and individuals.

Andrea Carlson Gielen expresses her gratitude to the Johns Hopkins Bloomberg School of Public Health for providing sabbatical time to plan this book and to the Center for Injury Research and Policy for the stimulating and nurturing environment that helped bring the book to fruition (grant R49CCR302486, National Center for Injury Prevention and Control, Centers for Disease Control). She is grateful for her mentors and colleagues at the center and in the health education field, in particular, Ellen MacKenzie, Eileen McDonald, Susan Baker, Stephen Teret, Ruth Faden, and Lawrence Green. She thanks her family—Price, Ryan, Matthew, Andrew, and her parents, Friede and Ted—for their lifelong encouragement and support.

David A. Sleet acknowledges H. H. Leonards and Ted at the Mansion for providing a creative environment to write and Tavricheskiy National University in Simferopol, Ukraine, for solace during many writing visits. He thanks many who have contributed to his own development in health psychology: Ralph Grawunder, Bob Kaplan, Lindsay Carter, David Jenkins, Lawrence Green, Don Iverson, Bruce Bigelow, Charles Watson, and the late Mayhew Derryberry, Marshall Becker, Herbert Spiegelberg, Ernst Jokl, and Lizette Peterson, whom he never got to thank personally while they were still alive. He thanks his wife, Louise Gobron, without whose entertaining company this book might have been written much earlier.

Ralph J. DiClemente acknowledges his family, his lovely wife, Gina Maria, and their beautiful daughter, Sahara Rae, for being the axis around which his world revolves. With their love, support, and encouragement, anything is possible.

Finally, we all thank Andy Pasternack, Seth Schwartz, Susan Geraghty, and the entire editorial staff at Jossey-Bass who encouraged us to write this book and helped bring it to completion. This book, which has been brewing in our minds for about eight years, might never have been published without their support.

January 2006

Andrea Carlson Gielen
Ellicott City, Maryland

David A. Sleet
Berkeley Lake, Georgia

Ralph J. DiClemente
Atlanta, Georgia

THE EDITORS

Andrea Carlson Gielen is professor in the Department of Health, Behavior and Society and director of the Center for Injury Research and Policy in the Department of Health Policy and Management at the Johns Hopkins Bloomberg School of Public Health. She has twenty-six years of public health experience, including as a health department practitioner and an academic researcher directing federally funded studies of health behaviors. For the Maryland Department of Health and Mental Hygiene, she directed Project KISS (Kids in Safety Seats), a comprehensive child passenger safety program that received a National Program of Excellence Award from the Society for Public Health Education. Her research focuses on interventions to prevent childhood injury and domestic violence, especially as they affect low-income, urban populations. Gielen's injury areas of special interest are home- and motor vehicle–related injuries in childhood, and current projects include evaluating theory-based computer-tailored kiosk interventions and a community-based, mobile safety center intervention. The Johns Hopkins Children's Safety Center and the CARES Mobile Safety Center, which were developed under grants that Gielen directed, are unique, interactive interventions bringing low-cost safety products and personalized education to families and communities. Gielen's research on domestic violence includes examining the relationship between human immunodeficiency virus risk and intimate partner violence risk among low-income, urban women and developing theory-based interventions to reduce these risks. She teaches courses in health education and health promotion, and behavioral sciences applications to injury prevention. Gielen serves on the editorial boards of *Health Education Research* and *Patient Education and Counseling.* She has served on technical advisory boards and as a consultant to a variety of governmental and private national and international organizations, including the American Academy of Pediatrics, the Centers for Disease Control and Prevention, Home Safety Council, and the World Health Organization. In 2002, Gielen received the Distinguished Career Award of the American Public Health Association's Public Health Education and Health Promotion Section.

David A. Sleet is the associate director for science in the Division of Unintentional Injury Prevention at the National Center for Injury Prevention and Control at the Centers for Disease Control and Prevention (CDC). He is the senior adviser to the division on matters of science and policy. Before joining CDC, he was professor of public health at San Diego State University in California, where he taught and conducted research in health psychology. He joined the National Highway Traffic Safety Administration as a research psychologist in the 1980s and directed the Road Accident Research Unit in Perth, Australia, in the 1990s. While in Australia, he developed the first distance learning course on injury prevention and developed a statewide injury control plan. As a research fellow in Finland, he conducted the first study in that country on air bag effectiveness and conducted sports injury research in Belgium. Sleet established the first International Working Group on Behavioral Science and Unintentional Injury Prevention. He was responsible for organizing the unintentional injury section of CDC's Injury Research Agenda and was coeditor of the 2004 *WHO World Report on Road Traffic Injury Prevention.* He is adjunct faculty at Curtin University (Perth, Australia) and on the teaching faculty of behavioral science and health education at the Rollins School of Public Health at Emory University in Atlanta. Sleet has contributed more than 150 articles, book chapters, and reports on injury prevention, health promotion, and preventive medicine. He is a recipient of the American Public Health Association's Derryberry Award for his outstanding contributions to theory and practice in public health, the Society for Automotive Engineering "best paper" award for identifying the challenges in traffic safety and public health, the ASTEPPHE Health Education Advocacy Award, and, with colleagues at CDC, he won the Secretary of HHS Excellence in Research Award for his work on preventing alcohol-impaired driving. He is a member of the American Psychological Association and a fellow of the American Academy of Health Behavior.

Ralph J. DiClemente is Charles Howard Candler Professor of Public Health in the Rollins School of Health (Department of Behavioral Sciences and Health Education) and Emory University School of Medicine (Department of Pediatrics, Division of Infectious Diseases, Epidemiology, and Immunology, and Department of Medicine, Division of Infectious Diseases, and Department of Psychiatry). He is also the associate director for prevention sciences, Emory/Atlanta Center for AIDS Research. DiClemente has had a diverse array of research experiences, serving in a county public health department, an ethnic minority community-based organization, and academic institutions. Much of his research is applied, specifically dedicated to reducing health disparities among women and children through the application of social and behavioral sciences theory, techniques, and methods. DiClemente is particularly well versed in designing programs that use peer-based models of implementation and are culturally and developmentally appropriate. He has been the recipient of a number of awards, including the Prevention Pioneer Award in HIV/AIDS from the Morehouse School of Medicine and the Georgia Department of Community Health, Office of Minority Health, in 2005, and the Society for Adolescent Medicine/Organon Pharmaceutical Visiting Professorship in Adolescent Research, in 1999.

THE CONTRIBUTORS

John P. Allegrante is senior professor of health education at Teachers College, Columbia University, where he has been a member of the faculty since 1979, and is president of the National Center for Health Education. He holds appointments as adjunct professor of sociomedical sciences at the Mailman School of Public Health of Columbia University and adjunct professor of behavioral science in medicine at the Weill Medical College of Cornell University. His current research interests include developing and testing novel behavioral and educational strategies that can improve health behavior and health outcomes in people with chronic disease. Allegrante is the lead coeditor of *Derryberry's Educating for Health: A Foundation for Contemporary Health Education Practice* (Jossey-Bass) and the author of numerous book chapters and journal articles in health education and health promotion. A past president and Distinguished Fellow of the Society for Public Health Education, he is currently associate editor of *Health Education Research*. He received the Distinguished Career Award from the American Public Health Association Public Health Education and Health Promotion Section in 2003.

Joseph L. Annest has worked in injury prevention and control since 1988 and is director, Office of Statistics and Programming, National Center for Injury Prevention and Control, CDC, Atlanta, Georgia. His interests are to improve emergency department-based injury surveillance systems, develop internationally accepted injury surveillance guidelines and standards, and improve the availability of injury

statistics. During the past decade, Dr. Annest is known most for his work in helping to establish the National Electronic Injury Surveillance System-All Injury Program and the Web-based Injury Statistics Query and Reporting System
(WISQARS) (http://www.cdc.gov/ncipc/wisqars) that provides national data on
fatal and nonfatal injuries in the United States.

James P. Bliss is associate professor and Ph.D. programs director of psychology at
Old Dominion University. Prior to his arrival there he was a tenured associate
professor and chair of the Psychology Department at the University of Alabama-
Huntsville. Over the past twelve years, he has pursued research effort in two primary areas. Beginning with his doctoral dissertation, Bliss has studied the
occurrence of alarm (and automation) mistrust. Specifically, he is interested in
what factors contribute to the development of mistrust and how designers and
trainers can optimize compliance to automated systems. The second broad area
includes the use of virtual environments for task training. Bliss has worked with a
number of research laboratories (including Boeing, the U.S. Army, and the National Aeronautics and Space Administration) to design and test the effectiveness
of virtual environments for training complex tasks such as firefighting, soldiering,
and navigating unfamiliar environments. Bliss has served as an expert witness in
a number of product liability cases involving warnings and alarms.

Jessica G. Burke is assistant professor in the Department of Behavioral and Community Health Sciences at the University of Pittsburgh Graduate School of Public Health. She earned her Ph.D. in social and behavioral sciences and M.H.S. in
international health from the Johns Hopkins Bloomberg School of Public Health,
where she holds appointments in the Department of Population and Family
Health Sciences and in the Center for Injury Research and Policy. Burke is a behavioral scientist whose work has concentrated on the health and well-being of
women and children and the reciprocal relationship of health, behavior, and environment. She employs both ethnographic and social epidemiologic techniques
to explore the multiple levels of influencing factors associated with maternal and
child health problems such as intimate partner violence, youth violence, low birth
weight, and preterm delivery.

Kathryn M. Clinton is a principal at Northport Associates with wide research, program development, and evaluation experience in the fields of education, road
safety, health promotion, and energy emergency planning. At Northport Associates, she has led or contributed to R&D projects across a range of safety and injury prevention initiatives, including road safety policy, health and safety behavior
change, driver education and improvement, senior drivers, and program evaluation. She has extensive experience in research methods including literature and sys-

tematic reviews, in-depth telephone and face-to-face interviewing techniques, focus groups, and jurisdiction surveys. She specializes in qualitative research applications. Prior to entering consulting, Clinton held senior government policy development and management positions in the transportation and energy sectors. She designed, implemented, and managed education programs for seat belt use among school-age children and their parents, drinking among young drivers, and fuel-efficient driving behaviors. She coauthored *The Human Collision,* one of Canada's most influential traffic safety education publications. She also developed government policy on contingency plans for oil shortages and directed the development of detailed plans and procedures for implementation in the event of a shortfall in oil supplies. Clinton has recently completed a Master of Public Health degree and is pursuing a Ph.D. in population health at the University of Ottawa, Canada.

David W. Coombs is associate professor emeritus in the Department of Health Behavior, School of Public Health, University of Alabama at Birmingham. He earned a B.A. degree from Notre Dame University and a doctoral degree in sociology at the University of Florida. During much of his career, Coombs worked and taught extensively in Central and South America. He has worked in suicide prevention and research for thirty years and is currently interested in the role of primary care providers in identifying and assessing potentially suicidal patients. Recently he has worked on identifying risk factors and correlates of suicidal behavior among young African American males. He is a member of the Alabama Task Force for Suicide Prevention. Coombs's work with that organization involves developing a comprehensive state plan for suicide prevention.

Alex E. Crosby is a medical epidemiologist in the Division of Violence Prevention in the National Center for Injury Prevention and Control of the Centers for Disease Control and Prevention in Atlanta, Georgia. His work involves descriptive and analytical research and community technical assistance in prevention of self-directed violence, interpersonal violence among adolescents, firearm-related injuries, and assaultive violence among minorities. He completed two residencies, the first in family practice and the second in general preventive medicine and public health. He received his B.A. in chemistry from Fisk University in Nashville, his M.D. from Howard University College of Medicine in Washington, D.C., and his M.P.H. in health policy and management from Emory University School of Public Health in Atlanta, Georgia.

Courtney Landau Fleisher is a pediatric psychologist at LaRabida Children's Hospital in Chicago, Illinois. She earned her B.A. at Bates College and her M.A. and Ph.D. at Kent State University. Fleisher's research interests include traumatic stress reactions following medical events and patient/family–provider communication in health care environments and addressing psychosocial issues in medical settings. Currently, Fleisher provides clinical services to children experiencing traumatic medical events and their families. She also consults with medical staff to facilitate interactions among members of the treatment team and families. Fleisher's present research investigates application of a systems-based trauma treatment model to an inpatient medical setting.

Kimberley Freire is a doctoral candidate in the Health Behavior and Health Education Department at the University of North Carolina (UNC) and a predoctoral fellow at UNC's Cecil G. Sheps Health Services Research Center. She also works at UNC's Injury Prevention Research Center on evaluation and violence prevention projects. Freire is particularly interested in adolescent health, women's health, violence prevention, and family-centered prevention efforts, as well as community-driven prevention initiatives. She currently works on a process evaluation for a program to improve access to domestic violence and sexual assault services for women with disabilities and as an instructor and evaluation team member for a Centers for Disease Control and Prevention national violence primary prevention training initiative (PREVENT). Her dissertation work examines how parenting style and alcohol-related parenting practices influence rural adolescents' alcohol use. Freire received her master's degree in public health in social and behavioral sciences from Boston University. Prior to coming to UNC, she worked as a program evaluator for the Massachusetts Department of Public Health in its adolescent health and injury prevention units.

E. Scott Geller has taught and conducted research as a faculty member in the Department of Psychology at Virginia Polytechnic Institute and State University, better known as Virginia Tech, for more than three decades. He has published widely on the development and evaluation of behavior change interventions to improve quality of life. He is a Fellow of the American Psychological Association, the American Psychological Society, and the World Academy of Productivity and Quality Sciences. He is past editor of the *Journal of Applied Behavior Analysis* (1989–1992), current associate editor of *Environment and Behavior* (since 1982), and current consulting editor for *Behavior and Social Issues*, the *Behavior Analyst Digest*, and the *Journal of Organizational Behavior Management*. He has received numerous awards for his work, including the University Alumni Award for Excellence in Research, Alumni Outreach Award for real-world applications of behavioral science, and the University Alumni Award for Graduate Student Advising.

Deborah C. Girasek is the director of social and behavioral sciences and associate professor in the Department of Preventive Medicine and Biometrics at the Uniformed Services University of the Health Sciences (USUHS) in Bethesda, Maryland. Prior to joining the USUHS faculty, Girasek served as the director of health communications at Memorial Sloan-Kettering Cancer Center in New York City and as senior adviser for communications to the deputy assistant secretary for health (disease prevention and health promotion) in Washington, D.C. Girasek's research focuses on the psychosocial aspects of unintentional injury prevention. She is a strong advocate of conducting needs assessments and applying evidence-based strategies. She earned a Ph.D. in social and behavioral sciences from the Johns Hopkins University School of Public Health and an M.P.H. from the University of Michigan School of Public Health.

Lawrence W. Green served on the public health and medical faculties at the University of California at Berkeley, Johns Hopkins, Harvard, University of Texas, the University of British Columbia, Emory, and now the University of California at San Francisco. He served the Carter administration as the director of the Office of Health Information, Health Promotion, Physical Fitness and Sports Medicine (now the Office of Disease Prevention and Health Promotion) with a central role in the first round of the Healthy People objectives for the nation in health promotion and disease prevention. He retired in 2004 as Distinguished Fellow/Visiting Scientist at the Centers for Disease Control and director of the Office of Science and Extramural Research. He is now adjunct professor in the Department of Epidemiology and Biostatistics at the University of California at San Francisco. Among his more than three hundred chapters, monographs, and articles, four of his books have been widely adopted as college texts, including *Health Program Planning* (4th edition with Marshall Kreuter, 2005). He is on the editorial boards of twelve journals in the health sciences, past president of the Society for Public Health Education, fellow and research laureate of the Academy of Health Behavior, and recipient of the Award for Excellence, Distinguished Career, and Mayhew Derryberry awards of the American Public Health Association. Green received his M.P.H. and Dr.P.H. from the University of California at Berkeley.

Dale W. Hanson is the Tom and Dorothy Cook Research Fellow in Public Health with the School of Public Health and Tropical Medicine at James Cook University of Australia. He graduated from Flinders University of South Australia in 1982 with a degree in medicine. Hanson initially worked as a community family physician before returning to the hospital system to train in emergency medicine. He was awarded a fellowship of the Australasian College for Emergency Medicine in 1996. He has since worked as staff emergency physician at Mackay Base Hospital in regional Queensland. Concerned with the high rate of injury he observed during his clinical practice, he developed an interest in injury research and safety promotion, completing a master's degree in public health and tropical medicine at James Cook University in 2000. His research interests include ecological models of safety promotion with a particular focus on inducing and sustaining change within community social systems. In 2002 the Australian Injury Prevention Network awarded him its biennial award for meritorious practice in injury prevention.

Erin Heiden is a doctoral student in the department of Community and Behavioral Health, College of Public Health, the University of Iowa (UI). She is currently an Occupational Injury Prevention Fellow, sponsored by NIOSH and the Heartland Center for Occupational Health and Safety. Her primary research interests are the evaluation of injury prevention interventions and the effects of disability and injuries in the workplace. She has worked at UI's Injury Prevention Research Center on various research projects and with the Iowa Safe Kids Coalition to educate legislators about the importance of upgrading Iowa's child passenger safety legislation.

Ralph Hingson is the director of the Division of Epidemiology and Prevention Research at the National Institute on Alcohol Abuse and Alcoholism and professor at the Boston University School of Public Health Center to Prevent Alcohol Problems Among Young People. He has authored or coauthored over 120 research articles. In recognition of his research contributions, the Robert Wood Johnson Foundation honored Hingson in 2001 with its Innovators Combating Substance Abuse Award. In 2002, he received the Widmark Award, the highest award bestowed by the International Council on Alcohol Drugs and Traffic Safety, of which he is currently president-elect. In 2003, Mothers Against Drunk Driving instituted the Ralph W. Hingson Research in Practice Annual Presidential Award, with Hingson honored as its first recipient.

Darrell Hudson is a doctoral student in the Department of Health Behavior and Health Education at the University of Michigan, School of Public Health. His primary research interests are youth violence prevention and the relationship between health and poverty among urban African Americans. Recently Hudson and several colleagues from the Department of Health Behavior and Health Education and the Flint Youth Violence Prevention Center produced a short documentary that addresses themes of youth violence and viable catalysts for violence prevention from the perspective of high school youth in Flint, Michigan. Hudson received his master of public health in health behavior and health education from the University of Michigan and completed his bachelor of arts degree at Morehouse College. Prior to coming to Michigan, he was a National Institutes of Health Intramural Training Award recipient and completed a one-year research fellowship at the National Institute of Drug Abuse.

Nancy Kassam-Adams is codirector of the Center for Pediatric Traumatic Stress and associate director for Behavioral Research at TraumaLink, both at the Children's Hospital of Philadelphia. She is a licensed psychologist with training in clinical and school psychology and twenty years of clinical experience with children, adults, and families in a variety of clinical settings. Kassam-Adams's research interests include traumatic stress, psychological aspects of emergency care and injury, research ethics, and measure development. Her current research focuses on posttraumatic stress in ill and injured children and their parents, and on developing screening and secondary prevention protocols for traumatic stress in health care settings.

Jennifer Lasenby is a doctoral student in the Psychology Department at the University of Guelph. She received her master's degree from the University of Toronto in human development and applied psychology. While in Toronto she worked with the Toronto Catholic District School Board and the Hospital for Sick Children's Learning Disabilities Research Program as a research assistant. Her dissertation research, which is funded by the Ontario Neurotrauma Foundation, focuses on how individual child factors such as personality attributes influence risk compensation and how this information can be helpful in developing intervention programs to identify individuals who will be most likely to engage in injury risk activities.

Karen Liller is associate dean for academic affairs and a tenured full professor specializing in children's injury prevention and health education at the University of South Florida College of Public Health. Liller holds undergraduate and graduate degrees in medical technology, technical education, curriculum and instruction, and public health. Her teaching, research, and service activities largely focus on health education and the prevention and control of children's unintentional injuries. She has been the recipient of a University of South Florida Faculty Excellence Award and a University Teaching Award for Excellence in Graduate Teaching. Liller has been the recipient of several national and state grants related to injury prevention and has published extensively on this topic. She served as the education director of the Deep-South Agricultural Health and Safety Center funded by the National Institute for Occupational Safety and Health. Through this grant, she established the Florida Farm Safety 4 Just Kids chapter. Liller is a member of several health education/health behavior and injury prevention professional associations and societies, including the American Academy of Health Behavior and the Eta Sigma Gamma national health education professional honorary. She serves on several prestigious advisory boards statewide and nationally that focus on health behavior and injury prevention.

Lawrence P. Lonero is principal at Northport Associates and has many years' experience in human factors R&D and administration aimed at motor vehicle injury prevention. He combines a background of graduate study in psychology and a lifelong interest in vehicles and driving. He is trained and experienced in advanced driving techniques for automobiles and motorcycles. He is an internationally recognized authority on the driving task and methods of influencing driver behavior. Prior to entering consulting, he held senior government positions in R&D, program management, and strategic management in transportation safety. He conducted R&D and policy development and managed the public information program that led to North America's first seat belt use law. He has been responsible for program development, evaluation, regulation, and administration of driver education, driver licensing, and driver improvement. He maintains a strong interest in safety strategy, policy development, and government relations. He has training and ongoing interest in regulatory theory and practice, as well as experience with policy development processes at provincial ministry and cabinet levels. He is a member of the Canadian Association Road Safety Professionals, the Transportation Research Board Committee on Operator Education and Regulation, the American Evaluation Association, and the judges' panel for the PACE Awards for Innovation in the Automotive Supply Industry.

John B. Lowe is professor and head of the Department of Community and Behavioral Health in the College of Public Health at the University of Iowa. Lowe received his doctorate in community health from the University of Texas Health Science Center, School of Public Health. He is a fellow of the Australia Health Promotion Association and a fellow of the American Academy of Health Behavior. Lowe also holds an honorary professorship at the University of Queensland, School of Population Health, and James Cook University in Australia. He is currently the principal investigator and director of the Centers for Disease Control and Prevention–funded Prevention Research Center of Iowa. Lowe is a member of the executive committee of the Iowa Injury Prevention Research Center and is director of the evaluation Core. His research interests are in injury prevention and cancer control and prevention. Lowe continues to focus on community development to make sustainable, long-term changes to promote health. He has received numerous grants from the National Institutes of Health, the Commonwealth of Australia, state and local groups, private foundations, and corporations. He is widely published and serves on a number of editorial boards of national and international journals.

Morag MacKay has been the director of Plan-it Safe, the child and youth injury prevention center at the Children's Hospital of Eastern Ontario in Ottawa since its establishment in July 1997. Since 1998, she has helped secure over $1.5 million in grants to support local research and program evaluation initiatives. MacKay has an undergraduate degree in nursing science and a graduate degree in medical science with a specialization in epidemiology. Her professional activities have largely focused on the prevention and control of children's unintentional injuries, and she has been involved in injury prevention projects in Canada at the national, provincial, and local levels. She is a founding member of the Canadian Collaborative Centres for Injury Prevention and Control and the Canadian Injury Research Network. Her contributions to the field over the past ten years have been in the areas of strategic planning for injury control, injury surveillance, education, research, program planning, and evaluation. MacKay is taking a two-year leave from her position at Plan-it Safe to pursue a Ph.D. and manage a project for the European Child Safety Alliance. The project, which involves working with eighteen countries in Europe on the development of national child safety action plans, brings together her areas of interest: surveillance, best practice, and policy development.

Ray Marks is associate director at the National Center for Health Education and adjunct associate professor of health education at Teachers College, Columbia University. In 2000, she was the recipient of a SOPHE/CDC Injury Prevention Fellowship Award. Marks has been an Andrew Stewart Research Scholar and a Province of Alberta Fellow in Canada, a John Dewey Scholar at Teachers College, and the recipient of a New York Arthritis Foundation Dissertation Research Fellowship Award. She has conducted numerous professional presentations worldwide, authored or coauthored many publications, and served as a consultant to numerous universities, research groups, and consortia across the globe in the areas of chronic arthritis management and prevention of arthritis-related disability. She currently cochairs the Society for Public Health Education Ethics Committee.

Eileen M. McDonald is an associate scientist at the Johns Hopkins Bloomberg School of Public Health in the Department of Health, Behavior and Society and a member of the core faculty of the Center for Injury Research and Policy in the Department of Health Policy and Management. Her research focuses on the application of innovative health education methods, health communication technology, and other hospital- and community-based interventions aimed at reducing pediatric injuries. Her work has involved the development and evaluation of the Johns Hopkins Children's Safety Center (CSC), a hospital-based safety resource center, and a community-based mobile version of the CSC. McDonald has developed injury prevention curricula and training for groups as diverse as day care providers in Philadelphia and the World Health Organization for use in schools of public health and medicine around the world. She has authored a nationally distributed guidebook for child safety and numerous research articles on injury prevention and health education topics. She codirects the school's master's degree training program in behavioral sciences and health education. She has received the Early Career Award and Mohan Singh Award from the American Public Health Association's Public Health Education and Health Promotion Section, as well as awards for teaching and mentoring.

Karen A. McDonnell is assistant professor of maternal and child health at the George Washington University School of Public Health and Health Services. She is a public health psychologist who has conducted research and published a number of peer-reviewed articles on intimate partner violence, its consequences, research needs, and future directions to be taken by the intervention community. She has worked with research and advocacy teams at the local and national levels to investigate the needs of abused women from countries throughout the world. McDonnell is particularly interested in investigating cultural factors associated with the experience of intimate partner violence. She earned her Ph.D. in social and behavioral sciences from the Johns Hopkins Bloomberg School of Public Health, where she currently holds appointments in the Women and Children's Health Policy Center of the Department of Population and Family Health Sciences and the Center for Injury Research and Policy in the Department of Health Policy and Management. Her injury research focuses on the psychosocial aspects of intimate partner violence and children's unintentional injury prevention and the integration of innovative qualitative and quantitative techniques for injury prevention research.

Susan Morrel-Samuels is the managing director of the Prevention Research Center of Michigan and Flint's Youth Violence Prevention Center at the University of Michigan School of Public Health. She has managed numerous projects relating to community health and health policy. These have included an assessment and plan for family and children's services in Kent County, Michigan; evaluations of the Michigan Partnership to Prevent Gun Violence and the Genesee County Neighborhood Violence Prevention Collaborative; and Youth Empowerment Solutions for Peaceful Communities. She codirected the Flint Photovoice project, an innovative research strategy using photography for community assessment. Morrel-Samuels teaches a course on youth violence at the University of Michigan School of Public Health. Prior to joining the University of Michigan, she was a program manager and trainer for Hawaii Healthy Start, a child abuse and neglect prevention program that has been widely replicated throughout the United States.

Barbara A. Morrongiello is a professor in the Psychology Department at the University of Guelph. She received her Ph.D. from the University of Massachusetts-Amherst after training in developmental psychology, and child clinical and pediatric health psychology. She has conducted extensive research to identify key factors that elevate children's risk of unintentional injury, with particular interest in understanding why school-age children make decisions to engage in play behaviors that can lead to injury and why parents of toddlers and preschool children make decisions that elevate young children's risk of injury at home. She is also involved in the application of these findings to support the development and evaluation of education and prevention programs to reduce the incidence of children's injuries at home, on playgrounds, and at school. She has numerous grants from the Social Sciences Research Council of Canada and the Canadian Institutes of Health Research, has published extensively, currently serves on the editorial boards of a number of journals, and has been awarded fellow status by the Developmental Psychology Division of the American Psychological Association.

Tonja Nansel is an investigator at the National Institute of Child Health and Human Development, Prevention Research Branch. Previously she was a psychiatric nurse in adolescent and adult units, an emergency room psychiatric nurse consultant, and a home health nurse and research/development coordinator. She then worked with Kansas State Extension Office of Community Health, facilitating various local and state community health promotion programming. She has taught courses in general psychology, health psychology, and research methods at Wichita State University. Nansel's current research focuses on the integration of prevention and health promotion interventions within the health care setting. Nansel received her bachelor of science in nursing from Fort Hays State University and her doctoral degree in community/clinical psychology from Wichita State University.

Patricia J. O'Campo is professor in public health sciences at the University of Toronto, Alma and Baxter Richard Endowed Chair in Inner City Health, and the Director at the Centre for Research on Inner City Health at the St. Michael's Hospital in Toronto. She is adjunct professor in the Department of Population and Family Health Sciences at the Johns Hopkins Bloomberg School of Public Health. O'Campo's research interests include social epidemiology focused on women's and children's health and health policy. She is active in many academic societies and is currently president of the International Society of Urban Health. Her scholarly and methodological contributions in the area of women's and children's health have been recognized by national organizations as she was given the Young Professional Award by the Maternal and Child Health Section of the American Public Health Association and later a mid-career award in research on Families and Children by the National Academy of Sciences. She has had a long-standing research interest in the determinants and prevention of partner violence against women. Other interests include welfare reform and women's health; prevention of HIV infection in women; perinatal outcomes with a particular focus on infant mortality and preterm birth prevention; and children's health and development.

Christopher P. Ogolla, currently a law student at Thurgood Marshall School of Law, was an Association of Schools of Public Health/Centers for Disease Control and Prevention Research fellow at the time of writing this book. He works in the Strategic Workforce Activity unit within the Office of Workforce and Career Development, CDC. Ogolla received his B.A. in anthropology from the University of Nairobi, Kenya, and both his M.A. in anthropology and M.P.H. from the University of Massachusetts, Amherst. Prior to coming to CDC, he worked for the New York State Department of Health as a public health representative, Division of Tuberculosis Control and Elimination, and as an adjunct faculty member in the Health and Society Program, State University of New York at Old Westbury. While at the New York State Department of Health, he also served as a health management development fellow, Office of Strategic Consulting and Organization Performance Enhancement.

Bryan E. Porter is associate professor and assistant chair of psychology at Old Dominion University in Norfolk, Virginia. His area of emphasis is behavioral community psychology, focusing on community problems and psychology's role in solving those problems. He has studied techniques for increasing driving safety, pedestrian safety, fire safety, and environmental action. He is a member of the International Association of Applied Psychology, for which he is the North American representative for Division 13 (Traffic and Transportation Psychology). Porter, as principal investigator, co-principal investigator, or research mentor, has received research funding from the Virginia Department of Motor Vehicles, Daimler-Chrysler Corporation, the Centers for Disease Control and Prevention, and the National Science Foundation. He has also worked to establish community partnerships to target driver and pedestrian safety in particular. His partners have included media, engineering, and enforcement agencies. The media regularly call on Porter to be an expert interviewee for various traffic safety issues. He has also assisted in Virginia public policy debates over traffic safety initiatives.

Carol W. Runyan is professor of health behavior and health education and of pediatrics at the University of North Carolina (UNC). Since 1989, she has been director of the UNC Injury Prevention Research Center. She has served as a member of the Centers for Disease Control and Prevention's Advisory Committee for Injury Prevention and Control and the U.S. Armed Forces Epidemiologic Board. She is a founding member of the board of directors of the National Association of Injury Control Research Centers and leads the National Training Initiative on Injury and Violence Prevention as well as the PREVENT Program, a national violence prevention training effort. Runyan's research has focused on injuries to adolescents, violence against women, home safety, and occupational injury as well as conceptual issues in injury control. She is the recipient of the Outstanding Service Award of the State and Territorial Injury Prevention

Directors Association, the Excellence in Science Award from the American Public Health Association Injury Control and Emergency Health Services Section, and the Secretary of Defense Metal for Outstanding Public Service, and she was inducted into the Johns Hopkins University Society of Scholars. She was educated at Macalester College, University of Minnesota, University of North Carolina, and Johns Hopkins University.

Frederic E. Shaw is a medical officer in the Public Health Law Program at the Centers for Disease Control and Prevention (CDC) in Atlanta, Georgia. He received his medical training at the University of Vermont College of Medicine, Burlington, the State University of New York-Downstate, New York City, and the Medical Center Hospital of Vermont. He studied law at Columbia and Harvard universities and is a member of the New Hampshire bar. At CDC, he trained in applied epidemiology in the Epidemic Intelligence Service and later served as a staff epidemiologist at the Hepatitis Branch, Division of Viral Diseases, National Center for Infectious Diseases. Prior to returning to CDC in 2001, he served as the New Hampshire state epidemiologist, New Hampshire Division of Public Health Services, Concord; staff counsel to the U.S. Senate Committee on Health, Education, Labor, and Pensions, Washington; assistant health commissioner for policy and planning at the Texas Department of Health, Austin; and as a private consultant. He works and writes in public health law.

Bruce Simons-Morton is chief of the Prevention Research Branch (PRB), Division of Epidemiology, Statistics, and Prevention Research, National Institute of Child Health and Human Development, NIH, where he directs an intramural research group at NIH devoted to child and adolescent health behavior. The PRB program of research focuses on preventing motor vehicle crashes among young drivers, preventing adolescent problem behavior, and promoting family management of childhood injury and disease. He is the author of the second edition of the textbook, *Introduction to Health Education and Promotion,* and has published over one hundred journal articles, books, and book chapters. Simons-Morton is a fellow of the American Academy of Health Behavior and previously was chair of the Public Health Education Section of the American Public Health Association and vice president of the Society of Public Health Educators. He was educated at San Diego State University (M.S.), the University of Northern Colorado (Ed.D.), and Johns Hopkins University (M.P.H.). Previously he held academic positions at Temple University, the University of Texas Medical Branch, and the University of Texas School of Public Health.

Nancy J. Thompson is associate professor of behavioral sciences and health education, jointly appointed in epidemiology, in the Rollins School of Public Health of

Emory University. Prior to her appointment at Emory, she spent fifteen years with the Centers for Disease Control and Prevention (CDC) as a statistician and epidemiologist. She has been working in the field of unintentional injury since the mid-1980s, publishing a number of articles related to injuries in youth, particularly sports injuries. Since 1993, she has worked closely with the Division of Unintended Injury Prevention of the National Center for Injury Prevention and Control, CDC. In this capacity, she authored *Demonstrating Your Program's Worth: A Primer on Evaluation for Programs to Prevent Unintentional Injury*, and also worked on models of behavior to increase the use of bicycle helmets, smoke alarms, and child safety seats. Thompson has taught courses in the behavioral sciences in public health, social behavior, behavioral theory, and behavioral epidemiology as well as research design, basic epidemiology, and statistics.

Lara B. Trifiletti is assistant professor in the Department of Pediatrics in the College of Medicine and Public Health at the Ohio State University and an investigator in the Center for Injury Research and Policy at the Columbus Children's Research Institute. Prior to joining the OSU faculty, Trifiletti was an assistant scientist in the Department of Health Policy and Management at the Johns Hopkins Bloomberg School of Public Health. She received a national award for her dissertation proposal from the Society for Public Health Education and U.S. Centers for Disease Control and Prevention. Her research interests in the field of public health broadly include social and behavioral sciences and child injury prevention and control. To date, her research has focused on the health of low-income children and the delivery of injury prevention counseling, with specific attention to injuries that occur in and around the home, as well as the delivery of injury prevention interventions in the pediatric emergency department and the community. Trifiletti received her M.A. in psychology from the Catholic University of America and Ph.D. in social and behavioral sciences from the Johns Hopkins Bloomberg School of Public Health.

Leigh Willis is assistant professor in the Department of Sociology and Institute of African-American Studies. Willis is a medical sociologist and a public health practitioner who earned his Ph.D. and M.P.H. from the University of Alabama, Birmingham. His areas of expertise are health (epidemiology, health education and promotion, program evaluation, health communication, intervention development); racial and ethnic studies (cultural competency); and popular culture (Internet, youth, urban, and various subcultures). Willis is also skilled in program evaluation, and cultural communication. He completed a two-year Association of Teachers of Preventive Medicine Fellowship in the Division of Violence Prevention at the Centers for Disease Control and Prevention. He has conducted studies and published works in the areas of STI/HIV risk, mental health, health disparities, substance abuse, violence prevention, and African American health.

Jingzhen Yang is assistant professor in the Department of Community and Behavioral Health, College of Public Health, University of Iowa, and a member of the University of Iowa Injury Prevention Research Center. She received her master's in public health from Indiana University at Bloomington and doctorate in health behavior and health education from University of North Carolina (UNC) at Chapel Hill. Prior to coming to the United States, she was associate professor at Suzhou University, China. While studying at UNC, Yang has worked with the biostatistical core of North Carolina Injury Prevention Research Center and engaged in several injury prevention research projects. Her doctoral work at UNC investigated intrapersonal, interpersonal, and organizational factors related to high school athletes' use of discretionary protective equipment (protective equipment not required by rules) and sport injury. Her current work has largely focused on youth sports injury prevention and control. In 2004, she received Best Paper Award in the Student Paper Competition of the Injury Control and Emergency Health Services Section of the American Public Health Association.

Marc A. Zimmerman is professor and chair in the Department of Health Behavior and Health Education in the School of Public Health at the University of Michigan. He is also a professor in psychology and the combined program in education and psychology, and a research scientist in the Center for Human Growth and Development. He received his Ph.D. in psychology from University of Illinois. Zimmerman is the director of the Centers for Disease Control (CDC)–funded Prevention Research Center of Michigan. He is also the principal investigator for the CDC-funded Youth Violence Prevention Center, a National Institute on Drug Abuse–funded longitudinal study designed to investigate adolescent resiliency, and a youth violence prevention program that involves youth in community change activities. Zimmerman is the editor of *Health Education and Behavior* and a member of the editorial board for *Health Education Research*. His primary research interests include application and development of empowerment theory and the study of adolescent health and resiliency. He has published on a wide variety of topics, including adolescent mental health, school outcomes, social relationships, racial identity, violence, sexual behavior, substance abuse, HIV/AIDS prevention, and empowerment theory.

INJURY AND VIOLENCE PREVENTION

CHAPTER ONE

Injury Prevention and Behavior

An Evolving Field

Andrea Carlson Gielen, David A. Sleet

Despite substantial gains in reducing some types of unintentional and violent injuries, these remain the leading cause of death from ages one to forty-four in the United States (Centers for Disease Control and Prevention, 2005). In fact, injuries are an increasing burden globally, with motor vehicle crashes projected to move from being the ninth leading cause of death in the world in 1990 to becoming the third leading cause of death by the year 2020 (Peden et al., 2004). Ironically, this projection comes at a time when we know more about effective prevention strategies than ever before. For example, the protective effect of seat belts, child auto restraint devices and bicycle helmets is irrefutable (National Highway Traffic Safety Administration, 2004; National Safe Kids Campaign, 2003; Marshall et al., 1998; Doll, Mercy, Bonzo, & Sleet, 2006). For these interventions, the challenge is to increase dissemination and adoption of preventive behaviors and practices. For other interventions less well researched, the challenges are in developing and testing promising interventions. In either case, the benefit of using, adapting, or applying behavior change theory, principles, and methods is clear.

There are numerous products, practices, and programs that can save lives, but many people have either not heard about them or have not accepted and

Portions of this section are reproduced with permission from Elsevier, Ltd., for Gielen A. C. (2002). Injury and violence prevention: A primer. *Patient Education and Counseling, 46,* 163–169.

adopted them. Many people do not see the need to change, do not perceive themselves to be at risk, or do not have access to affordable safety products or programs that could save their lives. Behavioral scientists can help remedy this situation.

In other cases, product or environmental redesign or new laws and regulations could benefit safety. For example, playgrounds could be designed in such a way as to reduce injury risk behaviors or minimize injury in a fall. Hazardous equipment at workplaces could be designed to minimize workers' unsafe behaviors and the likelihood of dangerous man-machine interactions. Here, roles for behavioral scientists include helping others to understand how to influence employers, city planners, product designers, and decision makers who have the authority to change the culture of safety. Studying the interaction among environments, products, and human behavior is an important role for behavioral scientists, as is facilitating the dissemination and adoption of best practices. Health psychology as a discipline has been slow to recognize this role in injury prevention, but this situation is improving (Spielberger & Frank, 1992; Sleet, Hammond, Jones, Thomas, & Whitt, 2004).

Just as behavioral scientists have made significant contributions to the prevention and control of other health-related behaviors (for example, human immunodeficiency virus and sexually transmitted diseases, asthma, overeating, smoking, and drug use), there are new opportunities to use their tools, skills, and concepts to address the problem of injuries. As DiLillo, Peterson, and Farmer (2002) point out, "More people are beginning to recognize that, for injury control to be effective, behavior must change among some groups, such as children, parents, legislators, manufacturers, and educators. . . . Furthermore, many of the constructs with which psychologists are most conversant (e.g. motivation, perception, learning) are thought by many to be the key determinants of injury-related behaviors" (p. 565).

In this chapter, we trace the development of injury prevention as a field and highlight the evolving role of behavior change. We start with a description of the magnitude of the injury problem in the United States, followed by a brief introduction to the principles of injury prevention. We conclude with a discussion and examples of behavior change that could reduce the toll of injuries.

The Injury Problem

Whether by violent or unintentional means, injury exacts a large toll on individuals, families, workplaces, and the community. Despite the presence of many effective interventions, there were more than 160,000 injury-related fatalities in the United States in 2002 (Centers for Disease Control and Prevention, 2005). In addition, in 2003, there were almost 30 million nonfatal incidents requiring emergency department care (Centers for Disease Control and Prevention, 2005). In too many of these situations, effective interventions existed but were not available to or not used by practitioners or other end users.

Because injuries and violence disproportionately affect the young, their impact on years of potential life lost (YPLLs) is great. By the year 2020, motor vehicle crashes are projected globally to rank second behind ischemic heart disease in YPLLs, ahead of cerebrovascular disease, cancer, and HIV. Violence and suicide rank eleventh and thirteenth, respectively. Disability-adjusted life-years (DALYs), a measure of the population burden of nonfatal injuries, projected for the year 2020, indicate that motor vehicle crashes, violence, and self-inflicted injuries will be in the top fifteen causes of DALYs (Murray & Lopez, 1996).

In the United States, unintentional injuries represent the first leading cause of death for individuals ages one to thirty-four and the fifth leading cause of death overall. Homicide and suicide figure prominently as well and, when they are combined with unintentional injuries, make injuries the leading cause of death for ages one to forty-four (Centers for Disease Control and Prevention, 2005). Years of potential life lost are greater for injuries than for any of the other leading causes of death in the United States.

Injury rates vary by geography, individual characteristics, and type of injury. For example, Fingerhut and Warner's analyses of U.S. data (1997) found the following:

- Unintentional injury death rates were higher in nonmetropolitan counties than in metropolitan counties, whereas the opposite was true for homicide rates.
- Injury death rates were higher for males than females in all age groups except infancy.
- Of violent crimes reported in the National Crime Victimization Survey, 43 percent were crimes against women, and women are more likely than men to be victimized by an intimate partner.
- For infants and children under age fifteen, motor vehicles, fires and burns, drowning, suffocation, and firearms accounted for 80 percent of all injury deaths.
- For males ages fifteen to twenty-four, the firearm death rate was 32 percent higher than the motor vehicle injury death rate.
- Among those over the age of seventy-five, three out of five injury hospitalizations were due to fractures, half of which were hip fractures, and for those over age eighty-five, falls caused one-third of all injury deaths.

A complete discussion of injury epidemiology is beyond the scope of this chapter. Interested readers are referred to existing textbooks (Barss, Smith, Baker, &

Mohan, 1998; Baker, O'Neill, Ginsburg, & Li, 1992; Robertson, 1992; Christoffel & Gallagher, 1999; McClure, Stevenson, & McEvoy, 2004) and national databases available online (Centers for Disease Control and Prevention, 2005; National Center for Health Statistics, 2005). (See Appendix this volume.)

The development of modern injury prevention is typically credited to the work of William Haddon (a physician and engineer) who, beginning in the late 1960s, pulled together efforts of Hugh DeHaven (a physiology researcher), John Gordon (an epidemiologist), and James Gibson (an experimental psychologist) and refined the definitional and conceptual issues related to injury (Christoffel & Gallagher, 1999). Injuries are defined as "any unintentional or intentional damage to the body resulting from acute exposure to thermal, mechanical, electrical, or chemical energy or from the absence of such essentials as heat or oxygen" (National Committee for Injury Prevention and Control, 1989, p. 4). Of these, mechanical or kinetic energy contributes the most to injuries and is a concept that the public and professionals in the field need to understand. The impact on the human body of kinetic energy that results from any number of events (falling, crashing a car, or being shot, for example) will be a function of the mass and velocity involved. Understanding the basics of this concept will help the new mother understand why holding her baby in her lap in a car is a dangerous idea. In a 35 mile per hour crash into a rigid object, a twenty-pound baby will travel with a force of as much as eight hundred pounds and would be ripped out of anyone's arms (Christoffel & Gallagher, 1999). The goal of vehicle crush zones, air bags, seat belts, and car seats is to reduce the impact of the crash on the human body by absorbing some of the energy from the crash, slowing the transfer of energy over a longer period of time, and distributing the crash forces over a larger area of the body (Barss et al., 1998). According to Stevenson, Ameratunga, and McClure (2004, p. 37), "The conceptualization of energy as the causal agent has been acclaimed as the essential explanation for the dramatic success of injury control over the last 40 years."

Injury Prevention

Injury prevention opportunities have historically been conceptualized in three ways: Haddon matrix and countermeasures, passive versus active strategies, and the three E's (education, ergonomics, and enforcement).

Haddon Matrix and Countermeasures

The Haddon Matrix classifies injury by phases and factors, as described here. First, Haddon identified three phases of the injury problem (Barss et al., 1998; see also Chapter Seven, this volume):

Pre-event: Before the crash (or other injury event). What affects the likelihood that it will occur?

Event: During the crash (or other injury event). What affects the likelihood that someone will be injured?

Postevent: After the crash (or other injury event). What affects the outcomes once an injury has occurred?

Second, each of these has host, agent and vehicle, and environmental factors that are relevant to the injury and offer many opportunities for prevention.

Haddon (Haddon & Baker, 1981) then identified ten countermeasures that would prevent or interrupt the transfer of energy:

- Eliminating the production of the hazard
- Reducing the amount of energy contained in the hazard
- Preventing the release of the hazard
- Modifying the rate or spatial distribution of the hazard
- Separating the hazard in time or space from those to be protected
- Separating the hazard from those to be protected by a material barrier
- Modifying the relevant basic qualities of the hazard
- Making individuals more resistant to the hazard
- Countering the damage already done by the hazard
- Stabilizing, repairing, and rehabilitating the individual damaged

These countermeasures do not link specifically to the different phases of the Haddon matrix, although there are countermeasures appropriate for each cell. For example, four-sided pool fencing would separate people from the hazard and thus work at the pre-event phase by modifying the physical environment. Of course, simply installing a four-sided fence (modifying the environment) is not the complete solution. To ensure the fence keeps out unauthorized visitors, it must be of sufficient height to ward off climbers, and the gate to the fence must be self-closing and self-latching. Even environmental countermeasures must account for behavioral interactions that might negate or reduce their effectiveness.

Passive Versus Active Strategies

Passive strategies are those that require no action on the part of the individual being protected (for example, shatter-resistant windshields), whereas active strategies require some individual action (for example, buckling a seat belt; Haddon & Baker, 1981). Passive strategies have consistently been given preference in developing injury prevention programs, largely due to their remarkable success in other areas of public health (for example, water fluoridation or vaccination) However, even air bags, once hailed as the penultimate passive strategy, require the concomitant use of active strategies: buckling the seat belt and seating children in the rear of the vehicle (Sleet, 1984; Gielen & Sleet, 2003). While passive strategies are still preferred for their obvious appeal, many require some active behavioral interaction (Gielen & Sleet, 2003; Sleet & Gielen, 2004). For example, the passive strategy of child-resistant caps on medicines requires caregivers to replace the caps; smoke alarm batteries must be changed; factory-set hot water heater temperatures must not be manually raised. Although passive, all of these intervention strategies require some human interaction to achieve their full safety potential.

The Three E's

The original concepts behind the three E's (education, ergonomics, and enforcement) was put forth in 1973 by Susan Baker in the tenth edition of Sartwell's *Preventive Medicine and Public Health* (Baker, 1973; Pearn, Nixon, & Scott, 2004). In 1989, the National Committee for Injury Prevention and Control adopted a similar paradigm, labeling these approaches as education, engineering, and enforcement. Table 1.1 summarizes suggested criteria for these three strategies to be effective.

TABLE 1.1. CRITERIA FOR EFFECTIVE USE OF INJURY PREVENTION STRATEGIES.

Education	Engineering	Enforcement
Audience must be:	Modification must be:	Law or regulation must be:
Exposed to the appropriate information	Effective and reliable	Widely known and understood by the public
Understand and believe the information	Compatible with the environment	Acceptable to the public
Have resources and skills to take action on the information	Result in products that dominate the marketplace	Probability (or perceived probability) of enforcement is high
Derive benefit (or perceive a benefit) from taking action	Acceptable to the public	Punishment is (or is perceived to be) swift and severe
Be reinforced to maintain the change over time	Easily understood by the public	
	Properly used by the public	

Source: Based on Sleet and Gielen (1998).

Education was the mainstay of early injury prevention efforts because it was consistent with an orientation to injury causation that focused on the individual's behavior. At the time, it was believed that information and education on risks of injury might be sufficient to change behavior. Educational approaches were also relatively inexpensive compared to more intensive efforts (Pearn et al., 2004; Stevenson et al., 2004). Historically, education referred simply to awareness or information campaigns. Early safety campaigns, which were largely ineffective, focused on preaching safety, arousing inappropriate levels of fear, and victim blaming (Gielen & Girasek, 2001). Just as the injury field was evolving, so too was the health behavior change field, and early injury prevention education did not incorporate scientific advances in learning or behavior change theory or what was known from health communication research. More recent educational approaches have met with greater success, most often when they incorporate improved access to recommended safety products, use theory-based approaches, and apply principles of community participation (DiGuiseppi & Roberts, 2000; Towner, Dowswell, Mackereth, & Jarvis, 2001; Klassen, MacKay, Moher, Walker, & Jones, 2000). As noted in Table 1.1, contemporary approaches to using education recognize that providing information is only one element. Addressing an audience's beliefs, skills, resources, and need for continued reinforcement are additional necessary elements.

Ergonomics, engineering, and product design refer to modifying the built environment, equipment, homes, toys, and clothes, and these strategies have met with much success. For example, safer highways and automobiles have been credited with being instrumental to the reduction in motor vehicle injuries in the United States (Bonnie, Fulco, and Liverman, 1999). Engineering changes that eliminate, reduce, or modify the transfer of energy are well illustrated in the numerous other successful injury prevention examples, among them child-resistant packaging of medications, smoke alarms, bicycle helmets, energy-absorbing surfaces, and flame-resistant child sleepwear. These strategies are wholly consistent with and underscore the importance of the scientific advances that led to appreciating energy transfer as the key causal factor in injury.

The relationship of these strategies to behavior is in some cases obvious (as in the consistent and proper use of the safety product) and less so in other cases (as in behavioral responses to safety features of vehicles or use of safety products). For efficacious engineering solutions to be effective for the larger population, they must be widely available, accepted, and properly used. For example, early safety enhancements in motor vehicles were often available only in expensive cars, leaving large segments of the population unprotected. Air bags provide another example: they must first be designed properly and then used properly to provide protection: the air bag on-off switch must be reset after use, belted passengers should sit twelve or more inches from the air bag, and small children should be seated in the back seat away from the air bag. These examples illustrate the notion of an active approach to passive protection.

Enforcement involves safety legislation and regulations that are used to modify products, environments, and individual behavior. Mandatory standards for products, roadways, and vehicle designs have been successful, despite often being controversial because of their cost to industry. For example, a device fitted to a disposable cigarette lighter to make it child resistant may cost the lighter industry from four to twelve cents per lighter, but may save two hundred burn deaths annually. Perhaps most relevant for this chapter is legislation that mandates certain personal behaviors, such as using seat belts, car seats, and motorcycle helmets. Safety legislation works but is often opposed because it interferes with individual freedoms. (Schieber, Gilchrist, & Sleet, 2000; see also Chapter Twenty, this volume). According to Pearn et al. (2004), legislation is typically the last strategy introduced and only after failed educational and voluntary ergonomic efforts to reduce a hazard. Legislative approaches require attention to issues of education, implementation, and enforcement so that the public is aware of and accepts the law. Although many safety laws are not consistently enforced and police often have considerable latitude in enforcement, widespread visible enforcement can increase public perceptions of the negative consequences of noncompliance (Gielen & Girasek, 2001).

Behavior Change and Injury Prevention

Behavior change is reemerging as an important element in injury prevention as our understanding of injury is now more complex and dynamic. The most recent Institute of Medicine report on injury (Bonnie, Fulco, and Liverman, 1999) highlighted psychosocial research as one of three promising areas for the injury field and recommended intensified research into "differences in risk perception, risk taking, and behavioral responses to safety improvements among different segments of the population, particularly among those groups at highest risk of injury" (p. 6). In addition, an even broader focus on behavior is relevant for several reasons, as previously described in Gielen and Girasek (2001).

First, legislative strategies often require behavioral compliance by those who are to be protected; examples are seat belt use and car seat use). Second, passive protection is often not absolute and requires behavioral adaptation by those who are to be protected. McLoughlin (1997) notes that air bags will continue to provide passive protection in crashes, "provided that vehicle occupants practice the necessary safe behaviors" (p. 245). Furthermore, even when new and safer products become available, existing unsafe products will still be in circulation and the public will need to modify or replace them. Baby cribs and walkers are good examples. Both have been made safer—cribs by reducing slat spacing and corner protrusions and walkers by eliminating the wheels—yet many older, unsafe ones are still available through hand-me-downs and yard sales. Finally, for some injury problems, technological or engineering solutions are not readily available or are unacceptable to the public. For example, there are numerous types of choking hazards for children, and it is infeasible, if not, impossible to redesign them all (Shield, 1997). Four-sided pool fencing is an example of an environmental modification that can meet with public resistance (Wintemute & Wright, 1990) because it interferes with the aesthetics of a residential pool. While the search for more and better passive protections continues, we must never lose sight of the human behavioral components.

The Haddon model, which has guided the field so effectively in terms of countermeasure conceptualization and development, may need to be extended and enriched to more adequately account for the importance of behavior on the effectiveness of countermeasures (Lonero et al., 1994; Gielen et al., 1992; Runyan, 1998). Behavior change, traditionally confined to only the first "E," education, is increasingly recognized as relevant to engineering, legislation, and enforcement. First, safety legislation frequently is used to modify individuals' safety behaviors. Second, policy and environmental modifications depend on the behavior of decision makers, and there is a critical need to better understand how to influence their behavior. Third, educating individuals to change their personal safety behaviors ignores the potential of also educating individuals to become change agents—to help advocate for and support policy and environmental modifications. Table 1.2 provides a summary of the relevant behavior change issues for the host, agent or vehicle, and environmental determinants of injury. (For a full discussion of these issues, see Gielen & Girasek, 2001.)

While the injury burden remains unacceptably high, there are notable successes in changing individual behavior. For example, the dramatic reduction in motor vehicle injuries and deaths has been declared one of the ten greatest public health accomplishments of the twentieth century (Centers for Disease Control and Prevention, 1999a). Although the number of vehicle miles traveled has multiplied ten times since the 1920s, the annual death rate has decreased 90 percent (Centers for Disease Control and Prevention, 1999b). Modifications to roadways and vehicles, increased use of seat belts and child safety seats, and decreased rates of drunk driving are the most frequently mentioned and well-documented reasons for the sharp decline in motor vehicle fatality rates (Centers for Disease Control and Prevention, 1999b; Nichols, 1994; Graham, 1993; Waller, 2001; Rivara & MacKenzie, 1999; Zwerling & Jones, 1999). Each of these successful interventions

TABLE 1.2. INTEGRATING BEHAVIOR CHANGE WITHIN THE EPIDEMIOLOGICAL FRAMEWORK FOR INJURY CONTROL.

	Host	Agent or Vehicle or Vector	Environment
Target audience for behavior change	At-risk individuals, public at large	Manufacturers, engineers, business leaders	Policymakers, law enforcement officials, engineers, media, health care providers
Behavior change goals	Modify personal risk behaviors; advocate for change in products, environments, and laws	Make safer products; make products easier to use safely; make safety products more accessible	Make safer environments; support and enforce safety legislation; promote public awareness and safety-enhancing social norms
Examples	Auto restraint use, drunk driving, use of safety products	Safer vehicles, child-resistant containers, smoke alarms	Safer highways, auto-restraint legislation, helmet legislation, media portrayals of injuries and risk behaviors

Source: Reproduced with permission from Gielen and Girasek (2001).

has important behavioral components. For example, the National Highway Traffic Safety Administration (2003) reports that the number of alcohol-related fatalities per year dropped from 26,000 in 1982 to 17,419 in 2002, and the alcohol-related fatalities per 100 million vehicle miles traveled declined from 1.46 in 1982 to 0.53 in 2002. In response to large-scale federal education programs, modest increases in voluntary seat belt use were observed: from 11 percent in 1980 to 15 percent in 1984 (Nichols, 1994). With mandatory seat belt legislation in place, overall national use rates have risen to 75 percent in 2002 (National Highway Traffic Safety Administration, 2004). By 1985 all fifty states (and the District of Columbia) had laws requiring the use of car safety seats (Nichols, 1994), and 99 percent of infants and 94 percent of toddlers are riding restrained (National Highway Traffic Safety Administration, 2004). These successes would not have been achieved had it not been for the use of a comprehensive, multidisciplinary approach that included strong behavioral science contributions. These advances also exemplify the importance of taking an ecological approach to injury prevention (see Chapter Six, this volume).

Another example focuses on the policy environment that changed dramatically with the introduction of laws requiring changes in the behaviors of restraint use and drunk driving. The organizational environments of workplaces changes with requirements for using seat belts when driving for the job. The inter- and intrapersonal influences on these behaviors have also changed. Individuals are aware of the need to buckle up and not drink and drive through a variety of influences: the media, pediatric counseling, school programs, and social norms, for example. Taken together, these influences have changed the behaviors of millions of people and dramatically influenced the prospects of improved motor vehicle safety. Regarding drunk driving, for example, Graham (1993, p. 524) noted that in a relatively short time, "changes in social norms, in part spurred by such citizen activist groups as MADD, have apparently achieved what many traffic safety professionals believed was virtually impossible: a meaningful change in driver attitudes and behaviors resulting in a reduction of traffic fatalities."

There is an increasing number of meta-analyses and systematic reviews of the literature on evaluated interventions for injury prevention, some of which are focused on specific behavior change goals or approaches. For example, the Cochrane Collaboration has published reviews on a variety of injury prevention topics (www.thecochranelibrary.com). The Centers for Disease Control and Prevention–supported Task Force on Community Preventive Services has conducted systematic reviews of interventions to reduce motor vehicle injuries (Task Force on Community Preventive Services, 2005). Childhood injury prevention strategies have also been systematically reviewed (Klassen et al., 2000; Bruce & McGrath, 2005; Chapter Twelve, this volume), as have health promotion approaches to injury prevention (Towner, Dowswell, Simpson, & Jarvis, 1996). Readers interested in more examples of successful behavior change interventions and in learning about future research needs are referred to these sources as well as to the many other chapters in this book.

Conclusion

This chapter has provided a brief overview of the connection between behavioral science and injury prevention, reviewed the injury problem, discussed the advances made in injury prevention through the use of well-established epidemiological principles and methods, and described the role of behavior change in advancing injury prevention goals. Over the past twenty years, there have been substantial advances in reducing injuries and notable improvements in some safety behaviors. There are also broader roles for behavioral science to play in injury prevention. For example, we need to develop a better understanding of and ability to intervene in behaviors of decision makers who affect public safety through the products they manufacture, the laws and regulations they pass and enforce, and the influential communications they deliver to the public through the media. We also need to build stronger alliances with the public, so that it becomes more aware of the opportunities for injury prevention and the policies and programs that serve communities to make everyone safer.

Models, theories, and behavior change strategies that can help reduce preventable injuries historically have been underfunded, underused, and underrepresented in injury prevention research and practice. Nevertheless, there has been growing interest in the application of behavioral science to injury prevention in recent years. For example, the Centers for Disease Control and Prevention has issued requests for proposals related to theory-based approaches to injury prevention. It has also provided funds to each of its injury control research centers around the country to conduct training and research specifically related to behavioral science and injury prevention. The theme of the American Psychological Association's 2001 initiative, "Psychology Builds a Healthy World," focused on the opportunity to improve health and prevent injuries through the contributions of psychology (Sleet, Hammond, Jones, Thomas, & Whitt, 2004). Prevention strategies for both violence and unintentional injuries were included in *Integrating Behavioral and Social Sciences with Public Health*, a collaborative initiative of the American Psychological Association and the American Public Health Association (Gielen & Girasek, 2001). At the 2002 World Conference on Injury Prevention and Control in Montreal, Canada, and again at the 2005 National Injury Prevention Conference in Denver, Colorado, special sessions on behavioral approaches to injury and violence prevention were included. Special issues of scholarly journals have been devoted to behavioral and educational aspects of injury and violence prevention (Gielen, 2002; Sleet & Bryn, 2003; Liller & Sleet, 2004), and systematic reviews of prevention strategies have highlighted the need for more effective educational approaches to behavior change and studies with enhanced rigor (Task Force on Community Preventive Services, 2005; Zaza et al., 2001; DiGuiseppi & Roberts, 2000).

Future challenges for behavior change in injury prevention include the application and testing of behavior change theories to different injury problems in diverse communities. Many examples of such applications are presented in this book. While legislation may have been credited with motivating many of the behavioral changes benefiting safety, the most successful examples have also involved education—not only to prepare the public but also to ensure that laws are not repealed or overturned. Although there is little evidence that education alone works to change behavior, it can be a powerful initiator of and reinforcer for change.

There are fewer examples of theory-based efforts to change safety behaviors voluntarily. Also, the population that has yet to adopt recommended or mandated safety behaviors can be expected to be more difficult to reach; they often represent subgroups of the population that have limited access to safety information and products. Little is known about the safety practices, beliefs, and needs of the many diverse groups of society, and it is unlikely that broad, general information campaigns alone will be successful in persuading them to adopt safety practices. Fortunately, such campaigns, once the mainstay of educational approaches in injury prevention, are less often used; instead tailored programs using well-researched and effective behavior change methods are employed (Nansel et al., 2002; Gentilello, Ebel, Wickizer, Salkever, & Rivara, 2005; McDonald et al., 2005; Gielen et al., 2002; Ebel, Koepsell, Bennett & Rivara, 2003).

This is an exciting time to examine injuries from a behavioral perspective. A substantial knowledge base for applying behavioral science to injury and violence prevention is developing, as evidenced by the scholarly work presented in the remainder of this book. Whereas injury prevention initiatives during the past forty years have tended to focus on the risk factors, the three E's, and passive solutions, strategies in the future are likely to focus increasingly on problems that require additional behavior change expertise. Applying the behavioral theories, methods, and approaches described in this book can go a long way toward understanding how and when behavior change can be facilitated to decrease injury.

References

Baker, S. P., (1973). Injury control, accident prevention and other approaches to reduction of injury. In P. D. Sartwell (Ed.), *Preventive medicine and public health* (10th ed.). New York: Appleton-Century-Crofts.

Baker, S. P., O'Neill, B., Ginsburg, M. J., & Li, G. (1992). *The injury fact book* (2nd ed.). New York: Oxford University Press.

Barss, P., Smith, G., Baker, S., & Mohan, D. (1998). *Injury prevention: An international perspective.* New York: Oxford University Press.

Bonnie, R. J., Fulco, C. E., & Liverman, C. T. (Eds.). (1999). *Reducing the burden of injury, advancing prevention and treatment.* Committee on Injury Prevention and Control, Institute of Medicine. Washington, DC: National Academy Press.

Bruce, B., & McGrath, P. (2005). Group interventions for the prevention of injuries in young children: A systematic review. *Injury Prevention, 11*(3), 143–147.

Centers for Disease Control and Prevention. (1999a, Apr. 2). Ten great public health achievements. *Morbidity and Mortality Weekly Report,* 241–243.

Centers for Disease Control and Prevention. (1999b, May 14). Motor vehicle safety: A 20th century public health achievement. *Morbidity and Mortality Weekly Report,* 369–374.

Centers for Disease Control and Prevention. (2005, July 6). *Web-based Injury Statistics Query and Reporting System (WISQARS).* www.cd.gov/ncipc/wisqars.

Christoffel, T., & Gallagher, S. S. (1999). *Injury prevention and public health, practical knowledge, skills, and strategies.* Gaithersburg, MD: Aspen.

Christoffel, T., & Teret, S. P. (1993). *Protecting the public: Legal issues in injury prevention.* New York: Oxford University Press, 1993.

DiGuiseppi, C., & Roberts, I. G. (2000). Individual level injury prevention strategies in the clinical setting. In R. E. Behrman (Ed.), *The future of children: Unintentional injuries in childhood* (pp. 53–82). Los Altos, CA: David and Lucile Packard Foundations.

DiLillo, D., Peterson, L., & Farmer, J. E. (2002). Injury and poisoning. In T. Boll (Ed.), *Handbook of clinical health psychology* (pp. 555–582). Washington, DC: American Psychological Association.

Doll, L., Mercy, J. A., Bonzo, S., & Sleet, D. A. (Eds.). (2006). *Handbook of injury and violence prevention.* New York: Springer

Ebel, B. E., Koepsell, T. D., Bennett, E. E., & Rivara, F. P. (2003). Use of child booster seats in motor vehicles following a community campaign: A controlled trial. *JAMA, 289*(7), 879–884.

Fingerhut, L. A., & Warner, M. (1997). *Injury chart book, health, United States, 1996–97.* Hyattsville, MD: National Center for Health Statistics.

Gentelillo, L. M., Ebel, B. E., Wickizer, T. M., Salkever, D. S., & Rivara, F. P. (2005). Alcohol interventions for trauma patients. *Annals of Surgery, 241*(4), 541–550.

Gielen, A. C. (Ed.). (2002). Injury and domestic violence prevention [Special issue]. *Patient Education and Counseling, 46.*

Gielen, A. C., & Girasek, D. C. (2001). Integrating perspectives on the prevention of unintentional injuries. In N. Schneiderman, J. Gentry, J. M. deSilva, M. Speers, & H. Fomes (Eds.), *Integrating behavioral and social sciences with public health.* Washington, DC: APA Books.

Gielen, A. C., McDonald, E. M., Wilson, M.E.H., Hwang, W. T., Serwint, J. R., Andrews, J. S., & Wang, M.C. (2002). The effects of improved access to safety counseling, products and home visits on parents' safety practices. *Archives of Pediatrics and Adolescent Medicine, 156*, 33–40.

Gielen, A. C., & Sleet, D. (2003). Application of behavior-change theories and methods to injury prevention. *Epidemiologic Reviews, 25*(1), 1–12.

Graham, J. D. (1993). Injuries from traffic crashes: Meeting the challenge. *Annual Review of Public Health, 14*, 515–543.

Haddon, W., & Baker, S. P. (1981). Injury control. In D. Clarke & B. MacMahon (Eds.), *Preventive and community medicine* (pp. 109–140). New York: Little, Brown.

Klassen, T. P., MacKay, M., Moher, D., Walker, A., & Jones, A. L. (2000). Community-based injury prevention interventions. *Future of Children, Unintentional Injuries in Childhood, 10*(1), 83–110.

Liller, K., & Sleet, D. A. (Eds.). (2004). Injury prevention [Special issue]. *American Journal of Health Behavior, 28*(Suppl. 1).

Lonero, L. P., Clinton, K., Wilde, G. J. S., Roach, K., McKnight, A. J., MacLean, H., Guastello, S. J., and Lamble, R. W. (1994). *The roles of legislation, education and reinforcement in changing road user behavior.* Toronto, Ontario, Canada: Safety Research Office, Safety Policy Branch, Ministry of Transportation.

Marshall, S. W., Runyan, C. W., Bangdiwala, S. I., Linzer, M. A., Sacks, J. J., & Butts, J. D. (1998). Fatal residential fires: Who dies and who survives? *JAMA, 279*(20), 1633–1637.

McClure, R., Stevenson, M., & McEvoy, S. (Eds.). (2004). *The scientific basis of injury prevention & control.* Melbourne, Australia: IP Communications.

McDonald, E. M., Solomon, B., Shields, W., Serwint, J. R., Jacobsen, H., Weaver, N. L., Kreuter, M., & Gielen, A. C. (2005). Evaluation of kiosk-based tailoring to promote household safety behaviors in an urban pediatric primary care practice. *Patient Education and Counseling, 58*, 168–181.

McLoughlin, E. (1997). From educator to strategic activist for injury control. *Injury Prevention, 3*, 244–246.

Murray, C.J.L., & Lopez, A. D. (1996). *The global burden of disease.* Cambridge, MA: Harvard University Press, World Health Organization, and World Bank.

Nansel, T. R., Weaver, N., Donlin, M., Jacobsen, H., Kreuter, M. W., & Simons-Morton, B. (2002). Baby, be safe: The effect of tailored communications for pediatric injury prevention provided in a primary care setting. *Patient Education and Counseling, 46,* 175–190.

National Center for Health Statistics. Retrieved June 26, 2005, from http://www.cdc.gov/nchs/.

National Committee for Injury Prevention and Control. (1989). *Injury prevention: Meeting the challenge.* New York: Oxford University Press.

National Highway Traffic Safety Administration. (2003, Dec.). *Initiative to address impaired driving.* Retrieved June 26, 2005, from www.nhtsa.dot.gov.

National Highway Traffic Safety Administration. (2004, June). *The national initiative for increasing safety belt use.* Retrieved June 26, 2005, from www.nhtsa.dot.gov.

National Safe Kids Campaign. (2003). Report to the nation: Trends in unintentional childhood injury mortality, 1987–2000. Retrieved Oct. 28, 2005, from http://www.usa.safekids.org/content_documents/nskw03_report.pdf.

Nichols, J. L. (1994). Changing public behavior for better health: Is education enough? *American Journal of Preventive Medicine, 10*(Suppl.), 19–22.

Pearn, J., Nixon, J., & Scott, I. (2004). An historical perspective. In R. McClure, M. Stevenson, & S. McEvoy (Eds.), *The scientific basis of injury prevention and control,* Melbourne, Australia: IP Communications.

Peden, M., Scurfield, R., Sleet, D., Mohan, D., Hyder, A., Jarawan, E., & Mathers, C. (Eds.). (2004). *World report on road traffic injury prevention.* Geneva: World Health Organization.

Rivara, F. P., & MacKenzie, E. J. (Ed.). (1999). Systematic reviews of strategies to prevent motor vehicle injuries. *American Journal of Preventive Medicine, 16*(Suppl.), 1–90.

Robertson, L. S. (1992). *Injury epidemiology.* New York: Oxford University Press.

Runyan, C. W. (1998). Using the Haddon matrix: Introducing the third dimension. *Injury Prevention, 4,* 302–307.

Schieber, R. A., Gilchrist, J., & Sleet, D. A. (2000). Legislative and regulatory strategies to reduce childhood unintentional injuries. *Future of Children, 10*(1), 137–163.

Shield, J. (1997). Have we become so accustomed to being passive that we've forgotten how to be active? *Injury Prevention, 3,* 243–244.

Sleet, D. (Ed.). (1984). Occupant protection and health promotion [Special issue]. *Health Education Quarterly, 11*(2).

Sleet, D. A., & Bryn, S. (Eds.). (2003). Injury prevention for children and youth [Special issue]. *American Journal of Health Education, 34*(Suppl. 5).

Sleet, D. A., & Gielen, A. C. (1998). Injury prevention. In S. Sheinfeld Gorin & J. Arnold (Eds.), *Health promotion handbook.* St. Louis, MO: Mosby.

Sleet, D. A., & Gielen, A. (2004). Behavioral approaches to injury prevention. In R. McClure, M. Stevenson, & S. McEvoy (Eds.), *The scientific basis of injury prevention and control* (pp. 214–232). Melbourne, Australia: ISA Press.

Sleet, D. A., Hammond, W. R., Jones, R. T., Thomas, N., & Whitt, B. (2004). Using psychology for injury and violence prevention in the community. In R. H. Rozensky, N. G. Goodheart, & W. R. Hammond (Eds.), *Psychology builds a healthy world: Opportunities for research and practice.* Washington, DC: American Psychological Association.

Spielberger, C. D., & Frank, R. G. (1992). Injury control: A promising field for psychologists. *American Psychologist, 47,* 1029–1030.

Stevenson, M., Ameratunga, S., & McClure, R. (2004). The rationale for prevention. In R. McClure, M. Stevenson, & S. McEvoy (Eds.), *The scientific basis of injury prevention and control*. Melbourne, Australia: IP Communications.

Task Force on Community Preventive Services. (2005). *The guide to community preventive services: What works to promote health?* New York: Oxford University Press.

Towner, E., Dowswell, T., Mackereth, C., & Jarvis, S. (2001). *What works in preventing unintentional injuries in children and young adolescents? An updated systematic review.* London: Health Development Agency.

Towner, E., Dowswell, T., Simpson, G., & Jarvis, S. (1996). *Health promotion in childhood and young adolescence for the prevention of unintentional injuries.* London: Health Education Authority.

Waller, P. F. (2001). Public health's contribution to motor vehicle injury prevention. *American Journal of Preventive Medicine, 21*(Suppl. 4), 1–2.

Wintemute, G. J., & Wright, M. A. (1990). Swimming pool owners' opinions of strategies for prevention of drowning. *Pediatrics, 85*, 63–69.

Zaza, S., Carande-Kulis, V. G., Sleet, D. A., Sosin, D. M., Elder, R. W., Shults, R. A., Dinh-Zarr, T. B., Nichols, J. L., & Thompson, R. S. (2001). Methods for conducting systematic reviews of the evidence of effectiveness and economic efficiency of interventions to reduce injuries to motor vehicle occupants. *American Journal of Preventive Medicine, 21*(4S), 23–30.

Zwerling, C., & Jones, M. P. (1999). Evaluation of the effectiveness of low blood alcohol concentration laws for younger drivers. *American Journal of Preventive Medicine, 16*(Suppl.), 76–80.

PART ONE

BEHAVIOR CHANGE
THEORIES AND MODELS

CHAPTER TWO

INDIVIDUAL-LEVEL BEHAVIOR CHANGE MODELS

Applications to Injury Problems

David A. Sleet, Lara B. Trifiletti, Andrea Carlson Gielen, Bruce Simons-Morton

In translating an ecological model into action programs, Glanz and Rimer (1995) describe three societal levels and the theories that are useful at each. First is the intrapersonal level, which refers to the influence of an individual's knowledge, attitudes, and beliefs on his or her behavior. Theories of cognition, perception, and motivation are relevant at the intrapersonal level. Second is the interpersonal level, which refers to how significant other people, such as family members, friends, and coworkers, influence an individual's behavior. Theories particularly relevant to interpersonal relationships include those related to social influences. Intrapersonal and interpersonal levels are often combined and labeled simply as individual-level theories. The third level is the community level, which considers organizational settings and their influences (for example, workplaces, schools, churches) and social and health policies (such as welfare reform). This chapter reviews individual-level models, and Chapters Four and Six review injury examples from the perspective of the community level. (Additional resources for injury prevention interventions in the community can be found in Rozensky, Johnson, Goodheart, & Hammond, 2003; and Doll, Mercy, Bonzo, & Sleet, 2006.)

Portions of this chapter were excerpted with permission from Oxford University Press from Gielen, A. C. and Sleet, D. (2003). Application of behavior-change theories and methods to injury prevention, *Epidemiologic Reviews, 25,* 65–76.

A complete review of the individual-level theories used in the field of health behavior change to address other health problems is beyond the scope of this chapter; interested readers are referred to other books (Nutbeam & Harris, 1999; Institute of Medicine, 2001) and reports (Smedley & Syme, 2000; Schneiderman, Speers, Silva, Tomes, & Gentry, 2001; Nigg, Allegrante, & Ory, 2002). Instead, we describe here several examples of well-respected individual-level behavior change theories or models that have been applied to an injury problem: the health belief model, theory of reasoned action and theory of planned behavior, transtheoretical model, the precaution adoption process model, protection motivation, and applied behavior analysis. Social cognitive theory, the most notable of the interpersonal theories, is discussed in Chapter Three. In this chapter, we provide a brief overview of the theories describing the key constructs, critically review the literature of injury problems addressed by the theories, and discuss the practical utility of the theories and future research needs.

The Use of Individual Behavior Change Theories in the Scientific Literature

The extent to which many of the individual behavior change models have been applied to the prevention of unintentional injuries was recently reviewed by Trifiletti, Gielen, Sleet, and Hopkins (2005). The authors conducted a systematic review to evaluate the published literature from 1980 to 2001 on behavioral and social science theory applications to unintentional injury prevention and control. Electronic database searches in PubMed and PsycINFO identified articles that combined theories or models and injury causes.

The authors reviewed seventy-one articles and discarded thirty-four of them because they did not specifically mention or address a theory, model, or related construct or because the article focused on an injury topic outside the defined inclusion criteria (for example, violence-related injuries). The findings revealed that several important theories commonly applied in interventions to change other health behaviors have never been applied to injury prevention. There were no examples where the transtheoretical model had been applied to injury prevention. Among all the articles identified, PRECEDE-PROCEED, which is a planning model, was cited most frequently (see Chapter Seven, this volume). The theory of reasoned action/theory of planned behavior and the health belief model were the next most frequently cited theories in use in injury prevention research.

When behavioral and social sciences theories and models were applied to injury topics, they were most frequently used to guide program design and implement or develop evaluation measures; few examples of theory testing were found. These results suggest that the use of behavioral and social sciences theories and models in unintentional injury prevention research is in its infancy and is only marginally represented in the mainstream peer-reviewed literature.

Like many other health problems, injury is not a discrete behavior but a complex set of behaviors. Many related preventive behaviors may be involved, like obtaining and wearing helmets, crossing the street safely, or using a booster seat correctly. If the behavioral research was plentiful, one would expect to find multiple studies using a variety of research methods to study injury prevention behavior. Using bicycle safety as an example, we would expect to find theory-based studies relating to the adoption and use of bicycle helmets, reflective apparel, bike flags, and safe bicycling behaviors and practices. Moreover, the impact of behavioral studies would be expected to vary among populations by age, ethnicity, and socioeconomic status to better inform intervention research. Unfortunately, little theory-based research of this type has been conducted and published on injury-related behaviors.

The lack of theory-based studies is troubling and indicates that behaviorally based injury prevention research has great potential for important contributions in the future. Injury prevention and behavioral and social sciences could benefit from greater collaborative research to enhance behavioral approaches to injury control. This could prove useful to practitioners and researchers alike.

In this chapter, we start by presenting the three relatively commonly employed theories, each concerned to great extent with perceptions about risk and the efficacy of preventive actions. The health belief model suggests that the likelihood of taking action is based on beliefs about the susceptibility and severity of the disease and the benefits of taking specific action. The theory of reasoned action and the related theory of planned behavior focus on intent and the influence of perceptions about subjective norms and attitudes toward the behavior. Protection motivation theory focused on the role of perceptions about risk and coping strategies on behavior. The theories in the second group are based on stages-of-change concepts. The transtheoretical model emphasizes five stages of change, from precontemplation to maintenance of behavior. The precaution adoption process model has seven stages, from awareness to maintenance. All of these theories rely heavily but not exclusively on principles of persuasive communications to achieve changes in stage. The last theory discussed, applied behavior analysis, focuses on antecedents, characteristics of the behavior, consequences that follow, and opportunities for identifying, creating, and controlling stimuli and reinforcement. Finally, we discuss a recent effort to integrate cognitive approaches to behavior change.

Health Belief Model

The health belief model (HBM) (Rosenstock, 1974; Janz & Becker, 1984; see Figure 2.1) was one of the earliest models developed in an effort to understand and explain health-related behavior. According to the model, health-related behavior is a function of four beliefs: beliefs about susceptibility to a condition, beliefs about the severity of that condition, beliefs that specific behaviors will reduce one's risk, and beliefs that the benefits outweigh the costs or barriers.

This model says that preventive behaviors are a function of individuals' beliefs about their susceptibility to the health problem, the severity of the health problem, the benefits versus costs of adopting the preventive behavior, and experiencing a cue to action. Later, the concept of self-efficacy was added to the model. Self-efficacy, a concept originally from Bandura's work (Bandura, 1989), is one's confidence in the ability to perform a specific behavior.

HBM has been used to study bicycle injuries (Gielen, Joffe, Dannenberg, Wilson, & Beilenson, 1994; Marsh, Connor, Wesolowski, & Grisoni, 2000; Lajunen & Rasanen, 2004), motor vehicle injuries (Brink, Simons-Morton, & Zane, 1989; Chesham, Rutter, & Quine, 1993), multiple injuries (Russell, 1991; Glik, Kronenfeld, & Jackson, 1991; Glik, Greaves, Kronenfeld, & Jackson, 1993;

FIGURE 2.1. HEALTH BELIEF MODEL.

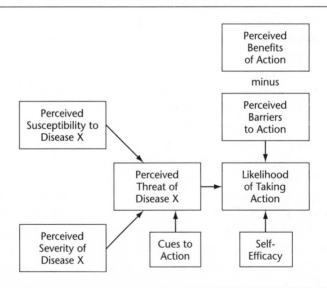

Source: Based on Rosenstock, Strecher, & Becker (1988).

Wortel, de Geus, & Kok, 1995; Smith, Sullivan, Bauman, Powell-Davies, & Mitchell, 1999), and other injuries such as occupational, recreational, and alcohol-related injuries (Peterson, Farmer, & Kashani, 1990; Wortel et al., 1995; Williams-Avery & MacKinnon, 1996; Wong and Seet, 1997; Sellstrom, Bremberg, Garling, & Hornquist, 2000; Arcury, Quandt, & Russell, 2002).

An illustration of this model in injury prevention comes from Peterson et al.'s study (1990) of the beliefs and safety practices of 198 parents with children ages eight to seventeen. She used a variation of the HBM to build formal predictions of how parents' attitudes influence their injury prevention teaching and environmental modifications. Parents were generally not very worried about injuries to their child (they had low perceived susceptibility). The HBM constructs most strongly associated with parental safety efforts were beliefs that their actions would be effective (benefits), a realistic appraisal of the costs of action (costs), and feeling knowledgeable and competent to perform the behaviors (efficacy). These results can be used to target educational messages and strategies to those variables associated with the desired behavioral outcomes. In this case, the authors suggest that interventions be directed toward increasing parents' beliefs about their child's susceptibility to injury while simultaneously increasing their competency to intervene. Health education methods and strategies are widely available for such interventions and in this case might include interpersonal or mediated communications using small media, such as informational brochures, or mass media, such as radio messages, to address perceived susceptibility and severity, skills training to increase perceived efficacy, and improved access to needed safety products to reduce barriers to action and compliance.

Protection Motivation Theory

Protection motivation theory (PMT) is concerned with the effects of information on attitudes and behavior (Rogers & Prentice-Dunn, 1997). In its simplest form, PMT suggests that action is unlikely unless individuals perceive that a threat is relevant and important. Therefore, persuasion is needed to increase people's perceptions about the threat of a particular problem so that they will seriously appraise possible strategies for coping. In short, threat appraisal and coping appraisal produce protection motivation. Protection motivation is the likelihood that the individual will engage in protective action. Threat appraisal includes perceived susceptibility, vulnerability, and anticipated consequences (outcome expectations) of the proposed protective action, while coping appraisal includes response efficacy (behavioral capability and self-efficacy). The primary causal pathway is that of predicting the occurrence of coping action in response to a particular threat.

Accordingly, when an individual perceives that a threat is important and personally relevant, the recommended action would provide useful protection, and is reasonably confident about taking the action, the motivation to initiate a coping action would be relatively high.

The theory states that as protection motivation increases, coping actions, whether adaptive or maladaptive, become increasingly likely. Accordingly, PMT suggests that persuasive communication may be effective to the extent it increases the salience of a threat and the acceptability of a suitable coping option. For example, parents may perceive that in general, teen driving is dangerous, but they may not realize that their own teenage child is at risk or that their management of their novice driver may reduce the risk of a motor vehicle crash. Viewed from the perspective of PMT, parents must be convinced that teen driving poses a personal and serious threat and that actions they could take would protect against this threat.

PMT has been used to study parental management of newly licensed teen drivers (Simons-Morton, Hartos, Leaf, & Preusser, 2005) and home-related injury prevention behaviors among parents of preschool children (Wortel et al., 1995).

Simons-Morton et al. (2005) described intervention effects on parent limits on novice teen driving during the first months of licensure, a period when crash rates are particularly high. Families were randomly assigned to intervention or comparison groups at the time the teen obtained a learner's permit. Comparison families received standard information on driving procedures and safety. Intervention families received the Checkpoints Program, a series of persuasive communications directed at risk appraisal and the benefits and normative aspects of parental restrictions on high-risk driving conditions by using the parent-teen driving agreement provided. Families who received the Checkpoints Program, compared with the control families, imposed significantly greater restrictions on teen driving privileges, including teen passengers and nighttime curfew. The intervention also produced changes in perceptions and expectations related to teen driving, which in turn promoted teen driving limits. The results of this study provide evidence that it is possible to alter perceptions through persuasive materials and that driving limits are mediated by changes in these perceptions.

Wortel and colleagues (1995) studied the behavioral determinants of eighteen parental safety measures. To select behavioral determinants, an attitude–social influence–self-efficacy/barriers model was used with the inclusion of variables from the HBM and the PMT. A written questionnaire was completed by 1,129 Dutch mothers of preschool children. Most safety measures were explained well by the same set of determinants. Main determinants for adopting or not adopting a safety measure were the mother's belief in the necessity of the safety measure according to the child's age, her belief about her partner's opinion on the necessity, and her belief about the success of taking the measure. Determinants of secondary importance were the mother's belief about the inconvenience and instrumentality of the safety measure; the perceived susceptibility had a minor or moderate influence on most measures. These results could be used to inform potentially persuasive messages, focused more on need and effectiveness and less on likelihood of an injury event.

Theory of Reasoned Action and Theory of Planned Behavior

The theory of reasoned action (TRA; Ajzen & Fishbein, 1980) and its successor, theory of planned behavior (TBP; Ajzen, 1988, 1991), are among the most frequently employed behavioral theories in health education, health promotion, unintentional injury prevention, and other areas of applied behavioral science (Figures 2.2 and 2.3). TPB includes all of the aspects of TRA, plus behavioral control; thus, in this section, we focus on TPB. A key concept in TPB is that beliefs and perceptions are primarily useful for predicting and influencing behavioral intention. Intention has been demonstrated in many studies to predict behavior, but not perfectly. Of course, intention does not always convert to action because things get

FIGURE 2.2. THEORY OF REASONED ACTION.

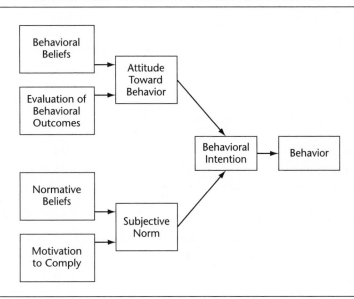

FIGURE 2.3. THEORY OF PLANNED BEHAVIOR.

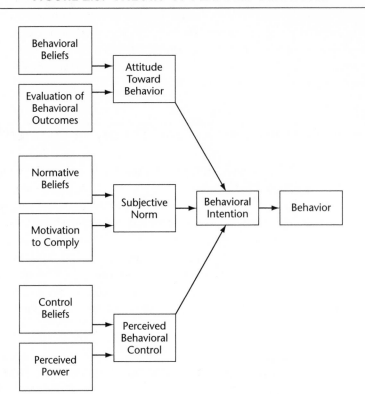

Source: Based on Ajzen (1991).

in the way. Sometimes there are barriers to intended action. At other times, opportunities to act may be rare or personal skill or confidence may be lacking.

For the most part, TPB does not concern itself particularly with issues of why intent does not always predict behavior. What it is concerned with are the beliefs and attitudes that predict intent. In particular, TPB is concerned with how attitudes toward the behavior, subjective norms, and perceived behavioral control predict intention. Attitudes are derived from measures of beliefs about the consequences of the behavior in question and the relative importance of these consequences to the individual. Subjective norms are derived from measures of beliefs about significant others' preferences and the individual's motivation to comply with their wishes. Perceived behavioral control relates to barriers and facilitators to taking action and includes elements of self-efficacy and behavioral capability.

It has become increasingly common for researchers to integrate TPB and social cognitive theory concepts (see also Chapter Three, this volume).

TRA/TPB has been used to study bicycle injuries (Gielen et al., 1994; Lajunen & Rasanen, 2004), motor vehicle injuries (Wittenbraker, Gibbs, & Kahle, 1983; Budd, North, & Spencer, 1984; Gielen & Radius, 1984; Parker, Manstead, Stradling, & Reason, 1992; Chesham et al., 1993; Thuen & Rise, 1994); multiple injuries (Glik et al., 1991; Russell, 1991; Gielen, Wilson, Faden, Wissow, & Harvilchuck, 1995; Wortel et al., 1995), and other injuries (Wong & Seet, 1997; Sellstroem, Bremberg, Garling, & Hornquist, 2000; Myers, 2002).

One example of how TRA was used was in a survey of parents' beliefs and practices regarding car safety seat use (Gielen, Eriksen, & Daltroy, 1984). A statewide, random-digit-dial survey of 406 parents of children five years old and younger was completed in an effort to better understand parents' use of car safety seats. The TRA was used as the conceptual framework for the survey instrument. The construct of attitude toward car seat use was found to be the single best variable for distinguishing between car seat users and nonusers. Consistent with the TRA, this variable consisted of responses to six items measuring beliefs about the consequences of the behavior (for example, using a car seat would be a hassle; the child would be better behaved in a car seat). Respondents who believed that their spouse would approve of using a car seat (a measure of subjective norm) were also more likely to report using one. These results can help inform the development of public and patient education materials by identifying salient messages and credible sources to deliver those messages. For example, media messages might communicate the ease with which car seat use becomes a habit with positive consequences such as child comfort and spouse approval.

Transtheoretical Model

The transtheoretical model (TM) incorporates constructs from several other models (Prochaska, DiClemente, & Norcross, 1992). This model is distinguished from TRA/TPB in its conceptualization of behavior change as a dynamic rather than static process, acknowledging that individuals differ in their readiness to change a behavior and that changes occur in discrete steps or stages over time (see Figure 2.4). There are typically five stages in this model: (1) precontemplative, not thinking about changing; (2) contemplative, aware and thinking about changing; (3) preparation, taking steps necessary for changing; (4) action, making the change for a short period of time; and (5) maintenance, having successfully changed the behavior, usually measured as six months or longer. This model includes the possibility of relapse to earlier stages, noting that maintained behavior change often occurs after a cyclical process of progressing and relapsing. One advantage of TM and other stage theory is their emphases on gradual cognitive and behavioral transitions, allowing programmers to target intervention and assess impact more narrowly and specifically to those relevant to each stage, thus providing a better match between intervention and measured outcomes. The most obvious example of the utility of the model is smoking, where an intervention may target contemplation, preparation, and trial of smoking cessation, maintenance of quitting, and relapse prevention.

The TM model has been used to describe men's ability to change their abusive behaviors (Brown, 1997; Daniels & Murphy, 1997) and describe abused women's safety behaviors and ability to end their abuse (Burke, Gielen, McDonnell, O'Campo, & Maman, 2001).

In Burke et al.'s qualitative (2001) study of women's descriptions of how they coped with and ended their abuse, there were clear examples of women moving from precontemplation (for example, not considering their partner's behavior toward them a problem, or labeling their experiences as abuse), to action (recognizing the abuse as a problem and taking some protective action, such as calling a shelter, contacting legal assistance, and moving out), to maintenance (having experienced no abuse or having been away from the partner for six months or more). The point of knowing what stage an individual is in with regard to a desired outcome is that it allows the interventionist to select and apply the most appropriate stage-matched intervention. For example, to move someone from precontemplation to contemplation, awareness-raising strategies such as information distribu-

FIGURE 2.4. TRANSTHEORETICAL MODEL: STAGES AND PROCESSES OF CHANGE.

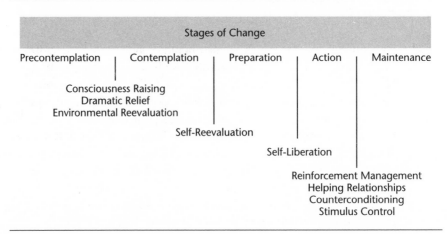

Source: Prochaska, DiClemente, and Norcross (1992). Reproduced with permission.

tion are recommended. To move someone from contemplation to preparation and action requires providing, identifying, and facilitating access to the necessary resources. (See Chapter Fifteen, this volume, for a fuller description of how the TM was applied to intimate partner violence.)

Precaution Adoption Process Model

The precaution adoption process model (PAPM), explains the adoption of health-related behavior as a developmental process through seven distinct behavioral stages that culminate in the adoption and maintenance of a precautionary behavior (Weinstein, 1988; Weinstein & Sandman, 1992). The current PAPM stages are: stage 1, unaware of precaution; stage 2, not engaged; stage 3, undecided; stage 4, not planning; stage 5, planning; stage 6, acting; and stage 7, maintenance. The goal of the PAPM is to explain the process by which an individual arrives at a decision to take action and translates that decision into action. The model has received increasing support for its usefulness in predicting health-related actions. It has been examined in seven studies of home radon testing as well as studies of osteoporosis and hepatitis B vaccination (Weinstein & Sandman, 1992; Blalock et al., 1996; Hammer, 1998). Glik et al. (1991) drew on the PAPM in her study of parents' risk perceptions related to a variety of childhood injuries. The stages proposed by the PAPM can be assessed by a series of questions to identify a person's adoption process. This simple and direct method for evaluating a person's stage makes this model highly desirable and suggests its usefulness in many settings.

The PAPM focuses on the psychological processes that occur within an individual. Factors such as social norms, risk perceptions, knowledge, and beliefs will likely influence whether a person adopts a particular behavior. Therefore, stages are defined by what a person may be thinking at each stage in the model rather than being defined by things external to the individual such as past behavior (Weinstein & Sandman, 2002). Weinstein and Sandman (2002) made two key points with regard to the various stages of development. First, people at different stages of the process behave differently. Second, different interventions and information or messages are needed at each stage to allow a smooth transition to the next stage. Knowing where in the change process an individual or group of individuals is allows one to develop more appropriately tailored persuasive message and intervention components. For example, moving people from earlier stages requires messages that heighten awareness of risk and precaution effectiveness, whereas moving people through the later stages requires messages that address access barriers. For example, a higher perceived likelihood of injury may be important in helping a parent who is undecided about getting a car safety seat move toward planning to purchase one, whereas easy access to a car safety seat may help move a parent who is already planning to purchase one into acting by purchasing a car safety seat.

The utility of stage-based models has been well articulated by the work of Prochaska, DiClemente, and Norcross (1992) in their stages of change model, as well as by Weinstein's own original development of the PAPM and testing of it with the behavior of home radon testing (Weinstein, Lyon, Sandman, & Cuite, 1998; Weinstein et al., 2002). The PAPM differs from the stages of change model and other traditional static models such as the health belief model in ways that make it particularly relevant for studying the adoption of safety practices. The model explicitly deals with both the hazard (for example, car accidents) and the precaution (car safety seats), arguing that individuals must first perceive a hazard of sufficient personal relevance before they are ready to hear messages about adopting a precaution. The PAPM does resemble another stage theory, the transtheoretical model; however, the similarities lie with the names given to the stages. Closer examination shows that the number of stages is not the same in the two theories, and even the stages with similar names are actually defined quite differently (Weinstein & Sandman, 2002).

Empirical data documenting parents' current safety practices (smoke alarm use, poison storage, and car safety seat use) and their readiness to adopt future practices has been examined using the PAPM in one study (Trifiletti, 2005), and two of the authors (Gielen, Trifiletti) are currently using it in an ongoing study funded by the National Institute of Child Health and Development (NICHD). These are the first studies to evaluate this model for its utility in understanding the adoption of parent safety behaviors related to childhood injury prevention. It is clear that smoke alarms, poison storage devices, and car safety seats help save lives; however, much remains to be known about how to encourage widespread adoption of these specific behaviors. A theory-based understanding of car safety seat use and how to influence the adoption of this behavior should support the development of persuasive and effective injury prevention interventions.

The following example is provided to illustrate the use of the PAPM for car safety seat use. In the first study (Trifiletti, 2005), parents with young children were asked to respond to a series of questions that assessed their PAPM stage for car safety seat use, smoke alarms, and poison storage. A staging algorithm was used to assign each respondent to one of seven stages (see Figure 2.5). The algorithm placed participants reporting "perfect" behavior in the highest stage (stage 7, maintenance): having the correct car safety seat for their child's age and weight, facing the correct direction, in the correct position in the car, and using it every time the child rides in the car. From this preliminary study, results indicated that staging could be done easily and quickly. Results showed parents to be in the highest stages with regard to the

FIGURE 2.5. PRECAUTION ADOPTION PROCESS MODEL
AND INTERVENTIONS: SMOKE ALARM EXAMPLE.

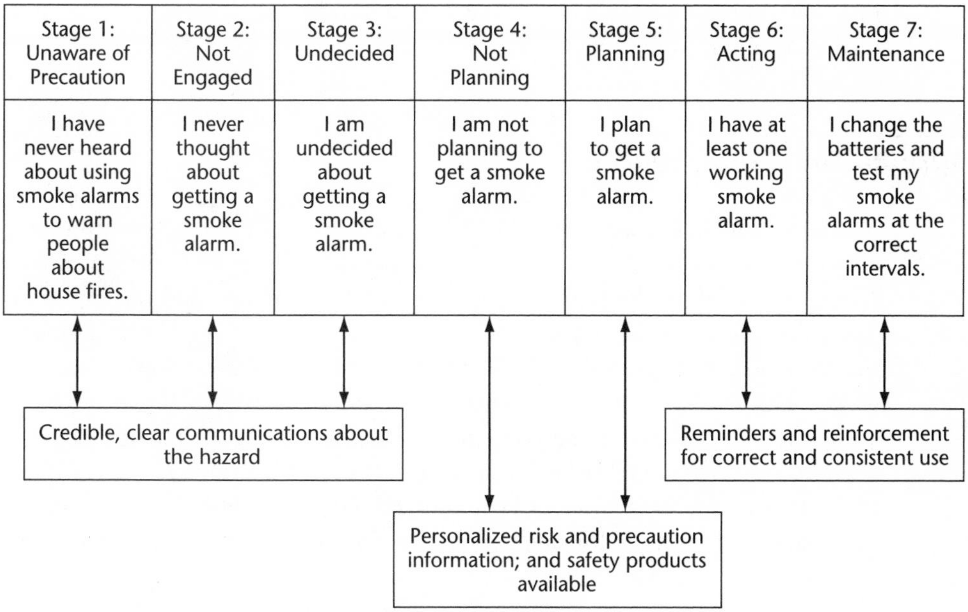

Stage 1: Unaware of Precaution	Stage 2: Not Engaged	Stage 3: Undecided	Stage 4: Not Planning	Stage 5: Planning	Stage 6: Acting	Stage 7: Maintenance
I have never heard about using smoke alarms to warn people about house fires.	I never thought about getting a smoke alarm.	I am undecided about getting a smoke alarm.	I am not planning to get a smoke alarm.	I plan to get a smoke alarm.	I have at least one working smoke alarm.	I change the batteries and test my smoke alarms at the correct intervals.

Credible, clear communications about the hazard

Reminders and reinforcement for correct and consistent use

Personalized risk and precaution information; and safety products available

Source: Based on Weinstein & Sandman (2002).

three safety behaviors (for example, 67 percent were in stage 7, maintenance for car seat use). All three safety behaviors were skewed to the higher stages.

Based on the results of this research and in consultation with the model's creator, Neil Weinstein, the new NICHD-funded study modified the PAPM stages to develop a more refined and realistic measure of the safety behaviors. Profiles were created to represent more specific behaviors. That is, car safety seat use as a practical matter is made up of four distinct behaviors, which we call profiles: profile 1, having a car safety seat; profile 2, having the correct car safety seat; profile 3, using the car seat every time; and profile 4, having the car seat installed or inspected by an expert. The same PAPM stages 1 through 7 are used to stage respondents within each profile. For example, a parent may have the correct car seat for his or her child (profile 3) but has never heard about using it every time (stage 1). This expanded profile and stage model is being tested in the Safety in Seconds Project. This NICHD-funded, randomized controlled trial involves nine hundred families with young children. Using PAPM profiles and stages, we assess parents' readiness to adopt home and motor vehicle safety behaviors. Parents are randomly assigned to receive a tailored Safety in Seconds feedback report that is specific to the individual's profile and stage (intervention group) or a personalized health magazine (control group). Primary outcome measures are changes in profile and stages over a four-month follow-up period.

Applied Behavior Analysis

The term *applied behavior analysis* (ABA) identifies a specific subfield within psychology that uses the technology of behavior modification and operant conditioning to facilitate change. Behavior is viewed as learned, and principles of stimulus control, feedback, reinforcement, and punishment shape the acquisition, maintenance, and extinction of behavior (Hovell, Elder, Blanchard, & Sallis, (1986). This model has a richer body of literature than many of the theories examined above, and has been used in many settings to change behavior (Margolis & Kroes, 1975). Applied behavior analysis seeks to understand and modify behavior by addressing the ABCs of behavior (antecedents, behaviors, consequences). For example, in studying drinking and driving behavior, behaviorists are interested in analyzing:

A Antecedents to the behavior, such as cues in the environment, social pressure of friends, or driving alone to a social function

B The Behavior itself, such as frequency of drinking, size of the drink, and time between drinking and driving

C Consequences that follow the behavior (both positive and negative), such as social attention or punishment for drinking and driving

Understanding the ABCs that control a behavior can help the behaviorist intervene by shaping behavior and the environment to yield change. Removing roadside billboards that remind drivers of drinking, increasing prompts and cues in the drinking environment that discourage drinking and driving, and selecting a designated driver can be used to modify the antecedents. Slowing the rate of alcohol consumption, patron refusal skills, server intervention in the drinking environment, and feedback from blood alcohol consumption meters can be used to modify the behavior. Social and peer support for not drinking and driving, positive feedback from bartenders or friends, and punishment for being caught for drinking and driving can be used to modify consequences (Sleet & Lonero, 2002; Grasek, Gielen, & Smith, 2002).

Multiple studies using applied behavior analysis to address safety behaviors have produced fairly consistent and positive results. Applications of these strategies in road safety have effectively increased the use of safety belts (Williams, Wells, & Farmer, 2002; Sleet, Hollenbach, & Hovell, 1986; Streff & Geller, 1986) and child restraints (Lonero et al., 1994), reduced vehicle speeding (Ragnarsson & Bjorgvinsson, 1991; Van Houten & Nau, 1983), improved child pedestrian safety (Thompson et al., 1998), bicycle helmet use (Thompson, Sleet, & Sacks, 2002), and crash avoidance (Ludwig, Geller, & Mawhinney, 2000; Hutton, Sibley, Harper, & Hunt, 2001). In other areas relevant to injury prevention, applied behavior analysis has been used to reduce children's fall-related behavior on playgrounds (Heck, Collins, & Peterson, 2001); improve fire escape behaviors and emergency response skills in the event of a residential fire (Holmes & Jones, 1996; Jones, vanHasselt, & Sisson, 1984; Jones, Ollendick, & McLaughlin, & Williams, 1989); change safety behaviors in a fire in public buildings (Leslie, 2001; Roberts, Fanurik, & Layfield, 1987); and modify other injury control behaviors (McKnight, 1990; Geller et al., 1990). This behavioral safety approach also has a strong history of use and success in promoting occupational health and safety (Krause, Hidley, & Hodson, 1990) and has been successfully applied to increase the use of personal protection devices such as hard hats and ear protection, reduce injuries on the job, and increase worker productivity and morale (Geller, 1998). (Chapter Fourteen, this volume, documents many of the practical uses for ABA in occupational settings.)

ABA can be applied to change one person's behavior (such as a juvenile's fire-starting behavior), a group at risk (such as factory workers), or the behavior of an entire community (such as accessing emergency services by telephoning 911). Use of brief interventions in counseling and feedback sessions, together with the application of sound behavior modification strategies, has also been successfully used to change injury-related risk behaviors and the risk of reinjury (Johnston, Rivara, Droesch, Dunn, & Copass, 2002; Hungerford & Pollock, 2002).

The target audience is not limited to individuals at risk. These approaches can also be applied to modifying the behavior of parents, legislators, medical personnel, managers, inventors, policymakers, and enforcers whose behavior influences large segments of the public. Little research has been undertaken to apply ABA to legislative and manufacturing behavior, to build safer cars and safer products, or to reinforce introduction and passage of strong pro-injury prevention legislation. Reinforcers inherent in the legislative and political arena often take precedence over what's good for public health.

Integrating Models at the Individual Level

The paucity of behavioral theories and models applied to injury problems is a dilemma similar to that faced by HIV/AIDS practitioners in the 1980s. At that time, the lack of attention to theory often led to ineffective prevention programs to respond to the pressing need for behavior modification among those at greatest risk for HIV infection (Mantell, DiVittis, & Auerback, 1997; Fishbein et al., 1991). There may be lessons from this early experience with HIV that may help shape behavioral interventions for injury control.

In 1991 the National Institute of Mental Health convened a theorists' workshop to bring together creators of behavioral theory to develop a unifying framework to facilitate applying behavioral theory to prevent HIV/AIDS (Fishbein et al., 1991). Their discussions led to an enumeration of five theories that, taken together, contain virtually all of the variables that have been used in attempts to understand and change a wide variety of human behaviors: health belief model (Janz & Becker, 1984) , social cognitive theory (Bandura, 1989), theory of reasoned action (Fishbein & Ajzen, 1975), theory of self-regulation and self-control (Kanfer & Kanfer, 1991), and theory of subjective culture and interpersonal relations (Triandis, 1980). After considering all five theories and their many variables, the theorists reached consensus on eight variables that appear to account for most of the variations in health-related behaviors: (1) intentions, (2) environmental barriers, (3) skills, (4) outcome expectancies (or attitude), (5) social norms, (6) self-standards, (7) emotional reactions, and (8) self-efficacy. It is likely that these same eight variables might also regulate and predict change in injury risk behavior (M. Fishbein, personal communication, Mar. 20, 2004).

Translating this guidance to action, Fishbein (Fishbein et al., 2001) concluded that for a person to perform a given behavior, one or more of the following generally must be present:

1. The person forms a strong, positive intention or makes a commitment to perform the behavior.
2. There are no environmental barriers that make it impossible to perform the behavior.
3. The person possesses the skills necessary to perform the behavior.
4. The person believes that the advantages of performing the behavior outweigh the disadvantages.
5. The person perceives more normative pressure to perform than not to perform the behavior.
6. The person perceives that performance of the behavior is consistent with his or her self-image or values.
7. The person's emotional reaction to performing the behavior is more positive than negative.
8. The person perceives that he or she has the capabilities to perform the behavior under different circumstances.

The first three factors are viewed as necessary and sufficient for producing any behavior, and the remaining five are viewed as modifying variables, influencing the strength and direction of intentions.

By way of a hypothetical example, we can apply these notions to the injury control behavior of testing the functionality of a residential smoke alarm: if a home owner is committed to testing the smoke alarm every month, has access to the alarms in the home, and has the skills necessary to test the alarm successfully, we would predict that there is a high probability he or she will perform the behavior. The probability that the individual will test the smoke alarm monthly would be predicted to increase even more if the home owner also believes that testing is worth the time and trouble, knows that all neighbors test their alarms, believes that testing is consistent with his or her values as a responsible home owner, has no negative emotional reaction to testing, and can test the alarms under different conditions in the home. According to this notion, the probability of testing monthly would be predicted to reach nearly 100 percent under these conditions.

To date, this integrated model has not been applied to this or any other injury-related behavior but holds promise as an innovative approach that may be useful for program development, at least until such time as sufficient research is available on specific theories as they relate to injury prevention. Adapting and integrating models such as these at the individual level for injury prevention behavior is just beginning; more work is needed to design, test, and evaluate interventions based on these behavioral models.

Conclusion

In this chapter, we have reviewed some of the most commonly used individual-level theories in health behavior change and described their application to injury prevention. In most cases, the studies were observational, designed to identify factors associated with injury-preventive behavior. In a few cases, theory was used to develop interventions that were evaluated in randomized trials, providing information about the theory and also evidence of program efficacy. Unfortunately, given the wide range of types of injuries and injury-preventive behaviors and the uniqueness of various target populations, it is difficult to draw conclusions about the utility of individual-level theories across the numerous areas in injury prevention. What is clear is that despite the wide range of studies in behavioral and social science in unintentional injury prevention published in the past twenty years (Sleet & Hopkins, 2004), there is still a paucity of published research using behavior change theories or models. The opportunity for additional research remains ample.

While evidence from a single study can provide useful information for practitioners about what variables to target or about program efficacy, only multiple studies and replications studies carried out on many different injury prevention behaviors and among different populations can lead to evidence for best practices.

What is needed is substantial research on both the determinants of behavior and the efficacy of behavior change interventions using behavioral science theories, methods, and applications. This information would fuel recommendations to practitioners about the most important variables to address and the program components that are most likely to succeed. Most noticeably absent from this body of literature are longitudinal study designs and mediator models of analysis, both of which would aid in understanding behavior over time and the influencing factors that account for any changes. Nevertheless, this brief review should enable practitioners and researchers in injury and violence prevention to more easily identify potentially useful theoretical approaches to any injury problem of interest.

References

Ajzen, I. (1988). *Attitudes, personality, and behavior.* Chicago: Dorsey Press.

Ajzen, I. (1991). The theory of planned behavior. *Organizational Behavior Human Decision Processes, 50,* 179–211.

Ajzen, I., & Fishbein, M. (1980). *Understanding attitudes and predicting social behavior.* Upper Saddle River, NJ: Prentice Hall.

Arcury, T. A., Quandt, S. A., & Russell, G. B. (2002). Pesticide safety among farmworkers: Perceived risk and perceived control as factors reflecting environmental justice. *Environmental Health Perspective, 2,* 233–240.

Bandura, A. (1989). Perceived self-efficacy in the exercise of personal agency. *Psychological Bulletin of the British Psychological Society, 10,* 411–424.

Blalock, S. J., DeVellis, R. F., Giorgino, K. B., DeVellis, B. M., Gold, D. T., Dooley, M. A., Anderson, J. J., & Smith, S. L. (1996). Osteoporosis prevention in premenopausal women: Using a stage model approach to examine the predictors of behavior. *Health Psychology, 15*(2), 84–93.

Brink, S. G., Simons-Morton, B. G., & Zane, D. (1989). A hospital-based infant safety seat program for low-income families: Assessment of population needs and provider practices. *Health Education Quarterly, 16,* 45–56.

Brown, J. (1997). Working toward freedom from violence: The process of change in battered women. *Violence Against Women, 3,* 5–26.

Budd, R. J., North, D., & Spencer, C. (1984). Understanding seat-belt use: A test of Bentler and Speckart's extension of the "theory of reasoned action." *European Journal of Social Psychology, 14,* 69–78.

Burke, J. G., Gielen, A. C., McDonnell, K. A., O'Campo, P., & Maman, S. (2001). The process of ending abuse in intimate relationships. *Violence Against Women, 7,* 1144–1163.

Chesham, D. J., Rutter, D. R., & Quine, L. (1993). Motorcycling safety research: A review of the social and behavioral literature. *Social Science and Medicine, 37,* 419–429.

Daniels, J. W., & Murphy, C. M. (1997). Stages and processes of change in batterers' treatment. *Cognitive Behavior and Practice, 4,* 123–415.

Doll, L., Bonzo, S., Mercy, J., & Sleet, D. (Eds.). (2006). *Handbook of injury and violence prevention.* New York: Springer.

Fishbein, M. (1995). Developing effective behavior change interventions: Some lessons learned from behavioral research. In T. E. Backer, S. L. David, & G. Soucy (Eds.),

Reviewing the behavioral science knowledge base on technology transfer. Washington, DC: U.S. Department of Health and Human Services.

Fishbein, M., & Ajzen, I. (1975). *Belief, attitude, intention, and behavior: An introduction to theory and research.* Reading, MA: Addison-Wesley.

Fishbein, M., Bandura, A., Triandis, H. C., Kanfer, F. H., Becker, M. H., & Middlestadt, S. E. (1991). *Factors influencing behavior and behavior change. Final report–Theorists workshop.* Washington, DC: National Institute of Mental Health.

Fishbein, M., Triandis, H. C., Kanfer, F. H., Becker, M., Middlestadt, S. E., & Eichler, A. (2001). Factors influencing behavior and behavior change. In A. Baum, T. A. Tevenson, & J. E. Singer (Eds.), *Handbook of health psychology.* Mahwah, NJ: Erlbaum.

Geller, E. S. (1998). *The psychology of safety.* Boca Raton, FL: CRC Press.

Geller, E. S., Berry, T., Ludwig, T., Evans, R. E., Gilmore, M. R., & Clarke, S. W. (1990). A conceptual framework for developing and evaluating behavior change interventions for injury control. *Health Education Research, 5*(2), 125–137.

Gielen, A. C., Eriksen, M. P., & Daltroy, L. H. (1984). Factors associated with the use of child restraint devices. *Health Education Quarterly, 11,* 195–206.

Gielen, A. C., Joffe, A., Dannenberg, A. L., Wilson, M.E.H., & Beilenson, P. L. (1994). Psychosocial factors associated with the use of bicycle helmets among children in counties with and without helmet use laws. *Journal of Pediatrics, 124,* 204–210.

Gielen, A. C., & Radius, S. (1984). Project KISS (Kids in Safety Seats): Educational approaches and evaluation measures. *Health Education, 15,* 43–47.

Gielen, A. C., Wilson, M. E., Faden, R. R., Wissow, L., & Harvilchuck, J. D. (1995). In home injury prevention practices for infants and toddlers: The role of parental beliefs, barriers, and housing quality. *Health Education Quarterly, 22,* 85–95.

Girasek, D. C., Gielen, A. C., & Smith, G. S. (2002). Alcohol's contribution to fatal injuries: A report on public perceptions. *Annals of Emergency Medicine, 39,* 622–652.

Glanz, K., & Rimer, B. K. (1995). *Theory at a glance: A guide for health promotion practice.* Bethesda, MD: National Cancer Institute.

Glanz, K., Rimer, B. K., & Lewis, F. M. (Eds.). (1997). *Health behavior and health education: Theory, research, and practice* (2nd ed.). San Francisco: Jossey-Bass.

Glik, D. C., Greaves, P. E., Kronenfeld, J. J., & Jackson, K. L. (1993). Safety hazards in households with young children. *Journal of Pediatric Psychology, 18,* 115–131.

Glik, D., Kronenfeld, J., & Jackson, K. (1991). Predictors of risk perceptions of childhood injury among parents of pre-schoolers. *Health Education Quarterly, 18,* 285–301.

Hammer, G. P. (1998). Factors associated with hepatitis B vaccine acceptance among nursing home workers. *Dissertation Abstracts International: Section B, The Sciences and Engineering, 59*(1-B), 182.

Heck, A., Collins, J., & Peterson, L. (2001). Decreasing children's risk taking on the playground. *Journal of Applied Behavior Analysis, 34,* 349–352.

Holmes, G. A., & Jones, R. T. (1996, First Quarter). Fire evacuation skills: Cognitive behavior versus computer-mediated instruction. *Fire Technology,* 51–64.

Hovell, M. F., Elder, J. P., Blanchard, J., & Sallis, J. F. (1986). Behavior analysis and public health perspectives: Combining paradigms to effect prevention. *Education and Treatment of Children, 9,* 287–306.

Hungerford, D. W., & Pollock, D. A. (Eds.). (2002). *Alcohol problems among emergency department patients: Proceedings of a research conference on identification and intervention.* Atlanta, GA: National Center for Injury Prevention and Control, Centers for Disease Control and Prevention.

Hutton, K. A., Sibley, C. G., Harper, D. N., & Hunt, M. (2001). Modifying driver behavior with passenger feedback. *Transportation Research Part F: Traffic Psychology and Behavior, 4,* 257–269.

Institute of Medicine. Committee on Health and Behavior. (2001). *Health and behavior: The interplay of biological, behavioral and societal influences.* Washington, DC: National Academy Press.

Janz, N. K., & Becker, M. H. (1984). The health belief model: A decade later. *Health Education Quarterly, 11*(1), 1–47.

Johnston, B. D., Rivara, F. P., Droesch, R. M., Dunn, C., & Copass, M. (2002). Behavior change counseling in the emergency department to reduce risk: A randomized, control trial. *Pediatrics, 110*(2), 267–274.

Jones, R. T., Ollendick, T. H., McLaughlin, K. H., & Williams, C. E. (1989). Elaborative and behavioral rehearsal in the acquisition of fire emergency skills and the reduction of fear of fires. *Behavior Therapy, 20,* 93–101.

Jones, R. T., vanHasselt, V. P., & Sisson, L. A. (1984). Emergency fire safety skills, *Behavior Modification, 8,* 59–78.

Kanfer, R., & Kanfer, F. H. (1991). Goals and self-regulation: Applications of theory to work settings. In M. L. Machr & P. R. Pintrich (Eds.), *Advances in motivation and achievement* (Vol. 7, pp. 287–326). Greenwich, CT: JAI Press.

Krause, T. R., Hidley, J. H., & Hodson, S. J. (1990). *The behavior-based safety process.* New York: Van Nostrand Reinhold.

Lajunen, T., & Rasanen, M. (2004). Can social psychological models be used to promote bicycle helmet use among teenagers? A comparison of the health belief model, theory of planned behavior and the locus of control. *Journal of Safety Research, 35*(1), 115–123.

Leslie, J. (2001). Behavioural safety: Extending the principles of applied behavioral analysis to safety in fires in public buildings. In *Proceedings of the Second International Symposium on Human Behavior in Fire* (pp. 1–10). London: Interscience Communications.

Lonero, L. P., Clinton, K. M., Wilde, G.J.S., Roach, K., McKnight, A. J., MacLean, H., Guastello, S. J., & Lamble, R. W. (1994). *The roles of legislation, education and reinforcement in changing road user behaviour.* Toronto, Ontario, Canada: Safety Research Office, Safety Policy Branch, Ministry of Transportation.

Ludwig, T. D., Geller, E. S., & Mawhinney, T. C. (Eds.). (2000). Intervening to improve the safety of occupational driving: A behavior change model and review of empirical evidence. *Journal of Organizational Behavior Management, 19,* 1–134.

Mantell, J. E., DiVittis, A. T., & Auerbach, M. I. (1997). *Evaluating HIV prevention interventions.* New York: Plenum.

Margolis, B. L., & Kroes, W. H. (Eds.). (1975). *The human side of accident prevention: Psychological concepts and principles which bear on industrial safety.* Springfield, IL: Charles C. Thomas Publisher.

Marsh, E., Connor, S., Wesolowski, K., & Grisoni, E. (2000). Preventing bicycle-related head trauma in children. *International Journal of Trauma Nursing, 6,* 117–122.

McKnight, A. J. (1990). Intervention with alcohol-impaired drivers by peers, parents and purveyors of alcohol. *Health Education Research, 5*(2), 225–236.

Myers, M. L. (2002). Tractor risk abatement and control as a coherent strategy. *Journal of Agricultural Safety and Health, 8*(2), 185–198.

Nigg, C. R., Allegrante, J. P., & Ory, M. (Eds.). (2002). Behavior Change Consortium (BCC). *Health Education Research: Theory and Practice* [Special issue], *17*(5), 493–690.

Nutbeam, D., & Harris, E. (1999). *Theory in a nutshell: A guide to health promotion theory.* New York: McGraw-Hill.

Parker, D., Manstead, A. S., Stradling, S. G., & Reason, J. T. (1992). Determinants of intention to commit driving violations. *Accident Analysis and Prevention, 24,* 117–131.

Parker, D., Manstead, A.S.R., Stradling, S. G., Reason, J. T., & Baxter, J. S. (1992). Intention to commit driving violations: An application of the theory of planned behavior. *Journal of Applied Psychology, 77,* 94–101.

Peterson, L., Farmer, J., & Kashani, J. H. (1990). Parental injury prevention endeavors: A function of health beliefs? *Health Psychology, 9,* 77–91.

Prochaska, J. O., DiClemente, C. C., & Norcross, J. C. (1992). In search of how people change: Applications to the addictive behaviors. *American Psychologist, 47*(9), 1102–1114.

Ragnarsson, R. S., & Bjorgvinsson, T. (1991). Effects of public posting on driving speed in Icelandic traffic. *Journal of Applied Behavioral Analysis, 24,* 53–58.

Roberts, M. C., Fanurik, D., & Layfield, D. A. (1987). Behavioral approaches to preventing childhood injuries. *Journal of Social Issues, 43*(2), 105–118.

Rogers, R. W., & Prentice-Dunn, S. (1997). Protection motivation theory. In D. D. Gochman (Ed.), *Handbook of health behavior research I: Personal and social determinants* (pp. 113–132). New York: Plenum Press.

Rosenstock, R. M. (1974). Historical origins of the health belief model. *Health Education Monographs, 2,* 328–335.

Rosenstock, I. M., Strecher, V. J., & Becker, M. H. (1988). Social learning theory and the health belief model. *Health Education Quarterly, 15*(2), 175–183.

Rozensky, R. H., Johnson, N. G., Goodheart, C. D., & Hammond, R. W. (2003). *Psychology builds a healthy world.* Washington, DC: American Psychological Association.

Russell, K. M. (1991). Development of an instrument to assess maternal childhood injury health beliefs and social influence. *Issues in Comprehensive Pediatric Nursing, 14,* 163–177.

Schneiderman, N., Speers, M. A., Silva, J. M., Tomes, H., & Gentry, J. H. (Eds.). (2001). *Integrating behavioral and social sciences with public health.* Washington, DC: American Psychological Association.

Sellstrom, E., Bremberg, S., Garling, A., & Hornquist, J. O. (2000). Risk of childhood injury: Predictors of mothers' perceptions. *Scandinavian Journal of Public Health, 28*(3), 188–193.

Simons-Morton, B. G., Hartos, J., Leaf, W. A., & Preusser, D. (2005). *Cognitive mediation of the effect of persuasive materials on parent-imposed driving limits of novice young drivers.* Manuscript submitted for publication.

Sleet, D. A., & Hopkins, K. N. (Eds.). (2004). *Bibliography of behavioral science research in unintentional injury prevention* [CD-ROM]. Atlanta, GA: Department of Health and Human Services, Centers for Disease Control and Prevention, National Center for Injury Prevention and Control. www.cdc.gov/pub-res/behavioral.

Sleet, D. A., Hollenbach, K., & Hovell, M. (1986). Applying behavioral principles to motor vehicle occupant protection. *Education and Treatment of Children, 9,* 320–333.

Sleet, D. A., & Lonero, L. (2002). Behavioral strategies for reducing traffic crashes. In L. Breslow (Ed.), *Encyclopedia of public health* (pp. 105–107). New York: Macmillan.

Smedley, B. D., & Syme, S. L. (Eds.). (2000). *Promoting health: Intervention strategies from social and behavioral research.* Washington, DC: National Academy Press.

Smith, B., Sullivan, E., Bauman, A., Powell-Davies, G., & Mitchell, J. (1999). Lay beliefs about the preventability of major health conditions. *Health Education Research, 14,* 315–325.

Streff, F. M., & Geller, E. S. (1986). Strategies for motivating safety belt use: The application of applied behavior analysis. *Health Education Research, 1,* 47–59.

Thompson, N. J., Sleet, D., & Sacks, J. J. (2002). Increasing the use of bicycle helmets: Lessons from behavioral science. *Patient Education and Counseling, 46,* 191–197.

Thomson, J. A., Ampofo Boateng, K., Lee, D. N., Grieve, R., Pitcairn, T. K., & Demetre, J. D. (1998). The effectiveness of parent in promoting the development of road crossing skills in young children. *British Journal of Educational Psychology, 68,* 475–491.

Thuen, F., & Rise, J. (1994). Young adolescents' intention to use seat belts: The role of attitudinal and normative beliefs. *Health Education Research, 9,* 215–223.

Triandis, H. C. (1980). Values, attitudes and interpersonal behavior. In H. E. How & M. M. Page (Eds.), *Nebraska Symposium on Motivation 1979* (pp. 197–259). Lincoln: University of Nebraska Press.

Trifiletti, L. B. (2005). *The utility of the precaution adoption process model for understanding car safety seat use.* Unpublished manuscript.

Trifiletti, L. B., Gielen, A. C., Sleet, D. A., & Hopkins, K. (2005, Jan. 4). Behavioral and social sciences theories and models: Are they used in unintentional injury prevention research? *Health Education Research (Advance Access),* 1–10.

Van Houten, R., & Nau, P. A. (1983). Feedback interventions and driving speed: A parametric and comparative analysis. *Journal of Applied Behavior Analysis, 16,* 153–281.

Weinstein, N. D. (1988). The precaution adoption process. *Health Psychology, 7*(4), 355–386.

Weinstein, N. D., Lyon, J. E., Sandman, P. M., & Cuite, C. L. (1998). Experimental evidence for stages of health behavior change: The precaution adoption process model applied to home radon testing. *Health Psychology, 17*(5), 445–453.

Weinstein, N. D., & Sandman, P. M. (1992). A model of the precaution adoption process: Evidence from home radon testing. *Health Psychology, 11*(3), 170–180.

Weinstein, N. D., & Sandman, P. M. (2002). The precaution adoption process model and its application. In R. J. DiClemente, R. A. Crosby, & M. C. Kegler (Eds.), *Emerging theories in health promotion practice and research.* San Francisco: Jossey-Bass.

Williams, A. F., Wells, J. K., & Farmer, C. M. (2002). Effectiveness of Ford's belt reminder system in increasing seat belt use. *Injury Prevention, 8,* 293–296.

Williams-Avery, R. M., & MacKinnon, D. P. (1996). Injuries and use of protective equipment among college in-line skaters. *Accident Analysis and Prevention, 28,* 779–784.

Wittenbraker, J., Gibbs, B., & Kahle, L. R. (1983). Seat belt attitudes, habits, and behaviors: An adaptive amendment to the Fishbein model. *Journal of Applied Social Psychology, 13,* 406–421.

Wong, T. Y., & Seet, B. (1997). A behavioral analysis of eye protection use by soldiers. *Military Medicine, 162,* 744–748.

Wortel, E., de Geus, G. H., & Kok, G. (1995). Behavioral determinants of mothers' safety measures to prevent injuries of pre-school children. *Scandinavian Journal of Psychology, 36,* 306–322.

CHAPTER THREE

THE APPLICATION OF SOCIAL COGNITIVE THEORY TO INJURY PREVENTION

Bruce Simons-Morton, Tonja Nansel

Overview of Social Cognitive Theory

Social cognitive theory (SCT) represents a revolutionary way of thinking that has had a major and sustained impact on the applied behavior sciences. It provides a comprehensive explanation of behavior, integrating elements of cognitive and operant theories. Importantly, it has become a dominant perspective guiding the development and evaluation of health promotion interventions, although it has been employed in surprisingly few injury prevention studies. The major advantage of SCT is that it provides a comprehensive theoretical explanation for behavior and introduces several key constructs that are readily understandable and adapt well to the development of intervention activities.

Psychoanalytic, trait, and related intrapsychic perspectives of behavior and psychopathology have been the predominant models guiding psychology for many years and remain prominent today among personality theorists, who assume that some characteristic inside a person accounts for motivation and behavior (Kazdin, 2001; Weiner, 1992). In contrast, classical principles of learning assume that motivation and behavior are primarily the product of the situational exposure (Hull, 1943). Essentially, the more a behavior is reinforced, the greater is the frequency or likelihood of its reoccurrence (Skinner, 1953). Today it is understood that both the environment and the individual are important determinants of behavior and are interactive rather than independent (Kazdin, 2001). Since the mid-1900s, the field of psychology has recognized that motivation is influenced by drive, personality, emotion, cognition, and past experience, as well as overt reinforcement (Weiner, 1992). Few would argue with the contention that individuals exhibit some consistencies in performance over time, suggesting inherent individual differences or traits. Accordingly, it takes less reinforcement to increase the frequency of some behaviors than others, and the effect of reinforcement on behavior varies from individual to individual (Kazdin, 2001). Moreover, it is becoming increasingly clear that the reinforcement of human behavior is much more complex than first indicated by rat maze research. It is not that the principles of operant conditioning are incorrect, but rather that human beings are cognitive creatures who can and do anticipate reinforcement and calculate the likelihood of reinforcement in any given situation (Weiner, 1992). They are also capable of generalizations about the likelihood of future events that are quite beyond other creatures. Consequently, the study of human behavior has shifted dramatically toward cognitive theories.

Julian Rotter (1954) provided the basis for social learning theory (of which SCT is a specific, if comprehensive, application) by introducing the idea of generalized expectancies as a way of understanding cognitive processing of anticipated reinforcement. Rotter suggested that people behave according to their cognitive expectations for reinforcement and not just according to actual reinforcement. While this seems obvious now, it was a breakthrough in thinking about how people evaluate stimuli. The perspective that people store their experiences cognitively helped explain how stimuli can influence behavior even in the absence of reinforcement. Rotter's concepts extended well beyond the idea that people remember being reinforced in similar situations, which had long been understood. He suggested that people, based on their experience and their cognitive interpretation of their experience, develop generalized expectations about the likelihood of being reinforced in any given situation. Finally it was clear that humans anticipate reinforcement and even in the absence of obvious reinforcement will behave as if being reinforced because they have been in the past and believe they may be again under similar circumstances.

Rotter's contributions to social learning theory were seminal for psychology. They fostered generations of enlightened theorists and researchers who, over the course of half a century, have advanced what are known as value expectancy theories to the point where a great deal is now understood about information processing and cognitive influences on complex human behaviors. Although cognition does not fully explain behavior (due to other important influences such as drive, personality, and environment), it is particularly important because it is highly amenable to change, even through common educational means.

Of the many important theorists who followed Rotter, Albert Bandura, the father of modern SCT, is certainly one of the most important. Bandura is credited with many important contributions to social learning theory, for example, the recognition that behavior could be learned and increased through the observation of others performing the behavior (Bandura, 1986). Thus, modeling became an important part of SCT. Bandura also noted that people could be reinforced vicariously by observing the experience of others (vicarious reinforcement). He introduced the concepts of efficacy and outcome expectations as key cognitive mediators of behavior (Bandura, 1982). Certainly, one of Bandura's most important contributions has been providing an overarching conceptualization of how environmental and cognitive factors influence behavior (Bandura, 1986). This monumental task of organizing the many conceptual pieces of the puzzle from classical learning theory, operant conditioning, and expectancy theories is a noble attempt to provide one grand unifying theory of behavior.

Description of Social Cognitive Theory

Initially, Bandura described his ideas about behavior within the prevailing context of social learning theory (Miller & Dollard, 1941). The term *social learning theory* has long been employed to describe a range of disparate concepts about social interactions and behavior. Eventually Bandura consolidated his ideas under a new term, *social cognitive theory*, and introduced and elaborated it in his landmark book, *Social Foundations of Thought and Action: A Social Cognitive Theory* (1986). Here Bandura synthesized an impressive array of studies and concepts in support of a social cognitive theory. Social cognitive theory, like social learning theory, emphasizes social influences on behavior. Moreover, Bandura's social cognitive theory is comprehensive, emphasizing both social and cognitive mediation of behavior and providing a cohesive conceptualization of the relationships between behavior, cognition, and the social and physical environment.

The grand concept of social cognitive theory is reciprocal determinism, also referred to as triadic reciprocity, shown in Figure 3.1. Accordingly, environment, behavior, and person are understood to be dynamically interrelated. Here the *environment* represents the external social and physical milieu. *Behavior* refers to actions, either intentional or not. *Person* refers to the individual cognitive, affective, and biological self. The environment influences behavior by providing context, opportunity, and reinforcement, which are processed by the person and acted on. Through action, behavior influences the environment, and this experience provides information that is processed and stored cognitively and emotionally by the person. Of course, each person processes information gathered from his or her

FIGURE 3.1. RECIPROCAL DETERMINISM.

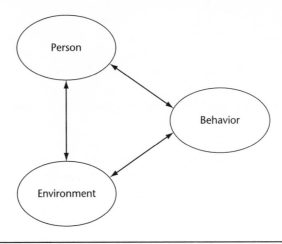

Source: Based on Bandura (1986).

behavior, the environment, and the interaction between behavior and the environment based on his or her unique self and past experiences. The constant and dynamic reciprocity of these three components makes them integral, such that a change in one component is associated with a change in the others.

Today the concept of reciprocal determinism is a generally accepted principle of many health behavior paradigms and has been an important stimulus for the development of multilevel programming in health promotion (Simons-Morton, Simons-Morton, Parcel, & Bunker, 1988; Simons-Morton, Brink, Lee, & Bunker, 1988; Simons-Morton & Simons-Morton, 1989; Simons-Morton, Parcel, Baranowski, O'Hara, & Forthofer, 1991; Simons-Morton, Greene, & Gottlieb, 1995; Simons-Morton, Haynie, Saylor, Davis, & Chen, 1999; Bartholomew, Parcel, Kok, & Gottlieb, 2001) and injury prevention (Simons-Morton, Brink, Lee, & Bunker, 1988; Simons-Morton & Simons-Morton, 1989; Simons-Morton, Hartos, & Haynie, 2002). In general, modern health promotion and injury prevention practice assume that each individual is more or less unique, that each learns from his or her behavior, and that behavior and person are shaped by the environment. Bandura elaborated on these ideas and placed them within a cohesive conceptualization.

Nonetheless, it is not the development of these concepts as much as their implications that are important here. Notably, each person is unique and therefore will not behave or react to the environment in exactly the same manner as another person. Each person has unique experiences, genetic makeup, and personality and has variable mood and cognitive capabilities and propensities. Therefore, people do not experience the common environment in the same way. Moreover, the environment is not a uniform context, encompassing the physical environment and the broader social setting, such as policy, neighborhood, school, as well as very specific social settings, such as family and peer relationships and interactions. Finally, while the environment affects behavior, behavior also affects the environment, providing unique feedback to the person and also creating a unique environment for each individual. Social cognitive theory takes into account the uniqueness of humans, but at the same time provides a common framework for understanding their behavior.

Social Cognitive Theory Constructs

One purpose of theory is to provide a context for various ideas and sources of evidence. The broad concept of reciprocal determinism brings together and allows us to better understand a number of important constructs that would otherwise be understood only within their own more limited contexts. SCT is richly described by Bandura (1986), and Baranowski, Perry, and Parcel (2002) have provided a succinct overview. Given the comprehensiveness of the theory, only a few of the more popular and easily understood constructs can be described in this chapter.

Environment. The broad physical and social environment sets the stage for behavior. The environment includes physical things, such as resources, equipment, and facilities, as well as policies, programs, and enforcement practices that influence behavior. Importantly, the environment encompasses social influences, including the profound influence of close others and the more subtle influence of general social norms. In general, the environment provides both opportunity and reinforcement.

Situation. The environment is not uniform in how it influences behavior, because people experience it in unique ways. The environment may seem to be supportive, but some people may not perceive it to be supportive. For example, car safety seat use is required by law for infants and toddlers, and low-cost loaner programs are widely available. However, some parents may perceive that their particular environment is not supportive of car safety seat use. They may perceive a lack of social support or that their routine use of several different vehicles makes car safety seat use too difficult.

Reinforcement. At the simplest level, reinforcement, the primary construct in operant conditioning, explains the frequency or likelihood of behavior. Positive reinforcement, or reward, is a response to a person's behavior that increases the frequency or likelihood that the behavior will occur again. For example, when parents regularly provide approval of their children's use of bicycle helmets, the frequency of their children's helmet use is likely to increase. Negative reinforcement increases behavior by withdrawal of something aversive when the desired behavior is performed. For example, a child may wear a bicycle helmet to stop his parents' nagging about it. But reinforcement is infinitely complex because people do not experience the same stimuli in the same way. For example, some children may avoid wearing bicycle helmets because their parents' nagging provides a valued source of interaction, and despite the intent and nature of the interaction, nagging in this case actually reinforces noncompliance. Also, the reinforcement that parents provide their children for wearing bicycle helmets may be less powerful than the reinforcement the children obtain from just not bothering, from the perception that their peers will approve of their not wearing helmets, or from their self-image as a free spirit or daredevil. Then again, it may be that parental admonishments about bicycle helmets are unheeded because they are not contingent, that is, parents impose no actual consequence for nonuse. It may be that children require substantial and sustained environmental reinforcement before they develop the habit of wearing bicycle helmets.

Some behaviors provide their own reinforcement, while others may require more frequent attention or the threat of more substantial consequences or the promise of incentives, at least for a time, if they are to be initiated and maintained. Of course, some consequences are more reinforcing than others. Material rewards, for example, greatly influence behavior and are often employed to get people to initiate the performance of a behavior that they might otherwise never try. Personal appeals and relations are also powerful sources of reinforcement (Kazdin, 2001). The Safety Belt Connection study (Simons-Morton, Brink, & Bates, 1987) demonstrated that it is possible to increase safety belt use among drivers at employee parking lots through reinforcement. Initially, belt users were provided immediate reinforcement in the form of inexpensive material incentives as they exited the parking lot. A few drivers at each lot were recruited to provide testimonials and serve as models on posters displayed in prominent locations. Group rates of weekly safety belt use were recorded on large thermometer-type signs located at the parking lot. The intervention resulted in significant and substantial increases in safety belt use rates.

Because reinforcement is complicated by cognitive interpretation, the same consequence does not affect each person's behavior in the same way or to the same extent. The task for behavioral scientists interested in understanding and influencing behavior is to better understand the nature of reinforcement and how the environment, both the proximal social environment and the more distal community and policy environment, can be shaped to reinforce health-promoting behavior and discourage health-damaging behavior.

Observational Learning. Another way people learn is by observing the behavior of others (Bandura, 1962). The process of learning through the observed experience of others occurs through both vicarious reinforcement and modeling. In vicarious reinforcement, people learn from the reinforcement experience of others. For example, skateboarders do not need to personally experience lacerations and broken bones to understand the importance of safety equipment because they can observe the experience of others. Of course, people do not always interpret the experience of others in the same way. Some witnesses of gruesome skateboard injuries may gain increased appreciation for safety equipment, while others witnessing the same events but who have somewhat different orientations may perceive that the injuries sustained without safety gear were an acceptable risk, that the injuries were avoidable, or that they are not personally vulnerable to such injuries. Sometimes a few key role models may greatly influence the view of an entire group. Wearing safety gear for skateboarding, for example, may depend on the behavior of certain influential members of the group whose behavior and attitudes influence the others, shaping the norms for the entire referent group. Thus, the use of safety gear may vary by location, group, and orientation.

Modeling is a form of observational learning. Observing a behavior performed by influential others can affect the perceptions of the observer about social norms and outcome expectations, thereby influencing behavior. Modeling is not only an important concept for understanding the general social environment and the influence of significant others on behavior, but also provides a useful method for changing behavior. For example, infant car seat use increases when hospital staff require that infants' first ride home be in a car safety seat, particularly when car safety seats can be obtained at the hospital (Brink & Simons-Morton, 1989); mothers are more likely to place their infants to sleep on the back when they observe hospital staff placing their infants on the back (Brenner et al., 2003); safety belt use among children is greater when parents buckle their own safety belts (Page, 1986); and bicycle helmet use among children may be more likely when parents serve as models for these behaviors.

Behavioral Capability. *Behavioral capability* is the SCT term for knowledge and skills. As every health educator knows, knowledge and skills are essential but not necessarily sufficient to promote the adoption and maintenance of health-promoting behaviors. Still, if a complex behavior is to be performed, the actor must be knowledgeable about the behavior and have relevant practical skill that would allow performance of the behavior under a variety of relevant conditions. This does not always mean that the person needs to be taught how to do things, because people also learn from doing. Many people figure out on their own how to install car seats, for example, but some people are better able to figure it out than others. Also, some people think they have figured it out but get it wrong, so there is sometimes a need in health education and injury prevention for specific instruction. It may often be the case that people develop skills, but not to the point of mastery, so they are able to perform the behavior under ideal but not actual circumstances. For example, in our research on adolescent problem behavior, where we teach middle school students social skills to enable them to deal with difficult peers and complex social situations, the difficulty many students have is being able to employ their new skills outside the classroom in situations that are dynamic and emotional (Simons-Morton, Haynie, Saylor, Crump, & Chen, 2004). Behavioral capability implies practical and useful understanding of knowledge that is essential for performing a skill or task under a range of practical situations.

Outcome Expectations and Expectancies. Outcome expectations are the anticipated consequences of behavior. This important SCT construct operationalizes Rotter's concepts about cognitive expectations for reinforcement. SCT posits that a person develops impressions about the likelihood of various responses to behaviors under consideration. Accordingly, people anticipate the consequences of their actions in advance of actually engaging in the behavior and sometimes in advance of encountering situations in which the behavior would be possible and relevant. Outcome expectations are developed primarily through actual and vicarious experience and are stored as memories and emotions. For example, a mother's expectations about the outcomes that are likely to result from installing a car seat and putting her young child in the seat are developed from past experience with car seats and from observing the car seat experience of others. Every possible outcome of an action may range from good to bad. Each person may perceive the likelihood of the possible outcomes differently and develop unique values or expectancies for those outcomes. Social influence features prominently in the development of outcome expectations. In our example of car seats, a mother may anticipate that her husband will be annoyed that securing the child is taking a long time. At the same time, the mother may be concerned that the child may be fussy while being installed, that she is in a hurry to get someplace, and that the child is likely to be safe, secure, and content while in the car seat. All of these outcomes may be likely, and the mother will value each, but not equally. In other words, she will not only expect certain outcomes but she will have different expectancies about each of these outcomes in various contexts. These expectancies, the value placed on each possible outcome, are factored into assumptions about their likelihood. The combination of expectations about the likelihood of the possible outcomes and their relative and absolute value determines the strength of influence on behavior.

Self-Efficacy. Self-efficacy is unique to SCT (Bandura, 1982, 1997), although many other theories have come to include a similar construct. Self-efficacy refers to a person's confidence in his or her ability to undertake a specific action successfully. It may be influenced by a person's specific capabilities and other individual factors, as well as by environmental facilitators and barriers. In our car seat example, the mother may develop different values regarding the possible outcomes depending on her confidence in her ability to deal with them. If she is confident that she can deal with her husband's impatience, her baby's fussiness, and the complexity of the car seat fittings, she may develop more positive outcome expectations and expectancies and be more likely to employ the car seat.

Self-efficacy is a central SCT construct as it relates not just to perceptions about specific capabilities but also to the exercise of self-influence in general, relating in important ways to the broad concepts of self-concept, self-esteem, and self-image. Self-efficacy is viewed as an essential aspect of intent (or personal agency, as Bandura refers to it). Accordingly, choice among alternative behaviors is partially the product of reflective thought about potential self-influence. A person's consideration of the extent to which he or she can influence a particular event or accomplish a particular outcome is a powerful aspect of their motivation. Of course, this is complicated. A mother struggling to buckle a child into a car safety seat or booster seat may persist to success only to the extent that she perceives herself capable not only of securing and settling the child, but also of managing an impatient husband or unbelieving mother and her own feelings of conflict about not holding her unhappy baby.

Other Constructs. SCT includes a wealth of other constructs too lengthy to describe here. However, the interested reader can expect to be well rewarded for reading Bandura's (1986, 1997) descriptions of self-control (and related self-regulation mechanisms), emotional arousal, moral judgment, modes of thought verification, and the like.

Application of Social Cognitive Theory to Injury Prevention

Although a considerable body of research has addressed demographic predictors of injury risk and protective behavior, few studies that examine social and cognitive determinants of injury behavior have been conducted, and most of these have not been theory driven. However, several studies have included an assessment of one or more constructs central to social cognitive theory. An examination of findings across these studies lends substantial support to the relevance of social cognitive theory.

Environmental influences are a consistent and important predictor of injury prevention behavior. Notably, the introduction of legislation is one of the most effective mechanisms for wide-scale adoption of safety behaviors (Schieber, Gilchrist, & Sleet, 2000) and has demonstrated effectiveness in reducing injury mortality in a variety of areas, particularly motor vehicle safety (Foss, Feaganes, & Rodgman, 2001; O'Toole, 2002; Beck, Mack, & Shults, 2004). Smaller-scale environmental factors also exert considerable influence. Several studies addressing workplace safety among manual laborers have shown a relationship between workplace safety climate (for example, management commitment to safety or corporate safety policies) and safety behavior or injury incidence (Gillen, Baltz, Gassel, Kirsch, & Vaccaro, 2002; Huang & Acton, 2004; Huang, Chen, Krauss, & Rogers, 2004; O'Toole, 2002; Rundmo & Hale, 2003; Varonen & Mattila, 2000). Reinforcement in the form of incentives and feedback has demonstrated efficacy in improving workplace safety conditions and reducing injury (McAfee & Winn, 1989), and the use of incentives to promote seat belt use has shown considerable effectiveness (Roberts, Alexander, & Knapp, 1990; Roberts & Fanurik, 1986; Roberts, Fanurik, & Wilson, 1988; Roberts & Turner, 1986; Simons-Morton et al., 1987). Another important environmental influence is the behavior of peers and family. For example, among a sample of high school students, friends' helmet use and parents' positive attitude toward helmet use were the strongest predictors of having and using a bicycle helmet (Lajunen & Rasanen, 2001). Friends' use of car seats and spouse's approval have been found to be associated with car seat use (Gielen, Eriksen, Daltroy, & Rost, 1984), and perceived norms of relatives and friends was shown to be an important determinant of mothers' injury prevention behaviors (Sellstrom & Bremberg, 1996). Environmental factors may also inhibit the performance of safety behaviors. For example, the presence of environmental barriers was associated with greater in-home safety hazards and fewer injury prevention practices among parents of young children (Gielen, Wilson, Faden, Wissow, & Harvilchuck, 1995; Russell & Champion, 1996).

Individual beliefs central to social cognitive theory have also consistently demonstrated a relationship with injury prevention behaviors. Greater self-efficacy has been found to be associated with a positive attitude toward safety rules (Grau, Martinez, Agut, & Salnova, 2002), parent teaching of safety skills (Peterson, Farmer, & Kashani, 1990, 1991), and fewer in-home safety hazards (Russell & Champion, 1996). Self-efficacy has been examined as an important outcome in injury prevention intervention studies targeting water heater thermostat temperatures (Cardenas & Simons-Morton, 1993) and falls among elderly persons (Huang & Acton, 2004). Risk perceptions and outcome expectations—beliefs that injury prevention behavior will result in specific positive outcomes or avoid specific negative outcomes—have been shown to be associated with various injury prevention behaviors, including car seat use (Gielen et al., 1984; Inder & Geddis, 1990), seat belt use (Trafimow & Fishbein, 1994; Thuen & Rise, 1994), parent teaching of safety skills (Peterson, Farmer, & Kashani, 1990, 1991), and bicycle helmet use (Weiss, Okun, & Quay, 2004).

Given SCT's utility for guiding intervention development and successful application across a range of health behaviors (Abrams & Follick, 1983; Parcel et al., 1987; Simons-Morton et al., 1991; Baranowski et al., 2000; Perry et al., 2000; Simons-Morton, Haynie, Saylor, Crump, & Chen, 2004), it is surprising that few injury prevention interventions have used SCT as the underlying theoretical framework guiding program development and implementation. SCT may be employed as the primary theory guiding intervention development or in conjunction with other theoretical perspectives. To illustrate the application of SCT to injury prevention, we first explore several conceptual applications and then present two case studies from our own work.

Conceptual Applications of SCT Constructs to Injury Prevention

In Table 3.1 we present the application of SCT constructs to three areas of injury prevention: car safety seats, workplace safety, and falls among the elderly. For each injury area, examples of the application of eight SCT constructs are provided. A review of the application of each construct illustrates the utility of SCT for both understanding behavior and the development of interventions to effect change.

The reader may note the ways in which behavior may be influenced at multiple levels and how the most appropriate or feasible constructs to target may vary across injury areas. For example, an examination of the application of SCT to workplace safety practices demonstrates the influence of the work environment on the observational learning and reinforcement provided to workers, and subsequently their behavioral capability, expectations, expectancies, and self-efficacy. The concept of reciprocal determinism is also evidenced across these applications. In preventing falls among the elderly, for example, one can see how influencing the person's behavior to install assistive devices would create a change in the environment that would affect future behavior. Similarly, a strength-training intervention would increase physical capability, resulting in a subsequent effect on individual behavior, further creating change in the person's self-efficacy.

Specific Applications of SCT to Injury Prevention Intervention Development

In the following sections we present two examples of injury prevention programs based on SCT. The first, Safe n' Sound, is a program designed to improve home injury prevention among parents of young children. The program seeks to affect

TABLE 3.1. APPLICATION OF SOCIAL COGNITIVE THEORY VARIABLES TO THREE INJURY AREAS.

Construct	Car Safety Seats (CSS)	Workplace Safety Practices	Prevention of Falls in Elderly
Environment	CSS regulations regarding standards for safety and use; mandatory use laws; enforcement practices; cost, availability of loaner, and reduced cost access; prevailing social values and norms	Occupational Safety and Health Administration regulations; enforcement policies; workplace safety policies; presence of workers' union; presence of safety officers; safety inspections; specific work site hazards; availability of safety equipment and information; presence of posted or verbal reminders	Existence of sidewalks, stairs, handrails; layout of home; environmental factors influencing lifetime diet and physical activity
Situation	Perceptions of laws, enforcement, relative advantages; cost; social values and norms	Job demands; safety training provided; coworkers' compliance with safety rules	Degree of strength and mobility, side effects of medications, living alone, instrumental social support, resources for assistive devices
Reinforcement	Consequences (actual or anticipated) of CSS use or nonuse	Supervisor recognition for safe workplace behavior	Responses to use or nonuse of assistive devices
Observational learning	Reinforcement that occurs from viewing others' use and the outcomes of others' use of CSS	Observed management response to other workers' safety concerns, safety behaviors, and injuries	Exposure to others using assistive devices and outcomes
Expectations	Anticipated positive and negative outcomes of using CSS	Anticipated positive and negative outcomes of implementing safety policies and practices	Anticipated positive and negative outcomes of assistive device use
Expectancies	The value placed on any anticipated given outcomes of CSS use	The value placed on any given anticipated outcome	The value placed on any given anticipated outcome
Behavioral capability	Ability to use CSS correctly	Ability to perform job tasks, identify hazards, negotiate with others	Ability to install and use assistive devices
Self-efficacy	Confidence in ability to use CSS correctly and consistently	Confidence in ability to implement safety policies and practices	Confidence in ability to perform activities of daily living without falling
Emotional coping	Strategies for dealing with emotional stimuli related to or competing with CSS use	Strategies for dealing with emotional responses influencing workplace safety behavior	Strategies for dealing with emotional response to need for assistive devices

key SCT variables through tailored persuasive messages. The second example, The Checkpoints Program, is designed to improve parental management of novice teen driving by fostering social norms, outcome expectations, and efficacy leading to limits on teen driving privileges.

Safe n' Sound. Unintentional injuries are the leading cause of preventable death and a major cause of morbidity among children ages one to five years in the United States (Centers for Disease Control and Prevention, 2004). Over 90 percent of these injuries occur in and around the home (Rivara, Calonge, & Thompson, 1989). The type and severity of injuries occurring during these years exhibit developmental patterns, reflecting changes in both exposure and developmental capabilities (Dowd, Keenan, & Bratton, 2002; Mazurek, 1994; Pickett, Streight, Simpson, & Brison, 2003; Scheidt et al., 1995). While considerable progress has been made in reducing the burden of injury, it is estimated that approximately one-third of childhood injury deaths are preventable (Philippakis et al., 2004).

Behaviors and devices for preventing in-home injuries in children at each stage are well known; however, they are used insufficiently (Gielen et al., 1995; Glik, Greaves, Kronenfeld, & Jackson, 1993; Gofin & Palti, 1991; Nansel et al., 2002). Various educational programs have been implemented in an attempt to increase injury prevention behavior, but the effectiveness of these has been less than optimal (Damashek & Peterson, 2002; DiGuiseppi & Roberts, 2000; Pless & Arsenault, 1987; Scheidt, 1988; Towner, 1995; Wortel, de Geus, Kok, & van Woerkum, 1994). Possibly, a program that provides education and targets key social cognitive constructs may result in greater behavior change.

Safe n' Sound was developed to increase injury prevention behaviors among parents of children age four and younger. The program was designed to address the most relevant and potentially malleable social cognitive determinants of pediatric injury prevention behavior (Table 3.2). Additional features of the program selected to increase effectiveness include delivery in the pediatric outpatient clinic, provision of individually tailored information based on current behaviors and beliefs, and reinforcement of information by the health care provider.

Safe n' Sound is a computerized assessment and tailored feedback system designed to provide parents with relevant and motivating injury prevention information. Parents complete an age-appropriate assessment of their current injury prevention practices on-screen. Responses are written to a database, and algorithms are used to determine (1) the two highest-priority injury prevention behavior changes and (2) injury prevention message content to provide. The selected messages are then printed to a blank template and provided to the parent.

The printed feedback provided to parents consists of three pages. The first page contains introductory and summary information, including messages tailored

TABLE 3.2. SOCIAL COGNITIVE THEORY APPLIED TO PARENTAL INJURY PREVENTION BEHAVIORS FOR YOUNG CHILDREN.

Construct	Definition	Measurement	Intervention Components
Environment	Physical structure of home; social norms regarding home safety practices	Perceived importance of injury prevention to physician; perceived peer norms for use of safety devices	Tailored introduction regarding importance of injury prevention as part of health care; parent testimonial regarding specific safety behaviors
Situation	Perceptions regarding injury prevention behaviors; perceived impediments to safety behaviors	Attitudes toward injury prevention; barriers to injury prevention behavior	Tailored message targeting attitudes competing with injury prevention behavior; provision of concrete step-by-step instructions for reducing risk
Reinforcement	Responses of others to safety and risk behaviors	Perceived importance of injury prevention to physician; perceived peer norms for use of safety devices	Praise for safety behaviors reported; message regarding importance to physician; parent testimonials
Observational learning	Observed safety and risk behaviors of others	Perceived peer norms for use of safety devices	Parent testimonial regarding decision to implement specific safety behaviors
Expectations	Anticipated outcomes of using safety devices or engaging in risk behaviors	Outcome expectations for risk and protective behaviors	Specific, targeted information (based on assessment data) about risks and benefits; parent testimonial demonstrating positive outcome
Expectancies	Values placed on anticipated outcomes	Outcome expectations for risk and protective behaviors	Message nesting importance of injury prevention within other important parenting concerns
Behavioral capability	Skills in implementing injury prevention practices	Current injury prevention practices	Provision of simple, concrete steps to implement injury prevention behavior
Self-efficacy	Confidence in ability to use safety devices and prevent child injury	Self-efficacy for preventing injuries	Parent testimonials structured as role modeling; introductory efficacy-building message
Emotional coping	Strategies for dealing with emotional stimuli related to injury prevention	Response to injury prevention messages	Message acknowledging difficulty of parenting; presentation of a limited number of priority changes (based on assessment data); focus on limited number of specific behaviors to keep child safe

to specific injury prevention beliefs and a summary of the individual's highest injury risk areas (falls, burns, poisoning, airway obstruction, drowning, and car safety). Pages 2 and 3 provide information on each of the two highest-priority injury prevention behavior changes. Education information includes sections with general information on the importance and relevance of the injury topic, specific information about the priority risk behavior, and specific steps to take to reduce risk. In addition, a brief testimonial by a parent describing why he or she decided to engage in the particular preventive behavior is provided.

An additional one-page summary is created for the health care provider, indicating the two priority injury prevention behavior changes. This concise summary allows the health care provider to reinforce the injury prevention provided and address any relevant questions or concerns the parent may have regarding the information or its implementation. The printout also includes several priority injury prevention behaviors the parent is already doing, allowing the health care provider to reinforce continuation of these behaviors.

The content and structure of Safe n' Sound were designed to have an impact on determinants of parents' injury prevention behavior as understood in relation to social cognitive theory. Nesting the program within the health care setting and providing messages indicating the importance of injury prevention to the health care provider create environmental stimuli to increase the salience and perceived importance of injury prevention behavior. Provision of information to health care providers was designed to increase provider discussion of injury prevention with parents, creating stronger social norms for injury prevention behavior. Parent testimonials in the printed feedback provide an opportunity for observational learning and may influence both perceived social norms and self-efficacy for injury prevention behavior. Specific information about risks to the child and benefits of the target injury prevention behavior is designed to increase positive outcome expectations for the preventive behavior. Parent-reported beliefs indicative of outcome expectations that inhibit injury prevention behaviors are individually addressed. In addition, the introduction nests injury prevention within the context of the many important responsibilities associated with parenting, to further increase expectancies regarding injury prevention behaviors. Finally, to facilitate emotional coping and reduce barriers to change, parents were provided with only two priority behavior changes and were given concrete, simple steps to achieve those changes.

Evaluation of a preliminary version of the program developed for a more restricted age range indicated that parents receiving the intervention demonstrated greater behavior change and a greater use of injury prevention practices than those receiving standard injury prevention information one month after the intervention (Nansel et al., 2002). Current (unpublished) analyses of data from implementation of the full Safe n' Sound program in multiple clinical sites also found greater behavior change after the intervention compared to receipt of standard injury prevention information, particularly among the lower-educated participants. Those receiving the intervention were also more likely to report behavior changes of greater complexity. However, despite the provision of a printed summary and prompt, provider communication with parents regarding injury prevention was minimal; thus, we were unable to determine the potential effect of systematic provider reinforcement of the injury prevention feedback.

Checkpoints Program to Prevent Motor Vehicle Crashes Among Young Drivers.
Motor vehicle crashes are the leading cause of death and disability among adolescents (Centers for Disease Control and Prevention, 1999). Newly licensed teens are at particular risk, and crash rates are especially elevated during the first six months and one thousand miles of independent driving (McCartt, Shabanova, & Leaf, 2003). The causes are well known and include young age at licensure, inexperience, and risk taking, particularly speeding and tailgating (Williams & Ferguson, 2002). Of these, inexperience appears to be the most important. Also, certain driving conditions increase risk, particularly teen passengers, night, and unfamiliar roads. Alcohol, of course, greatly increases the risk of a crash among young drivers and is highly associated with severe crashes (Williams & Ferguson, 2002).

Graduated driver licensing (GDL) is a successful policy innovation that has been adopted by most states over the past two decades. GDL has a three-step licensing process, with an extended supervised practice period, followed by a provisional period when teens can drive without supervision but not after midnight and, in at least one state, with a limited number of teen passengers. Typically, teens can obtain a full, unrestricted license at age eighteen as long as they maintain a good driving record. GDL has been shown to reduce crashes among teen drivers. Some analysts (McKnight & Peck, 2002) have found that most of the crash benefits of GDL come from the prolonged supervised practice period, which serves to delay licensure by some months, thereby reducing exposure somewhat. Foss and Goodwin (2003) indicated that GDL is largely passive because police generally do not ticket for infractions unless in conjunction with another violation. Others (Simons-Morton & Hartos, 2003a, 2003b) have pointed out that GDL empowers parents to manage teen driving. Unfortunately, while most parents do impose modest restrictions on their newly licensed teens, these limits tend not to be those that improve safety and are not maintained for very long (Hartos, Eitel, Haynie, & Simons-Morton, 2000; Hartos, Eitel, & Simons-Morton, 2001).

The goal of the Checkpoints Program is to increase parental management of teen driving during the extremely dangerous early months of licensure (see Table 3.3). The Checkpoints Program consists of a videotape, *Who Wants to Be a Driver?* persuasive newsletters, and the Checkpoints Parent-Teen Driving Agreement. The video and newsletters are designed to increase outcome expectations for the parent-teen driving agreement and self-efficacy for negotiating and maintaining an agreement during for the first twelve months of licensure. The program is essentially based on a persuasive communications approach. Viewed through the prism of protection motivation theory, the materials were designed to increase threat appraisal regarding teen driving and coping appraisal regarding the utility of the parent-teen driving agreement as a way of managing risk. SCT constructs were employed to improve the salience of the messages, particularly to emphasize the relative advantages of adopting a parent-teen driving agreement, promote efficacy, and convey the normative nature of parental management practices. Accordingly, the video and newsletters included information about how dangerous driving is during the early months of licensure, emphasizing that inexperience is largely to blame rather than intentional risk-taking behavior, so all inexperienced teens are at risk. The video follows the successful experience of several families (models) as they employ the Checkpoints Parent-Teen Driving Agreement with their newly licensed adolescent. The idea is to convey positive outcome and efficacy expectations for adopting driving limits during the early months of teen licensure. Each newsletter highlights specific teen driving risks, provides suggestions for parental management, includes testimonials from parents and teens, and encourages the adoption and maintenance of the Checkpoints Parent-Teen Driving Agreement. The Checkpoints Program has been evaluated in several randomized trials.

In one Maryland State Department of Motor Vehicle (DMV) licensing office, we recruited families when the teen successfully tested for a provisional (independent driving but not after midnight) driving license. At the DMV, consent and baseline information were collected, and families were exposed to the video, *Who Wants to Be a Driver?* (The dialogue was included in captions at the bottom of the screen to facilitate understanding even in a noisy environment.) A research assistant then provided the family with the Checkpoints Parent-Teen Driving Agreement and provided the following brief verbal admonishment: "Many families have found it helpful and effective to establish an agreement in writing about teen driving privileges. This is the Checkpoints Parent-Teen Driving Agreement. I strongly encourage you complete this agreement right away." The evaluation of this study indicated a significant effect on teen driving privileges that lasted for at least four months after licensure but declined to nonsignificance at nine months (Simons-Morton, Hartos, & Beck, 2003, 2004).

In another study conducted in Connecticut, the Checkpoints Program was implemented at the time of the learner's permit. Families were recruited at multiple state licensing offices and randomized to the Checkpoints Program or the comparison group. The families in the Checkpoints Program received by mail the video and a series of newsletters, one every month or so over the permit period

TABLE 3.3. SOCIAL COGNITIVE THEORY APPLIED TO PARENTAL MANAGEMENT OF TEEN DRIVERS.

Construct	Definition	Measurement	Intervention Components (newsletter, video, personal persuasion)
Environment	Driver licensing laws and enforcement; social values and norms regarding driving and parental management practices	GDL policies; perceive norms for parent limits on teen drivers; risk perceptions	Family models; information about risk; testimonials; information about risk
Situation	Perceptions of licensing laws and enforcement; social values and norms regarding driving and parental management practices	Perceive norms for parent limits on teen drivers; expected limits; risk perceptions	Family models; information about risk; testimonials; information about risk
Reinforcement	Responses to parental restrictions that increase the maintenance of driving restrictions	Outcome expectations; expected limits	Family models reinforced by no accidents and teen acceptance of limits; police and other authorities reward model families; information about risk
Observational learning	Increased restrictions or maintenance of restrictions from vicarious reinforcement	Outcome expectations; expected limits	Family models reinforced by no accidents and teen acceptance of limits; police and other authorities reward model families
Expectations	Anticipated positive and negative outcomes of initiation and maintenance of restrictions	Outcome expectations; expected limits	Information about risk and benefits
Expectancies	Values placed on anticipated outcomes of restrictions	Outcome expectations; expected limits	Information about risk and benefits
Behavioral capability	Skills in negotiation and maintaining restrictions	Expected limits	Instructions for use of the parent-teen driving agreement
Self-efficacy	Confidence in ability to negotiate and maintain restrictions	Self-efficacy	Families model effective negotiation
Emotional coping	Strategies for dealing with emotional stimuli related to or competing with restrictions	Expected limits	Families model improved emotional coping from completing driving agreement

and first six months of licensure. Just before licensure, the family received the Checkpoints Parent-Teen Driving Agreement. This study found that the Checkpoints Program significantly increased parent-imposed driving limits lasting up to twelve months after licensure (Simons-Morton, Hartos, & Leaf, 2002; Simons-Morton, Hartos, Leaf, & Preusser, 2005). Recent analyses indicate that this effect was mediated by changes in risk perception and outcome expectations (Simons-Morton, Hartos, Leaf, & Preusser, in press).

Each of the studies evaluating the efficacy of the Checkpoints Program had unique characteristics. The first study was conducted in Maryland where GDL has been in place for many years, and the recent policies that strengthened GDL were heavily promoted. It would be expected that parents would be more amenable to the Checkpoints Program in a GDL state (Simons-Morton & Hartos, 2003b). Also, in this study, the program was delivered personally by a knowledgeable research assistant at the time of licensure when independent driving was imminent. In the Connecticut study, the newsletters prepared families during the learning period to anticipate parent-imposed licensure limits. However, Connecticut does not have a GDL policy, and the program was delivered passively through the mail. While a great deal needs to be learned about how best to foster greater parental management of teen drivers, the results of the limited research show that it is possible to increase risk perceptions and outcome expectations for parental management through either passive or active delivery of persuasive communications, leading to increased limits on teen driving.

Conclusion

SCT is a grand theory of behavior that incorporates cognition and operant aspects of behavior. Reciprocal determinism suggests that behavior, environment, and person interact dynamically. The environment shapes behavior, and behavior provides consequences and also shapes the environment. The cognitive and affective aspects of the person interpret and store experience uniquely. SCT posits that skill and outcome and efficacy expectations are central cognitive determinants of behavior. SCT fits well with other theories, and it is not uncommon in practice for SCT to be paired with another cognitive theory. SCT is prominent in the development and elaboration of meta-theories of behavior. Given the long-standing focus of injury prevention on environment-person interaction, SCT would seem to be an ideal theory to guide injury prevention research and practice. Yet SCT has been underused in injury prevention research and is employed much less often than in other areas of health promotion and disease prevention. Indeed, for areas such as cardiovascular disease prevention and substance use prevention, SCT is the preeminent theoretical perspective for research and practice.

Nevertheless, SCT has usefully guided research across several areas of injury prevention, and the potential for its application to a range of injury problems is vast.

References

Abrams, D. B., & Follick, M. J. (1983). Behavioral weight-loss intervention at the worksite: Feasibility and maintenance. *Journal of Consulting and Clinical Psychology, 51,* 226–233.

Bandura, A. (1962). Social learning through imitation. In R. R. Jones (Ed.), *Nebraska Symposium on Motivation.* Lincoln: University of Nebraska Press.

Bandura, A. (1982). Self-efficacy mechanism in human agency. *American Psychologist, 37,* 122–147.

Bandura, A. (1986). *Social foundations of thought and action: A social cognitive theory.* Upper Saddle River, NJ: Prentice Hall.

Bandura, A. (1997). *Self-efficacy: The exercise of control.* New York: Freeman.

Baranowski, T., Davis, M., Resnicow, K., Baranowski, J., Doyle, C., Lin, L. S., Smith, M., & Wang, D. T. (2000). Gimme 5 fruit, juice, and vegetables for fun and health: Outcome evaluation. *Health Education and Behavior, 27,* 96–111.

Baranowski, T., Perry, C., & Parcel, G. (2002). How individuals, environments, and health behavior interact: Social cognitive theory. In K. Glanz, B. Rimer, & F. Lewis (Eds.), *Health behavior and health education: Theory, research, and practice* (pp. 165–184). San Francisco: Jossey-Bass.

Bartholomew, L. K., Parcel, G. S., Kok, G., & Gottlieb, N. H. (2001). *Intervention mapping.* Mountain View, CA: Mayfield.

Beck, L. F., Mack, K. A., & Shults, R. A. (2004). Impact of primary laws on adult use of safety belts—United States, 2002. *Journal of the American Medical Association, 291*(19), 2310–2311.

Brenner, R. A., Simons-Morton, B. G., Bhaskar, B., Revenis, M., Das, A., & Clemens, J. (2003). Infant-parent bed sharing in an inner-city population. *Archives of Pediatrics and Adolescent Medicine, 157*(1), 33–39.

Brink, S. G., & Simons-Morton, B. G. (1989). Evaluation of a hospital-based car safety seat education and loan program for low-income mothers: The Car Seat Connection. *Health Education Quarterly, 16*(1), 45–56.

Cardenas, M. P., & Simons-Morton, B. G. (1983). The effect of anticipatory guidance on mothers' self-efficacy and behavioral intentions to prevent burns caused by hot tap water. *Patient Education and Counseling, 21,* 117–123.

Centers for Disease Control and Prevention. (1999). Motor vehicle safety—A twentieth century public health achievement. *Morbidity and Mortality Weekly Report, 48,* 369–374.

Centers for Disease Control and Prevention. National Center for Injury Prevention and Control. (2004). *Injury fact book 2001–2002.* Retrieved Oct. 30, 2004, from http://www.cdc.gov/ncipc/fact_book/.

Damashek, A., & Peterson, L. (2002). Unintentional injury prevention efforts for young children: Levels, methods, types, and targets. *Developmental and Behavioral Pediatrics, 23*(6), 443–455.

DiGuiseppi, C., & Roberts, I. G. (2000). Individual-level injury prevention strategies in the clinical setting. *Future of Children, 10*(1), 53–82.

Dowd, M. D., Keenan, H. T., & Bratton, S. L. (2002). Epidemiology and prevention of childhood injuries. *Critical Care Medicine, 30*(11), S385–S391.

Foss, R. D., Feaganes, J. R., & Rodgman, E. A. (2001). Initial effects of graduated driving licensing on 16-year-old driver crashes in North Carolina. *JAMA, 286,* 1588–1592.

Foss, R., & Goodwin, A. (2003). Enhancing effectiveness of graduated driver licensing legislation. *Journal of Safety Research, 34,* 79–84.

Gielen, A. C., Eriksen, M. P., Daltroy, L. H., & Rost, K. (1984). Factors associated with the use of child restraint devices. *Health Education Quarterly, 11*(2), 195–206.

Gielen, A. C., Wilson, M.E.H., Faden, R. R., Wissow, L., & Harvilchuck, J. D. (1995). In-home injury prevention practices for infants and toddlers: The role of parental beliefs, barriers, and housing quality. *Health Education Quarterly, 22*(1), 85–95.

Gillen, M., Baltz, D., Gassel, M., Kirsch, L., & Vaccaro, D. (2002). Perceived safety climate, job demands, and coworker support among union and nonunion injured construction workers. *Journal of Safety Research, 33,* 33–51.

Glik, D. C., Greaves, P. E., Kronenfeld, J. J., & Jackson, K. L. (1993). Safety hazards in households with young children. *Journal of Pediatric Psychology, 18*(1), 115–131.

Gofin, R., & Palti, H. (1991). Injury prevention practices of mothers of 0 to 2 year olds: A developmental approach. *Early Child Development and Care, 71,* 117–126.

Grau, R., Martinez, I. M., Agut, S., & Salanova, M. (2002). Safety attitudes and their relationship to safety training and generalized self-efficacy. *International Journal of Occupational Safety and Ergonomics, 8*(1), 23–35.

Hartos, J. L., Eitel, P., Haynie, D. L., & Simons-Morton, B. G. (2000). Can I take the car? Relations among parenting practices and adolescent problem driving practices. *Journal of Adolescent Research, 15*(3), 352–367.

Hartos, J. L., Eitel, P., & Simons-Morton, B. G. (2001). Do parent-imposed delayed licensure and restricted driving reduce risky driving behaviors among newly licensed teens? *Prevention Science, 2*(2), 111–120.

Huang, T. T., & Acton, G. J. (2004). Effectiveness of home visit falls prevention strategy for Taiwanese community-dwelling elders: Randomized trial. *Public Health Nursing, 21*(3), 247–256.

Huang, Y. H., Chen, P. Y., Krauss, A. D., & Rogers, D. A. (2004). Quality of the execution of corporate safety policies and employee safety outcomes: Assessing the moderating role of supervisor safety support and the mediating role of employee safety control. *Journal of Business and Psychology, 18*(4), 483–506.

Hull, C. L. (1943). *Principles of behavior.* Englewood Cliffs, NJ: Appleton-Century-Crofts.

Inder, T., & Geddis, D. C. (1990). Factors influencing the use of infant car restraints. *Accident Analysis and Prevention, 22*(3), 297–300.

Kazdin, A. E. (2001). *Behavior modification in applied settings* (6th ed.). Belmont, CA: Wadsworth Press.

Lajunen, T., & Rasanen, M. (2001). Why teenagers owning a bicycle helmet do not use their helmets. *Journal of Safety Research, 32,* 323–332.

Mazurek, A. (1994). Pediatric injury patterns. *International Anesthesiology Clinics, 32*(1), 11–25.

McAfee, R. B., & Winn, A. R. (1989). The use of incentives/feedback to enhance work place safety: A critique of the literature. *Journal of Safety Research, 20,* 7–19.

McCartt, A. T., Shabanova, V. I., & Leaf, W. A. (2003). Driving experience, crashes, and traffic citations of teenage beginning drivers. *Accident Analysis and Prevention, 35*(3), 311–320.

McKnight, A. J., & Peck, R. C. (2002). Graduate driver licensing: What works? *Injury Prevention, 8*(suppl. 2), ii32–ii38.

Miller, N. E., & Dollard, J. (1941). *Social learning and imitation.* New Haven, CT: Yale University Press.

Nansel, T. R., Weaver, N., Donlin, M., Jacobsen, H., Kreuter, M. W., & Simons-Morton, B. (2002). Baby, be safe: The effect of tailored communications for pediatric injury prevention provided in a primary care setting. *Patient Education and Counseling, 46,* 175–190.

O'Toole, M. (2002). The relationship between employees' perceptions of safety and organizational culture. *Journal of Safety Research, 33,* 231–243.

Page, R. M. (1986). Role of parental example in preadolescents' use of seat belts. *Psychological Reports, 59*(pt. 2), 985–986.

Parcel, G. S., Simons-Morton, B. G., O'Hara, N. M., Kolbe, L. J., Baranowski, T., & Bee, D. E. (1987). School health promotion and cardiovascular health: An integration of institutional change and social learning theory intervention. *Journal of School Health, 57*(4), 150–156.

Perry, C. L., Williams, C. L., Komro, K. A., Veblem-Mortensone, S., Forster, J. L., Bernstein-Lachter, R., Pratt, L. K., Dudovitz, B., Munson, K. A., Farbakhsh, K., Finnegan, J., McGovern, P. (2000). Project Northland High School intervention: Community action to reduce adolescent alcohol use. *Health Education and Behavior, 27,* 29–49.

Peterson, L., Farmer, J., & Kashani, J. H. (1990). Parental injury prevention endeavors: A function of health beliefs? *Health Psychology, 9*(2), 177–191.

Peterson, L., Farmer, J., & Kashani, J. H. (1991). The role of beliefs in parental injury prevention efforts. In J. H. Johnson & S. B. Johnson (Eds.), *Advances in child health psychology.* Gainesville: University of Florida Press.

Philippakis, A., Hemenway, D., Alexe, D. M., Dessypris, N., Spyridopoulos, T., & Petridou, E. (2004). A quantification of preventable unintentional childhood injury mortality in the United States. *Injury Prevention, 10,* 79–82.

Pickett, W., Streight, S., Simpson, D., & Brison, R. J. (2003). Injuries experienced by infant children: A population-based epidemiological analysis. *Pediatrics, 111*(4 Pt. 1), 365–370.

Pless, I. B., & Arsenault, L. (1987). The role of health education in the prevention of injuries to children. *Journal of Social Issues, 43*(2), 87–103.

Rivara, F. P., Calonge, N., & Thompson, R. S. (1989). Population-based study of unintentional injury incidence and impact during childhood. *American Journal of Public Health, 79,* 990–994.

Roberts, M. C., Alexander, K., & Knapp, L. G. (1990). Motivating children to use safety belts: A program combining rewards and "Flash for Life." *Journal of Community Psychology, 18*(2), 110–119.

Roberts, M. C., & Fanurik, D. (1986). Rewarding elementary schoolchildren for their use of safety belts. *Health Psychology, 5*(3), 185–196.

Roberts, M. C., Fanurik, D., & Wilson, D. R. (1988). A community program to reward children's use of seat belts. *American Journal of Community Psychology, 16*(3), 395–407.

Roberts, M. C., & Turner, D. S. (1986). Rewarding parents for their children's use of safety seats. *Journal of Pediatric Psychology, 11*(1), 25–36.

Rotter, J. B. (1954). *Social learning and clinical psychology.* Upper Saddle River, NJ: Prentice Hall.

Rotter, J. B. (1966). Generalized expectancies for internal versus external control of reinforcement. *Psychological Monographs, 80*(1), 1–28.

Rundmo, T., & Hale, A. R. (2003). Managers' attitudes towards safety and accident prevention. *Safety Science, 41,* 557–574.

Russell, K. M., & Champion, V. L. (1996). Health beliefs and social influence in home safety practices of mothers with preschool children. *Journal of Nursing Scholarship, 28*(1), 59–64.

Scheidt, P. C. (1988). Behavioral research toward prevention of childhood injury. *American Journal of Diseases of Children, 142,* 612–617.

Scheidt, P., Harel, Y., Trumble, A., Jones, D. H., Overpeck, M. D., & Bijur, P. E. (1995). The epidemiology of nonfatal injuries among US children and youth. *American Journal of Public Health, 85*(7), 932–938.

Schieber, R., Gilchrist, J., & Sleet, D. A. (2000). Legislative and regulatory strategies to reduce childhood unintentional injuries. *Future of Children, 10*(1), 111–136.

Sellstrom, E., & Bremberg, S. (1996). Perceived social norms as crucial determinants of mother's injury-preventive behaviour. *Acta Paediatrica, 85*(6), 702–707.

Simons-Morton, B. G., Brink, S. G., & Bates, D. (1987). The effectiveness and cost effectiveness of persuasive communications and incentives in increasing safety belt use: The Safety Belt Connection Project. *Health Education Quarterly, 14*(2), 167–179.

Simons-Morton, B. G., Brink, S. G., Lee, R., & Bunker, J. (1988). Unsafe in any season: Injury control in beachfront communities. *Family and Community Health, 11*(1), 17–27.

Simons-Morton, B. G., Brink, S. G., Simons-Morton, D. G., Parcel, G. S., McIntyre, R. M., Chapman, M., & Longoria, J. (1989). An ecological approach to preventing injuries due to drinking and driving. *Health Education Quarterly, 16*(3), 397–411.

Simons-Morton, B. G., Greene, W. A., & Gottlieb, N. (1995). *Introduction to health education and health promotion* (2nd ed.). Prospect Heights, IL: Waveland Press.

Simons-Morton, B. G., & Hartos, J. (2003a). How well do parents manage young driver crash risks? *Journal of Safety Research, 34*, 91–97.

Simons-Morton, B. G., & Hartos, J. L. (2003b). Improving the effectiveness of counter measures to prevent motor vehicle crashes among young drivers. *Journal of Health Education, 34*(5), S57–S61.

Simons-Morton, B. G., Hartos, J. L., & Beck, K. (2003). The persistence of effects of a brief intervention on parental restrictions of teen driving privileges. *Injury Prevention, 9,* 142–146.

Simons-Morton, B. G., Hartos, J. L., & Beck, K. (2004). Increased parent limits on teen driving: Positive effects from a brief intervention administered at the motor vehicle administration. *Prevention Science, 5*(2), 101–111.

Simons-Morton, B. G., Hartos, J., & Haynie, D. (2002). Application of authoritative parenting to adolescent health behavior. In R. DiClemente, R. Crosby, & M. Kegler (Eds.), *Emerging theories and models in health promotion research and practice: Strategies for improving practice* (pp. 109–122). San Francisco: Jossey-Bass.

Simons-Morton, B. G., Hartos, J., & Leaf, W. A. (2002). Promoting parental management of teen driving though persuasion: Impact of the Checkpoints Program on immediate outcomes. *Injury Prevention, 8*(suppl. 2), 24–38.

Simons-Morton, B. G., Hartos, J., Leaf, W. A., & Preusser, D. (2005). The persistence of effects of the Checkpoints Program on parental restrictions of teen driving privileges. *American Journal of Public Health, 95*(3), 447–452.

Simons-Morton, B. G., Hartos, J., Leaf, W. A., & Preusser, D. (in press). Cognitive mediation of the effect of persuasive materials on parent-imposed driving limits of novice young drivers. *Journal of Adolescent Research.*

Simons-Morton, B. G., Haynie, D., Saylor, K., Crump, A. D., & Chen, R. (2004). The effects of the Going Places Program on early adolescent substance use and anti-social behavior. *Prevention Science, 5*(2), 101–111.

Simons-Morton, B. G., Haynie, D., Saylor, K., Davis, A. D., & Chen, R. (2005). Evaluation of the Going Places Program: Impact and mediation of program outcomes. *Health Education and Behavior, 32*(2), 227–241.

Simons-Morton, B. G., Lerner, N., & Singer, J. (2005). The observed effects of teenage passengers on the risky driving behavior of teenage drivers. *Accident Analysis and Prevention, 37*(6), 973–982.

Simons-Morton, B. G., Parcel, G. P., Baranowski, T., O'Hara, N., & Forthofer, R. (1991). Promoting a healthful diet and physical activity among children: Results of a school-based intervention study. *American Journal of Public Health, 81*(8), 986–991.

Simons-Morton, B. G., & Simons-Morton, D. G. (1989). Controlling injuries due to drinking and driving: The context and functions of education. In *The Surgeon General's Workshop on Drunk Driving: Background papers*. Washington, DC: U.S. Department of Health and Human Services.

Simons-Morton, D. G., Simons-Morton, B. G., Parcel, G. S., & Bunker, J. F. (1988). Influencing personal and environmental conditions for community health: A multilevel intervention model. *Family and Community Health, 11*(2), 25–35.

Skinner, B. F. (1953). *Science and human behavior.* New York: Macmillan.

Thuen, F., & Rise, J. (1994). Young adolescents' intention to use seat belts: The role of attitudinal and normative beliefs. *Health Education Research, 9*(2), 215–223.

Towner, E.M.L. (1995). The role of health education in childhood injury prevention. *Injury Prevention, 1,* 53–58.

Trafimow, D., & Fishbein, M. (1994). The importance of risk in determining the extent to which attitudes affect intentions to wear seat belts. *Journal of Applied Social Psychology, 24*(1), 1–11.

Varonen, U., & Mattila, M. (2000). The safety climate and its relationship to safety practices, safety of the work environment and occupational accidents in eight wood-processing companies. *Accident Analysis and Prevention, 32,* 761–769.

Weiner, B. (1992). *Human motivation: Metaphors, theories, and research.* Thousand Oaks, CA: Sage.

Weinstein, N. D. (1988). The precaution adoption process. *Health Psychology, 7*(4), 355–386.

Weiss, J., Okun, M., & Quay, N. (2004). Predicting bicycle helmet stage-of-change among middle school, high school, and college cyclists from demographic, cognitive, and motivational variables. *Journal of Pediatrics, 145*(3), 360–364.

Williams, A. F., & Ferguson, S. A. (2002). Rationale for graduate licensing and the risks it should address. *Injury Prevention, 8*(Suppl. 2), ii9–ii16.

Wortel, E., de Geus, G. H., Kok, G., & van Woerkum, C. (1994). Injury control in pre-school children: A review of parental safety measures and the behavioral determinants. *Health Education Research, 9*(2), 201–213.

CHAPTER FOUR

Community Models and Approaches for Interventions

Andrea Carlson Gielen, David A. Sleet, Lawrence W. Green

The injury prevention field's long tradition of effectively using community-wide approaches reflects its commitment to passive protection and to interventions that protect whole populations. In this sense, community interventions in injury control have had a different connotation from that which may be most familiar to health promotion professionals. They share with health promotion an emphasis on ways to protect populations through policy and environmental changes such as safer automobile and roadway designs and safe surfacing installed on playgrounds, to protect entire communities of people without relying on changes in individuals' behaviors. In other instances, communitywide approaches in both injury prevention and other areas of health promotion have tried to change the behavior of large groups of individuals. Examples in injury control include seat belt and car seat legislation, as well as campaigns to promote bicycle helmet use and safe routes to school. It is on this latter approach to community intervention that behavior change theory can be most usefully applied and that is the focus of this chapter. What theory, research, and experience in other areas of

Portions of this chapter were first published in Gielen, A. C., & Sleet, D. (2003). Application of behavior-change theories and methods to injury prevention. *Epidemiologic Reviews, 25,* 65–76; and based on Sleet, D., & Gielen, A. C. (2004). Developing injury interventions: The role of behavioral science. In R. McClure, M. Stevenson, & S. McEvoy (Eds.), *The scientific basis of injury prevention and control.* Melbourne, Australia: IP Communications. Reproduced with permission.

health promotion bring more substantially to injury prevention in this realm is the use of community-based (in addition to communitywide) approaches.

Definition of Community

Although *community* has been variously defined, it is commonly understood to mean a geographical area with defined boundaries and governance, or, more generally, it may be used to describe a group with shared characteristics, interests, values, and norms (Minkler & Wallerstein, 2003). For interventionists, an important feature of communities is that they are dynamic, changing in demographic profile and in response to social, political, and economic events. A distinguishing characteristic of communitywide interventions is that they seek change across an entire population, not solely among high-risk subgroups (Chamberlin, 1988; Shea & Basch, 1990). Green and Kreuter (2005) also distinguish between community interventions and interventions in communities, which are usually channel specific or setting based, such as mass media, school, work site, or medical care. Given these changing meanings of *community*, it might be equally fitting to substitute "population-level models and approaches for intervention" for the title and topic of this chapter.

But Coggan and Bennett (2004) note that community-based injury prevention "occurs when people and organizations collaborate as communities to design and implement strategies to promote safety, reduce the incidence and/or severity of injury in their population, and reduce the prevalence of injury determinants in the community" (p. 349). Collaboration bridges some of the communitywide and community-based elements of programs that depend on multiple organizations and individuals within the community. They go on to highlight the need for multiple strategies, including environmental change, awareness raising, education, and behavior change, the scope of which is consistent with the conclusions drawn from reviews of community intervention evaluations described in the next section. The inclusion of complementary and mutually reinforcing individual-, organizational-, and population-level interventions makes *community*, rather than *population*, the term of choice for this chapter.

Background

Reviews of community interventions for injury prevention are becoming increasingly common (Gielen & Collins, 1993; Klassen, MacKay, Moher, Walker, & Jones, 2000; Turner, McClure, Nixon, & Spinks, 2004, 2005; Turner, Spinks,

McClure, & Nixon, 2004; Nixon, Spinks, Turner, & McClure, 2004; Spinks, Turner, McClure, & Nixon, 2004; Spinks, Turner, Nixon, & McClure, 2005). In addition, the formation of the U.S. Task Force on Community Preventive Services and its systematic reviews have contributed to our knowledge of effective population interventions (Zaza et al., 2000; Shults et al., 2001; Dinh-Zarr et al., 2001; Zaza, Sleet, Thompson, Sosin, & Bolen, 2001). Community interventions for injury prevention are a global phenomenon. At the end of 2005, there were 96 World Health Organization Safe Communities worldwide (Spinks, Turner, Nixon, & McClure, 2005), the U.S. Safe Kids Campaign has established a Safe Kids Worldwide Campaign, and at least thirteen programs have been identified in Australia and New Zealand where community models and theories have been used frequently for injury prevention (Moller, 1995; National Safety Council of Australia, 1992; Jeffs, Booth, & Calvert 1993; Day, Ozanne-Smith, Cassell, & McGrath, 1997).

Use of Behavior Change Theory

Particularly relevant for this chapter is the role of behavior and social change theory in development of the community intervention strategies and methods. Klassen et al. (2000) describe a few examples in which concepts from social learning theory were used; for example, bicycle helmet and car seat interventions demonstrated the importance of peer pressure and modeling by others (see Chapter Three, this volume). They also suggest the health belief model (see Chapter Two, this volume) and PRECEDE (with at least twenty-four published applications in injury control; see Chapter Seven, this volume; www.lgreen.net; Gielen & McDonald, 2002; Green & Kreuter, 2005) as useful models for community intervention. Each of the Community Preventive Service Task Force systematic reviews (www.TheCommunityGuide.org) starts with a logic model that describes how the community-level interventions (for example, laws regulating drinking and driving and use of restraints) are presumed to work through shaping environments and individual perceptions (Shults et al., 2001; Dinh-Zarr et al., 2001; Zaza, Sleet, Thompson, Sosin, & Bolen, 2001). Both Klassen et al. (2000) and Gielen and Collins (1993) note that successful community interventions appear to incorporate principles from community organization models, including community involvement and ownership of the interventions. This is also consistent with the Swedish and WHO Safe Communities model that many international examples apply and includes organizing cross-sectoral planning groups or coalitions; reliance on existing local community networks; coverage of all ages, environments, and injury types; empowerment of the socially weak; and continuous tracking of high-risk environments and groups for intervention (Svanstrom, 1999; Coggan & Bennett, 2004; see also Chapter Six, this volume).

Importance of Social Norms

Another concept related to change at the community level is social norms, which are frequently invoked in discussions of community interventions. Social norms is a concept from social psychology that refers to implicit rules or standards inferred by individuals from the behavior they observe or expectations they assume in their social milieu and that guide their own behavior; they can be descriptive (how most people behave) or injunctive (how others think one should behave) (Lewis, DeVellis, & Sleath, 2002). Although there is increasingly more interest and descriptive research into social norms as they relate to injury behaviors (see, for example, Taylor & Sorenson, 2004; Fabiano, Perkins, Berkowitz, Linkenbach, & Stark, 2003; Salazar, Baker, Price, & Carlin, 2003; Cheng et al., 2003), there is little consensus on how norms should be conceptualized or measured (Lewis et al., 2002) and no body of literature that empirically describes efforts to change social norms regarding some injury-related behavior. Perhaps the most noteworthy example in injury prevention is drinking and driving (Graham, 1993). As Graham (1993) describes it, "Changes in social norms, in part spurred by such citizen activist groups as MADD [Mothers Against Drunk Driving], have apparently achieved what many traffic safety professionals believed was virtually impossible: a meaningful change in driver attitudes and behaviors resulting in a reduction of traffic fatalities" (p. 524). For more about social norms, see Lewis et al. (2002) and Cialdini and Trost (1999). See also Eriksen and Green (2002) for a review of the tobacco control experience with the denormalization of smoking in public places, which has been more extensively documented than the denormalization of binge drinking or normalization of the designated driver, seat belt use, or bicycle helmet use.

Purpose of This Chapter

We now turn our attention to the community theories and models that are the focus of this chapter. Specifically, we focus on diffusion of innovations, community organization, community mobilization, and community-based participatory research. We hope that this review will provide readers with information on how these models and approaches can help in building injury prevention programs with and for communities. We conclude with thoughts on future research needs to improve community interventions.

Diffusion of Innovations

A symposium celebrating the fortieth anniversary of the publication of *Diffusion of Innovations* (Rogers, 2003) described it as "one of the most cited books in the social sciences" (Moseley & Rogers, 2004, p. 149). The diffusion model is a communication model that defines diffusion as the "process through which an innovation, defined as an idea perceived as new, spreads via certain communication channels over time among the members of a social system" (Rogers, 2004, p. 13). It is a special type of communication, in that the messages are about a new idea, and it is a type of social change defined as the process by which change occurs in the structure and function of a social system (Haider & Kreps, 2004; Rogers, 1995).

Adoption of Innovations

The cumulative adoption of an innovation among the people within a social system has been found to follow a predictable pattern over time: the S-shaped diffusion curve (Figure 4.1), which is consistent across a wide variety of innovations, much as it was found to be with the spread of Mendelian characteristics and epidemic diseases in the nineteenth century. Distinguishing characteristics of population subgroups that adopt an innovation at earlier or later stages in the adoption curve have been identified, as have communication channels and messages that reach and influence those earlier or later adopters. The categories of adopters are identified roughly by standard deviations from the mean time of adoption in a population (Figure 4.2): innovators, early adopters, early majority adopters, late majority adopters, late adopters, and laggards. To reach these different segments of a community, communication messages typically move from more informational to more motivational from early to later adopters and from less intensive or interpersonal to more intensive; later adopters usually need special attention to reducing barriers to adoption (for example, resources and other enabling factors). For example, once seat belts were available in all vehicles, early wearers responded to public education about the benefits of seat belts, whereas later adopters started buckling up only when seat belt laws were promulgated; there is still a proportion of the population not wearing seat belts who would be considered laggards in the diffusion model, though their reasons might be more socioeconomic than motivational, as the epithet might imply.

Characteristics of the innovation itself also make it more or less likely to be adopted. These include features such as its complexity; compatibility with the audience's beliefs, values, and practices; its observability; and its perceived relative advantage. Continuing with the seat belt example, its use was not complex but was initially perceived as incompatible, and its perceived relative advantage was low. Once laws were passed, the observability of its use and changes in perceived relative advantage probably contributed to more rapid adoption. Why laggards do not buckle up may be due to a variety of factors, such as lack of resources to retrofit old vehicles with seat belts or to different normative behavior among this subgroup of the population or social isolation from the earlier adopters.

FIGURE 4.1. BELL-SHAPED FREQUENCY CURVE AND THE S-SHAPED CUMULATIVE CURVE FOR AN ADOPTER DISTRIBUTION.

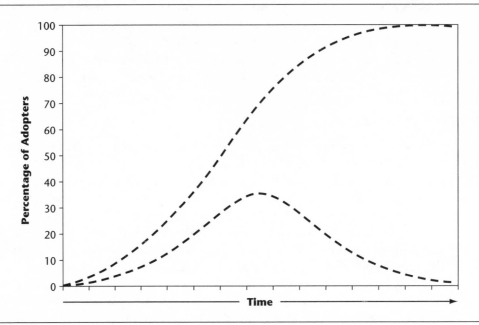

Note: Both curves are for the same data: the adoption of an innovation over time by the members of a social system. But the bell-shaped curve shows these data in terms of the number of individuals adopting each year, whereas the S-shaped curve shows these data on a cumulative basis.

Source: Reproduced with permission of The Free Press, a Division of Simon & Schuster Adult Publishing Group, from *Diffusion of Innovations,* Third Edition by Everett M. Rogers. Copyright © 1996 by Everett M. Rogers. Copyright © 1962, 1971, 1983 by The Free Press. All rights reserved.

Since the diffusion model's formulation as an explanatory model by rural sociologists studying the adoption of hybrid seeds through Agricultural Extension Services in the first half of the twentieth century (Ryan & Gross, 1943), Rogers (2004) continued to refine the model. He cites several important additions:

- A *critical mass,* the point when enough individuals have adopted an innovation so that further diffusion becomes self-sustaining
- *Networks,* a means of better understanding how new ideas spread through interpersonal channels
- *Reinvention,* the process through which a new idea is changed by its adopters during the diffusion process

The model has been adapted and widely applied in public health since the family planning and immunization campaigns of the 1960s (Derryberry, 1971;

FIGURE 4.2. ADOPTER CATEGORIZATION ON THE BASIS OF INNOVATIVENESS.

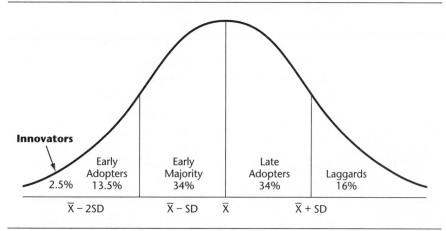

Note: The innovativeness dimension, as measured by the time at which an individual adopts an innovation, is continuous. However, this variable may be partitioned into five adopter categories by standard deviations from the average time of adoption.

Source: Reproduced with permission from Rogers, E. M. *Diffusion of innovations* (4th ed.). New York: Free Press, 1995.

Green, 1970) and, later, the cardiovascular community trials (Green, 1975) and other chronic disease prevention programs (Green, Gottlieb, & Parcel, 1991; Johnson, Green, Frankish, MacLean, & Stachenko, 1996).

Key Elements

Using the diffusion model for program planning can involve five key elements according to Oldenberg and Parcel (2002): innovation development, dissemination, adoption, implementation, and maintenance. This model is particularly relevant to injury prevention because many effective innovations have been developed (for example, seat belts, car seats, bike helmets, smoke alarms), yet we have not achieved anything close to universal coverage of the population. *Dissemination* refers to the communication channels and systems that are best for diffusing the innovation to its intended audience. *Adoption* refers to the uptake of the innovation by the target audience and involves their knowledge of the innovation and their decision making about its use. *Implementation* is the initial use of the innovation in practice, and *maintenance* refers to ongoing implementation and continued use of the innovation in practice.

Applications in Injury Prevention

An example of how the diffusion of innovations five-stage framework is being used in injury prevention is a current CDC/NCIPC-funded evaluation project of one of the authors (A.C.G.) in Baltimore, Maryland. In this project, we are using a mobile safety center (MSC) to disseminate known effective child safety products and safety education to low-income, urban communities. The MSC is a forty-foot vehicle outfitted to look like a home environment, with interactive educational safety exhibits, fire safety and injury prevention educators, and low-cost safety products. Working in partnership with a community clinic, the Baltimore City Fire Department, and other organizations, we are using qualitative and quantitative methods to study the dissemination process at the levels of the participating organizations and the individuals the MSC is intended to serve.

Adoption is being assessed by interviewing key stakeholders about their awareness of and participation in the MSC initiative and by surveying clinic patients to determine if they have heard about the MSC from the clinic or elsewhere, if they have used its services, and if not, why not. Implementation is being evaluated by using a variety of process evaluation measures on the MSC itself, such as visit feedback surveys and daily tracking of visitors and services provided. Outcome evaluation will compare the adoption, implementation, and maintenance of safety practices over time between families who do and do not visit the MSC. Efforts to maintain the MSC itself as a service to the community are also being documented.

A second example comes from a recent meta-analysis of the effect of mediated health communication campaigns on behavior change in the United States (Snyder et al., 2004). In this study, the concept of adoption of innovations was used to classify the behavioral outcomes (the innovations) of campaigns by their adoption goals: starting a desirable behavior, preventing an undesirable behavior, or ceasing an undesirable behavior. They also classified behaviors according to the rate of behavioral compliance before the campaign started (that is, location on the diffusion curve). Comparisons were made across campaigns targeting seven behaviors: seat belt use, oral health, alcohol use reduction, heart disease prevention, smoking, mammography and cervical cancer screening, and sexual behaviors. The five studies focused on seat belt use demonstrated an average change of 15 percent in seat belt use, which was the largest effect size found. Among the four campaigns to reduce alcohol consumption, which is also relevant to many injury problems, the average change in alcohol behaviors was 7 percent. These improvements could have a sizable effect on a population basis. Enforcement messages and baseline rates of the target behavior are both related to campaign effect sizes, but how they are related specifically to seat belt use could not be determined from this study and needs further research. This type of research is helpful to campaign planners, because it helps set realistic program goals, and to evaluation researchers, because it allows them to develop sample size estimates.

Community Organization

Community organization models emphasize the active participation and development of communities to strengthen self-reliance in planning, evaluating, and solving health and social problems (Minkler & Wallerstein, 1997). Bracht, Kingsbury, and Rissel (1999) define community organization as the purposeful effort to "activate a community to use its own social structures and any available resources that are decided on primarily by community representatives and that are generally consistent with local values" (p. 86) to accomplish community goals. The newer definitions blur the earlier distinction between community organization and community development, which was seen to place greater emphasis on participation, use of indigenous resources, and development of self-reliance. Community organization has tended in the past to encompass these and a variety of alternatives for community planning and action that are less dependent on participation, indigenous resources, or self-reliance (Rothman & Tropman, 1987).

Early commentaries on the importance of community interventions in injury control described the difference between communitywide interventions and community-based programs (Gielen & Collins, 1993) and suggested that the effectiveness of communitywide programs could be enhanced by treating the community as the source for programs rather than simply the site in which programs are placed (McLoughlin, Vince, Lee, & Crawford, 1982). Among the types of community organization models are community organizing, community building, and Braithwaite's community organization and development model (Braithwaite, Bianchi, & Taylor, 1994; Minkler & Wallerstein, 2003). (Readers interested in the historical development of this area of health promotion practice and more details on the distinctions between models are referred to Minkler & Wallerstein, 2003, and Rothman & Tropman, 1987, on early classification of models for practice.)

One example of a successful community organization effort in injury control is the Injury Free Coalition for Kids initiative that started with the Harlem Hospital Injury Prevention Program in New York (Davidson et al., 1994; Durkin, Laraque, Lubman, & Barlow 1999). In the mid-1980s, injury surveillance was used to identify the causes of injury to children and adolescents living in low-income neighborhoods surrounding the hospital. In response to compelling evidence of the injury problem, a multidisciplinary lay-professional coalition was formed to develop and implement prevention programs, which included new educational programs, safe play areas, and supervised activities for children. Some of the specific program components were playground renovations; a Safety City, a model of a city environment used to teach and practice safety; window guard legislation for high-rise apartments; art, dance, and sports programs; and free bicycle helmets. From 1983 to 1995, hospital admissions due to injury decreased by 55 percent overall, 46 percent for pedestrian injury, 50 percent for playground injuries, and 46 percent for violence-related injuries (www.IFCK.org). Although total injuries also declined in the comparison community, the declines in the intervention community were most noticeable in specific injuries and age groups targeted by the program (Davidson et al., 1994).

Community Mobilization

The term *community mobilization* has been used to refer to efforts to involve community members in activities ranging from defining needs for prevention to obtaining community support for a predesigned prevention program (Treno & Holder, 1997). Mobilization usually emphasizes changing the social and economic structures that influence injury risk. Treno and Holder (1997) note that mobilization can include elements of both bottom-up (or grassroots) and top-down (leader-initiated) strategies; the difference between these two strategies is in who defines the problems and decides on solutions. In the former, it is the community members themselves, and in the latter, it is an authority or expert who is not necessarily identified with the community (external or self-appointed community leader). Limitations arise using either strategy exclusively: grassroots involvement is essential but may not be sufficient if, for example, community organizations have competing priorities or lack expertise in defining effective interventions. Alternatively, top-down approaches may have limited sustainability if community organizations and leaders are not supportive and engaged (Treno & Holder, 1997). Because community leaders understand their local culture, politics, and traditions better than outsiders do, their participation is essential for tailoring imported prevention programs to local needs. The balance between bottom-up and top-down approaches can be situation specific: "Community is, ideally, a level of collective decision making appropriate to the urgency and magnitude of the problem, the cost and technical complexity of the solutions required, the culture and traditions of shared decision making, and the sensitivity and consequences of the actions required of people after the decision is made" (Green, 1999, p. 82).

In Treno and Holder's Community Trials Project (1997), "mobilization is the purposeful organization of community members to implement and support policies that will reduce alcohol involved trauma" (p. 175), and a community-science partnership was formed. The overarching conceptualization of how this project addresses the alcohol-injury connection is environmental, focusing on how changing the social and structural contexts of alcohol use can effectively modify individual behavior (Holder et al., 1997). Prevention policies and activities that were to be implemented were those supported by research evidence, and communities were asked to customize and prioritize their initiatives depending on local concerns and interests. Specific components of the mobilization effort were directed toward responsible beverage service, drinking and driving, under-age drinking, and alcohol access. Coalitions, task forces, and media advocacy were used to raise awareness and support for effective policies among the public and relevant decision makers (Holder et al., 1997). In an evaluation of the impact of the mobilization efforts, Holder and colleagues compared intervention communities with control communities and demonstrated significant reductions in the following indicators: 6 percent in the reported quantity of alcohol consumed, 51 percent in driving over the legal alcohol limit, 10 percent in nighttime injury crashes, 6 percent in alcohol-related crashes, and 43 percent in alcohol-related assault injuries seen in emergency departments.

Cross-Cutting Concepts and Principles

For all types of community-level interventions, there are certain principles of practice that are embodied in the various theories or models presented previously. These include empowerment, community capacity, and participation and relevance. These concepts are described in more detail in this section.

Empowerment

The concept of empowerment was demonstrated in the Harlem Hospital and the Community Trials programs through the use of coalitions and task forces to foster community ownership and participatory problem solving (Minkler & Wallerstein, 1997). According to Fawcett et al. (1995), "Community empowerment is defined broadly: the process of gaining influence over conditions that matter to people who share neighborhoods, workplaces, experiences or concerns" (p. 679). This notion, which some call a theory, operates at multiple and interrelated levels, including individuals, organizations, and communities (Fawcett et al., 1995; Speer, Jackson, & Peterson, 2001; Zimmerman, 1995; Minkler & Wallerstein, 2003). The importance of empowerment has been discussed in much of the domestic violence literature, especially in feminist and gender politics analyses of intimate partner violence (see, for example, Stark, 1990; Campbell & Campbell, 1996; Peled,

Eisikovits, Enosh, & Winstok, 2000; Jewkes, 2002). Empowerment also undergirds much of the Safe Communities work, as seen, for example, in the Harstad Injury Prevention Study by Ytterstad and Sogaard (1995; see also Chapter Six, this volume).

Community Capacity

Various notions of building the self-reliance of communities have merged into the current literature on community capacity building. Most of these derive from a recognition that grants, technical assistance, and other external stimuli, resources, and support cannot be counted on for more than a few years at best. The earliest representations of community capacity building were inherent in the community development model (Smith, Baugh Littlejohns, & Thompson, 2001). It has gained political favor during periods of fiscal conservatism and decentralization of government (Chaskin, Brown, Venkatesh, & Vidal, 2001). Its most recent incarnation has been in relation to notions of social capital and training, mobilizing, or empowering indigenous health workers, resources, and local volunteers or community leaders (Eng, Parker, & Harlan, 1997; Norton, McLeroy, Burdine, Felix, & Dorsey, 2002; Poland, 2000).

Participation and Relevance

Principles that derive from a community organization model and are reflected by the experience of community approaches to injury prevention, such as those of the Harlem Hospital and the Community Trials programs described previously, include the principles of participation and relevance (Green & Kreuter, 1999). The principle of participation states that behavior change will be greatest when those whose behavior or circumstances are to be changed are directly involved in intervention planning and decision making. The principle of relevance states that change will be greatest when community organizers "start where the people are" and engage community members for their knowledge of what matters to the population at risk. By working with coalitions and task forces and supporting community tailoring of program components, both of these principles were observed. These principles are also very evident in the Safe Communities movement (Svanstrom, 1999).

Community-Based Participatory Research

Several of the examples presented in this chapter provide support for another relatively new movement in public health research and practice: community-based participatory research (CBPR) (Green & Mercer, 2001; Minkler & Wallerstein,

2003). While participatory research is increasingly being advocated for dealing with a multitude of public health problems, it is perhaps especially important for problems that relate to individual behavior. To implement and evaluate policies and programs that attempt to change personal behavior requires extreme sensitivity to the ethical issues surrounding the protection of individual autonomy. By engaging communities in needs assessment and decision making about program design and evaluation, which is at the heart of CBPR, program planners are more likely to adopt strategies that are consistent with the core values of the community and society. The syntheses of highly controlled research on what works in injury prevention produce recommended best practices, but these are unlikely to be widely adopted by practitioners and communities unless they see them as relevant to their communities. Participatory research ensures a greater opportunity for research to be made relevant and to be perceived as relevant to the community's needs and circumstances.

Conclusion

Community intervention work has a long and rich history in injury prevention and health promotion. While this has led to demonstrable successes, some of which were described above, it has also resulted in numerous different terminology that may obfuscate the commonalities across the approaches being used. From a practical perspective, it may be useful to take an overarching view of these different models, theories, and concepts and simply describe the necessary components of community-level interventions:

> Given reasonable resources, the chances are that a community intervention will succeed if the practitioner (1) builds from a base of community ownership of the problems and the solution, (2) plans carefully, (3) uses sound theory, meaningful data and local experience as a basis for problem decisions, (4) knows what types of interventions work best for specific populations and circumstances, and (5) has an organizational and advocacy plan to orchestrate multiple intervention strategies into a complementary, cohesive program [Green & Kreuter, 2005, p. 261].

Other practical considerations include the time and capacity needs involved in successful community intervention. Coggan and Bennett (2004) note that "it is important that funders of community-based injury prevention programs are mindful of the time commitment required to achieve change at the community level, and the importance of encouraging community-based injury prevention capacity and capabilities" (p. 356). The capacity of communities to participate in planning, implementation, and evaluation of community programs is critically important, especially for long-term sustainability of effective programs.

Evaluation methods for demonstrating effectiveness of community-based injury prevention programs remain challenging, and there continues to be debate about the use of the traditional randomized controlled trial versus other research models and sources of evidence that may be more appropriate for community-level interventions (Victoria, Habicht, & Bryce, 2004). What makes this more than a debate about design and methodology is the recognition that randomized and other highly controlled conditions of trials cannot be imposed on free-living communities, and to the extent that such controls have been imposed in previous research makes that research less generalizable and relevant to other communities (Green, 2001; Green & Ottoson, 2004; Wandersman, 2003).

The principles of community intervention are particularly relevant to injury prevention because they can help shape effective programs, regardless of whether the desired outcomes are individual behaviors or environmental modifications or both. By engaging our intended audiences as partners and using the tenets and theories outlined in this chapter, we can more powerfully communicate both personal protection messages and the demand for safer environments. It is in this latter application that advocacy skills and political science theory can be effectively applied, a relatively untapped potential for future collaborations between social and behavioral scientists and injury prevention professionals.

References

Bracht, N., Kingsbury, L., & Rissel, C. (1999). A five-stage community organization model for health promotion, empowerment and partnership strategies. In N. Bracht (Ed.), *Health promotion at the community level: New advances* (2nd ed.). Thousand Oaks, CA: Sage.

Braithwaite, R. L., Bianchi, C., & Taylor, S. E. (1994). Ethnographic approach to community organization and health empowerment. *Health Education Quarterly, 21*(3), 407–416.

Campbell, J. C., & Campbell, D. W. (1996). Cultural competence in the care of abused women. *Journal of Nurse Midwifery, 41*(6), 457–462.

Chamberlain, R. W. (1988). *Beyond individual risk assessment: Community wide approaches to promoting the health and development of families and children.* Washington, DC: National Center for Education in Maternal and Child Health.

Chaskin, R. J., Brown, P., Venkatesh, S., & Vidal, A. (2001). *Building community capacity.* New York: Aldine de Gruyter.

Cheng, T. L., Brenner, R. A., Wright, J. L., Sachs, H. C., Moyer, P., & Rao, M. (2003). Community norms on toy guns. *Pediatrics, 111*(1), 75–79.

Cialdini, R. B., & Trost, M. B. (1999). Social influence: Social norms, conformity, and compliance. In D. T. Gilbert, S. T. Fiske, & G. Lindzey (Eds.), *Handbook of social psychology* (4th ed., pp. 151–192). New York: McGraw-Hill.

Coggan, C., & Bennett, S. (2004). Community-based injury prevention programs. In R. McClure, M. Stevenson, & S. McEvoy (Eds.), *The scientific basis of injury prevention and control* (pp. 347–358). Melbourne, Australia: IP Communications.

Davidson, L. L., Durkin, M. S., Kuhn, L., O'Connor, P., Barlow, B., & Heagarty, M. C. (1994). The impact of Safe Kids/Healthy Neighborhoods Injury Prevention Program in Harlem, 1988–1991. *American Journal of Public Health, 84*(4), 580–586.

Day, L. M., Ozanne-Smith, J., Cassell, E., & McGrath, A. (1997, July). *Latrobe Valley Better Health Project: Evaluation of the injury prevention program, 1992–1996.* Victoria, Australia: Accident Research Center.

Derryberry, M. (1971). Education in the health aspects of family planning. *Pacific Health Education Reports, 2,* 16–50.

Derryberry, M. (2004). Education in the health aspects of family planning. In J. P. Allegrante & D. A. Sleet (Eds.), *Derryberry's educating for health* (pp. 291–338). San Francisco: Jossey-Bass.

Dinh-Zarr, T. B., Sleet, D. A., Shults, R. A., Zaza, S., Elder, R. W., Nichols, J. L., Thompson, R. S., & Sosin, D. M. Task Force on Community Preventive Services (2001). Reviews of evidence regarding interventions to increase the use of safety belts. *American Journal of Preventive Medicine, 21*(4 Suppl), 48–65.

Durkin, M. S., Laraque, D., Lubman, I., & Barlow, B. (1999). Epidemiology and prevention of traffic injuries to urban children and adolescents. *Pediatrics, 103*(6), 1–8.

Eng, E., Parker, E. A., & Harlan, C. (Eds.). (1997). Lay health advisors: A critical link to community capacity building [Special issue]. *Health Education and Behavior, 24,* 407–510.

Eriksen, M. P., & Green, L. W. (2002). Progress and next steps in reducing tobacco use in the United States. In F. D. Scutchfield & C. W. Keck (Eds.), *Principles of public health practice* (2nd ed., pp. 351–363). Albany, NY: Delmar Thompson.

Fabiano, P. M., Perkins, H. W., Berkowitx, A., Linkenbach, J., & Stark, C. (2003). Engaging men as social justice allies in ending violence against women: Evidence for a social norms approach. *Journal of American College Health, 52*(3), 105–112.

Fawcett, S. B., Paine-Andrews, A., Francisco, V. T., Schultz, J. A., Richter, K. P., Lewis, R. K., Williams, E. L., Harris, K. J., Berkley, J. Y., Fisher, J. L., & Lopez, C. M. (1995). Using empowerment theory in collaborative partnerships for community health and development. *American Journal of Community Psychology, 23*(5), 677–697.

Gielen, A. C., & Collins, B. (1993). Community-based interventions for injury prevention. *Family and Community Health, 15*(4), 1–11.

Gielen, A. C., & McDonald, E. M. (2002). Using the PRECEDE/PROCEED planning model to apply health behavior theories in health promoting program planning. In K. Glanz, B. K. Rimer, & L. Lewis (Eds.), *Health behavior and health education* (3rd ed., pp. 409–436). San Francisco: Jossey-Bass.

Graham, J. D. (1993). Injuries from traffic crashes: Meeting the challenge. *Annual Review of Public Health, 14,* 515–543.

Green, L. W. (1970). Identifying and overcoming barriers to the diffusion of knowledge about family planning. *Advances in Fertility Control, 5,* 21–29.

Green, L. W. (1975). Diffusion and adoption of innovations related to cardiovascular risk behavior in the public. In A. J. Enelow & J. B. Henderson (Eds.), *Applying behavioral science to cardiovascular risk.* New York: American Heart Association.

Green, L. W. (1999). Health education's contributions to public health in the twentieth century: A glimpse through health promotion's rear-view mirror. *Annual Review of Public Health, 20,* 67–88.

Green, L. W. (2001). From research to "best practices" in other settings and populations. *American Journal of Health Behavior, 2*(25), 165–178.

Green, L. W., Gottlieb, N. H., & Parcel, G. S. (1991). Diffusion theory extended and applied. In W. Ward & F. M. Lewis (Eds.), *Advances in health education and promotion* (vol. 3). London: Jessica Kingsley Publishers.

Green, L. W., & Kreuter, K. W. (1999). *Health promotion planning: An educational and environmental approach* (3rd ed.). Mountain View, CA: Mayfield.

Green, L. W., & Kreuter, M. W. (2005). *Health program planning: An educational and ecological approach* (4th ed.). New York: McGraw-Hill.

Green, L. W., & Ottoson, J. M. (2004). From efficacy to effectiveness to community and back: Evidence-based practice vs. practice-based evidence. In R. Hiss, L. W. Green, M. H. Chin, B. J. DeVinney, L. J. Fine, S. A. Garfield, R. E. Glasgow, R. Kuczmarski, S. Malozowski, & K.M.V. Narayan (Eds.), *From clinical trials to community: The science of translating diabetes and obesity research.* Conference proceedings, Jan. 12–13. Bethesda, MD: National Institutes of Health.

Green, L. W., & Mercer, S. L. (2001). Can public health researchers and agencies reconcile the push from funding bodies and the pull from communities? Community-based participatory research. *American Journal of Public Health, 91*(12), 1926–1943.

Haider, M., & Kreps, G. L. (2004). Forty years of diffusion of innovations: Utility and value in public health. *Journal of Health Communication, 2004, 9,* 3–12.

Harborview Injury Prevention and Research Center. (n.d.). Best Practices. Retrieved Oct. 28, 2005, from http://depts.washington.edu/hiprc/practices/index.html.

Heck, A., Collins, J., & Peterson, L. (2001). Decreasing children's risk taking on the playground. *Journal of Applied Behavior Analysis, 34*(3), 349–352.

Holder, H. D., Gruenewal, P. J., Ponicki, W. R., Treno, A. J., Grube, J. W., Saltz, R. F., Voas, R. B., Reynolds, R., Davis, J., Sanchez, L., Gaumont, G., & Roeper, P. (2000). Effect of community-based interventions on high-risk drinking and alcohol related injuries. *JAMA, 284*(18), 2341–2347.

Holder, H. D., Saltz, R. F., Grube, J. W., Voas, R. B., Gruenewalk, P. J., & Treno, A. J. (1997). A community prevention trial to reduce alcohol-involved accidental injury and death: Overview. *Addiction, 92*(Suppl. 2), 155–171.

Jeffs, D., Booth, D., & Calvert, E. (1993). Local injury information, community participation and injury reduction. *Australian Journal of Public Health, 17,* 365–72.

Jewkes, R. (2002). Intimate partner violence: Causes and prevention. *Lancet, 359,* 1423–1429.

Johnson, J. L., Green, L. W., Frankish, C. J., MacLean, D. R., & Stachenko, S. (1996). A dissemination research agenda to strengthen health promotion and disease prevention. *Canadian Journal of Public Health, 87*(Suppl. 2), S5–S10.

Klassen, T. P., MacKay, J. M., Moher, D., Walker, A., & Jones, A. L. (2000). Community-based injury prevention interventions. *Future of Children: Unintentional Injuries in Childhood, 10*(1), 83–110.

Lewis, M. A., DeVellis, B. M., & Sleath, B. (2002). Social influence and interpersonal communication in health behavior. In K. Glanz, B. K. Rimer, & F. M. Lewis (Eds.), *Health behavior and health education* (3rd ed., pp. 240–264). San Francisco: Jossey-Bass.

McLoughlin, E., Vince, C., Lee, A., & Crawford, J. (1982). Project Burn Prevention: Outcome and implications. *American Journal of Public Health, 72,* 241–247.

Minkler, M., & Wallerstein, N. (1997). Improving health through community organization and community building. In K. Glanz, F. M. Lewis, & B. K. Rimer (Eds.), *Health behavior and health education: Theory, research, and Practice* (2nd ed., 241–269). San Francisco: Jossey-Bass.

Minkler, M., & Wallerstein, N. (2003). *Community-based participatory research for health.* San Francisco: Jossey-Bass.

Moller, J. (1995). An introduction to community-based injury prevention. In J. Ozanne-Smith & F. Williams (Eds.), *Injury research and prevention: A text.* Victoria: Monash University Accident Research Center.

Moseley S. F., & Rogers, E. (2004). Diffusion of innovations theory: Its utility and value in public health. *Journal of Health Communication, 9,* 149–154.

National Committee for Injury Prevention and Control. (1989). Injury prevention: Meeting the challenge. *American Journal of Preventive Medicine, 5,* 8.

National Safety Council of Australia. (1992). *Community-based injury prevention: A practical guide.* Cowandilla, South Australia: National Safety Council of Australia.

Nixon, J., Spinks, A., Turner, C., & McClure, R. (2004). Community-based programs to prevent poisoning in children 0–15 years. *Injury Prevention, 10,* 43–46.

Norton, B. L., McLeroy, K. R., Burdine, J. N., Felix, M.R.J., & Dorsey, A. M. (2002). Community capacity: Concept, theory, and methods. In R. J. DiClemente, R. A. Crosby, & M. C. Kegler (Eds.), *Emerging theories in health promotion practice and research: Strategies for improving public health* (pp. 194–227). San Francisco: Jossey-Bass.

Oldenburg, B., & Parcel, G. S. (2002). Diffusion of innovations. In K. Glanz, B. K. Rimer, & F. M. Lewis (Eds.), *Health behavior and health education* (3rd ed., pp. 312–334). San Francisco: Jossey-Bass.

Peled, E., Eisikovits, Z., Enosh, G., & Winstok, Z. (2000). Choice and empowerment for battered women who stay: Toward a constructivist model. *Social Work, 45*(1), 9–25.

Poland, B. D. (2000). Social capital, social cohesion, community capacity, and community empowerment: Variations on a theme? In B. D. Poland, L. W. Green, & I. Rootman (Eds.), *Settings in health promotion: Linking theory and practice* (pp. 301–307). Thousand Oaks, CA: Sage.

Rogers, E. M. (1996). *Diffusion of innovations* (4th ed.). New York: Free Press.

Rogers, E. M. (2003). *Diffusion of innovations* (5th ed.). New York: Free Press.

Rogers, E. M. (2004). A prospective and retrospective look at the diffusion model. *Journal of Health Communication, 9*(1), 3–19.

Rothman, J., & Tropman, J. E. (1987). Models of community organization and macro practice: Their mixing and phasing. In F. M. Cox, J. Erlich, J. L. Rothman, & J. E. Tropman (Eds.), *Strategies of community organization* (4th ed., pp. 3–26). Itasca, IL: F. E. Peacock.

Ryan, B., & Gross, N. C. (1943). The diffusion of hybrid seed corn in two Iowa communities. *Rural Sociology, 8*(1), 15–24.

Salazar, L. F., Baker, C. K., Price, A. W., & Carlin, K. (2003). Moving beyond the individual: Examining the effects of domestic violence policies on social norms. *American Journal of Community Psychology, 32*(3–4), 253–264.

Shea, S., & Basch, C. E. (1990). A review of five major community-based cardiovascular disease prevention programs. Part II: Intervention strategies, evaluation methods, and results. *American Journal of Health Promotion, 4,* 279–287.

Shults, R. A., Elder, R. W., Sleet, D. A., Nichols, J. L., Alao, M. O., Carande-Kulis, V. G., Zaza, S., Sosin, D. M., & Thompson, R. S. Task force on community preventive services. (2001) Reviews of evidence regarding interventions to reduce alcohol-impaired driving. *American Journal of Preventive Medicine, 21*(Suppl. 4), 66–88.

Smith, N., Baugh Littlejohns, L., & Thompson, D. (2001). Shaking out the cobwebs: Insights into community capacity and its relation to health outcomes. *Community Development Journal, 36,* 30–41.

Snyder, L. B., Hamilton, M. A., Mitchell, E. W., Kiwanuka-Tondo, J., Flemin-Milici, F., & Proctor, D. (2004). A meta-analysis of mediated health communication campaigns on behavior change in the United States. *Journal of Health Communication, 9*, 71–96.

Speer, P. W., Jackson, C. B., & Peterson, N. A. (2001). The relationship between social cohesion and empowerment: Support and new implications for theory. *Health Education and Behavior, 28*(6), 716–732.

Spinks, A., Turner, C., McClure, R., & Nixon, J. (2004). Community based programs targeting all injuries for children. *Injury Prevention, 10*(3), 180–185.

Spinks, A., Turner, C., Nixon, J., & McClure, R. (2005). The "WHO Safe Communities" model for the prevention of injury in whole populations. *The Cochrane Database of Systematic Reviews, 2*, CD004445.

Stark, E. (1990). Rethinking homicide: Violence, race, and the politics of gender. *International Journal of Health Services, 20*(1), 3–26.

Svanstrom, L. (1999). *Evidence-based injury prevention and safety promotion—A review of concepts and studies.* Stockholm: Karolinska Institute, Department of Public Health Sciences.

Taylor, C. A., & Sorenson, S. B. (2004). Injunctive social norms of adults regarding teen dating violence. *Journal of Adolescent Health, 34*(6), 468–479.

Treno, A. J., & Holder, H. D. (1997). Community mobilization: Evaluation of an environmental approach to local action. *Addiction, 92*(Suppl. 2), 173–187.

Turner, C., McClure, R., Nixon, J., & Spinks, A. (2004). Community-based programmes to prevent pedestrian injuries in children 0–14 years: A systematic review. *Injury Control and Safety Promotion, 11*(4), 231–237.

Turner, C., McClure, R., Nixon, J., & Spinks, A. (2005). Community-based programs to promote car seat restraints in children 0–16 years—A systematic review. *Accident Analysis and Prevention, 37*(1), 77–83.

Turner, C., Spinks, A., McClure, R., & Nixon, J. (2004). Community-based interventions for the prevention of burns and scalds in children. *Cochrane Database Systematic Reviews, 3*, CD004335.

Victoria, C. G., Habicht, J. & Bryce, J. (2004). Evidence-based public health: Moving beyond randomized trials. *American Journal of Public Health, 94*(3), 400–405.

Wandersman, A. (2003). Community science: Bridging the gap between science and practice with community-centered models. *American Journal of Community Psychology, 31*, 227–242.

Ytterstad, B., & Sogaard, A. J. (1995). The Harstad Injury Prevention Study: Prevention of burns in small children by a community-based intervention. *Burns, 21*(4), 259–266.

Zaza, S., Lawrence, R. S., Mahan, C. S., Fullilove, M., Fleming, D., Isham, G. J., & Pappaioanou, M. (2000). Scope and organization of the Guide to Community Prevention Services. *American Journal of Preventive Medicine, 18*(Suppl. 1), 27–34.

Zaza, S., Sleet, D. A., Thompson, R. S., Sosin, D. M., & Bolen, J. C. (2001). Reviews of evidence regarding interventions to increase use of child safety seats. *American Journal of Preventive Medicine, 21*(Suppl. 4), 31–47.

Zimmerman, M. A. (1995). Psychological empowerment: Issues and illustrations. *American Journal of Community Psychology, 23*, 581–599.

CHAPTER FIVE

HEALTH RISK COMMUNICATION AND INJURY PREVENTION

Deborah C. Girasek

To the uninitiated, communicating with the public about injury risks would seem to be straightforward. Surely we all want to avoid hazards and take precautions that will keep us safe. In practice, risk communication turns out to be a complicated business. Our understanding of how to explain injury hazards and increase compliance with safety recommendations is not well developed. That is because there have been few well-designed studies of communication interventions in the field of injury control. Many related bodies of knowledge are contained in the scientific literature, however, which can inform our efforts to prevent injury deaths and disability.

Risk Communication Science

Risk communication as a field has evolved on two dimensions: at the level of the individual and that of the community. Much of what is known about how individuals perceive and react to risk-related information was contributed by social psychologists (Finnegan & Viswanath, 1997). Our understanding of public assessments of hazards, and governmental responses to potential threats, is rooted primarily in the realm of environmental health. In the waning decades of the twentieth century, government officials, corporate leaders, and practitioners of the so-called hard sciences were frustrated by what they perceived as the public's overreaction to environmental hazards that posed statistically insignificant risks. Cognitive psychologists studying this phenomenon established that risks had qualitative as well as quantitative dimensions in the eyes of the lay public. Historically, corporations and civic bodies had either ignored the former or dismissed them as irrational. Officials, for example, would chide audiences that they were taking a greater risk driving to the meeting than living next to an environmental hazard. Such behavior only fueled community outrage and increased the distance between opposing parties (Sandman, 1989). Risk comparisons that are based solely on epidemiological data are not complex enough to predict the psychological assessments that citizens make when they feel threatened. There are multiple descriptions of the qualities that make some hazards less tolerable to the public, but here are some of the most frequently cited concepts: dread, familiarity, immediacy of effect, voluntariness, controllability, catastrophic potential, equity, severity of consequences, threat to future generations, and level of knowledge (Lowrance, 1976; Slovic, 2000b). Risk communicators note also that some events hold power as signals, portending future threats on the horizon (Slovic, 2000a). An important philosophical contribution of risk communication is the notion that lay risk perceptions are to be respected rather than merely tolerated. As explained above, lay perceptions typically differ from those of public health professionals because they are more multidimensional, not because they are based on ignorance.

Does Risk Communication Science Have Application to Injury Control?

In the light of its nascent context, the guidance that emerged from the psychometric school of risk communication science focused predominantly on allaying community concerns. By reversing its logic, however, we may find clues to why society focuses relatively few resources on injury prevention. Table 5.1 examines the outrage potential inherent in the major types of fatal injuries. The descriptions listed in column 1 are adapted from Sandman (1991), who differentiates between primary (more influential) and secondary components The Y (Yes) notations are the product of my—albeit subjective—analysis of whether the public generally associates that characteristic with a given type of injury event. For example, Sandman refers to certain threats as memorable if they have the power to evoke dramatic images in the minds of the public, whether due to personal experience or media portrayals. I conjecture that murders, fatal fires, and motor vehicle crashes might possess this trait, in contrast to fatal falls (which often involve an elderly victim falling to the floor in her own home) and poisonings (which often involve a young adult who overdoses on drugs unintentionally).

Table 5.1 summarizes multiple such analyses, which suggest that the injury threat suffers generally from a paucity of the qualitative characteristics that risk communication has associated with public concern and action. Through framing, however, it may be possible to change how these hazards are perceived or portrayed in the media. For example, by documenting that a community's playground was not constructed according to current standards, perhaps we could increase parental perceptions that a vulnerable population's safety is being controlled by others. The effect of such manipulations, however, has not been tested. Consequently they should be evaluated with an eye to both intended and unintended consequences.

Let me extend the playground example. If our reframing efforts were successful, a group of parents might be spurred to organize and approach politicians to demand better enforcement of health and safety regulations. Perhaps community volunteers or local journalists could conduct ongoing monitoring of park conditions. The performance ratings of public officials who manage departments of recreation could be linked to how well their facilities fare on safety inspections. But if a park's equipment were brought up to code and that caused parents to believe that children could now play safely without adult supervision, injuries might increase. Or if there were insufficient funds to support increased enforcement but media coverage of the playground's substandard condition raised liability concerns for the municipality, perhaps the park would be closed. That could result in fewer injuries but also less physical activity for neighborhood children. Or they could put themselves at increased risk for pedestrian injuries by walking to a more distant park. Savvy advocates could anticipate and forestall many of these untoward developments. The message for readers, though, is not to be subjective or shortsighted in determining whether risk communication efforts are serving the public as intended.

Consult Experts and the Lay Public When Developing Communications

One clear lesson from the field of risk communication is that public perceptions should be formally assessed before, and integrated into, campaigns that deal with injury risk and safety precautions. Some of the professional concerns that have been raised about lay beliefs in the field of modern injury control have not held up to scientific scrutiny. One example has to do with the word *accident*. For the last few decades of the twentieth century, national and international safety advocates lamented the public's persistent use of that term:

> The magnitude of the automotive injury problem in the pediatric population remains as great as it is largely because of the perpetuation of a societal ethic that automotive injuries are accidents. The word accident suggests that the

TABLE 5.1. INJURY'S POTENTIAL TO INVOKE PUBLIC OUTRAGE.

Primary Hazard Components	Motor Vehicle Crashes	Suicide	Falls	Poisoning	Homicide	Fires/Burns	Drowning	Suffocation/Choking
Coerced/involuntary exposure					Yes			
Industrial/unnatural	Yes			Yes	Yes			Yes
Exotic/unfamiliar								
Memorable (conjures up dramatic image)	Yes				Yes	Yes		
Dreaded death/consequences						Yes		
Catastrophic (kills many people all at once)						Yes		
Unknowable/poorly understood by science								
Hazard is controlled by others					Yes			
Unfair distribution of hazard's costs and benefits					Yes	Yes		
Morally relevant/sociallyrepugnant								
Untrustworthy sources (those with ulterior motives)				Yes				
Unresponsive process (source of hazard is notaccountable)	Yes				Yes			

Secondary components						
Vulnerable populations at most risk	Yes			Yes	Yes	Yes
Delayed (versus acute) effects						
Substantial risk to future generations						
Victims identifiable (versus statistical)			Yes	Yes	Yes	
Totally preventable (versus only reducible)						
Few benefits (victims perceived to have taken foolish risk)		Yes	Yes	Yes		
Media attention			Yes	Yes	Yes	
Opportunities for collective action						

Source: Adapted from Sandman (1991).

injury event was determined by fate and, therefore, was unpredictable and unavoidable [Rosenberg, Rodriguez, & Chorba 1990, p. 1086].

Another critical element in understanding injuries in America [is] the extent to which their occurrence is affected by people's attitudes. Perhaps the most pervasive of these—what Haddon, Suchman, and Klein called the last folklore subscribed to by rational men—is the belief that injuries are accidents [National Committee for Injury Prevention and Control, 1989, p. 12].

The most important reason for this delay in the use of science to control injuries, and one which persists to some degree even today, is the sense of fatalism towards trauma. Injuries are still called accidents . . . [Rivara, 2001, p. 3].

The term *accident* has been banned by the U.S. National Highway Traffic Safety Administration (National Highway Traffic Safety Administration, 1997), as well as the *British Medical Journal* (Davis & Pless, 2001). At meetings of injury control professionals, audiences have been known to hiss if an invited speaker from another field inadvertently included the word in his or her remarks. Little attention was paid to a 1990 report by Eichelberger, Botschall, Feely, Harstad, and Bowman, which found no difference in parental perceptions of whether most childhood injuries were preventable, regardless of whether they were characterized as having resulted from an accident. In 1996, I addressed this issue by fielding a national random-digit-dialed telephone survey that assessed adult interpretations of the word *accident*. Eighty-three percent of respondents associated preventability with the term (Girasek, 1999). Scores of studies have now established that most adults believe a majority of accidents and injuries are preventable (Chiappone & Kroes, 1979; Colver, Hutchinson, & Judson, 1982; Duan, 2004; Green, 1997; Hooper, Coggan, & Adams, 2003; Hu, Wesson, Parkin, & Rootman, 1996; Roberts, Smith, & Bryce, 1995). This example is relevant not only because it illustrates that communication opportunities were wasted trying to overcome a misperception that never existed. More important, if we consider findings from risk communications studies, injury control professionals may have been hammering home a characteristic of the injury hazard that reduces public support for their cause. Studies have found that people are less likely to pay for government programs that prevent deaths from which victims could have protected themselves and less likely to support regulation of such hazards (Mendeloff & Kaplan, 1989; Beggs, 1984; Slovic, 1987). This issue illustrates the importance of conducting formative and summative evaluations of communication efforts.

Another finding that is important for injury control professionals to understand is that people find higher levels of risk to be acceptable if they are associated with activities that are perceived to be highly beneficial (Slovic, 2000a). This seems likely to contribute to public tolerance of the high social costs associated with certain products (alcohol and motor vehicles, for example). Affect and worldviews have also been shown to influence public acceptance of risk (Slovic, 2000a). For example, people with fatalistic orientations to life are generally more supportive of nuclear power. The data related to affect suggest that our positive and negative views on hazards may precede and influence risk perceptions rather than be their product. These phenomena have been shown to operate on expert perceptions as well, but when professionals present risk information to the public, such factors are generally not considered or discussed. Most often we present statistics, which form the basis of our recommendations. There is abundant evidence to suggest, however, that laypeople have trouble understanding the laws of probability and following logic when interpreting numeric estimates of risk (Weinstein, 1999). For example, they may estimate the likelihood of dying from a disease to be higher than their likelihood of developing the disease. (For a discussion of how visual displays can have an impact on risk perceptions, see Lipkus & Hollands, 1999.)

A promising alternative to presenting risk information in the form of data or graphical representations of data is to explore contextualized approaches to risk communication (Rothman & Kiviniemi, 1999). Advocates of this strategy present people with information they can use to determine the personal relevance of a particular health threat. That information can relate to the risk's antecedents (for example, its risk factors or behaviors) or consequences (for example, its symptoms or outcome). The underlying premise is to help people imagine that the negative outcome could happen to them and be able to understand how that might occur.

Health Communication

Communication theory has been applied more widely in public health generally than in injury prevention specifically, and like risk communication science, it also emphasizes the value of message testing and evaluation (Rice & Atkin, 1989). The Centers for Disease Control and Prevention (1999) defines *health communication* as the study and use of communication strategies to inform and influence individual and community decisions that enhance health. Studies that have evaluated the impact of health communication campaigns demonstrate their effectiveness, as well as their limits. Such program components can help increase knowledge and awareness, change attitudes or communicate norms, remind ready participants to take action, or demonstrate simple skills (McKenzie & Smeltzer, 2001). In isolation, however, it is generally not realistic to expect communication material to cause sustained behavior change. Human behavior results from complex interactions. Injuries in particular have been shown to increase and decrease based on the manipulation of factors that are external to individuals at risk, such as product engineering, highway design, and state legislation. (Chapters One, Twenty, and Twenty-One, this volume, go into more detail on these topics.)

Acknowledgment of this situation should not, however, be interpreted as decreasing the importance of communication. To the contrary, it expands the range of audiences to whom we might hope to communicate effectively. Manufacturers, architects, engineers, legislators, law enforcement authorities, retailers, school officials, journalists, attorneys, medical professionals, and injury survivors all have a role to play in injury control (Gielen & Girasek, 2001; Christoffel & Gallagher, 1999; Girasek, 2005). Increasing their awareness of this fact, and their knowledge of how they can contribute to injury prevention, are appropriate goals of a communication campaign. It has been noted that those who make decisions that put whole populations in danger are rarely the targets of risk communication campaigns (Wagenaar, 1992). All of this is not to suggest that the individuals we hope to protect are not appropriate foci for communication efforts. First, we know that policymakers are influenced by the public (Jason & Rose, 1984; Lowenstein, Koziol-McLain, Satterfield, & Orleans, 1993; Page & Shapiro, 1992). Also, the public's policy preferences can be influenced by exposure to effectiveness data (Schenck, Runyan, & Earp, 1985). Similarly, high levels of compliance with legal interventions are generally not seen without publicity that alerts the community to the new law or sanction.

Most products are accompanied by instructions that describe safe use. In the case of safety products, consumers need to know that they exist, how and why they should be used, and where they can be obtained. Finally, there are many types of injuries—such as bathtub drowning and airway obstruction among children—that rely primarily on adult supervision. Such behaviors, which take place in the privacy of a family's home, can be influenced only by persuasion and education. The need to communicate risk and risk reduction strategies is central to the work of injury control professionals.

Many of the health behavior theories that have received strong empirical support include a component that is related to risk communication. The health belief model (HBM), for example, posits that a person is unlikely to adopt a preventive recommendation unless he or she believes that it is effective, that the negative health event could happen to him or her, and that it would have consequences that are severe enough to merit the cost of taking the precaution (Strecher & Rosenstock, 1997). These elements of perceived personal susceptibility and consequence severity are also central to Weinstein's precaution adoption process (PAP) Model (Weinstein, 1988; Weinstein & Sandman, 2002). Both the HBM and the PAP tell us that protective behaviors should be portrayed as easy and desirable or at least worthy of their price (that is, cost and inconvenience). The benefits communicated to the target audience may relate to health, or to other intangibles that they value, such as social acceptance or reduced anxiety. A recent qualitative study of Mexican immigrants living in southern California, for example, found that one of their primary motivations for wearing a seat belt was to avoid being noticed by law enforcement officials (Arce, Dinh-Zarr, & Sherrets, 2004). Identifying salient issues for communities can be one important purpose for conducting a precampaign needs assessment.

An early analysis of seat belt nonuse demonstrates why it is sometimes necessary to add legal risks to those inherent in unsafe behavior (driving without wearing a passenger restraint). Slovic, Fischhoff, and Lichtenstein (1978) posited that repeated safe driving experiences teach us that the probability of being seriously injured or killed on any given car trip is extremely low. When choosing from among the virtually endless list of hazards from which we could protect ourselves, people naturally ignore those that seem to be highly improbable (Slovic, 2000a). According to Slovic, our discomfort with uncertainty causes us to deny it. He says people tend to dichotomize risks into those that are so small that they can be safely ignored or so large that they should clearly be avoided.

This work was an extension of research that demonstrated that people are more likely to insure against small losses with high probability than large losses that occur infrequently (Slovic, Fischhoff, & Lichtenstein, 1978). The authors note that societal institutions have been driven to mandating insurance coverage. They recommend that proponents of protective behaviors targeted to low-probability events present risk in a cumulative fashion (that is, the probability of a negative event over a lifetime of the activity in question). What we are trying to overcome with this strategy is people's tendency to extrapolate from their own experience, a phenomenon that may cause them to under- or overestimate personal risk. We know that people who are familiar with a consumer product are less likely to read or follow its warning labels (DeJoy, 1999a). Research into the effects of personal experience has produced results that are often surprising (Weinstein, 1989). For example, feelings of vulnerability following a negative experience are not widely generalized and may be short-lived.

As directed by the HBM, we should assess the benefits and barriers that people associate with the precaution we are recommending in addition to exploring the dangers they associate with the risk activity. A scared person who adopts an ineffective precaution is no better off than the person who remains uninformed. At least one national study has been conducted in the United States to identify injury prevention measures that are perceived to be effective (Girasek & Gielen, 2003). It showed, for example, that smoke detectors are highly regarded. Having such knowledge in advance of a communication campaign could free up space and airtime for messages about ease of smoke detector use (if that was perceived as a barrier) rather than precaution effectiveness. The precaution adoption process model (Weinstein & Sandman, 2002) provides guidance on the mix of messages that should be addressed, depending on an audience's placement on the spectrum between hazard awareness and precaution adoption (see also Chapter Two, this volume).

Message is just one of five variables that can be manipulated to affect the outcome of the communication process. Expanding on Hovland's information processing model (Flay, DiTecco, & Schlegel, 1980; Bettinghaus, 1986), McGuire (1989) has proposed that source, channel, receiver, and destination can also have powerful influences on a campaign's effectiveness. For example, sources that are perceived as credible, attractive, and powerful are more persuasive than those with the opposite characteristics. *Channel* includes medium choices, such as whether to choose words or images to convey messages. *Receiver* refers to the audience, and we have already established the importance of assessing their needs and tailoring communications to them. Finally, *destination* relates the campaign's target. Are we asking people to take some immediate action or aspiring to long-term behavior change? Those input or independent variables constitute the elements of our communication, according to McGuire.

McGuire (1989) describes twelve outputs or behavior substeps that must be evoked for successful persuasion to occur:

- Exposure to the communication
- Attending to the communication
- Being interested in the communication
- Understanding it
- Acquiring skill from it
- Agreeing with it
- Storing its content
- Being able to retrieve that information
- Knowing when to retrieve the information
- Behaving in accord with the information
- Being reinforced for that action
- Consolidating what was experienced in this process

This communication-persuasion model demonstrates the complexity involved in moving people from being audience members to actors who can contribute effectively to their own protection.

Fear Appeals

To communicate risk of any negative consequence, we may find ourselves in the position of generating anxiety or fear among a population. From both effective and ethical perspectives, it is important to couple such affect with a reassuring recommendation. That is, we are obliged to follow fear-inducing messages with steps people can take to reduce their vulnerability. Our recommendations should be based on empirical evidence, and the audience we are trying to reach should have access to the safety program or device we are promoting. Even with these prerequisites in place, fear is a complicated emotion to manipulate if our goal is to motivate protective action. It has generally been accepted that fear operates according to an inverted U-shaped curve. That is, people are unlikely to take action against a threat that does not scare them but will be paralyzed or retreat into psychological denial if we raise their anxiety beyond a motivating level. Empirical support for this line of reasoning is far from conclusive (Will & Geller, 2004), however, in part because it is difficult to know where messages actually fall on the hypothetical range of fear arousal (DeJoy, 1999b).

Sources of Bias

We all possess a repertoire of psychological defense mechanisms that may serve us well in terms of maintaining our self-esteem and navigating the uncertainties inherent in the human experience. Health communicators must overcome some of these biases, however, if they are to make audiences feel susceptible to injuries and accidents. One of the most relevant for our practice has been identified by Weinstein as the optimistic bias. Numerous studies have demonstrated that people tend to erroneously judge their own risk to be less than that of others (Weinstein, 1988). The erroneous aspect of this construct is important, because it means the high-risk subgroups we seek to reach are unlikely to agree with our assessment of their vulnerability. Weinstein and Klein (1995) have also demonstrated that it is difficult to debias audiences by mere manipulation of descriptions of the risk factors.

An additional source of bias that affects risk perceptions are mental heuristics. Heuristics are rules or mental shortcuts we all use to make decisions and judgments easier (Slovic, Fischoff, & Lichenstein, 2000). The availability heuristic causes people to think that an event is more likely to occur if it is easy for them to envision. While likelihood of occurrence and top-of-mind recall are often correlated, other characteristics of events may cause them to persist in our consciousness (for example, images of an airliner crashing into a skyscraper). This heuristic can actually operate in favor of injury control professionals in that it causes people to overestimate the frequency of dramatic causes of death like accidents, homicide, and natural disasters (Lichtenstein, Slovic, Fishchoff, Layman, & Combs, 1978).

One aspect of heuristics that can work for or against our efforts is the fact that laypeople (and technical experts) are overly confident about the accuracy of their risk-related judgments (Slovic, Fischoff, & Lichenstein, 2000). This phenomenon probably contributes to the persistence of people's beliefs despite conflicting evidence. Messages that depart too dramatically from an audience's baseline views are unlikely to be perceived as credible to them (Perloff, 1993). We also know that communications that trigger counterarguing, that is, thoughts that disagree with the material being presented, make audiences more resistant to persuasive messages in the future. This phenomenon has been shown to occur when individuals are presented with information that threatens to increase their risk perceptions or decrease their self-esteem (Aspinwall, 1999).

If a needs assessment indicates that the public does not hold strong views, there is considerable evidence that their beliefs can be influenced by how risk data are framed (Slovic, 2000a). Again, this points to the need to pretest alternative versions of key messages. Face-valid measures taken to decrease risk perceptions have been shown to backfire in actual practice (Slovic, 2000a). An analogy intended to depict small magnitude, for example, could provide an image for the public that makes it easier to envision.

While the sources of bias that we have discussed up to this point act across populations, certain subgroups have been shown to share risk perceptions that differ from those of the public at large. Males, for example, consistently rate the risks associated with a variety of activities as being smaller than do females (Slovic, 2000c; DeJoy, 1999a; Soori, 2000; Ey et al., 2000). Of particular interest is the fact that this phenomenon may be related to issues of social and political power. More detailed analyses of data from U.S. populations, for example, have shown that it is driven largely by the perceptions of white men, even when income and education were held constant (Slovic, 2000c). Although we do not know precisely how these beliefs might alter male risk-taking proclivity, we do know that men experience higher rates of injuries than females in every culture. One might hypothesize that men's reduced sense of vulnerability causes them to take greater risks.

Risk Communication Can Be Risky Business

The possibility that people may increase risk taking in response to feeling safer is an example of an unintended consequence that could be triggered by an injury prevention campaign. Closely related concerns relate to speculations that parents may become less vigilant once they believe they have reduced their children's injury risk (for example, by teaching them to swim or installing a pool fence; Carey, Chapman, & Gaffney, 1994; Morrongiello & Major, 2002). Theories of risk compensation and risk homeostasis have generated decades of debate. Hedlund (2000) summarized this history and suggested guidelines to assess whether a safety measure is at risk for triggering a compensatory increase in risk behavior. He identified visibility, which relates to whether the public has been made aware of new protections, as one of several key factors to be taken into consideration. This line of reasoning illustrates how communication could be perceived as contributing to increased risk taking. If you accept the premise that people might use a product more dangerously in response to safety enhancements and you inform users that such modifications have been made, then you should monitor subsequent changes in behavior.

Zuckerman (1994) has speculated that there is a subgroup of the population that seeks experiences that are novel, intense, and varied. Thrill and adventure seeking in particular have been associated with risky driving practices (Jonah, 1997). If a high proportion of the audience we are trying to reach possesses this characteristic, they might actually be drawn to experiences portrayed as dangerous.

Several studies of communication campaigns have reported a so-called boomerang effect on young people (DeJoy, 1999a). Male high school students, for example, were more likely to dive into shallow water after a sign was posted at a pool prohibiting such behavior (Goldhaber & deTurck, 1989). Sensation seeking is conceptualized as a personality trait, but the effect just described could have been triggered by reactance. This phenomenon occurs in response to a perceived restriction of freedom or imposition of external control (Janis & Rodin, 1979). Adolescence may be a developmental phase in which such reactions are more likely to occur. The widely accepted notion that teenagers consider themselves to be immortal, however, has not received much empirical support (Cohn, MacFarlane, Yanez, & Imai, 1995). Newer research on the brain development of adolescents (Giedd, 2004) is likely to contribute to a better understanding of their capabilities to use risk and risk-reduction information effectively.

Gray and Ropeik (2002) feel that risk communicators need to put more emphasis on helping the public put their fears in perspective. They refer, for example, to people who drove in the wake of the September 11, 2001, terrorist attacks rather than flying, an objectively safer option. As the psychometric paradigm has taught us, such public reactions should not be characterized as irrational. Rather they should be acknowledged as a potential unintended consequence of fear-inducing events. Chronic anxiety can also produce health effects and diminish quality of life.

Another potentially negative consequence of an injury prevention campaign could be the stigmatization of injury victims—either by blaming them for their plight (Girasek, 1999) or depicting injury outcomes in a manner that devalues people with disabilities (Wang, 1992). If we paint a particularly negative picture of the at-risk person, it is also possible that members of the audience may not identify with this portrayal and may not feel susceptible to the threat in question. This explanation was offered for the failure of one prevention broadcast that was intended to increase awareness of the dangers associated with holiday driving. Investigators concluded that the way they framed alcohol involvement resulted in the viewers seeing others (for example, drunken drivers) as the causers and main victims of accidents (Naisbett, 1961). It has been shown that optimistic bias is more likely to operate when people possess a stereotypical victim in their minds (Berry, 2004). If members of the audience were persuaded to identify with a negative portrayal of risk takers (as being foolish, for example) concerns have been raised about possible damage to their self-efficacy (Aspinwall, 1999); see Chapters Two and Three, this volume, for discussion of this important psychological construct.

All of these findings reiterate the importance of conducting formative and summative evaluations of safety campaigns that include the measurement of negative as well as positive outcomes.

Warnings and Signage

Injury prevention has often relied on warning labels and signage to inform people of hazards and precautions. It is likely that we will rely more and more on brief messages or icons to communicate dangers and how to avoid them because society is increasingly fast-paced, with little time for reading. In the future, increasing amounts of information may be displayed on small screens such as those incorporated into handheld communication devices. There is also growing concern about low levels of literacy, and in our increasingly diverse population many people may not be fluent in English.

When a message is restricted to a few words or an icon, clear communication is even more challenging. An influential study of this phenomenon in the product safety world was conducted with adults shopping for toys (Langlois et al., 1991). The research team found that 44 percent of subjects would buy a toy labeled "Recommended for 3 and up" for a child between the ages of two and three, primarily because they thought that the age on the label referred to a child's developmental level. Conversely, only 5 percent of respondents reported that they would buy that toddler a toy that was labeled "Not recommended for below 3—small parts." The more effective label served one of a warning's most important functions: to cue a target audience to remember safety knowledge they already possess (Laughery & Hammond, 1999). A subject who did not know that small parts posed a choking hazard might not have avoided the dangerous toy despite the improved label.

More extensive warnings can be designed to provide new hazard information or instructions for using a product safely. Increasing the length of a communication does not ensure clarity, however. A study of child safety seat instructions, for example, found them to be written at a level that exceeded the literacy skills of most U.S. parents (Wegner & Girasek, 2003). The U.S. Consumer Product Safety Commission has developed a useful guide for manufacturers that want to improve the quality and readability of their product instructions (Smith, 2003).

One clear finding of the warning literature is that perceived hazardousness—perceived severity in particular—is predictive of warning effectiveness (DeJoy, 1999a). This is why it is recommended that product labels feature graphic language about a product's most serious potential risks. Manufacturers hoping to sell more products, however, may be reluctant to highlight such information. Also, the boomerang effect may be triggered if attempts to raise perceived threat are not matched by assurances of precaution efficacy (DeJoy, 1999b).

Little attention has been devoted to studying positive framing of safety messages—that, is telling people what they stand to gain rather than lose when taking an injury control measure (DeJoy, 1999b). We do know, however, that when other types of risk information were presented positively (for example, the risk of surviving a cancer therapy versus the risk of dying from it), subjects were much more likely to choose the treatment option (Bennett & Calman, 1999).

Signs are also used, particularly in the field of traffic safety, to alert members of the public to potential risks. Studies into the effectiveness of such communications have established the following elements as critical (adapted from Mazis & Morris, 1999):

- Audience attention must be captured. Use signs at key points of product use or purchase.
- Make signs conspicuous. Try large, pointed signs in red or yellow.
- Minimize visual clutter around the warning sign.
- Use signal words like *Danger* or *Caution*. Symbols and pictographs can also help.
- Use simple messages since they must be read quickly.
- Tailor or personalize the address whenever possible.

Ethical treatment of this topic calls for mention of the fact that warning signs or labels should represent just one component of a safety system (Laughery & Hammond, 1999). The ultimate protection comes from designs that engineer the hazard out of a product or activity. Risk communicators should ask whether protection at that level has been maximized before they agree to take part in a public awareness campaign. A related guideline would be to consider whether we can make precaution adoption more convenient rather than just trying to convince people that the cost of compliance is justified. A number of studies have shown that manipulation of the effort or discomfort associated with carrying out a safety recommendation can increase or decrease compliance dramatically (DeJoy, 1999a, 1999b).

These findings provide support for the health belief model, which has been discussed earlier (see also Chapter Two, this volume). Signs can also serve as a cue to action. Social cognitive theory, particularly the power of modeling to influence precaution adoption, has also received strong empirical support in the warning literature (Silver & Braun, 1999; see also Chapter Three, this volume).

The theoretical models and scientific findings discussed in this chapter can be used to design more effective risk communication or help us understand why so many risk communications fail to motivate behavior change. A thoughtful analysis by Harrell (2003), for example, sheds light on why the signs he tested in grocery shopping carts had no effect on the behavior of the adults responsible for protecting the young children who had accompanied them to the store. The signs communicated statistical risk information, and an order ("Do Not Allow Your Children to . . ."). Shopping cart–related injuries are unlikely to occur, and 95 percent of those that do require no medical attention. Shopping carts are familiar to U.S. adults. No natural contingencies exist in the grocery store environment to punish high-risk activity. Few other families model safe behavior. While the adult is busy selecting merchandise, she is expected to monitor her bored child continuously because he is in an environment that has been designed for adult users. Of note is Harrell's observation that the majority of children who were protected from falling out of the shopping cart because they walked beside it stood on the edge of the cart, thereby risking its tipping. This scenario illustrates the limits of communication tools and the importance of designing such materials within a context that has been analyzed from the user's perspective.

Despite this discussion of the challenges inherent in designing brief warnings, there is evidence that such communication can cause target audiences to adopt safer behavior (Silver & Braun, 1999). For example, the presence of signs has been shown to increase the use of protective equipment, including seat belts, and to reduce dangerous practices. It is our hope that the guidance provided in this chapter will increase readers' ability to use warnings to such ends.

The Future

There have been calls throughout this chapter to collect data before, during, and after communication campaigns to measure whether the resources and efforts have been well spent. The necessity of confirming that we did not injure audiences in our attempt to prevent future injuries has also been noted. From a larger perspective, we need to share lessons learned with each other because injury risk communication is a young science.

It is encouraging that cross-disciplinary collaboration seems to be on the increase. Injury epidemiologists and engineers see increasing value in partnerships with behavioral and social scientists. Such interactions allow the injury control community to integrate relevant findings from the fields of environmental health (such as risk communication) and clinical psychology (such as posttraumatic stress disorder). Similarly, public health professionals who focus on increasing physical activity levels are interested in understanding how to incorporate injury prevention into their programs. Such cross-fertilization can only strengthen the impact and reach of all parties.

Technological advances have brought another promising avenue for future risk communication research and programming. Strecher, Greenwood, Wang, and Dumont (1999) have written convincingly that interactive multimedia offer many advantages over traditional health communication channels. Their interactive nature generates greater engagement on the part of learners using them. Their ability to use graphic images and animation may mean they can communicate complex concepts like interactions more effectively than print or aural media. Such special effects may also make them appealing to the next generation of potential injury victims. They can measure message comprehension and provide feedback in real time. Perhaps most important, they allow tailoring of information and presentation format according to a user's preferences, perceptions, and risk profile. Their potential for bidirectional communication is highly compatible with this chapter's emphasis. Society must invest in increasing access to such technologies, however, and learning how to optimize their use before their contribution to risk communication can be fully realized.

Unfortunately, not all modern developments represent progress. At the dawn of a new century, terrorism has emerged as a global threat to the public's health. It can take the form of biological, radiological, chemical, or more traditional forms of attack, all of which could be classified as intentional injury events. Preparations for dealing with this newly recognized threat must involve the medical and public health communities, law enforcement and military organizations, as well as a myriad of private sector players such as information technology firms, chemical manufacturers, and the airline industry. It is encouraging that our campaign to ensure a secure homeland has not neglected the importance of risk communication. The New York Academy of Medicine, for example, has conducted important research into how the public might react to government instructions issued in the wake of a terrorist attack (Lasker, 2004). The results suggest that most people would not report to a smallpox vaccination site if directed to, and 40 percent would not shelter in place for the recommended period following a dirty bomb explosion. This well-designed investigation explored public objections to official recommendations. Such information should prove extremely valuable to government officials who are responsible for safeguarding citizens in the event of another terrorist attack. Undoubtedly, tomorrow will bring new public health threats, with communication challenges to match. In this dynamic environment, it is vital to learn from the professionals who have come before us and to listen to the public who will stand before us, asking for protection.

References

Arce, C., Dinh-Zarr, T. B., & Sherrets, D. (2004, Nov.). *Driving with God's license: An exploration of Mexican immigrant drivers' attitudes and behavior with a focus on belt use.* Poster presented at the American Public Health Association Conference, Washington, DC.

Aspinwall L. G. (1999). Introduction of section: Persuasion of cancer risk reduction: Understanding responses to risk communications. *Journal of the National Cancer Institute Monographs, 25,* 88–93.

Beggs, S. D. (1984). *Diverse risks and the relative worth of government safety programs: An experimental survey* (Rep. No. 700). Washington, DC: U.S. Environmental Protection Agency, Economic Analysis Division.

Bennett, P., & Calman, K. (1999). *Risk communication and public health.* New York: Oxford University Press.

Berry, D. (2004). *Risk communication and health psychology.* Bristol, PA: Open University Press.

Bettinghaus, E. P. (1986). Health promotion and the knowledge—attitude—behavior continuum. *Preventive Medicine, 15,* 475–491.

Carey, V., Chapman, S., & Gaffney, D. (1994). Children's lives or garden aesthetics? A case study in public health advocacy. *Australian Journal of Public Health, 18*(1), 25–32.

Centers for Disease Control and Prevention. Office of Communication. HealthCommKey. (1999, May). *The role of health communication in disease prevention and control.* http://www.cdc.gov/od/hcomm/rolehcomm.html.

Chiappone, D. I., & Kroes, W. H. (1979). Fatalism in coal miners. *Psychological Reports, 44,* 1175–1180.

Christoffel, T., & Gallagher, S. S. (1999). *Injury prevention and public health.* Gaithersburg, MD: Aspen.

Cohn, L. D., MacFarlane, S., Yanez, C., & Imai, W. K. (1995). Risk-perception. Differences between adolescents and adults. *Health Psychology, 14*(3), 217–222.

Colver, A. F., Hutchinson, P. J., & Judson, E. C. (1982). Promoting children's home safety. *British Medical Journal, 285,* 1177–1180.

Davis, R. M., & Pless, I. B. (2001). BMJ bans accidents: Accidents are not unpredictable. *British Medical Journal, 322,* 1320–1321.

DeJoy, D. M. (1999a). Attitudes and beliefs. In M. S. Wogalter, D. M. DeJoy, & K. R. Laughery (Eds.), *Warnings and risk communication.* Philadelphia: Taylor & Francis.

DeJoy, D. M. (1999b). Motivation. In M. S. Wogalter, D. M. DeJoy, & K. R. Laughery (Eds.), *Warnings and risk communication.* Philadelphia: Taylor & Francis.

Duan, L. (2004, June). *A survey on unintentional childhood injury pattern and awareness in three cities in China.* Paper presented at the Seventh World Conference on Injury Prevention and Safety Promotion, Vienna, Austria.

Eichelberger, M. R., Botschall, C. S., Feely, H. B., Harstad, P., & Bowman, L. M. (1990). Parental attitudes and knowledge of child safety: A national survey. *American Journal of Diseases of Children, 144,* 714–720.

Ey, S., Kesges, L. M., Patterson, S. M., Hadley, W., Barnard, M., & Alpert, B. S. (2000). Racial differences in adolescents' perceived vulnerability to disease and injury. *Journal of Behavioral Medicine, 23*(5), 421–435.

Finnegan, J. R., & Viswanath, K. (1997). Communication theory and health behavior change: The media studies framework. In K. Glanz, F. M. Lewis, & B. K. Rimer (Eds.), *Health behavior and health education: Theory, research and practice* (2nd ed.). San Francisco: Jossey-Bass.

Flay, B. R., DiTecco, D., & Schlegel, R. P. (1980). Mass media in health promotion: An analysis using an extended information processing model. *Health Education Quarterly, 7*(2), 127–147.

Giedd, J. N. (2004). Structural magnetic resonance imaging of the adolescent brain. *Annals of the New York Academy of Sciences, 1021,* 77–85.

Gielen, A. C., & Girasek, D. C. (2001). Integrating perspectives on the prevention of unintentional injuries. In N. Schneiderman, M. A. Speers, J. M. Silva, H. Tomes, & J. H. Gentry (Eds.), *Integrating behavioral and social sciences with public health.* Washington, DC: American Psychological Association.

Girasek, D. C. (1999). How members of the public interpret the word *accident. Injury Prevention, 5,* 19–25.

Girasek, D. C. (2005). Advice from bereaved parents: On forming partnerships for injury prevention. *Health Promotion Practice, 6,* 207–213.

Girasek, D. C., & Gielen, A. C. (2003). The effectiveness of injury prevention strategies: What does the public believe? *Health Education & Behavior, 30*(3), 287–304.

Goldhaber, G. M., & deTurck, M. A. (1989). A developmental analysis of warning signs: The case of familiarity and gender. In *Proceedings of the Human Factors Society. 33rd Annual Meeting* (Vol. 2, pp. 1019–1023). Santa Monica, CA: Human Factors and Ergonomics Society.

Gray, G. M., & Ropeik, D. P. (2002). Dealing with the dangers of fear: The role of risk communication. *Politics and Public Health, 21,*106–116.

Green, J. (1997). *Risk and misfortune: A social construction of accidents.* London: University College London.

Harrell, W. A. (2003). Effect of two warning signs on adult supervision and risky activities by children in grocery shopping carts. *Psychological Report, 92,* 889–898.

Hedlund, J. (2000). Risk business: Safety regulations, risk compensation, and individual behavior. *Injury Prevention, 6,* 82–90.

Hooper, R., Coggan, C. A., & Adams, B. (2003). Injury prevention attitudes and awareness in New Zealand. *Injury Prevention, 9*(1), 42–47.

Hu, X., Wesson, D., Parkin, P., & Rootman, I. (1996). Pediatric injuries: Parental knowledge, attitudes and needs. *Canadian Journal of Public Health, 87*(2), 101–105.

Janis, I. L., & Rodin, J. (1979). Attribution, control, and decision making: Social psychology in health care. In G. C. Stone, F. Cohen, & N. E. Adler (Eds.), *Health psychology.* San Francisco: Jossey-Bass.

Jason, L. A., & Rose, T. (1984). Influencing the passage of child passenger restraint legislation. *American Journal of Community Psychology, 12*(4), 485–495.

Jenni, K. E., & Loewenstein, G. (1997). Explaining the identifiable victims effect. *Journal of Risk and Uncertainty, 14,* 235–257.

Jonah, B. A. (1997). Sensation seeking and risky driving: A review and synthesis of the literature. *Accident Analysis and Prevention, 29*(5), 651–665.

Langlois, J. A., Wallen, B. A., Teret, S. P., Bailey, L. A., Hershey, J. H., & Peeler, M. O. (1991). The impact of specific toy warning labels. *JAMA, 265*(21), 2848–2850.

Lasker, R. D. (2004). *Redefining readiness: Terrorism planning through the eyes of the public.* New York: New York Academy of Medicine.

Laughery, K. R., & Hammond, A. (1999). Overview. In M. S. Wogalter, D. D. DeJoy, & K. R. Laughery (Eds.), *Warnings and risk communication.* Philadelphia: Taylor & Francis.

Lichtenstein, S., Slovic, P., Fishchoff, B., Layman, M., & Combs, B. (1978). Judged frequency of lethal events. *Journal of Experimental Psychology: Human Learning and Memory, 4,* 551–578.

Lipkus, I. M., & Hollands, J. G. (1999). The visual communication of risk. *Journal of the National Cancer Institute Monographs, 25,* 149–163.

Lowenstein, S. R., Koziol-McLain, J., Satterfield, G., & Orleans, M. (1993). Facts versus values: Why legislators vote against injury control laws. *Journal of Trauma, 35*(5), 786–792.

Lowrance, W. W. (1976). *Of acceptable risk: Science and the determination of safety.* San Francisco: William Kaufmann.

Mazis, M. B., & Morris, L. A. (1999). Attention capture and maintenance. In M. S. Wogalter, D. M. DeJoy, & K. R. Laughery (Eds.), *Warnings and risk communication.* Philadelphia: Taylor & Francis.

McGuire, W. J. (1989). Theoretical foundations of campaigns. In R. E. Rice & C. K. Atkin (Eds.), *Public communication campaigns* (2nd ed.). Thousand Oaks, CA: Sage.

McKenzie, J. F., & Smeltzer, J. L. (2001). *Planning, implementing and evaluating health promotion programs: A primer* (3rd ed.). Needham Heights, MA: Allyn & Bacon.

Mendeloff, J. M., & Kaplan, R. M. (1989). Are large differences in lifesaving costs justified? A psychometric study of the relative value placed on preventing deaths. *Risk Analysis, 9,* 349–363.

Morrongiello, B. A., & Major, K. (2002). Influence of safety gear on parental perceptions of injury risk and tolerance for children's risk-taking. *Injury Prevention, 8,* 27–31.

Naisbett, H. J. (1961). The great holiday massacre. *Traffic Safety, 58,* 12–15, 36, 48–49.

National Committee for Injury Prevention and Control. (1989). *Injury prevention: Meeting the challenge.* New York: Oxford University Press.

National Highway Traffic Safety Administration. (1997). Crashes aren't accidents' campaign. *NHTSA Now, 3*(11), 1–2.

Page, B. I., & Shapiro, R. Y. (1992). *The rational public: Fifty years of trends in American policy preferences.* Chicago: University of Chicago Press.

Perloff, R. M. (1993). *The dynamics of persuasion.* Mahwah, NJ: Erlbaum.

Rice, R. E., & Atkin, C. K. (1989). *Public communication campaigns* (2nd ed.). Thousand Oaks, CA: Sage.

Rivara, F. P. (2001). An overview of injury research. In F. P. Rivara, P. Cummings, T. D. Koepsell, D. C. Grossman, & R. V. Maier, (Eds.), *Injury control: A guide to research and program evaluation.* Cambridge, MA: Cambridge University Press.

Roberts, H., Smith, S. J., & Bryce, C. (1995). *Children at risk? Safety as a social value.* Bristol, PA: Open University Press.

Rosenberg, M. L., Rodriguez, J. G., & Chorba, T. L. (1990). Childhood injuries: Where we are. *Pediatrics, 86,* 1084–1091.

Rothman, A. J., & Kiviniemi, M. T. (1999). Treating people with information: An analysis and review of approaches to communicating health risk information. *Journal of the National Cancer Institute Monographs, 25,* 44–51.

Sandman, P. M. (1989). Hazard versus outrage in the public perception of risk. In V. T. Covello, D. B. McCalum, & M. T. Pavlova (Eds.), *Effective risk communication: The role and responsibility of government and nongovernment organizations.* New York: Plenum.

Sandman, P. M. (1991). *Risk = Hazard and outrage: A formula for effective risk communication* [Video]. Available from American Industrial Hygiene Association: Fairfax, VA.

Schenck, A. P., Runyan, C. W., & Earp, J.A.L. (1985). Seat belt use laws: The influence of data on public opinion. *Health Education Quarterly, 12*(4), 365–377.

Silver, N. C., & Braun, C. C. (1999). Behavior. In M. S. Wogalter, D. M. DeJoy, & K. R. Laughery (Eds.), *Warnings and risk communication.* Philadelphia: Taylor & Francis.

Slovic, P. (1987). Perception of risk. *Science, 236,* 280–285.

Slovic, P. (2000a). Informing and educating the public about risk. In P. Slovic (Ed.), *The perception of risk.* Sterling, VA: Earthscan.

Slovic, P. (2000b). Introduction and overview. In P. Slovic (Ed.), *The perception of risk.* Sterling, VA: Earthscan.

Slovic, P. (2000c). Trust, emotion, sex, politics and sciences: Surveying the risk assessment battlefield. In P. Slovic (Ed.), *The perception of risk.* Sterling, VA: Earthscan.

Slovic, P., Fischhoff, B., & Lichtenstein, S. (1978). Accident probabilities and seatbelt usage: A psychological perspective. *Accident Analysis and Prevention, 10,* 281–285.

Slovic, P., Fischhoff, B., & Lichtenstein, S. (2000). Rating the risks. In P. Slovic (Ed.), *The perception of risk.* Sterling, VA: Earthscan.

Smith, T. P. (Ed.). (2003, Oct.). *Manufacturer's guide to developing consumer product instructions.* Washington, DC: U.S. Consumer Product Safety Commission.

Soori, H. (2000). Children's risk perception and parents' views on levels of risk that children attach to outdoor activities. *Saudi Medical Journal, 21*(5), 455–460.

Strecher, V. J., Greenwood, T., Wang, C., & Dumont, D. (1999). Interactive multimedia and risk communication. *Journal of the National Cancer Institute Monographs, 25,* 134–139.

Strecher, V. J., & Rosenstock, I. M. (1997). The health belief model. In K. Glanz, F. M. Lewis, & B. K. Rimer (Eds.), *Health behavior and health education: Theory, research and practice* (2nd ed.). San Francisco: Jossey-Bass.

Wagenaar, W. A. (1992). Risk taking and accident causation. In J. F. Yates (Ed.), *Risk-taking behavior.* Hoboken, NJ: Wiley.

Wang, C. (1992). Culture, meaning and disability: Injury prevention campaigns and the production of stigma. *Social Science and Medicine, 35*(9), 1093–1102.

Wegner, M. V., & Girasek, D. C. (2003). How readable are child safety seat instructions? *Pediatrics, 111*(3), 588–591.

Weinstein, N. D. (1988). The precaution adoption process. *Health Psychology, 7*(4), 355–386.

Weinstein, N. D. (1989). Effects of personal experience on self-protection behavior. *Psychological Bulletin, 105,* 31–50.

Weinstein, N. D. (1999). What does it mean to understand a risk? Evaluating comprehension of risk comprehension. *Journal of the National Cancer Institute Monographs, 25,* 15–20.

Weinstein, N. D., & Klein, W. M. (1995). Resistance of personal risk perceptions to debiased interventions. *Health Psychology, 14*(2), 132–140.

Weinstein, N. D., & Sandman, P. M. (2002). The precaution adoption process model. In K. Glanz, B. K. Rimer, & F. M. Lewis (Eds.), *Health behavior and health education* (3rd ed., pp. 121–143). San Francisco: Jossey-Bass.

Will, K. E., & Geller, E. S. (2004). Increasing the safety of children's vehicle travel from effective risk communication to behavior change. *Journal of Safety Research, 35,* 263–274.

Zuckerman, M. (1994). *Behavioural expression and biosocial basis of sensation-seeking.* Cambridge, MA: University of Cambridge Press.

CHAPTER SIX

ECOLOGICAL MODELS FOR THE PREVENTION AND CONTROL OF UNINTENTIONAL INJURY

John P. Allegrante, Ray Marks, Dale W. Hanson

We generally accept the notion that optimal health status and high quality of life enable humans to lead productive lives and contribute to the overall social and economic stability of society. Achieving the utopian ideal of optimal health, however, is not a simple task. The task is made complex because health is not merely a product of individual biological, psychological, and behavioral factors; it is the sum of collective social conditions and the nexus of transactions that is created when people interact with the environment in which they live, work, and play. Simply knowing the pathological causes of a disease or unintentional injury is not enough to achieve the goal of improving health status (Haignere, 1999). Improving health and preventing unintentional injury require attention to the entire social system.

Despite a history dating back to John Snow, whose intervention to stem the 1854 cholera epidemic in London demonstrated the importance of social systems for maintaining human health (Centers for Disease Control and Prevention, 2004), a pervasive ideology of individualism has increasingly colonized public health science and practice (Lomas, 1998). Much of our thinking about health and disease causation has been dominated from almost the start of the twentieth century by the prevailing medical model (Engel, 1977). By extension, injury prevention has been conceptualized as a biomedical construct in which injury is perceived to be a physical event resulting from the sudden release of environmental energy that produces tissue damage in an individual. This reductionist perspective is not only narrow and ill conceived, it overlooks the importance of the psychological, environmental, and sociocultural factors as individual and collective contributory determinants of injury.

William Haddon, the father of modern injury prevention, prophetically introduced the concept of ecological injury prevention with publication of his seminal paper, "On the Escape of Tigers: An Ecological Note" (Haddon, 1970). Until then, individual behavior was perceived to be the preeminent cause of an accident. But Haddon argued it did not follow that changing individual behavior was the most effective means by which to prevent injury. In the context of the prevailing epidemiological model of causation in which the agent, host, and environment interact, he highlighted the opportunities for harm reduction through redesign of the physical environment. Moreover, he argued that by preventing or dissipating the adverse release of energy, it was possible to minimize the chance of injury without necessarily preventing the accident (Haddon, 1980). By doing so, Haddon precipitated a major paradigm shift from accident prevention to injury prevention.

Now, three decades later, much has been achieved on the strength of this change in paradigm. Health promotion has embraced an ecological perspective on health that realizes the importance of both the physical and social environments and the interaction of the individual with the environment. Mounting evidence suggests that the social and economic environments exert profound and lasting effects on health status and on the incidence, prevalence, and severity of disease and unintentional injury (Laflamme, 2001; Petridou & Tursz, 2001). However, despite evidence suggesting that influences outside the individual play an important role in determining health, the application of this knowledge has not yet been a major focus of intervention policy in the context of the prevention and control of unintentional injury. Perhaps we need to revisit Haddon's original thinking, reappraise the best opportunities for harm reduction within the ecological framework, and ask whether we can capitalize on what has been achieved through reengineering the physical environment by going a step further and simultaneously reengineering the social environment (Hanson et al., 2005).

In this chapter, we describe the potential of the ecological model for understanding the antecedent causes of unintentional injuries and guiding intervention for their prevention and control. First, we briefly review the scope and impact of unintentional injuries. Second, we review the origins and conceptualize the elements of the ecological model, using the injury iceberg as a useful metaphor for understanding the multiple levels of intervention required in an ecological approach to injury. We conclude with some applications of the ecological model to the prevention and control of unintentional injury and community safety promotion.

Scope and Impact of Unintentional Injuries

According to the U. S. National Academy of Sciences (2003), unintentionial injury is under-recognized as a major public health problem. Regardless of gender, race, or economic status, injuries are a leading cause of premature death for people of all ages in the United States and other nations with advanced economies.

Deaths due to unintentional injury are only part of the picture. Millions of Americans are injured each year and survive. Sustaining an injury not only causes temporary pain and inconvenience for many; for some, a single injury can result in lifelong disability, chronic pain, and a profound change in the individual's lifestyle. However, although scientific advances and medical technologies have significantly improved the overall health status of advanced nations in the past forty years, unintentional injuries continue to threaten the health of millions. This is largely due to the fact that injury prevention and control have not been perceived as a major public health issue. Rather, injuries have been viewed as unavoidable accidents that are part of everyday life.

A large body of epidemiological and medical research, however, shows that injuries, unlike accidents, do not occur by chance. The science of injury prevention has clearly demonstrated that injuries, and the events leading up to them, are not random. Like disease, the risk of injury follows a predictable pattern. Studying these patterns has made it possible to prevent injuries from occurring and has the potential to decrease injury-related death, disability, and financial burden (Krug, 1999).

Two types of unintentional injury constitute much of the burden of injury-related death and disability in the United States and in most other nations with advanced economies: injuries due to falls and road traffic injuries that result from motor vehicle crashes. These two mechanisms of unintentional injury, both of which have complex antecedents, suggest an array of potential prevention and control strategies that can be aimed at the individual, as well as at the environmental setting in which these injuries occur. Thus, strategies that target both the individual and the environment are more likely to be successful in lowering the prevalence of injuries than any single preventive strategy.

Injuries Due to Falls

Data on injuries due to falls in the United States show that falls are the leading cause of injury deaths among people sixty-five years and older and that one in every three Americans sixty-five years old or older falls each year (Cesari et al.,

2002). Of those who fall and survive, 20 to 30 percent suffer moderate to severe injuries that often reduce mobility and limit independence (Sattin et al., 1990). Falls also result in hip fractures, which have devastating impacts on survival and health outcome among the elderly (Marks, Allegrante, MacKenzie, & Lane, 2003) and increase the risk of premature death (Alexander, Rivara, & Wolf, 1992). Preliminary data for 2003 show that over fifty-eight thousand people, most of whom are elderly, will have died (an age-adjusted rate of 19.9 per 100,000) from fall-related injuries (Hoyert, Kung, & Smith, 2005). Falls are also the leading cause of nonfatal unintentional injuries and emergency department visits for children between the ages of zero and fourteen (Barnes, Adams, & Schiller, 2001). Each year in the United States, falls among this age group account for an estimated 2.5 million emergency department visits (Centers for Disease Control and Prevention, 2005b). In addition to the costs in terms of physical disability, the direct economic costs of treating fall-related injuries are substantial (Englander, Hodson, & Terregrossa, 1996).

A growing body of research evidence now indicates that among the elderly, factors likely to contribute to initial and subsequent falls and fall-related injuries include physical frailty, muscle weakness (Branch, Katz, Kneipmann, & Papsidero, 1984; Tinetti, Speechley, & Ginter, 1988), visual impairments, use of psychoactive medications, and difficulties with gait and balance (Sorock, 1988; Tinetti & Speechley, 1989; Tinetti, Doucette, Claus, & Marottoli, 1995; Wolfson, Judge, Whipple, & King, 1995). In addition to these individual predisposing factors, environmental risk factors for falling include slippery floor surfaces, uneven floors, poor lighting, loose rugs, unstable furniture, obstacles, and objects on floors (Speechley & Tinetti, 1990). Among children, fall-related risk factors are similarly multidimensional for falls from windows and beds and falls that occur on the playground (Dal Santo, Goodman, Glik, & Jackson, 2004). Such falls are due to a combination of human and environmental factors. Thus, what emerges from the epidemiological research that has been conducted to date is that the etiology of falls is sufficiently complex to warrant a falls prevention model that addresses both environmental factors, such as the physical setting in which people live, and individual determinants, such as the physiological and physical status of the individual and behaviors that place the individual at risk for a fall. Multifactorial intervention approaches have shown promise in reducing the risk of falling in community settings (Tinetti et al., 1994; Tinetti & Speechley, 1991).

Road Traffic Injuries

Although road traffic death rates declined dramatically throughout the twentieth century, motor vehicle crashes are the leading cause of injury mortality in the United States for people aged one to thirty-four. The Centers for Disease Control and Prevention (CDC) reports that more than 41,000 people die on the nation's roads and highways, with more than 3 million suffering nonfatal injuries (Centers for Disease Control and Prevention, 2005a). Of those who died in motor vehicle crashes, 5,586 were teenagers, 2,055 were children, and nearly 8,000 were sixty-five years of age and older. Annually, this results in approximately 500,000 hospitalizations and over 4 million visits to the emergency department. Moreover, motor vehicle–related deaths and injuries account for more than $150 billion in costs each year.

Like falls, motor vehicle crashes and their associated injuries have multiple determinants; however, because of the weak behavioral technologies of the past, efforts to prevent injuries have largely focused on passive approaches. Nonetheless, with the decline in the potential for further engineering improvements, it has become clear that in addition to other considerations, behavioral modification is essential to effective road safety (Lonero & Clinton, 1997).

Because of the evidence from a wide variety of studies that have shown that even the simplest behavior is determined by a complex mix of biological, psychological, and sociocultural factors, the consensus among experts is that behavior change is most likely to occur in the context of comprehensive, multisectoral, participative, and socially supportive interventions (Lonero & Clinton, 1997). Road safety interventions thus need to incorporate an ecological approach (a mix of behavioral, environmental, and policy approaches) if we are to continue to make progress in the prevention of motor vehicle crashes and associated injuries.

The Ecological Model

Concepts underlying the ecological model date back to the early twentieth century when Park, Burgess, and McKenzie (1925) are believed to have coined the term *human ecology*, extrapolating the theoretical paradigm of plant and animal ecology to the study of human communities. More recently, Last (1995) defined *ecology* as "the study of relationships among living organisms and their environment" (p. 52), while *human ecology* refers to the "study of human groups as influenced by environmental factors, including social and behavioral factors" (p. 52).

Interventions that simultaneously influence multiple levels and multiple settings of an ecological system may be expected to lead to greater and longer-lasting changes in health outcomes (Cohen & Swift, 1999). This notion is supported by emerging data indicating that multiple determinants account for premature deaths occurring in the United States and other advanced economies. McGinnis, Williams-Russo, and Knickman (2002) have attempted to enumerate and quantify these determinants. They have estimated that genetic predisposition accounts for 30 percent of early deaths; social circumstances, 15 percent; environmental factors, 5 percent; behaviors, 40 percent; and shortfalls in medical care for 10 percent of all premature deaths. It follows, then, that the most effective interventions to address multiple influences occur at multiple levels (Smedley & Syme, 2000).

Despite growing acceptance of the multiple determinants of health, according to Stokols (1992, 1996), health promotion programs often lack a clearly specified theoretical foundation or are based on narrowly conceived conceptual models that fail to take into account the individual's interactions with the physical and social environments. This perspective has grown out of rich history and conceptual background that underlies contemporary thinking about ecological models and is grounded in both psychology (Sells, 1969) and the science of public health (Sallis & Owen, 2002). For example, B. F. Skinner's work (1953) showing how the environment could shape animal behavior, Kurt Lewin's concept (1966) of ecological psychology and environmental forces, and Albert Bandura's notion (1977) of reciprocal determinism and person-environment interactions in social learning theory all constitute psychology's recognition of the multiple influences of the environment on human behavior.

Although the ecological approach was inherent in Snow's decision to take the handle off the Broad Street pump and thus constitutes the first true application of ecological thinking in public health, Edward Rogers (1960) was one of the first to advance the conceptual and potentially pragmatic value of ecological models in organized public health efforts. This ecological perspective—especially as applied to changing health behavior—was furthered by Moos (1980), Green and McAlister (1984), and McLeroy, Bibeau, Steckler, and Glanz (1988). As noted by McLeroy et al., "The purpose of an ecological model is to focus attention on the environmental causes of behavior and to identify environmental interventions" (1988, p. 366) that can be used to improve health. Green and Kreuter (2005) have expanded on this by proposing a socioecological program planning model of health promotion where health and safety can be interpreted in the context of the whole (ecological) system. There are three dimensions to this system: (1) the individual and his or her behavior, (2) the physical environment, and (3) the social environment. According to Green and Kreuter, each dimension can be analyzed at five levels:

1. The *intrapersonal level,* which is concerned with characteristics of the individual, that is, his or her knowledge, skills, life experience, attitudes, and behaviors as they interface with the environment and society.
2. The *interpersonal level,* which refers to the immediate physical environment and social networks in which an individual lives, including family, friends, peers, and colleagues and coworkers.
3. The *organizational level,* which refers to commercial organizations, social institutions, associations, clubs, and other mediating structures. They have structures, rules, and regulations enabling them to pursue specific objectives and

have direct influence over the physical and social environments maintained within their organization.

4. A *community*, which may be defined in both structural and functional terms. Structurally, a community can be defined within geographical or political boundaries. Functionally, a community may share demographic, cultural, ethnic, religious, or social characteristics, with its members having "a sense of identity and belonging, shared values, norms, communication and helping patterns" (Green & Kreuter, 2005, p. 256).

5. *Societies*, which are larger systems, often defined along political boundaries, possessing the means to distribute resources and control the lives and development of their constituent communities.

To better understand the multiple levels of intervention required in an ecological approach to injury prevention and control, Hanson and colleagues (2005) have proposed a visual metaphor, the *injury iceberg*, showing the relationship of the individual to the physical and social environment and levels of intervention (Figure 6.1).

The individual is, metaphorically speaking, the tip of the iceberg—just one part of a complex ecological system with many levels. While the individual may be the most visible component of this system, important determinants of their behavior and environmental risk are "hidden below the waterline." Attempts to modify the risk of injury at one level in isolation (for example, individual behavior) will be resisted by the rest of the system, which will attempt to maintain its own internal stability (homeostasis). Syme and Balfour (1998) have observed that "it is difficult to expect that people will change their behavior easily when many forces in the social, cultural, and physical environment conspire against such change. If successful behavior modification programs are to be developed to prevent disease, more attention will need to be given not only to the behavior and risk profiles of individuals, but also to the environmental context in which people live" (p. 796). Such a statement constitutes a strong argument for ecological approaches to change.

The socioecological paradigm emphasizes the dynamic interface among the three dimensions—the individual, the physical environment, and the social environment—acting at five levels: intrapersonal, interpersonal, organizational, community, and societal. They provide the ecological context in which the individual acts. Each level is built on the foundation of a "deeper" level. As these deeper levels become larger and exercise more inertia, it becomes more difficult to change them. But once changed, these levels are more likely to sustain the desired outcome (Swerissen, 2004). This ecological model provides a complex web of causation and creates a rich context for multiple avenues of intervention. It can be used to map the key links in an accident sequence, identifying upstream latent failures, along

FIGURE 6.1. INJURY ICEBERG ECOLOGICAL MODEL.

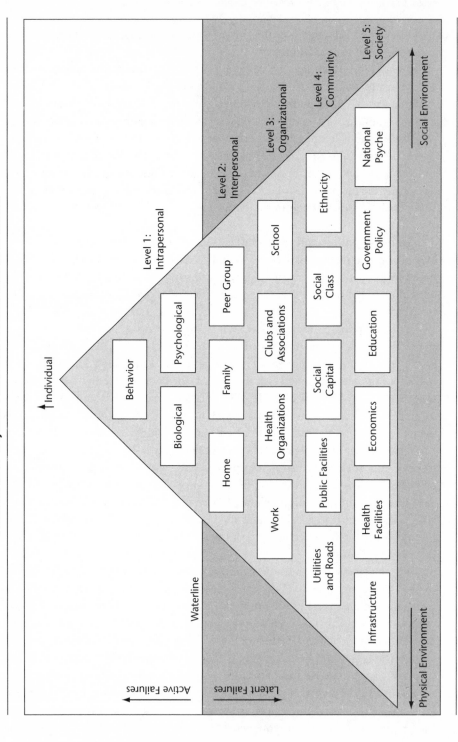

Source: From "The Injury Iceberg: An Ecological Approach to Planning Sustainable Community Safety Interventions," by D. Hanson, J. Hanson, P. Vardon, K. McFarlane, J. Lloyd, R. Muller, et al., 2005, *Health Promotion Journal of Australia, 16* (1), p. 6. Copyright © 2005 by the *Health Promotion Journal of Australia.* Reprinted by permission.

with the more obvious downstream active failures. Identifying the most strategic links thus ensures effective action.

Applications of the Ecological Model in Health Promotion and Injury Prevention and Control

Now that there are ecological models of health promotion, behavior modification, and identified potential strategies for intervention, the ultimate challenge remains: applying what we have learned in the real world. The transition from researching what works (efficacy) to researching how to make it work in a complex social setting (effectiveness) is not as straightforward as many assume (Howat, Cross, & Sleet, 2004). At the heart of the problem is how researchers and practitioners address the problem of complexity conceptually and methodologically (Glasgow, Lichtenstein, & Marcus, 2003). An ecological construct of injury causation is necessarily complex.

Efficacy trials test whether an intervention does more good than harm when administered under optimum conditions (Flay, 1986). To ensure internal validity, contextual factors are carefully controlled. A standardized intervention program is delivered in a uniform fashion to a specific, and usually homogeneous, target audience. Isolating the experimental variable from the influence of contextual factors can elucidate a clear relationship between the control and experimental variable. Effectiveness trials test whether an intervention does more harm than good in real-world conditions. Here the focus is on ensuring external validity. The population tested is unlikely to be homogeneous, and the outcome of the trial may be influenced by many extraneous contextual factors (Glasgow et al., 2003). Efficacy research may offer little insight into the practical challenges of implementation in a community social system if it has conceptually avoided the impact of contextual factors on outcome. Thus, if injury prevention is the science of controlling context, safety promotion is the art of managing context.

While the use of behavioral and social science theories in the context of injury prevention and control has been limited to a selected few (Trifiletti, Gielen, Sleet, & Hopkins, 2005), there has been increasing interest in ecological models in population health and safety promotion (Gielen & Sleet, 2003). A number of published studies have demonstrated the growing importance of this approach in a range of areas of health promotion. For example, recent studies designed to promote physical activity (MacDougall, Cooke, Owen, Willson, & Bauman, 1997; Sallis, Bauman, & Pratt, 1998; Sallis et al., 2001); improve health status of low-income, multiethnic women (Peterson et al., 2002); stimulate environmental change to support physical activity and dietary behavior change among adolescents in schools (Dzewaltowski, 1997; Dzewaltowski, Estabrooks, & Johnston, 2002); and prevent obesity among young people (Booth et al., 2001; Davison & Birch, 2001; Longjohn, 2004) have all used a broad ecological framework with which to design intervention strategy that addresses the health problem under study at the individual, familial, community, and societal levels. The application of the ecological model in injury prevention and control has shown the most promise in falls injury prevention, road traffic injury prevention, and community safety promotion.

Falls Injury Prevention

In addition to the prevention of road traffic injury, there is increasing support for the application of multifactorial interventions that target at-risk populations in reducing falls among both children and adults (Marks & Allegrante, 2004). A good example of a multifaceted community-based program for reducing the incidence of falls injury in the elderly is that published recently by Clemson et al. (2004). This group studied the impact of improving individual falls self-efficacy and lower limb balance and strength, while improving home and communal environmental and behavioral safety. Attention to regular visual screening and medication reviews was encouraged. Compared to a control group, the intervention group experienced a 31 percent reduction in falls. A similar home-based intervention to prevent falls among community-dwelling frail older people that included a home environmental assessment, the facilitation of any recommended changes, and training in the use of adaptive equipment reduced falls rates, especially among previously frequent fallers (Nikolaus & Bach, 2003).

A number of studies have demonstrated that multifaceted community-based approaches are more effective than single-strategy intervention approaches (for example, Dyer et al., 2004; Huang & Acton, 2004). Moreover, an ecological approach that focuses on the multiple causative factors that put people at risk for falls, as well as health promotion policies that foster high-quality screening and intervention programs, are indicated. As outlined in the ecological model, the need to train personnel, who can implement preventive interventions and risk assessment processes, as well as counsel individual clients, will also be required if we are to reduce falls. Moreover, legislation to optimize safety in the home and its environment and adequate medical coverage and funding for counseling are needed for achieving successful preventive outcomes (Marks & Allegrante, 2004).

Road Traffic Injury Prevention

There is general consensus that single interventions do not have the same impact as multiple interventions in efforts to reduce or prevent injury. Health promotion approaches to road traffic injury prevention have been advocated for this reason

(Sleet, 1984; Sleet, Wagenaar, & Waller, 1989). Indeed a CDC report describing motor vehicle safety as one of the twentieth century's important public health achievements strongly suggested that this was due to the fact that the interventions that were successful in improving motor safety were those that were designed to account for the multiple risk factors involved in motor vehicle injuries (Centers for Disease Control and Prevention, 1999; Dellinger, Sleet, & Jones, in press; Gielen & Sleet, 2003). The changes held responsible for the improvements in motor safety included legislative policies, educational programs, and changes in the physical and social environment (Gielen & Sleet, 2003; see also Chapters Ten and Eleven).

As early as 1989, Simons-Morton et al. (1989) proposed that taking an ecological perspective of individuals within their social and physical environments, a diagnostic framework identifying factors associated with drinking and driving injuries, and applying a conceptual intervention model with multiple components and four phases, plus evaluation criteria for societal and practice settings, would prove beneficial. This has been subsequently supported by Howat, Sleet, Elder, and Mayock (2004). These investigators have suggested that while health education interventions alone may not be effective for preventing alcohol-related traffic injury, ecological approaches may be beneficial. This is because in ecological intervention approaches, each intervention builds synergistically on the strengths of every other one. More specifically, given the complexity of issues that have an impact on driving under the influence of alcohol, ecological approaches to reducing alcohol-impaired driving that use all four components of the health promotion model proposed by Howat and his colleagues are likely to be especially effective. Lonero and Clinton (1997) listed four broad classes of tools with which to influence driver behavior: legislation, enforcement, education, and reinforcement. Moreover, the World Health Organization (WHO), in its report on preventing road traffic injuries (Peden et al., 2004), focuses on a systems approach to prevention, including the interaction among its elements—vehicles, roads, and road users and their physical, social, and economic environments.

There are five main elements of the ecological model in injury prevention and control:

1. Unintentional injury is determined by many different factors.
2. Behavior that leads to unintentional injury has both situational and psychological influences.
3. There are powerful sociological and environmental factors influencing injury.
4. Because safety is an ecological concept, determined by the relationship between an individual and his or her physical and social environment (Hanson, Vardon, & Lloyd, 2002b), prevention programs need to be sufficiently comprehensive to account for the dynamic interface between these dimensions.

5. Interventions must address beliefs, attitudes, behaviors, and environmental factors and involve community stakeholders in finding their own solutions.

Community Safety Promotion

To focus solely on the biomedical concept of injury prevention is to misunderstand the fundamental nature of the human experience, and hence how the positive state of "safety" is achieved. Maurice et al. (2001) define *safety* as "a state in which hazards and conditions leading to physical, psychological, or material harm are controlled in order to preserve the health and well-being of individuals and the community" (p. 237). The United Nations, in its 1994 report on human development, has asserted that safety and security is a fundamental human right and an essential condition for the sustainable development of societies (United Nations Development Program, 1994). Safety is as much concerned with the subjective dimension—the perception of safety—as it is with the objective dimension—the absence of injury. It is as much concerned with the community in which individuals reside as it is with the behavior of the individuals who comprise the community. Thus, it is evident that safety is a psychological, sociological, and environmental phenomenon, as much as it is physiological. As such, safety is inherently an ecological concept (Labonte, 1991).

Moller (2004) states, "The community-based model for injury prevention is an explicit approach to achieving reductions in the incidence of injury at the population level by the application of multiple countermeasures and multiple strategies in the context of community defined problems and community owned solutions" (p. 1). Thus, community-based safety promotion is not a single intervention but rather a set of processes that are implemented simultaneously and synergistically in the hope of promoting safety in a specific community. In each community, the mix and type of interventions used will differ because communities differ (Moller, 1991, 2004). Effectively managing context by implementing the most appropriate mix of strategies to address the specific injury problems faced by an individual community is the critical factor determining the success of community-based interventions. Most important, the community must be involved in the process of defining the problem, identifying practical solutions, and mobilizing the resources necessary to implement and sustain the solution (Coggan & Bennett, 2004). Few would dispute this principle, but a real shift toward community empowerment has been hard to achieve. While it is easy for politicians, bureaucrats, and senior researchers to "talk the talk," it is more difficult for them to "walk the walk" when this entails sharing control over the social or research agenda and especially difficult when it involves surrendering absolute control over the assignment of resources.

The reality is that power is asymmetrical, especially for poor or disenfranchised communities. In an era of financial accountability, economic rationalism, and aggressive competition for funding, short-term, project-based funding is the norm. Projects come and go depending on their ability to secure and maintain ongoing funding. This perpetuates a cycle of dependency in which short-term political agendas assume more importance than long-term community development. Professionally driven, externally initiated, and exogenously funded interventions have the potential to exacerbate this dependency if they do not build community capacity, encourage self-sufficiency, and foster self-efficacy in the prioritized target community (Hanson, Vardon, & Lloyd, 2002c).

We should not overlook the research implications of sharing control with a community coalition. In the context of community-based participatory research, this means a researcher has no innate right to set the parameters of a community effectiveness study; rather, this must be negotiated with the community (Green & Mercer, 2001). Stated another way, researchers must learn to work with community contextual factors rather than against them. However, researchers can have a significant influence on the community agenda. Communities appreciate and respect timely, relevant, and credible scientific information. Access to local injury surveillance data is a powerful tool for focusing the agenda of community safety promotion coalitions on strategic epidemiological issues (Hanson et al., 2003; Hanson, Vardon, & Lloyd, 2002a).

If population gains in health and safety are to be achieved and sustained, then this is contingent on the identification, mobilization, and development of local resources (McLeroy, Norton, Kegler, Burdine, & Sumaya, 2003). Outcomes dependent on external resources are vulnerable. The solution is to maximize the capacity of a community to institutionalize and maintain an outcome within its own "ecosystem" (Hanson et al., 2005). Eva Cox (1995) has identified four types of community resources that enable such capacity:

Financial capital: The economic resources available to a community. While clearly important, it is frequently overemphasized at the expense of other forms of capital.

Physical capital: The natural environment and man-made resources (for example, buildings and equipment) available to a community.

Human capital: The skill and knowledge of the individuals contained within a community.

Social capital: The "features of social organization such as networks, norms, and trust that facilitate co-ordination and co-operation for mutual benefit" (Putnam, 1995, p. 67).

Despite the controversy regarding the definition and operationalization of social capital (Labonte, 1999; Lin, 1999), the concept does highlight the important fact that a community is more than the sum of its parts and that the way communities organize and mobilize their social resources is an important resource in itself. Different types of social capital have been identified by Putnam (1995):

- The societal norms that define the community's expectations of the behavior of individuals and organizations within the community
- The ability of individuals and organizations within a community to form relationships of trust and thereby work collaboratively to identify and solve health, environmental, and sociological problems.
- The strength and effectiveness of individual, organizational, and social networks contained within a community (Hanson, Muller, & Durrheim, 2005)

Lin (1999) has suggested that the type of social capital necessary to maintain desirable social behaviors is different from the type of social capital necessary to change them. Social capital based on group cohesion (societal norms and community expectations of acceptable behavior) is useful to maintain desirable behavior (Hanson, Muller, & Durrheim, 2005). For example, wearing seat belts is now normative behavior. In the United States, seat belt use increased from 11 percent in 1981 to 68 percent in 1997 (Centers for Disease Control and Prevention, 1999). Drunk driving is also increasingly perceived to be socially unacceptable (Isaacs & Schroeder, 2001). While legislation and enforcement have undoubtedly contributed to this change in community standards, changes in community standards have meant that aggressive legislation and enforcement of child restraint, seat belt laws, and drunk-driving laws is considered politically acceptable by majorities of the American population.

In contrast, the type of social capital necessary to induce change is different in quality. Rather than being a function of group cohesion, it is a function of relationships that span boundaries and thereby induce change by producing social, political, and bureaucratic leverage (Hanson, Muller, & Durrheim, 2005; Burt, 2001; Granovetter, 1973). Here, individuals—whether political champions (for example, William Haddon as director of the U.S. National Highway Safety Bureau), consumer health advocates (for example, Ralph Nader in his "Unsafe at Any Speed" campaign of the 1960s), or community activists (for example, Doris Aitken, founder of Remove Intoxicated Drivers and Candy Lightner, founder of Mothers Against Drunk Driving)—can be important agents of change (Isaacs & Schroeder, 2001). This is because of the strategic relationships such individuals are able to build with others in the community and the way they use these relationships to advocate for organizational, social, and structural change (Pitt & Spinks, 2004).

WHO Safe Communities

Safe Communities is an approach to injury prevention and safety promotion that is supported by the World Health Organization (WHO, 2005; Svanstrom, 1999). The safe community model seeks to understand injury and intervene at a community level. By involving people in finding their own solutions to community problems, the community aims to be a catalyst for environmental, structural, sociological, and political change. This empowers the community, and ultimately individuals within a community, to change their environment and their behaviors to reduce the risk of injury and increase the perception of safety. It is therefore an ecological paradigm of safety promotion (Hanson, Vardon, & Lloyd, 2002b). WHO-designated Safe Communities are demonstration communities, which others can model when seeking to establish their own community safety programs. There are currently ninety-six WHO-designated Safe Communities (WHO Collaborating Center on Community Safety Promotion, 2005). Communities are assessed for WHO designation based on six indicators, designed to encourage best practice in safety promotion:

1. An infrastructure based on partnerships and collaborations, governed by a cross-sectoral group that is responsible for safety promotion in their community
2. Long-term, sustainable programs covering both genders and all ages, environments, and situations
3. Programs that target high-risk groups and environments and programs that promote safety for vulnerable groups
4. Programs that document the frequency and causes of injury
5. Evaluation measures to assess their programs, processes, and the effects of change
6. Ongoing participation in national and international Safe Communities Networks

Spinks, Turner, Nixon, and McClure (2005) conducted a systematic review of the WHO Safe Communities approach on behalf of the Cochrane Collaboration. They identified seven community-controlled evaluations using population-based injury morbidity and mortality data. These studies were conducted in four countries from two geographical regions: Scandinavia (Sweden and Norway) and Australasia (Australia and New Zealand). Although the authors concluded that the WHO model is effective in reducing injuries in whole populations, important methodological limitations were present in all studies. Perhaps this is not surprising given the methodological, organizational, political, and financial challenges of conducting large, robust studies of this type.

Programs conducted in Scandinavia demonstrated stronger population outcomes than those conducted in Australasia. Falkoping, a city in Sweden demonstrated a 23 percent decrease in all injury morbidity rates at the time the community coalition was active (Schlep, 1987). Motala, also a city in Sweden, demonstrated a 13 percent reduction in injury rates (Timpka, Lindqvist, Schelp, & Ahlgren, 1999). Harstad, (a city in Norway), produced significant reductions in child burns and scalds, and traffic injury rates (Ytterstad, 2003; Ytterstad, Smith, & Coggan, 1998). In New Zealand, the Waitakere Safe Communities Project documented a significant reduction in child injury admission rates, but was unable to demonstrate a significant reduction in hospitalization rates for all ages and all injuries (Coggan, Patterson, Brewin, Hooper, & Robinson, 2000). In Australia, the Shire of Bulla (later to become the Hume Safe Communities) was unable to demonstrate a significant reduction in injury rates (Ozanne-Smith, Day, Stathakis, & Sherrard, 2002). The Latrobe Valley Better Health Injury Prevention Program (Day, Ozanne-Smith, Cassel, & Li, 2001) was able to demonstrate reductions in age-standardized emergency department presentation rates using a quasi-experimental design (6,594 per 100,000 persons in the first year of the program to 4,821 in the final year), but there was no control community, and this study did not fulfill the selection criteria for the Cochrane Review.

No studies were identified of WHO Safe Communities in poorer countries, so any generalization of these results to the international community must be undertaken with caution. However, Spinks et al. (2005) conclude it is time to conduct an appropriately funded and rigorously conducted global multicommunity trial of the Safe Communities approach.

Conclusion

This chapter began by highlighting injury prevention as a biomedical construct based on a reductionist view that injury is a physical event resulting from a sudden release of environmental energy producing tissue damage in an individual. Such a conceptualization of injury underestimates the effect of environmental and social contextual factors on population-level injury outcomes and narrows the possibilities for the design and effectiveness of intervention. Injury prevention and control and the promotion of safety have physical, psychological, and sociological dimensions and thus should be considered an ecological concept.

To better understand that concept, Hanson's injury iceberg is a useful metaphor for an ecological system of injury causation. In this system, the individual is just the tip of the iceberg, the most visible and identifiable component of a complex system in which the individual interacts with the physical and social environment. The most enduring means to reduce an individual's risk of injury in such a system is to systematically address the physical and social environmental factors hidden beneath the waterline, which ultimately shape individual and social behaviors that give rise to injury.

While much has been achieved in the past fifty years, we face a new frontier of challenges in the prevention and control of injury at the outset of the twenty-first century. The epidemiological evidence is converging to tell us that social influences have profound impact on population health and injury outcomes. We must use this evidence to attack the problem of the social and environmental determinants of injury with the same energy, urgency, and intellectual rigor that our predecessors attacked the physical determinants of injury in the late 1900s. This will provide fertile new ground to advance injury prevention and control in the future. However, we must accept that current reductionistic scientific methods have limitations in their ability to deal with the complexity of socioecological systems. Scientists, administrators, and practitioners need to move out of the complacency of their comfort zone and embrace research tools, theories, methodologies, and types of evidence and safety promotion practice that can accommodate, elucidate, and manage this complexity. Some of these techniques already exist; others are yet to be developed and tested.

References

Alexander, B. H., Rivara, F. P., & Wolf, M. E. (1992). The cost and frequency of hospitalization for fall-related injuries in older adults. *American Journal of Public Health, 82,* 1020–1023.

Bandura, A. (1977). *Social learning theory.* Upper Saddle River, NJ: Prentice Hall.

Barnes, P. M., Adams, P. F., & Schiller, J. S. (2001). Summary health statistics for the U.S. population: National Health Interview Survey. *Vital Health Statistics, 10*(217), 1–82.

Booth, S. L., Sallis, J. F., Ritenbaugh, C., Hill, J. O., Birch, L. L., Frank, L. D., Glanz, K., Himmelgreen, D. A., Mudd, M., Popkin, B. M., Rickard, K. A., St Jeor, S., & Hays, N. P. (2001). Environmental and societal factors affect food choice and physical activity: Rationale, influences, and leverage points. *Nutrition Reviews, 59,* S21–S39.

Branch, L. G., Katz, S., Kneipmann, K., & Papsidero, J. A. (1984). A prospective study of functional status among community elders. *American Journal of Public Health, 74,* 266–268.

Burt, R. (2001). The social capital of structural holes. In M. F. Guillen, R. Collins, P. England, & M. Meyer (Eds.), *Economic sociology at the millennium* (pp. 202–247). New York: Russell Sage Foundation.

Centers for Disease Control and Prevention. (1995). Injury-control recommendations: Bicycle helmets. *MMWR Morbidity and Mortality Weekly Report, 44*(RR-1), 1–17.

Centers for Disease Control and Prevention. (1999). Motor vehicle safety: A 20th century public health achievement. *MMWR Morbidity and Mortality Weekly Report, 48*(18), 369–374.

Centers for Disease Control and Prevention. (2004). 150th anniversary of John Snow and the pump handle. *MMWR Morbidity and Mortality Weekly Report, 53*(34), 783.

Centers for Disease Control and Prevention. (2005a). *Community-based interventions to reduce motor vehicle-related injuries: Evidence of effectiveness from systematic reviews.* http://www.cdc.gov/ncipc/duip/mvsafety.htm.

Centers for Disease Control and Prevention. (2005b). Falls and hip fractures among older adults. http://www.cdc.gov/ncipc/factsheets/falls.htm.

Cesari, M., Landi, F., Torre, S., Onder, G., Lattanzio, F., & Bernabei, R. (2002). Prevalence and risk factors for falls in an older community-dwelling population. *Journals of Gerontology Series A: Biological Sciences and Medical Sciences, 57,* M722–M726.

Clemson, L., Cumming, R. G., Kendig, H., Swann, M., Heard, R., & Taylor, K. (2004). The effectiveness of a community-based program for reducing the incidence of falls in the elderly: A randomized trial. *Journal of the American Geriatric Society, 52,* 1487–1494.

Coggan, C., & Bennett, S. (2004). Community-based injury prevention programs. In R. McClure, M. Stevenson, & S. McEvoy (Eds.), *The scientific basis of injury: Prevention and control* (pp. 347–358). Melbourne, Australia: IP Communications.

Coggan, C., Patterson, P., Brewin, M., Hooper, R., & Robinson, E. (2000). Evaluation of the Waitakere Community Injury Prevention Project. *Injury Prevention, 6,* 130–134.

Cohen, L., & Swift, S. (1999). The spectrum of prevention: Developing a comprehensive approach to injury prevention. *Injury Prevention, 5,* 203–207.

Cox, E. (1995). *A truly civil society.* Boyer Lectures, Australian Broadcasting Commission, Sydney, Australia.

Dal Santo, J. A., Goodman, R. M., Glik, D., & Jackson, K. (2004). Childhood unintentional injuries: Factors predicting injury risk among preschoolers. *Journal of Pediatric Psychology, 29,* 273–283.

Davison, K. K., & Birch, L. L. (2001). Childhood overweight: A contextual model and recommendations for future research. *Obesity Reviews, 2,* 159–171.

Day, L. M., Ozanne-Smith, J., Cassell, E., & Li, L. (2001). Evaluation of the Latrobe Valley Better Health Injury Prevention Program. *Injury Prevention, 7,* 66–69.

Dellinger, A. M., Sleet, D. A., & Jones, B. (in press). Public health achievement in motor vehicle safety in the 20th century. In J. Ward & C. Warren (Eds.), *Silent victories: Public health triumphs of the twentieth century.* New York: Oxford University Press.

Dyer, C.A.E., Taylor, G. J., Reed, M., Dyer, C. A., Robertson, D. R., & Harrington, R. (2004). Falls prevention in residential care homes: A randomized controlled trial. *Age and Aging, 33,* 596–602.

Dzewaltowski, D. A. (1997). The ecology of physical activity and sport: Merging science and practice. *Journal of Applied Sport Psychology, 9,* 254–276.

Dzewaltowski, D. A., Estabrooks, P. A., & Johnston, J. A. (2002). Healthy youth places promoting nutrition and physical activity. *Health Education Research, 17,* 541–551.

Engel, G. (1977). The need for a new medical model: A challenge for biomedicine. *Science, 196,* 129–136.

Englander, F., Hodson, T. J., & Terregrossa, R. A. (1996). Economic dimensions of slip and fall injuries. *Journal of Forensic Science, 41,* 733–746.

Flay, B. (1986). Efficacy and effectiveness trials (and other phases of research) in the development of health promotion programs. *Preventive Medicine, 15,* 451–474.

Gielen, A. C., & Sleet, D. (2003). Application of behavior change theories and methods to injury prevention. *Epidemiologic Reviews, 25,* 65–76.

Glasgow, R., Lichtenstein, E., & Marcus, A. (2003). Why don't we see more translation of health promotion research to practice? Rethinking the efficacy-to-effectiveness transition. *American Journal of Public Health, 93,* 1261–1267.

Granovetter, M. (1973). The strength of weak ties. *American Journal of Sociology, 78,* 1360–1380.

Green, L. W., & Kreuter, M. W. (2005). *Health program planning: An educational and ecological approach* (4th ed.). New York: McGraw-Hill.

Green, L. W., & McAlister, A. L. (1984). Macro intervention to support health behavior: Some theoretical perspectives and practical reflections. *Health Education Quarterly, 11,* 323–338.

Green, L. W., & Mercer, S. L. (2001). Can public health researchers and agencies reconcile the push from funding bodies and the pull from communities? *American Journal of Public Health, 91,* 1926–1929.

Haddon, W. (1970). On the escape of tigers: An ecological note. *American Journal of Public Health, 60,* 2229–2235.

Haddon, W. (1980). Advances in the epidemiology of injuries as a basis for public policy. *Public Health Reports, 95,* 411–421.

Haignere, C. S. (1999). Closing the ecological gap: The public/private dilemma. *Health Education Research, 14,* 507–518.

Hanson, D., Hanson, J., Vardon, P., McFarlane, K., Lloyd, J., Muller, R., & Durrheim, D. (2005). The injury iceberg: An ecological approach to planning sustainable community safety interventions. *Health Promotion Journal of Australia, 16*(1), 5–15.

Hanson, D., Hart, K., McFarlane, K., Carter, A., Hockey, R., & Miles, E. (2003). Addressing childhood injury in Mackay: A safe communities initiative. *Injury Bulletin, 77,* 1–6.

Hanson, D., Muller, R., & Durrheim, D. (2005). *Documenting the development of social capital in a community safety promotion coalition using social network analysis.* International Conference on Engaging Communities, Brisbane, Australia, Aug. 14 to 17. Retrieved Oct. 19, 2005, from http://www.engagingcommunities2005.org/abstracts/S32-hanson-d.html.

Hanson, D., Vardon, P., & Lloyd, J. (2002a). Becoming Queeensland's first safe community: Considering sustainability from the outset. In R. Muller (Ed.), *Reducing injuries in Mackay, North Queensland* (pp. 35–52). Warwick, Queensland, Australia: Warwick Educational Publishing.

Hanson, D., Vardon, P., & Lloyd, J. (2002b). Collection of NDS-IS level 2 injury surveillance data in regional Queensland. In R. Muller (Ed.), *Reducing injuries in Mackay, North Queensland* (pp. 1–16). Warwick, Queensland: Warwick Educational Publishing.

Hanson, D., Vardon, P., & Lloyd, J. (2002c). Safe communities: An ecological approach to safety promotion. In R. Muller (Ed.), *Reducing injuries in Mackay, North Queensland* (pp. 17–34). Warwick, Queensland, Australia: Warwick Educational Publishing.

Howat, P., Cross, D., & Sleet, D. (2004). Introduction: Section V—program development, implementation and evaluation. In R. McClure, M. Stevenson, & S. McEvoy (Eds.), *The scientific basis of injury prevention and control* (pp. 261–265). Melbourne: IP Communications.

Howat, P., Sleet, D., Elder, R., & Mayock, B. (2004). Preventing alcohol-related traffic injury: A health promotion approach. *Traffic Injury Prevention, 5,* 208–219.

Hoyert, D. L., Kung, H. C., & Smith, B. L. (2005). Deaths: Preliminary data for 2003. *National Vital Statistics Reports, 53*(15), 1–48.

Huang, T. T., & Acton, G. J. (2004). Effectiveness of home visit falls prevention strategy for Taiwanese community-dwelling elders: Randomized trial. *Public Health Nursing, 21,* 247–256.

Isaacs, S. L., & Schroeder, S. A. (2001). Where the public good prevailed. *American Prospect, 12*(10), 1–10.

Krug, E. (1999). *Injury: A leading cause of the global burden of disease.* Geneva, Switzerland: World Health Organization, Department for Disability/Injury Prevention and Rehabilitation.

Labonte, R. (1991). Econology: Integrating health and sustainable development. Part one: Theory and background. *Health Promotion International, 6,* 49–65.

Labonte, R. (1999). Social capital and community development: Practitioner emptor. *Australian and New Zealand Journal of Public Health, 23,* 430–433.

Laflamme, L. (2001). Explaining socio-economic differences in injury risks. *Injury Control and Safety Promotion, 8,* 149–153.

Last, J. (1995). *A dictionary of epidemiology* (3rd ed.). New York: Oxford University Press.

Lewin, K. (1966). *Principles of topological psychology* (F. Heider & G. M. Heider, Trans). New York: McGraw-Hill. (Original work published 1936)

Lin, N. (1999). Building a network theory of social capital. *Connections, 22,* 28–51.

Lomas, J. (1998). Social capital and health: Implications for public health and epidemiology. *Social Science and Medicine, 47,* 1181–1188.

Lonero, L. P., & Clinton, K. M. (1997). Objectives for behavioral safety programs. Retrieved Dec. 2004 from http://www.drivers.com/article/302.

Longjohn, M. M. (2004). Chicago project uses ecological approach to obesity prevention. *Pediatric Annals, 33,* 62–63.

MacDougall, C., Cooke, R., Owen, N., Willson, K., & Bauman, A. (1997). Relating physical activity to health status, social connections and community facilities. *Australia and New Zealand Journal of Public Health, 21,* 631–637.

Marks, R., & Allegrante, J. P. (2004). Falls prevention programs for older ambulatory community dwellers: From public health research to health promotion policy. *Soz Praventivmed, 49,* 171–178.

Marks, R., Allegrante, J. P., MacKenzie, C. R., & Lane, J. M. (2003). Hip fractures among the elderly: Causes, consequences and control. *Ageing Research Reviews, 2,* 57–93.

Maurice, P., Lavoie, M., Laflamme, L., Svanstrom, L., Romer, C., & Anderson, R. (2001). Safety and safety promotion: Definitions for operational developments. *Injury Control and Safety Promotion, 8,* 237–240.

McGinnis, J. M., Williams-Russo, P., & Knickman, J. R. (2002). The case for more active policy attention to health promotion. *Health Affairs, 21,* 78–93.

McLeroy, K. R., Bibeau, D., Steckler, A., & Glanz, K. (1988). An ecological perspective on health promotion programs. *Health Education Quarterly, 15,* 351–377.

McLeroy, K. R., Norton, B. L., Kegler, M. C., Burdine, J. M., & Sumaya, C. V. (2003). Community based interventions. *American Journal of Public Health, 93,* 529–533.

Moller, J. (1991). Community based interventions: An emerging dimension of injury control models. *Health Promotion Journal of Australia, 1,* 51–55.

Moller, J. (2004). Reconsidering community based interventions. *Injury Prevention, 10,* 1–3.

Moos, R. H. (1980). Social-ecological perspectives on health. In G. C. Stone, F. Cohen, & N. E. Adler (Eds.), *Health psychology: A handbook.* San Francisco: Jossey-Bass.

National Academy of Sciences. (2003). *Reducing the burden of injury: Advancing prevention and treatment.* Washington, DC: National Academy of Sciences.

Nikolaus, T., & Bach, M. (2003). Preventing falls in community-dwelling frail older people using a home intervention team (HIT): Results from the randomized Falls-HIT trial. *Journal of the American Geriatric Society, 51,* 300–305.

Ozanne-Smith, J., Day, L., Stathakis, V., & Sherrard, J. (2002). Controlled evaluation of a community based injury prevention program in Australia. *Injury Prevention, 8*(1), 18–22.

Park, P., Burgess, E., & McKenzie, R. (1925). *The city.* Chicago: University of Chicago Press.

Peden, M., Scurfield, R., Sleet, D., Mohan, D., Hyder, A. A., Jarawan, E., & Mathers C. (Eds.). (2004). *World report on road traffic injury prevention.* Geneva, Switzerland: World Health Organization.

Peterson, K. E., Sorensen, G., Pearson, M., Hebert, J. R., Gottlieb, B. R., & McCormick, M. C. (2002). Design of an intervention addressing multiple levels of influence on dietary and activity patterns of low-income, postpartum women. *Health Education Research, 17,* 531–540.

Petridou, E., & Tursz, A. (2001). Socio-economic differentials in injury risk. *Injury Control and Safety Promotion, 8,* 139–142.

Pitt, R., & Spinks, D. (2004). Advocacy. In R. McClure, M. Stevenson, & S. McEvoy. (Eds.), *The scientific basis of injury prevention and control* (pp. 303–317). Melbourne, Australia: IP Communications.

Putnam, R. (1995). Bowling alone: America's declining social capital. *Journal of Democracy, 6,* 65–78.

Rogers, E. S. (1960). *Human ecology and health: An introduction for administrators.* New York: Macmillan.

Sallis, J. F., Bauman, A., & Pratt, M. (1998). Environmental and policy interventions to promote physical activity. *American Journal of Preventive Medicine, 15,* 379–397.

Sallis, J. F., Conway, T. L., Prochaska, J. J., McKenzie, T. L., Marshall, S. J., & Brown, M. (2001). The association of school environments with youth physical activity. *American Journal of Public Health, 91,* 618–620.

Sallis, J. F., & Owen, N. (2002). Ecological models. In K. Glanz, F. M. Lewis, & B. K. Rimer (Eds.), *Health behavior and health education: Theory, research, and practice* (3rd ed., pp. 462–484). San Francisco: Jossey-Bass.

Sattin, R. W., Lambert, H., DeVito, C. A., Rodriguez, J. G., Ros, A., Bacchelli, S., Stevens, J. A., & Waxweiler, R. J. (1990). The incidence of fall injury events among the elderly in a defined population. *American Journal of Epidemiology, 131,* 1028–1037.

Schlep, L. (1987). Community intervention and changes in accident pattern in a rural Swedish municipality. *Health Promotion, 2,* 109–125.

Sells, S. B. (1969). Ecology and the science of psychology. In E. P. Willems & H. L. Raush (Eds.), *Naturalistic viewpoints in psychological research* (pp. 15–30). New York: Holt, Rinehart, and Winston.

Simons-Morton, B. G., Brink, S. G., Simons-Morton, D. G., McIntyre, R., Chapman, M., Longoria, J., & Parcel, G. S. (1989). An ecological approach to the prevention of injuries due to drinking and driving. *Health Education Quarterly, 16,* 397–411.

Skinner, B. F. (1953). *Science and human behavior.* New York: Macmillan.

Sleet, D. A. (Ed.). (1984). Occupant protection and health promotion [Entire issue]. *Health Education Quarterly, 11*(2).

Sleet, D. A., Wagenaar, A. C., & Waller, P. F. (Eds.). (1989). Drinking, driving, and health promotion. [Entire issue]. *Health Education Quarterly, 16.*

Smedley, B. D., & Syme, S. L. (2000). *Promoting health: Intervention strategies from social and behavioral research.* Washington, DC: National Academy Press.

Sorock, G. S. (1988). Falls among the elderly: Epidemiology and prevention. *American Journal of Preventive Medicine, 4,* 282–288.

Speechley, M., & Tinetti, M. (1990). Assessment of risk and prevention of falls among elderly persons: Role of the physiotherapist. *Physiotherapy Canada, 42,* 75–79.

Spinks, A., Turner, C., Nixon J., & McClure, R. (2005). The "WHO Safe Communities" model for the prevention of injury in whole populations. *Cochrane Database of Systematic Reviews, 2,* CD004445.pub2. DOI: 10,1002/14651858.CD004445.pub2.

Stokols, D. (1992). Establishing and maintaining healthy environments: Towards a social ecology of health promotion. *American Psychologist, 47,* 6–22.

Stokols, D. (1996). Translating social ecological theory into guidelines for community health promotion. *American Journal of Health Promotion, 10,* 282–298.

Svanstrom, L. (1999). *Evidenced-based injury prevention and safety promotion—A review of concepts and studies.* Stockholm, Sweden: Karolinska Institute, Department of Public Health Sciences.

Swerissen, H. (2004). Australian primary care policy in 2004: Two tiers or one for Medicare? *Australia and New Zealand Health Policy, 1,* 2.

Syme, S. L., & Balfour J. L. (1998). Social determinants of disease. In R. Wallace, B. D. Doebbeling, & J. M. Last (Eds.), *Maxcy-Rosenau-Last public health and preventive medicine* (14th ed., pp. 795–810). Stamford, CT: Appleton and Lange.

Timpka, T., Lindqvist, K., Schelp, L., & Ahlgren, M. (1999). Community-based injury prevention: Effects on health care utilization. *International Journal of Epidemiology, 28,* 502–508.

Tinetti, M. E., Baker, D. I., McAvay, G., Claus, E. B., Garrett, P., Gottschalk, M., Koch, M. L., Trainor, K., & Horwitz, R. I. (1994). A multifactorial intervention to reduce the risk of falling among elderly people living in the community. *New England Journal of Medicine, 331,* 821–827.

Tinetti, M., Doucette, J., Claus, E., & Marottoli, R. (1995). Risk factors for serious injury during falls by older persons in the community. *Journal of the American Geriatrics Association, 43,* 1214–1221.

Tinetti, M. E., & Speechley, M. (1989). Prevention of falls among the elderly. *New England Journal of Medicine, 320,* 1055–1059.

Tinetti, M. E., & Speechley, M. (1991). Multiple risk factor approach to prevention of falls. In R. Weinruch, E. C. Hadley, & M. G. Ory (Eds.), *Reducing frailty and falls in older persons* (pp. 126–132). Springfield, IL: Charles C. Thomas.

Tinetti, M. E., Speechley, M., & Ginter, S. F. (1988). Risk factors for falls among elderly persons living in the community. *New England Journal of Medicine, 319,* 1701–1707.

Trifiletti, L. B., Gielen, A. C., Sleet, D. A., & Hopkins, K. (2005, Jan. 4). Behavioral and social sciences theories and models: Are they used in unintentional injury prevention research? *Health Education Research, 20*(3), 298–307.

United Nations Development Program. (1994). *Human development report 1994: New dimensions of human security.* Retrieved March 7, 2005, from http://www.undp.org/reports/global/1994/en/.

WHO Collaborating Center on Community Safety Promotion. (2005). *Safe communities network members.* Retrieved Oct. 19, 2005, from http://www.phs.ki.se/csp/who_safe_communities_network_en.htm.

Wolfson, L., Judge, J., Whipple, R., & King, M. (1995). Strength is a major factor in balance, gait, and the occurrence of falls. *Journal of Gerontology, 50A,* 64–67.

Ytterstad, B., Smith, G. S., & Coggan, C. A. (1998). Harstad injury prevention study: Prevention of burns in young children by community based intervention. *Injury Prevention, 4,* 176–180.

Ytterstad, B. (2003). The Harstad Injury Prevention Study: A decade of community-based traffic injury prevention with emphasis on children. Postal dissemination of local injury data can be effective. *International Journal of Circumpolar Health, 62,* 61–74.

CHAPTER SEVEN

PLANNING MODELS

PRECEDE-PROCEED and Haddon Matrix

Kimberley Freire, Carol W. Runyan

Program planning has been likened to preparing for travel (Green & Kreuter, 2005; Gielen & McDonald, 2002). Travelers use maps, guidebooks, previous experiences, and experts to determine a best route and key stops along the journey. The traveler might imagine the ideal trip, prioritize what must be done, consider logistics and practical issues, and decide how to maximize time and money. The actual journey rarely mirrors the imagined one. Nonetheless, the traveler may consider her trip successful if she reaches most of her itinerary stops, learns more about a new culture, and feels more confident about preparing for future travel. Program planning, like preparing for a trip, is a process where key stakeholders make decisions about where to go and how to get there. Program plans should specify an intervention pathway and a means by which planners can assess progress.

Today, planners who work outside research organizations are rarely required to forge uncharted territory. Evidenced-based practices and a broad array of social and behavioral theories are widely disseminated. Injury professionals have developed databases on many, although not all, injury topics. Furthermore, injury priorities have been defined by national collaboratives, and planners can access a great deal of information online.

This chapter considers the state of the art in both health promotion and injury prevention planning. Health promotion emphasizes a theory-driven, ecological approach to defining public health problems and their solutions. Injury prevention and control increasingly includes behavior change approaches, while maintaining even greater focus on traditional macrolevel strategies such as policies and regulations, which have been the mainstay of interventionists in the field for several decades. Perhaps most important, federal and other funding sources have increasingly urged programs to select best practices, which are strategies that have been rigorously evaluated, or promising practices, for which there is some evidence of success. The primary purpose of this chapter is to describe a planning approach to injury intervention that incorporates myriad sources of evidence, including theoretical constructs and frameworks, scientific data, and information from key stakeholders. A secondary purpose of the chapter is to illustrate how social and behavioral theories help planners frame injury problems and select effective solutions.

Injury Background

Injury prevention practitioners rely on a diverse set of intervention approaches, which historically have included education, regulation, legislation, and litigation. These approaches are directed at changing a wide array of environments and behaviors at multiple levels of an ecological framework. Injury professionals often have worked most effectively in applying measures focused on modifying physical environments through passive interventions that do not require individual effort to be effective (for example, employing safer highway, home, factory, or playground designs) or making changes in products that result in passive protection (for example, shatterproof glass, air bags in automobiles, and changing the characteristics of firearms so that young children cannot squeeze the trigger). These types of approaches usually require policy or regulatory intervention. Efforts to advocate for changes in the broader social environment often result in policy-level changes (for example, availability of safe child care, taxes on alcohol sales) but may also require broad programmatic efforts to change social norms (for example, the designated driver campaign and efforts to reduce harsh physical punishment of children).

In addition, the intervention options include strategies for modifying the behaviors of individuals at risk or those who influence others' behaviors and environments, such as health care providers, teachers, parents, or law enforcement officers (Wilson, Baker, Teret, Shock, & Garbarino, 1991). Furthermore, strategies that target environmental injury risks also involve behaviors, for example, actions by legislators, regulatory agency leaders, and corporate boardroom executives. Even litigation for safety involves decisions on the part of attorneys, judges, and juries, who must be persuaded to make specific choices. Hence, behavioral strategies are part of all types of planned injury prevention interventions.

Planning for Injury Prevention

Just as different guidebooks can bring travelers to the same key sites and feature the same preparations, so can different planning models assist planners in program and evaluation development. However, various planning approaches have been developed from work with specific populations or on particular health issues. That is, planners should consider how adaptable a particular planning model is to injury prevention and the intended audience (Green & Kreuter, 2005). For injury professionals, the best planning model will likely allow planners to easily integrate the language and methods familiar to the field into a systematic approach to decision making.

Two specific planning models are described in this chapter. The Haddon matrix brings together basic public health concepts of agent-host-environment interaction with the notions of intervening at different phases of the injury process by designating when interventions have their effects either to prevent potentially injurious events from happening or to minimize damage during or after an event (Haddon, 1972, 1980). The matrix facilitates broad thinking about the panoply of approaches to injury prevention and intervention. As with Haddon's other framework, the ten countermeasures (Runyan, 1998; Gielen, 1992; Haddon, 1973), the matrix easily allows thinking about strategies aimed at the kinds of passive changes that are directed at altering physical environments and the kinds of products that can cause injury. Alternatively, PRECEDE-PROCEED emphasizes multilevel intervention strategies to influence health-related behaviors and environments. The model delineates a process for examining and prioritizing behaviors and environmental factors that influence health outcomes—injuries in this case.

Haddon's matrix and PRECEDE-PROCEED share some common features that are well suited to many injury efforts. Specifically, they (1) focus on a population-based approach but allow high-risk group strategies, (2) provide a framework to organize and prioritize risk factors and risk conditions, and (3) allow integration of behavioral theories, scientific evidence, and input from the intended audience in the decision-making process. One important way the models differ is how they refer to risks: Haddon's matrix refers to risks (of which behavior is one) that occur at different phases of an injury-producing process with a primary aim being injury reduction, whereas PRECEDE-PROCEED refers to behavioral and environmental risks for specific causes of injury morbidity and mortality. The general planning process presented at the end of this chapter builds on the strengths of both models while considering the real-world circumstances in which planners develop programs. Injury professionals who have never taken a planning course or have little program development experience will likely benefit from learning the two models presented in this chapter in more detail (Green & Kreuter, 1992, 2005; Runyan, 2003; Gielen & McDonald, 2002; Runyan, 1998; National Committee for Injury Prevention and Control, 1989; Green, Wilson, & Bauer, 1983; Gielen, 1992; Haddon, 1972, 1973, 1980).

The Importance of Planning

Planning is essential to intervention development. All planners, in conjunction with other key decision makers, must decide how to use available resources to best address a specified problem. This presents the planner with various practical and ethical issues along the way, and planning models are heuristics that facilitate the decision-making process.

Returning to the travel analogy, a program plan is like a travel itinerary that details the proposed journey. A plan addresses key questions about a proposed program including, but not limited to:

- Destination: Where do we want to go?
  What is the injury problem we should address?
- Direction: Which way should we go?
  How do we move toward program goals?
  On which risk factors and conditions of the injury problem should we focus?
  Who should benefit from the program (for example, the general population or high-risk groups)?
- Evaluation and accountability: Did we get to where we wanted to go?
  Did the program implement the program as intended?
  What was the quality of the intervention implementation?
  Did the program achieve its stated goals? If so, how? If not, why?
  How can the program demonstrate its effect on processes, structures, health, and social outcomes?
  What constitutes good evidence?
- Replicability: How can we get there again?
  How can future programs achieve similar results or model best practices?
- Ethical considerations: Who do we leave behind? What are the potential harms?
  Does the program represent the best use of resources?
  What injury problems or populations do not benefit from the program?
  What harm may come from selected intervention strategies?

Key Features of Program Planning

Some features of program planning transcend any particular model. The features we discuss are not an exhaustive list and are not exclusive to injury prevention and control programs. Rather, they comprise, in our view, a planning approach that reflects current trends and principles in the field of public health. This approach requires planners to work collaboratively with communities and other interested parties, build on past successes, support decisions with evidence, and demonstrate success through evaluation.

National, State, and Local Priorities

Many planners work in agencies where injury prevention and control priorities are based on national, state, and local objectives. Examples are Healthy People 2010 (U.S. Department of Health and Human Services, 2000) and the National Center for Injury Prevention and Control Research Agenda (National Center for Injury Prevention and Control, 2002). The Institute of Medicine, National Research Council, and surgeon general also have published topic-specific reports (Institute of Medicine, 2001, 2002; U.S. Department of Health and Human Services, 2001; National Research Council, 1996) on injury control while *Reducing the Burden of Injury* (Bonnie, Fulco, & Liverman, 1999) urged overall better integration of research knowledge into practice. In addition, the State and Territorial Injury Prevention Directors' Association (2003) has developed *Safe States*, a document designed to provide the basic structure of a state injury program. Some states have developed their own planning priorities based on local data. All of these resources can help planners better understand the general context for their developing programs.

Evidence-Based Approach

The terms *best practices, promising practices,* and *best processes* are now part of the planning and health promotion lexicon and the standards on which many planners will be required to base, at least in part, their programmatic decisions. Green and Kreuter (2005) describe best practices as interventions that have been rigorously evaluated and ideally applied across various populations. In contrast, they term "promising practices" those that show some indication of success, for example, changes in risk factors of behaviors or injuries. A work site program designed to reduce on-the-job injuries may demonstrate that in its first year, participating organizations implemented new safety policies and practices. The organizational behavior change is a good indicator that injuries will be reduced, but it will take at least three years to gather enough data to assess a statistically significant difference between intervention and control organizations.

Planners who follow best processes, according to Green and Kreuter (2005), use their skills and tools to assess the particular circumstances of the intended audience members, including their social and built environments. (Green, 2001). By this means, they can select intervention strategies that are most appropriate for the intended audience.

Involving Key Stakeholders Early and Often

One of a planner's most important roles is to coordinate individuals and groups with an interest in the program and its consequences. Planners must first identify key stakeholders and then determine who should influence which decisions. The intended audience is always an important group for planners to consider from the beginning of the process. In addition, a planning team with diverse expertise can be an important resource for individuals who are responsible for keeping the process moving.

Social and Behavioral Theories

Planners can use social and behavioral theories throughout program development. Theories, in conjunction with scientific evidence and input from the intended audience, help planners define, clarify, and support decisions about priorities and intervention strategies.

Gielen and McDonald (2002) use their Safe Home program to provide examples of theories that can be used at each level of the social ecological framework and their relevance to each phase of PRECEDE-PROCEED planning. Green and Kreuter (2005) also describe how both micro- and macrolevel theories fit into planning processes. Although the Haddon matrix is silent on the issue of behavioral theory, it reflects an ecological approach to intervention strategy selection (see Chapter Six, this volume). Therefore, planners can use theory to inform decisions about items within each cell of a Haddon matrix. Theories, and their application to practice, are a type of evidence that explains the relationship between personal (for example, behaviors, attitudes, skills) and environmental factors (for example, social networks, built environment, policies) and injury outcomes. Most theories used in public health, and in particular those covered in this book, have been applied across health topics and tested in intervention studies. In addition, theories usually represent aspects of human (cognitive, physical, affective), relational (social support), and community and societal functioning that generalize across multiple settings and outcomes. Therefore, planners often can make strong arguments for selecting risk factors represented by theoretical constructs, even if the factors have been studied in a different injury problem from the one the program intends to address. For example, health professionals have applied the health belief model (see Chapter Two, this volume) to injury problems. The model's perceived susceptibility construct, when applied to injury, posits that people's beliefs about their chances of suffering a particular injury influence their decisions to engage in injury prevention behaviors. Planners who apply it to motor vehicle–related pedestrian injuries may decide that any strategy to change pedestrian walking behaviors should influence individuals' perceived susceptibility for motor vehicle related injury. That is, low perceived susceptibility to pedestrian injury is both an explanatory construct of pedestrian behavior and a risk factor for pedestrian injuries.

Planners can use theories to develop a conceptual model of the program. Some injury professionals use planning models and specific theories to guide program development by explicitly linking intervention activities to theoretical constructs that the program intends to change (Trifilleti, Gielen, Sleet, & Hopkins, 2005). A theory-based approach to planning strengthens the planner's rationale for selecting particular strategies by making explicit the program assumptions about how each activity will lead to changes in risk factors and conditions or have a direct impact on the injury outcome (Buchanan, 1998). Sometimes planners develop a logic model or conceptual picture that illustrates the links between program activities and intended changes, such as risk factors, behaviors, and injury events. Planners also can use theoretical constructs to define evaluation measures. For example, a pedestrian safety program that intends to heighten individuals' perceived susceptibility to motor vehicle injury could ask individuals about their beliefs regarding the likelihood of being injured while walking before and after an intervention is implemented to assess changes in perceived susceptibility.

Theoretical models also can inform the planning process by explicating approaches or specific strategies to organize communities, introduce new ideas (innovations), collaborate with key stakeholders, and take numerous other actions that planners will likely coordinate. Many of these frameworks are not specific theories, but they are theory-informed approaches and principles that arise from both practice and scholarly work.

A Population or Universal Approach

Public health, in name and principle, is a population-based field. Planners who begin the planning process with a universal or population-based orientation will consider how to reach whole communities of people with appropriate prevention strategies. Although behavioral approaches in one sense focus on individual-level change, the collective behavior of families, organizations, and communities that alters social norms and structures also is a critical focus for intervention. This point is probably best articulated by Geoffrey Rose in his sentinel work (Rose, 1985, 1992). Rose posits that shifting the population distributions of diseases and injuries has a greater impact on reducing morbidity and mortality than focusing on the distribution tail, or highest-risk group. Sometimes a comprehensive approach that includes both universal and high-risk group strategies is appropriate. Often there is more to gain from environmental-level interventions that provide universal protection (such as building safer highways) rather than focusing on high-risk drivers. However, many programs remain centered on only high-risk group strategies, often with an emphasis on individual behavior change.

Program Goals and Objectives

Health goals and objectives are the foundation of program planning. A program goal is a general statement about the health or quality-of-life outcome the program aims to achieve. For example, an intervention that addresses injuries to adolescents within a work setting may have a stated goal: to improve the quality of work conditions for adolescent workers through fair and safe organizational practices. Program objectives specify the information set forth in the program goals. Objectives should tell exactly who benefits from the program, what will change, and by how much and when (Green & Kreuter, 2005). For example, a program aimed at youth farmworkers may have the following objective: the rate of occupational injuries (*what*) among farmworkers, aged seventeen and under (*who*), will be reduced by 20 percent (*how much*) during the first year (*by when*). By addressing the four key components of objectives, the planner defines the target of change and a way to assess the program impact.

Program Evaluation

Often planners wait until they have specific intervention activities before they think about evaluation. However, both program activities and evaluation, which is critical to every program, hinge on the program's stated goals and objectives. Planners who integrate evaluation development from the beginning of their planning are able to incorporate data collection activities into the design. They also are better able to make informed decisions about how to allocate resources to distinct program components and to develop a useful feedback loop.

PRECEDE-PROCEED Overview

During the 1980s, injury professionals began to use PRECEDE as a framework to address injury problems. Project KISS (Kids in Safety Seats) used PRECEDE to identify behaviors linked to motor vehicle injuries among children and to develop relevant educational strategies (Eriksen & Gielen, 1983; Gielen & Radius, 1984). In 1987, Sleet introduced PRECEDE as a diagnostic tool in injury prevention (Sleet, 1987). And *Injury Prevention: Meeting the Challenge* (National Committee for Injury Prevention and Control, 1989) was the first injury book to mention PRECEDE as a framework for identifying interventions, citing Eriksen and Gielen's earlier work (1983) on child safety seats. Then Gielen (1992) integrated Haddon's matrix and countermeasures with PRECEDE's framework, which was the first effort at bridging traditional injury control concepts and strategies with health education approaches. During the past two decades, researchers and practitioners have used PRECEDE (and eventually PROCEED) to address myriad injury problems (see lgreen.net and Trifiletti, Gielen, Sleet, & Hopkins, 2005, for reviews of published articles).

The PRECEDE phases guide planners through gathering information to define and prioritize health and quality-of-life issues, behavioral factors, and environmental factors and their related risk factors and conditions. At the end of PRECEDE, planners move to PROCEED by assessing administrative, regulatory, and political circumstances that will influence program implementation. Finally, planners consider intervention and evaluation strategies at each level of the ecological framework by reviewing best and promising practices relevant to the program goals and objectives. Although these steps are described as a linear process, in reality the planning is more of an iterative process in which resources and best practices are considered simultaneously to inform the selection of high-priority targets for change.

Some strengths of PRECEDE-PROCEED are its ecological framework, wide application across injury topics, population- and evidenced-based approach, integration of theory, and emphasis on cultural sensitivity (Trifiletti, Gielen, Sleet, & Hopkins, 2005; Cross, Hall, & Howat, 2003; Hendrickson & Becker, 1998; Becker, Hendrickson, Sherry, & Shaver, 1998; Howat, Jones, Hall, Cross, & Stevenson, 1997; Stevenson, Iredell, Howat, Cross, & Hall, 1999; Jones & Macrina, 1993; Eriksen & Gielen, 1983).

PRECEDE-PROCEED focuses mostly on preimplementation phases of program development. Green and Kreuter (2005) provide additional guidance for developing and delivering intervention activities in their fourth edition.

Two guiding principles of program planning remain from the first through the latest (fourth) edition of Green and Kreuter's book (2005) and the PRECEDE-PROCEED model: (1) an ecological and educational approach and (2) an emphasis on community context and intended audience participation in setting priorities (see Figure 7.1).

Social Assessment

Social diagnosis is an assessment of the intended audience's values, priorities, norms, and community situation. Planners should elicit information from intended audience members about social values and needs related to their quality of life (refer to Green & Kreuter, 2005, for information-gathering techniques). Quality of life refers to individuals' or groups' beliefs about how their needs are being satisfied and whether they have opportunities to pursue happiness and fulfillment (Green & Kreuter, 2005). The relationship between health and quality of life is reciprocal, making it critical to understand an audience's perceptions about their quality of life.

FIGURE 7.1. PRECEDE-PROCEED PLANNING MODEL.

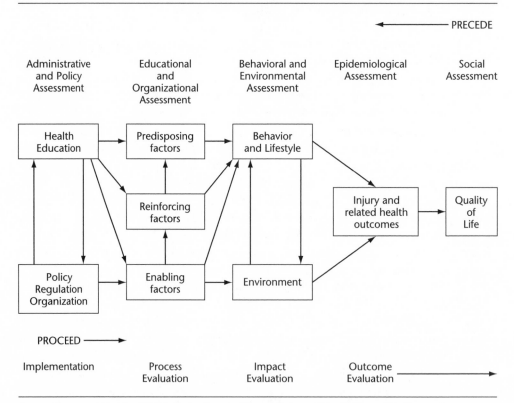

Source: Green and Kreuter (2005). Reproduced with permission of The McGraw-Hill Companies.

Consequently, the planning process begins with the participation of the intended audience. Audience participation helps planners develop programs that are relevant to intended groups; tailored to different community segments (to maximize the program's reach); and considerate of environmental context, including cultural norms, historical events, and social circumstances of intended program participants. Intended audience member participation can vary from sharing information to joining the planning team, with myriad variations in between. Community-based participatory research (see Chapter Four, this volume), where community members and health professionals jointly implement and evaluate a community program, is one model of full audience member participation. Other types of participation include advisory committees, key informants, community data collectors, and topic-specific experts.

Planners can use community-level theories and organizing frameworks to better understand community concepts and to develop an approach to the intended audience (see Chapter Four, this volume, for community-level theories, and Green & Kreuter, 2005, and Gielen & MacDonald, 2002, for explanations of community-level theories integrated with PRECEDE-PROCEED).

Epidemiological Assessment

The epidemiological diagnosis is a review of scientific data on the injury problem and the intended audience. This step and the social diagnosis can occur simultaneously as an iterative process, where planners integrate information streams and more precisely define the injury problem and intended audience. Planners trained in injury prevention and control are probably well acquainted with basic epidemiological concepts. Planners less familiar with the fundamentals of epidemiology can refer to Green and Kreuter's overview for the planner (2005) or one of the numerous texts on the subject (Rothman, 2002; Kelsey, Whittemore, Evans, & Thompson, 1996).

Behavioral and Environmental Assessment

During this step, planners identify behavioral and environmental factors that influence the selected injury problem and quality of-life-issues affected by injury. (The epidemiological diagnosis and behavioral and environmental diagnosis have been combined into one step in the fourth edition of Green and Kreuter's *Health Program Planning: An Educational and Ecological Approach.*) Injury professionals use various terms to refer to factors associated with injury. Green and Kreuter generally use *determinants of health.* Like others, they alternately use terms such as *antecedents, correlates, behavioral risk factors (individual), and environmental risk conditions.* For consistency, we use *risk factors* throughout the chapter to refer to both individual and environmental injury influences.

Planners can use information gathered during the social and epidemiological diagnoses to prioritize injury behavioral and environmental factors based on their importance and changeability. Some aspects of important behavioral and environmental factors include high prevalence (for example, common presence of toxic household products is an environmental factor for child poisonings), strong association between the factor and injury outcome (for example, bicycle helmet use and head injury reduction), and intended audience perceptions (for example, community beliefs that neighborhood violence is the most important issue affecting their safety). Some behavioral and environmental factors may be common and strongly associated with injury but may be less amenable to change through a program activity. For example, toddlers' exploration of their environment is a normal part of development and generally encouraged by adults. Exploratory behaviors in young children, such as tasting and feeling new substances found within the home, are less amenable to change than parental behaviors (such as safely storing household chemicals and monitoring children) and especially environmental factors (for example, having adequate locks on cabinets) that could reduce child poisonings.

Educational and Organizational Assessment

Planners further specify injury risks by considering factors that influence prioritized behavioral and environmental factors, and assess risk factors that will inhibit or promote change in priorities. PRECEDE-PROCEED delineates three types of risk factors or conditions: predisposing, enabling, and reinforcing factors. Social and behavioral science theories can help planners identify factors that directly influence behaviors or may indirectly influence behaviors through mechanisms such as social support, social networks, and community norms. Theories also provide evidence to support planners' decisions about which factors are most important and changeable.

Predisposing factors are characteristics of the individual that influence motivation to change. Qualities such as developmental stage, knowledge, attitudes, and values all affect how individuals perceive a program and the intended behavior change. For example, parents who believe that harsh corporal punishment is the best way to discipline a young child will likely have discipline practices that inflict more injury on their children than parents with different beliefs about physical discipline. Similarly, policymakers who believe that motorcycle helmet use is an important public safety issue are more likely to sponsor mandatory helmet legislation than those who believe that individuals have the right to choose their safety measures.

Enabling factors are the skills and resources necessary to facilitate behavioral and environmental change. For example, a program intended to increase bicycle helmet use should address the intended audience's ability to access helmets (resources) as well as properly fit helmets before riding (skill). Enabling factors also include environmental conditions such as availability of safe bike paths and motor vehicle traffic density along bike routes.

Reinforcing factors provide negative and positive feedback that affects behavior maintenance. Social relationships, such as peer, family, and coworker networks, are common sources of feedback and emotional support. At a community level, having common norms and social support among parents about safe driving practices may be a useful means of encouraging safe driving behaviors among their teenagers. Social policies and community norms can also reinforce behaviors. For example, the presence of policies prohibiting or encouraging off-campus school lunch for high school students may alter the risks of some types of crashes involving young drivers (Stone & Runyan, 2005).

Administrative and Policy Assessment

During this step, planners carefully consider how administrative policies and regulations, organizational climates, and political agendas will affect program implementation, depending on the intended program settings. Once planners identify appropriate program settings, they are ready to consider the facilitating factors and barriers to implementing the program. Organizational characteristics, such as leadership, organizational climate, and administrative policies, influence how well a program can be implemented and how well individuals in the organization will receive program activities. Social norms, political networks, and neighborhood resources are some examples of community-level characteristics that influence program success. Planners can use organizational and community-level theories to identify potential resources and barriers that will likely influence program implementation.

Determining Intervention and Evaluation Strategies

PRECEDE-PROCEED assumes that planners who have followed the systematic process laid out in the first five steps will have rich information to develop intervention and evaluation strategies. Different interventions are required for changing the predisposing, reinforcing, and enabling factors, which is why it is important to identify these risk factors before committing to a particular intervention strategy or methods. There are numerous guides to intervention development referenced by Green and Kreuter (2005).

Most important, PRECEDE-PROCEED approaches intervention development from an evidence-based perspective. First, planners match broad intervention components to their prioritized ecological levels. For example, a planner may focus on individuals, organizations, and communities to address falls among older adults in assisted living facilities. The broad intervention components may include resident education (individual), built environment modifications (individual and organizational), and community organizing (community) to lobby the town for safer pathways of travel between the residence and local businesses. Next, planners map tested best practices to their selected intervention components. Finally, planners pool information on promising practices and input from the intended audience to fill in program activity gaps.

Review of PRECEDE-PROCEED Research

Injury professionals have used PRECEDE-PROCEED to conceptualize injury problems, develop prevention programs, and define data collection measures (see lgreen.net and Trifiletti, Gielen, Sleet, & Hopkins, 2005). Injury professionals have most commonly used the PRECEDE portion of the model. Notable examples of how the full model has been applied to intervention development can be found for programs to reduce motor vehicle injuries (Simons-Morton et al., 1989; Sleet, 1987), home injuries (Gielen & McDonald, 2002), child pedestrian–related injuries (Howat et al., 1997), and low back injuries among postal workers (Daltroy et al.,1993). In addition, some injury professionals have integrated social and behavioral science theories with PRECEDE-PROCEED to enhance their conceptual framework or guide intervention strategies (Farley & Vaez, 2003; Wong, 1997; Wortel, deGeus, Kok, & van Woerkum, 1994; Gielen & Radius, 1984).

In addition, Chaney, Hunt, and Schulz (2000) used PRECEDE to summarize their review of school violence to identify quality-of-life (for example, feeling safe at school), injury (for example, death or injury resulting from violent acts), behavioral (for example, bringing weapons to school, physical fights), and educational (the predisposing, enabling, and reinforcing factors of the identified behaviors) priorities. Similarly, Frankish (2001) used PRECEDE to develop a conceptual model of suicide and its determinants and to guide recommendations for prevention efforts. Others have used only the predisposing, enabling, and reinforcing constructs to characterize important factors for intervention efforts and evaluation measures (Trifiletti, Gielen, Sleet, & Hopkins, 2005; Sugg & Thompson, 1999; Hall-Smith & Davis, 1998; Hendrickson & Becker, 1998). For example, Hall-Smith and Davis (1998) found that clinicians' knowledge of how to identify battered women, skills on how to care for these patients, and beliefs about the appropriateness of addressing domestic violence in a health care setting were predisposing factors that influenced whether and how clinicians addressed domestic violence. These factors, as well as reinforcing and enabling factors, were then included in a survey of clinicians on how they address domestic violence with their patients (that is, their behaviors). The authors linked intervention recommendations to the factors they found were most influential on clinicians' treatment of battered women.

Clearly, PRECEDE has been a useful framework for health professionals to conceptualize both unintentional and intentional injury problems. What is less clear, based on published work, is the extent to which planners use the model to guide the process of developing injury prevention programs and their respective evaluations. Few injury programs that have used PRECEDE seem to have included intended audience members during the planning process (social diagnosis), with some notable exceptions (Howat et al., 2001; Hall-Smith & Davis, 1998; Daltroy et al., 1993; Gielen & Radius, 1984). Furthermore, authors rarely discuss if or how they have integrated social and behavioral theory with the model's constructs (noted exceptions include Cross et al., 2003; Howat et al., 1997). For example, parents' beliefs about their ability to properly install a child safety seat, as predicted by social-cognitive theory (Chapter Three, this volume), could be a predisposing factor for parents' actual behavior.

Overview of Haddon's Matrix and the Third Dimension

William Haddon, a pioneer in injury control, developed two complementary models to guide injury prevention planning. Both are premised on the concepts of public health and derive from an understanding that injury results from the transfer of various types of energy to the human host—for example, mechanical energy in the case of blunt or piercing trauma, thermal energy for burns, and chemical energy in poisonings or chemical burns (Haddon, 1980). The ability to derive intervention ideas is predicated on understanding the injury process as a sequence of events involving interactions among the person affected (the host), the agent (energy) delivered (for example, an inanimate object such as a car, firearm, or the surface of a playground), or a vector (for example, a parent who shakes a baby causing unintentional harm, an assailant who fires a handgun at his spouse, or another participant in a contact sport whose tackle results in an energy exchange strong enough to break a limb). The other elements that contribute to the injury event are the physical and social environments in which the process occurs and which interact with the other elements to result in a traumatic event. The physical environment, for example, includes the structure of the home environment, the surface of the playground or nature of the equipment itself, or characteristics of the roadway. In contrast, the social environment consists of the multiple levels of the social-ecological model from interpersonal interactions (such as between husband and wife, parent and child, teenage peers, or worker and employer) as well as those involving broader social institutions (such as workplace organizations, religious organizations, schools, or political institutions) and the broader sociocultural environments of specific ethnic groups or communities, as well as the broader culture of a whole country or global environment. Norms, policies, laws, and activities within these various social environmental levels influence whether certain types of injury events will happen and how they take place, as well as the severity of the consequences. For example, policies about alcohol taxation or sales to minors, as well as social norms about drinking and driving, will influence the occurrence of the many types of injury that are associated with inebriation, while those affecting emergency care influence injury consequences. The integration of the social ecological framework (Bronfenbrenner, 1979) with the basic concepts of the public health model and Haddon's models is described more fully by Runyan (2003).

The Haddon Matrix

The Haddon matrix is used in two ways. One is to conceptualize the risk factors associated with a given injury problem (see Table 7.1 for an example). The matrix draws on the concepts of public health that define the major categories of risk: the host; the agent and its delivery mechanism through a vehicle or vector; and the social and physical environments. The rows of the matrix address the phases in the injury process at which risks might have their influence or at which given interventions can have an effect. These are defined as pre-event (before the injury-producing event occurs), event (at the time of the actual injury-producing event), and postevent referring (the time period after the event has occurred).

When used to help think about risk factors, the cells are used to depict those characteristics of the factors (host; agent, vehicle, or vector; physical environment; and social environment) that are influential in the occurrence of injury. Risk elements are placed into the rows corresponding to the time in the injury sequence at which they are influential. Those placed in the pre-event row are influential at that stage in determining whether an event occurs. At the event phase, risk factors are influential in altering the occurrence or severity of injuries during the event itself; and at the postevent phase, risk factors might be listed that affect the process of recovering from injuries that occur during the event. This way of using

TABLE 7.1. HADDON MATRIX APPLIED TO UNDERSTANDING RISK FACTORS FOR OCCUPATIONAL FALL INJURIES IN CONSTRUCTION WORK.

	Factors			
Phases	Host (Worker)	Agent/Vehicle/Vector (Equipment)	Physical Environment (Work Site)	Social Environment (Employer Practices and General Culture)
Pre-event	Drowsiness, carelessness, not trained to use equipment properly	Equipment not properly maintained	Work area that is crowded, slippery, dark, not shielded from weather	Management that emphasizes speed over safety, poor supervision and training of workers
Event (fall)	Refusal to wear protective gear (for example, safety harnesses or hard hats)	Equipment without safety shut-off devices or means of escape	Hazards that exacerbate event (for example, sharp objects onto which falling worker lands)	Lack of training, lack of safety equipment provided
Postevent	Lack of knowledge of how to signal for help	Equipment not easily removed once person is caught	Clutter prohibiting rescue, no clear directions at work site for emergency medical service to follow	Inaccessible or no 911 system; lack of training on how to handle emergencies

Source: Based on Haddon (1980).

the matrix to depict risk factors is compatible with the PRECEDE-PROCEED ideas about assessing predisposing, enabling, and reinforcing factors.

The second way in which the Haddon matrix is used is to develop ideas about injury interventions (Table 7.2). In this, the more common use, the matrix helps the user identify interventions directed at changing the factors associated with injury (the columns) according to when in the injury process those changes are likely to have their influence (the rows), as elaborated by Runyan (1998). By using the Haddon matrix at the stage of choosing an intervention approach, the planner can set out the array of intervention options and then carefully assess which to choose applying Runyan's third dimension (1998) criteria and theories of individual and organizational and social change, as urged by Green and Kreuter (2005) and others (Gielen & McDonald, 2002).

Using the Haddon Matrix

As a first step in completing the matrix, the planner defines the injury problem and then determines what constitutes "the event" so it is clear what is pre-event and what is postevent. For example, is a fall event defined as the moment the person trips on the stairs, or is it the point at which the person hits the floor? If the event is the former, then keeping the person from tripping is a pre-event strategy and having handrails to grab once tripping occurs is an event strategy. If the event is the latter, then reduction of both tripping hazards and handrails is a pre-event strategy, while ensuring that hip protectors are worn is an event strategy. Which way one defines this matters less than being clear about what is the event for purposes of developing multiple intervention ideas.

The second step is to define the columns in the matrix, being clear about the host as the person at risk of injury. This is sometimes confusing because the target of the intervention may be a third party who is intended to help protect a vulnerable person or "host." For example, if an infant is the one to be protected from brain injury due to harsh shaking, one may devise an educational intervention for the parent, but the vulnerable person is still the child. It is also important to clearly identify the other columns as well: identifying what the agent is and the vehicles or vectors that transmit the energy (for example, handguns and knives might both be thought of as vehicles used in assaults by teenage gang members, the vectors). Some problems will have only vehicles (inanimate means of delivering energy), while others will have only vectors (animate delivery means, such as a biting dog) or both vehicles and vectors (for example, a drunk driver and his or her vehicle). The physical environment should be identified; for example, it might be the entire home in the case of a house fire, a particular stretch of roadway associated with traffic crashes, or a particular part of a factory or playground that one wants

TABLE 7.2. HADDON MATRIX APPLIED TO ADDRESSING SAFETY FOR OCCUPATIONAL FALL INJURIES IN CONSTRUCTION WORK.

	Factors			
	Host (Worker)	Agent/Vehicle/Vector (Equipment)	Physical Environment (Work Site)	Social Environment (Employer Practices and General Culture)
Phases				
Pre-event	Train workers in correct procedures; wear properly fitting, slip-resistant shoes; avoid alcohol	Well-constructed scaffolding; lighter-weight tools that are carried to heights	Proper shading to reduce glare; slip-resistant surfaces	Train personnel to be better supervisors; foster culture of safety with incentives and regular safety inspections; use spotters to watch work flow and spot hazards
Event (fall)	Ensure proper use of safety devices (for example, safety harnesses, hard hats) through training, monitoring, enforcement	High-quality safety harnesses	Remove hazards on fall landing surfaces; cushioned landing surfaces for workers working at heights	Ensure that workers are not working alone at heights
Postevent	Teach all workers cardio-pulmonary resuscitation	Ensure easily removable equipment when extraction and rescue required	Use markers to make work site easy to locate by rescue personnel	Ensure adequate access to emergency care on site; provide good insurance to cover rehabilitation care

Source: Based on Haddon (1980).

to make safer. And the elements of the social environment should be considered from the standpoint of multiple levels within the social-ecological framework (see Chapter Six, this volume), including interpersonal (examples are parenting style, peer relationships, or supervisor-employee relationship), organizational (for example, work site; school or religious organizational policies, programs, and doctrine), sociocultural (such as ethnic, religious, political), or cultural expectations (practices and norms about issues such as workplace safety, child discipline, gender roles, acceptability of weapon carrying or speeding).

Filling in the matrix can be done by an individual planner, but is probably best done by a group as part of a creative brainstorming process. Runyan (1998) argues that diverse groups will likely arrive at more innovative ideas if they are allowed to brainstorm without critiquing ideas as they emerge. Individuals with specific expertise on an aspect of the model's rows (for example, someone knowledgeable about postevent treatment systems) or columns (perhaps an expert in the design of traffic patterns) may be less willing to think creatively and derive ideas that they know to be currently technologically infeasible within their own area of expertise, but they may be very good at suggesting ingenious ideas about some other area where they are not constrained by their knowledge or the practicalities of implementation. Doing the matrix in a group also allows one person's ideas, placed on a board or flip chart by a facilitator, to stimulate the thinking of others as part of an iterative process of filling in the cells with as many ideas as possible in a relatively short amount of time.

Once the matrix is filled in, the third dimension (Figure 7.2) comes into play as a means of helping practitioners decide which potential ideas to pursue to the implementation phase. The criteria proposed on the third dimension are derived from literature in policy analysis as elements to consider in making choices about policy and program options. To use the third dimension, think about what values are important in the development and implementation of interventions in the specific setting in which the intervention is to be applied, taking into account cultural considerations. This process will benefit from working with members of the community using strategies of community participatory research and community organization and development (Chapter Four, this volume; Minkler & Wallerstein, 2002) in which community members have the opportunity to participate in the problem definition and planning process. This type of participation is useful at several points in the process. There are multiple ways to engage community members, including helping to define the problem, suggesting strategies using the Haddon matrix, defining values important to completing the third dimension of the matrix, and synthesizing the information to determine which interventions to apply and how.

FIGURE 7.2. HADDON MATRIX WITH THE THIRD DIMENSION.

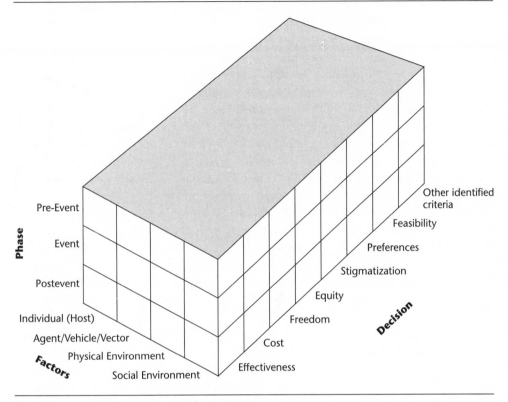

Source: Runyan (1998). Reproduced with permission.

Once key value criteria are identified, the task becomes one of examining selected strategies within the matrix for analysis with regard to the selected value criteria. It is hard to imagine a situation in which effectiveness would not be one of the criteria. However, even effectiveness is not always clear-cut depending on the body of evidence that has been generated about a given problem and approaches to intervening. Sometimes interventionists have to use less solid scientific evidence about effectiveness than they would like and instead apply their own judgment, based on theory, logic, and evidence about related issues or programs, to guess at the potential effectiveness of an intervention strategy, returning to concepts of best practices and best processes discussed earlier in the chapter.

Other criteria will be more variable depending on the situation, but key criteria that often are considered in public health and other social interventions include equity, cost, freedom, stigmatization, preferences of the community, and feasibility. (Each is defined briefly here; for more extensive discussion, see Margolis & Runyan, 1983; Runyan, 1998, 2003.)

Equity concerns issues of fairness and relates to whether one is trying to achieve horizontal equity (treating everyone equally), as with a universal approach, or give special treatment to those with greatest vulnerability or fewest resources (for example, high-risk groups such as children or residents of disadvantaged neighborhoods). This latter type is referred to as vertical equity.

Cost is frequently a critical component of decision making but can be thought of in several ways. For example, one might consider the trade-offs in costs of the problem (medical care and lost years of productivity associated with serious head injury to an injured adolescent driver, for example) against the costs of developing an intervention program (implementing and enforcing a graduated driver licensing system).

Freedom concerns the types of restrictions that certain types of interventions impose—for example, restrictions on freedoms that are associated with risk behaviors such as the freedom to ride a motorcycle without a helmet or freedom to brandish a gun in public. This factor also refers to freedom from risk situations, such as freedom to walk in a well-lighted neighborhood with less fear of crime or freedom to be protected from driving on the road with drunk drivers. While freedom restriction is subjective, evidence can be collected about the extent to which the public views certain freedoms as more or less important so as to gauge the extent to which restriction of those freedoms is acceptable or unacceptable.

Stigmatization refers to the extent to which the policy or program intentionally or unintentionally stigmatizes a certain group. For example, car seat loaner programs or home visitation programs for families below a certain income level may inadvertently stigmatize them if they have to self-identify as poor or otherwise at high risk in order to receive assistance.

Preferences of the community refers to the way in which the community at large, as well as given members, particularly influential members, view the problem and its solution. It relates to community will to approach a problem and the resources the community is willing to bring to bear to address it. In this way, it relates closely to how the community views the attributes of interventions with respect to all the other factors, like cost, equity, stigmatization, and freedom. Evidence to assess preferences comes from various types of data collection, such as community forums, focus groups, surveys, key informant interviews, and other processes used to conduct community needs assessments.

Feasibility can encompass either technological feasibility or political feasibility, based on preferences of the community or key decision makers. It is best to leave this consideration until the end so as not to rule out good ideas too early in the process. Innovations to overcome feasibility constraints can sometimes be developed to facilitate ideas that are otherwise well regarded. But if an idea is discarded as infeasible early in the process, its other attributes may never have a chance to be fully considered. Evidence for feasibility also comes from technological sources as well as assessments of community preferences and political barriers often made through focus groups, interviews of key leaders, review of similar decision processes and policies in the same jurisdiction or organization, or review of editorials in newspapers, to name just a few examples.

Applying Haddon's Matrix and PRECEDE-PROCEED to Injury Prevention Planning Efforts

Haddon's matrix and PRECEDE-PROCEED are compatible in many ways, but differ in how they conceptualize injury problems and solutions. Injury program planners may find that one or the other model provides better guidance at certain points. For example, Haddon's matrix reflects the episodic (versus chronic) nature of injury events and organizes strategies accordingly. PRECEDE-PROCEED offers a systematic way to approach behaviors and their antecedents. Planners may pick one or use components of each model to suit their planning needs and injury problem.

Regardless of the specific models, health professionals consistently use a set of action steps to guide their planning efforts. Therefore, we end our planning discussion by proposing and explaining how injury professionals can integrate the strengths of Haddon's matrix and PRECEDE-PROCEED to achieve their planning goals. Following is description of a planning process that incorporates the key ideas about planning presented at the beginning of the chapter (see Figure 7.3). For each step, we describe how Haddon's matrix or PRECEDE-PROCEED, or both, can facilitate planning. Table 7.3 provides an example of how to use components of Haddon's matrix and PRECEDE-PROCEED to address a specific injury problem.

Organize a Planning Team with Diverse Expertise

Planning usually works best when key stakeholders engage in the process early. Organizing a planning team is one way to garner support and resources from individuals and groups that can contribute to a successful program. Some team members may participate throughout the process, and others may contribute their complementary expertise for certain planning activities. At a minimum, a planning team should include members with expertise in the injury topic, evaluation, knowledge of the intended audience (or someone who is willing to learn more

FIGURE 7.3. PLANNING PROCESS THAT INTEGRATES
HADDON'S MATRIX AND PRECEDE-PROCEED.

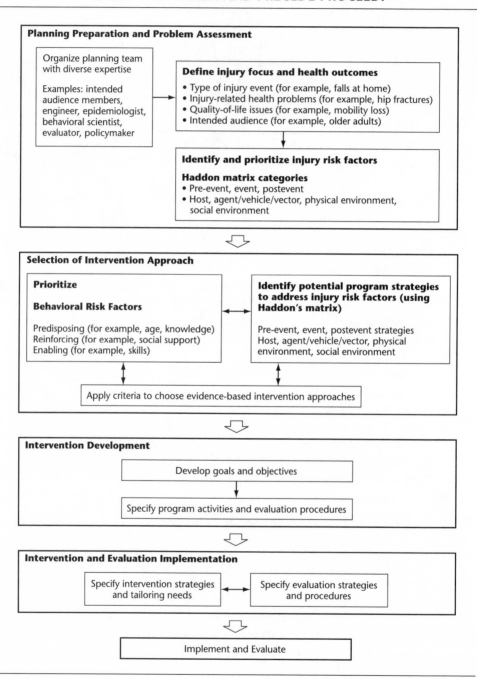

about the population), and someone who is willing to take responsibility for keeping the process moving. Often a program coordinator becomes the primary planner, who develops time lines, facilitates collaboration, and manages the day-to-day planning work.

By the end of this step, the developing program should have a team of committed people who are responsible for guiding the process and completing planning tasks, as well as some clarity about who will play what roles on the team.

Define Injury Focus and Health Outcomes

Injury prevention planners must decide on the injury problems to address and then specify how injuries affect morbidity and mortality for the intended audience. In some cases, planners determine the financial costs associated with injuries. PRECEDE-PROCEED's social and epidemiological diagnosis steps can guide planners through gathering epidemiological and health services data, as well as information from intended audience members.

In reality, when planners begin to review research in a particular injury area, they often review epidemiological and program evaluation studies simultaneously. In addition, planning teams may begin to formulate intervention ideas from the beginning of the process.

By the end of this step, planners should have a defined injury topic area and desired health outcomes.

Identify and Prioritize Injury Risk Factors

During this step, planners can use epidemiological and social data, as well as theory, to array all known risk factors and conditions associated with the injury problem. Haddon's matrix provides a useful way to organize risk factors for injury occurrence and severity by pre-event, event, and postevent. Individual behaviors will likely be among the risk factors, which can be examined using PRECEDE's predisposing, enabling, and reinforcing constructs. The caution here is not to limit consideration to only one type of risk factor, such as behavior or environment, but to consider all the elements in the social ecology of the problem contributing to event occurrence and whether injuries will occur during an event. Planners can rank risk factors based on their importance and changeability, described earlier in the chapter and in PRECEDE's behavioral and environmental diagnosis.

As planners begin to brainstorm intervention strategies, they may choose to consider how injury risk factors affect the behaviors of individuals in the intended audience and others who influence injury risk, such as policymakers, legislators, and work site managers. Figure 7.3 represents the iterative process of identifying intervention strategies and behavioral risk factors and applying value criteria.

TABLE 7.3. EXAMPLE: CHILD MOTOR VEHICLE SAFETY.

Planning Step	Child Motor Vehicle Safety
Organize a planning team with diverse expertise	Program coordinator Car safety expert (for example, pediatrician) Department of Transportation representative University program evaluator Local health department representative Parent residing in community of interest Law enforcement officer
Define injury focus and health outcomes	Injury focus: child injuries sustained from motor vehicle crashes Health outcomes: death, injuries that result in emergency department visits
Identify and prioritize injury risk factors	Improper restraint* Lack of driver restraint use* Driver intoxication Poor access to restraints High-severity crashes in certain roadway segments Lack of enforcement of child restraint use* Incompatibility of restraint system and car design Lack of hospital AND pediatrician guidance
Prioritize behavioral risk factors	Improper Restraint (example of prioritized behavior) *Predisposing* Parent knowledge about proper restraint* Parents' beliefs about their abilities to properly install a car seat* Parents' beliefs that restraint will prevent or lessen motor vehicle injury Parents' attitudes about driver restraint use *Enabling* Access to child car seats Parent skills to properly install car seat Cheap access to car seats *Reinforcing* Checkpoints to examine child restraint use Driver's car restraint use Health provider's counseling about car restraint use

Identify potential program strategies to address injury risk factors and conditions	Event Phase	Host (Children)	Agent/Vehicle (Child Restraint System in Car)	Physical Environment (Motor Vehicle)	Social Environment (Family, Community, Political)
	Pre-event	Educate parents and children about proper child restraint use	Design and provide age- and size-appropriate restraints that are easy to install and operate correctly	Ensure car has functioning seat belts	Provide cheap or free access to seats in community Improve health provider's counseling about child restraints

Apply criteria to select program strategies	Effectiveness: strong evidence to education and car seat give-away strategies; good cooperation from enforcement officials Community preferences: parents' desire for loaner programs in specific accessible settings Cost: costs of running loaner programs relative to costs for medical expenses associated with injury Equity, stigmatization: enough seats to be available to all, regardless of level of income
Develop goals and objectives	Example long-term goal: To reduce the number of child deaths and injuries that result from motor vehicle crashes. Example short-term outcome objective: By the end of the program's first year, 80 percent of parents who participate in hospital education and receive an age-appropriate car seat will properly restrain their infant every time the child rides in a motor vehicle.
Specify program activities and evaluation procedures	*Program activities:* Parent education prior to hospital discharge; health provider education, reminders, incentives (for example, insurance reimbursement) Car seat loaner program Car inspection and seat installation *Evaluation activities:* In-person parent interviews at baseline; inspection of seat installation at three, six, and twelve months Written parent survey at three, six, and twelve months; in-depth interviews with trained law enforcement officers
Implement and evaluate program activities	Will specify the implementation procedures and protocols Will use evaluation information to refine, sustain, and disseminate program

Note: An asterisk indicates a prioritized item.

Because the Haddon matrix does not provide a means to explicitly link behaviors and other risk factors identified in various cells, planners can use the PRECEDE conceptual model to organize risk factors and examine how predisposing, enabling, and reinforcing factors relate to behaviors.

By the end of this step, planners should be able to specify which risk factors of the defined injury problem are most important to address.

Prioritize Behavioral Risk Factors

Planners can organize risk factors well suited for behavior change strategies using PRECEDE's predisposing, reinforcing, and enabling constructs. Behaviors can refer to actions by individuals in the intended audience, but often they can refer to policymakers, legislators, employers, and others who influence various communities and structures that have an impact on injury events. Therefore, understanding behavioral factors can help planners develop strategies at all levels of an ecological framework and for all types of interventions that can be generated using the Haddon matrix (see the next step). This step and the next can be performed in either order, and it may be helpful to cycle through these two steps more than once so that each process benefits from the other so as not to limit thinking to behavioral risk factors.

By the end of this step, planners should be able to define factors that influence injury-related behaviors and determine which factors are important to address.

Identify Potential Program Strategies to Address Injury Risk Factors and Conditions

This step allows planners to think broadly about possible solutions before applying real-world filters that may inhibit creativity. Planning teams often develop intervention ideas early in the process and by using an organizing framework can help planners maintain an ecological and universal view of their developing program. In addition, planning teams can solicit input from key stakeholder groups, such as intended audience members, policymakers, and municipal government agencies, to develop a comprehensive view of possible strategies.

Haddon's matrix systematizes intervention brainstorming by providing distinct categories that reflect the chronology and influences of injury events. The matrix organizes creative thinking about a range of options for addressing the problem. PRECEDE's predisposing, reinforcing, and enabling constructs can also help planners identify and organize intervention options at this stage. Planners may choose to perform this step and the prior one in the reverse order or move back and forth between them several times before settling on an approach.

By the end of this step, planners should have a comprehensive list of potential intervention strategies they can apply to their defined injury problem.

Apply Criteria to Select Program Strategies

Once planners have imagined the possible, they can begin to refine their intervention approach by applying criteria that will help them make evidence-based decisions about strategy selections. Evidence can include evaluation studies, theoretical support, intended audience values, and practical circumstances. Haddon's third dimension, described above, includes many criteria that planners may consider. In addition, PRECEDE-PROCEED's social diagnosis and administrative, policy, and regulatory assessment provide guidance on how to use collected information to apply to planning decisions. Planners can also reference Green and Kreuter's general discussion (2005) of an evidence-based approach and related case studies.

By the end of this step, planners should know which values are most relevant and important in a setting and be able to apply and explain the criteria they used to make their intervention strategy selections.

Develop Goals and Objectives

Goals and objectives are the best way for planners to synthesize and articulate the theory, science, and practice that informed their planning decisions thus far. Programs may have few overall goals, but each intervention activity should link to at least one measurable objective. Therefore, the planning team can assess whether the program achieved its stated objectives as measures of the programs success. (Program evaluation is discussed in more detail in Chapter Nine, this volume.)

Specify Program Activities and Evaluation Procedures

At this point, planners are ready to specify intervention activities that will achieve the program objectives. They can use one or more of the intervention development models that provide specific instruction on how to develop intervention activities (Green & Kreuter, 2005).

Implement and Evaluate Program Activities

Program implementation includes sets of procedures and actions that define the intervention. Planners begin to roll out intervention strategies and evaluate progress. Evaluation is an important part of an evidence-based approach because planners can collect information on what works and what does not.

Conclusion

Program planning is a creative and systematic process whereby key decision makers work together to address injury problems and their consequences. Like travelers preparing for a trip, planners make decisions based on relevant information, experience, and consultation with others. Injury planners may be most successful when they use an approach that incorporates best practices, social and behavioral science theory, intended audience participation, and conceptual models derived from the injury field.

References

Becker, H., & Hendrickson, S. L., Sherry, L., & Shaver, L. (1998). Nonurban parental beliefs about childhood injury and bicycle safety. *American Journal of Health Behavior, 22,* 218–227.

Bonnie, R. J., Fulco, C. E., & Liverman, C. T. (Eds). (1999). *Reducing the burden of injury: Advancing prevention and treatment.* Washington, DC: National Academy Press.

Bronfenbrenner, U. (1979). *The ecology of human development.* Cambridge, MA: Harvard University Press.

Buchanan, D. R. (1998). Beyond positivism: Humanistic perspectives on theory research in health education. *Health Education Research, 13*(2), 439–450.

Chaney, J. D., Hunt, B. P., & Schulz, J. W. (2000). An examination using the PRECEDE model framework to establish a comprehensive program to prevent school violence. *American Journal of Health Studies, 16*(4), 199–204.

Cross, D., Hall, M., & Howat, P. (2003). Using theory to guide practice in children's pedestrian safety education. *American Journal of Health Education, 34*(Suppl. 5), S42–S47.

Daltroy, L. H., Iverson, M. D., Larson, M. G., Ryan, J., Zwerling, C., Fossel, A. H., Liang, M. H. (1993). Teaching and social support: Effects on knowledge, attitudes, and behaviors to prevent low back injuries in industry. *Health Education Quarterly, 20*(1), 43–62.

Eriksen, M. P., & Gielen, A. C. (1983). The application of health education principles to automobile child restraint programs. *Health Education Quarterly, 10*(1), 30–55.

Farley, C. L., & Vaez, M. (2003). Bicycle helmet campaigns and head injuries among children. Does poverty matter? *Journal of Epidemiology and Community Health, 57*(9), 668–672.

Frankish, J. C. (2001). Crisis centers and their role in treatment: Suicide prevention versus health promotion. *Death Studies, 18,* 327–339.

Gielen, A. C. (1992). Health education and injury control: Integrating approaches. *Health Education Quarterly, 19*(2), 203–218.

Gielen, A. C., & McDonald, E. M. (2002). Using the PRECEDE-PROCEED planning model to apply health behavior theories. In K. Glanz, B. K. Rimer, & F. M. Lewis (Eds.), *Health behavior and health education: Theory, research and practice* (3rd ed., pp. 409–436). San Francisco: Jossey-Bass.

Gielen, A. C., & Radius, S. (1984). Project KISS (Kids in Safety Belts): Educational approaches and evaluation measures. *Health Education, 15,* 43–47.

Green, L. W. (2001). From research to "best practices" in other settings and populations. *American Journal of Health Behavior, 25*(3), 165–178.

Green, L. W., & Kreuter, M. W. (1999). *Health program planning: An educational and ecological approach* (3rd ed.). Mountain View, CA: Mayfield.

Green, L. W., & Kreuter, M. W. (2005). *Health program planning: An educational and ecological approach* (4th ed.). New York: McGraw-Hill.

Green, L. W., Wilson, R. W., & Bauer, K. G. (1983). Data required to measure progress on the objectives for the nation in disease prevention and health promotion. *American Journal of Public Health, 73*, 18–24.

Haddon, W. (1972). A logical framework for categorizing highway safety phenomena and activity. *Journal of Trauma, 12*, 193–207.

Haddon, W. (1973). Energy damage and the ten countermeasure strategies. *Journal of Trauma, 12*, 321–331.

Haddon, W. (1980). Advances in the epidemiology of injuries as a basis for public policy. *Public Health Reports, 95*, 411–421.

Hall-Smith, P., & Davis, M. (1998). Changing the health care response to battered women: A health education approach. *Family and Community Health, 20*(4), 1–18.

Hendrickson, S. G., & Becker, H. (1998). Impact of a theory based intervention to increase bicycle helmet use in low-income children. *Injury Prevention, 4*(2), 126–131.

Howat, P., Cross, D., Iredall, H., Stevenson, M., Gibbs, S., Officer, J., & Dillon, J. (2001). Community participation in road safety: Barriers and enablers. *Journal of Community Health, 26*(4), 257–269.

Howat, P., Jones, S., Hall, M., Cross, D., & Stevenson, M. (1997). The PRECEDE PRO-CEED model: Application to planning a child pedestrian injury prevention program. *Injury Prevention, 3*(4), 282–287.

Institute of Medicine. (2001). *Confronting chronic neglect: The education and training of health professionals on family violence.* Washington, DC: National Academy Press.

Institute of Medicine. (2002). *Reducing suicide: A national imperative.* Washington, DC: National Academy Press.

Jones, C. S., & Macrina, D. (1993). Using the PRECEDE model to design and implement a bicycle helmet campaign. *Wellness Perspectives: Research, Theory and Practice, 9*, 68–75.

Kelsey, J. L., Whittemore, A. S., Evans, A. S., & Thompson, W. D. (1996). *Methods in observational epidemiology* (2nd ed.). New York: Oxford University Press.

Margolis, L., & Runyan, C. W. (1983). Accidental policy: An analysis of the problem of unintended injuries in childhood. *American Journal of Orthopsychiatry, 53*(4), 629–644.

Minkler, M., & Wallerstein, N. B. (2002). Improving health through community organization and community building. In K. Glanz, B. K. Rimer, & F. M. Lewis (Eds.), *Health behavior and health education: Theory, research and practice* (3rd ed., pp. 279–311). San Francisco: Jossey-Bass.

National Center for Injury Prevention and Control. (2002). *CDC injury research agenda.* Atlanta: Centers for Disease Control and Prevention.

National Committee for Injury Prevention and Control. (1989). *Injury prevention: Meeting the challenge.* New York: Oxford University Press.

National Research Council. (1996). *Understanding violence against women.* Washington, DC: National Academy Press.

Rose, G. (1985). Sick individuals and sick populations. *International Journal of Epidemiology, 14*, 32–38.

Rose, G. (1992). *The strategy of preventive medicine.* New York: Oxford University Press.

Rothman, K. (2002). *Epidemiology: An introduction.* New York: Oxford University Press.

Runyan, C. W. (1998). Using the Haddon matrix: Introducing the third dimension. *Injury Prevention, 4,* 302–307.

Runyan, C. W. (2003). Back to the future: Revisiting Haddon's conceptualization of injury epidemiology and prevention. *Epidemiologic Reviews, 25,* 60–64.

Simons-Morton, B. G., Brink, S. G., Simons-Morton, D. G., McIntyre, R., Chapman, M., Longoria, J., & Parcel, G. (1989). Ecological approach to the prevention of injuries due to drinking and driving. *Health Education Quarterly, 16*(3), 397–411.

Sleet, D. A. (1987). Health education approaches to motor vehicle injury prevention. *Public Health Reports, 102,* 606–607.

State and Territorial Injury Prevention Directors' Association. (2003). *Safe states.* Retrieved April 1, 2005, from http://www.stipda.org/s-pubs/ss03.pdf.

Stevenson, M., Iredell, H., Howat, P., Cross, D., & Hall, M. (1999). Measuring community/environmental interventions: The child pedestrian injury prevention project. *Injury Prevention, 5,* 26–30.

Stone, L. M., & Runyan, C. W. (2005). High school off-campus lunch policies and adolescent motor vehicle crash risks. *Journal of Adolescent Health, 36*(1), 5–8.

Sugg, N. K., & Thompson, R. S. (1999). Domestic violence and primary care. *Archives of Family Medicine, 8,* 301–306.

Trifiletti, L. B., Gielen, A. C., Sleet, D. A., & Hopkins, K. (2005). Behavioral and social science theories and models: Are they used in unintentional injury and prevention research? *Health Education Research, 20*(3), 298–307.

U.S. Department of Health and Human Services. (2000). *Healthy people 2010.* Retrieved April 1, 2005, from http://www.healthypeople.gov/Document/HTML/Volume2/15Injury.htm.

U.S. Department of Health and Human Services. (2001). *Youth violence: A report of the surgeon general.* Retrieved April 1, 2005, from http://www.surgeongeneral.gov/library/youth violence/default.htm.

Wilson, M. H., Baker, S. P., Teret, S. P., Shock, S., & Garbarino, J. (1991). *Saving children.* New York: Oxford University Press.

Wong, T. Y. (1997). Behavioral analysis of eye protection use by soldiers. *Military Medicine, 162*(11), 744–748.

Wortel, E., deGeus, G. H., Kok, G., & van Woerkum, C. (1994). Injury control in pre-school children: A review of parental safety measures and the behavioural determinants. *Health Education Research, 9*(2), 201–213.

PART TWO

RESEARCH AND ASSESSMENT METHODS FOR BEHAVIOR CHANGE INTERVENTIONS

CHAPTER EIGHT

STUDY METHODS FOR UNDERSTANDING INJURY BEHAVIOR

Nancy J. Thompson

One of the first tasks in assessing an injury-related behavior problem in a community is to determine how frequently, when, where, and among whom the problem is occurring. The process of identifying the frequency of the behavior by time, place, and person is usually called *descriptive study*. Associating the behavior with other factors that are measured at the same time as the behavior, such as knowledge or attitudes, is usually called *correlational study*. From a correlational study, we cannot determine whether the other factors cause the behavior, because we cannot determine which came first. Despite this limitation, descriptive and correlational studies are time- and cost-efficient methods of assessing a community's needs, understanding a safety behavior, and identifying behavior change options. As a result, they are commonly used to develop injury prevention programs.

In addition to descriptive and correlational studies, there are study designs that allow us to determine factors that were present before a behavior took place. These methods are useful in establishing cause-and-effect relationships, because causes must precede effects in time. If the potential causal factor is something protective we are offering to the population, like training caregivers in the correct way to install child safety seats, we can randomly expose people to the factor and study its effect on subsequent behavior. This is called an *intervention study*. (Intervention studies are covered in greater detail in Chapter Ten, this volume.) If the factor is something that we did not offer, that is, a factor that occurred on its own, such as past hospitalization for an injury, we can study its effect on subsequent behavior using cohort or case control methodology. Cohort studies and case control studies are sometimes referred to as *observational methods* because we study factors as they occurred without our intervention.

Suppose we wanted to measure the relationship of the factor of past experience of bicycle-related injury to the subsequent behavior of bicycle helmet–wearing cohort or case control methods. A cohort study would begin with a naturally occurring group of people, such as a community or school, who did not already wear helmets. This group would be divided into those with and without the factor of interest, that is, a past experience of bicycle-related injury, and followed forward in time to observe their subsequent helmet-wearing behavior. In contrast, case control studies would begin with people with and without the behavior (those who do and do not wear helmets) and look back into their history for evidence of the factor of interest: bicycle-related injuries.

For several reasons, cohort and case control methods are not often used in the study of injury behavior. Cohort studies require following a naturally occurring group of people, like a community. Thus, they frequently require following large numbers of people. In addition, these people must be followed long enough to observe the outcome of interest (in this case, a behavior change), which can sometimes take years. As a result, cohort studies are often logistically difficult and costly. This is not true of case control studies, since both the factor of interest and the behavior have both already occurred. As a result, it is much more common to use case control methodology to establish a relationship between a factor and an outcome. In the case of injury behavior, however, the factors we are most interested in studying are theoretical constructs that may lead to the behavior. For example, guided by the theory of reasoned action, we would want to know if behavioral intentions or attitudes were associated with injury behavior. Unfortunately, it is rarely possible to look backward in someone's history to accurately assess theoretical constructs, for example, to determine the person's prior intentions or attitudes. For this reason, case control studies are not often useful in the study of psychosocial contributors to injury behavior.

Because intervention studies are covered in Chapter Ten and cohort and case control studies are rarely used in the study of injury behavior, the remainder of this chapter focuses on descriptive and correlational (cross-sectional) studies. There are a number of data collection methods that can be used to collect descriptive and correlational information about injury-related behaviors. These are generally divided into qualitative methods and quantitative methods. Qualitative methods are designed to gain detailed insight about the subject at hand, usually from a limited number of persons. Qualitative data usually address the "why" and "how" of some phenomenon, whereas quantitative data usually address the "how much" and "how many." Qualitative methods are not designed to produce information that can be generalized to a larger population or to test hypotheses, but rather to give an in-depth look at the problem—its possible causes and potential solutions—and to generate hypotheses. The three most commonly used qualitative methods are individual interviews, focus groups, and participant observation. In contrast to qualitative methods, quantitative methods are designed to gather information from a larger number of persons, with the goal of generalizing results to an entire population of interest or to test hypotheses. The most common quantitative methods of collecting descriptive and correlational information are through surveys and observations.

The following sections describe in detail each of these data collection methods, including their strengths and limitations. Examples of studies using the methodologies are also provided as examples of the specific procedures used.

Collecting Qualitative Information

In this section, the most commonly used methods for collecting qualitative information are reviewed (see Table 8.1).

Individual Interviews

In individual interviews, information is gathered by asking questions directly of community members or other persons of interest and recording their answers verbatim (Rubin & Rubin, 1995; Thompson & McClintock, 1998). The questions are designed to get the respondent talking. For this reason, the questions are open-ended, and response choices are not proposed. An example of an open-ended question is: "What would you say are some of the main reasons that people do not test their smoke alarms?" Participants' responses are recorded verbatim, usually transcribed, and analyzed by reviewing the content of the transcriptions.

Among the main advantages of individual interviews are that the person gathering the information can follow the respondent's lead and learn about the issue from the respondent's perspective. Major disadvantages include the time and resources it takes to interview participants individually, transcribe their responses, and review the transcriptions in depth.

Studies have employed individual interviews in a variety of populations to assess a multitude of injury-related behavioral factors. For example, after identifying safe and unsafe behaviors from analyses of injury records, Cooper, Phillips,

TABLE 8.1. QUALITATIVE METHODS AT A GLANCE.

Method	Advantages	Disadvantages
Individual interviews	Easier to schedule than focus groups	Number of interviews increases the cost and time
	Can include questions about sensitive topics	One-on-one format may increase respondent's pressure to give "desirable" responses
	Can clarify responses by probing information that arises during the interview	
Focus groups	One person's contributions can serve as a trigger or reminder for other people's input	Can be difficult to schedule
	Group members can support one another (particularly useful if the group differs in some way from the facilitator)	Hard to convene in rural areas or where population is dispersed
		Requires space for a group
		Sensitive topics are not appropriate for group discussion
Qualitative observation	Eliminates relying on participants' reports	Time-consuming
	Findings not restricted to questions asked	Difficult to observe concurrent events
	In participant-observation, the observer has firsthand experience of participating	Presence of observer may alter the events, but this is less likely with participant-observation

Sutherland, and Makin (1994) conducted in-depth interviews with seventy-two employees of a construction plant to validate the behaviors identified and identify other critical safety behaviors that contributed to injury in the construction industry. Using a markedly different population, Peterson (1999) conducted interviews with ninety-six children, ages two to thirteen at the time of injury, to assess their recall of a medically treated injury event two years after the event. And in a third population, Gould, Udry, Bridges, and Beck (1997) conducted qualitative interviews with twenty-one U.S. Ski Team members who suffered season-ending injuries to identify factors that were perceived to facilitate recovery.

Girasek (2003) employed individual interviews to determine how parents who had lost children to accidental injuries three to five years earlier felt about participating in campaigns as advocates for injury prevention. Parents were identified through the office of the state medical examiner. The interviews, conducted in private, lasted one to two hours. Questions assessed the parents' exposure to previous campaigns, whether they had ever been asked to participate in a similar campaign, and whether they would agree to do so at varying levels of commitment (for example, providing a photo of their child or telling their story in a local setting). They also inquired about reasons someone in the parents' situation might or might not choose to participate in such activities. Parents identified barriers to participation, including acute grief in the early period following the death. They also identified benefits to participation, including saving children's lives and saving other parents from bereavement.

Focus Groups

Focus groups are another means of collecting qualitative information. This method is similar to individual interviewing in that open-ended questions are asked and responses are recorded verbatim. In focus groups, however, the questions are asked of groups of people, usually with about six to eight participants (Krueger, 1994; Thompson & McClintock, 1998). This allows the responses of one person to stimulate the thinking of the others in the group. Focus groups can be more cost-effective than individual interviews, but the logistics of gathering six to eight respondents in one place can sometimes be more difficult. In addition, this method is not effective if the topic is one for which group members' responses are likely to be guarded in the presence of other group members.

Like individual interviews, focus groups have also been used to assess a variety of behavioral factors associated with injury, as the following examples indicate. Kidd, Scharf, and Veazie (1996) conducted focus groups of farmers and their spouses to identify types and circumstances of farm injuries and strategies for preventing these injuries. A causal model was developed using information from six focus groups and validated using an additional three focus groups. Haslam, Sloane, Hill, Brooke-Wavell, and Howarth (2002) conducted three focus groups among persons ages sixty-five to seventy-nine to assess their knowledge of safety on stairs. While the participants recognized that use of alcohol and medications may increase the likelihood of falling, they did not appear to recognize when they are at increased personal risk. Stutts and Wilkins (2003) used focus group methodology to explore the feasibility of offering on-road driving evaluations for older drivers. The focus groups were conducted with three types of stakeholders: five focus groups of driver educators, two of occupational therapists, and one of physicians. Information solicited included the potential value of on-road evaluations, how they should be structured, how they might be marketed, and who should offer them. All groups acknowledged the differences in driving evaluations for youth versus the aging.

Howland et al. (1989) conducted focus groups of fourth, fifth, and sixth graders in Massachusetts as a preliminary step in understanding bicycle helmet–wearing behaviors. Among the forty-two participants, five (12 percent) owned bicycle helmets. When asked how someone looks when wearing a bike helmet, positive responses such as "smart" and "safe" were most frequent. Only a minority of students gave negative responses such as "stupid" or "being a sissy." In contrast, few of the students had positive feelings about wearing helmets. Most thought their peers would call them names. Some students distinguished between wearing a helmet for racing versus regular use, finding the former more acceptable. Attitudes toward helmets were also influenced by the helmet design and color, with black and bright colors being better accepted. Most of the students did not consider head injury among the possible outcomes of a bicycle crash until they were prompted. The fourth-, fifth-, and sixth-grade children in the focus groups expressed support for helmet laws. They believed that such laws would reduce the peer pressure they experience, since everyone would have to wear helmets.

Qualitative Observation

Qualitative observation occurs when the individual gathering the information is present for the events of interest and records his or her observations. The recording of information is usually done in detail using supporting field notes. Sometimes the event of interest is videotaped, and several observers independently record their observations as they view the videotape.

Participant-observation occurs when the individual gathering the information actually is or becomes part of the group of interest (that is, a participant) for the purpose of observing the group members' behavior (Jorgensen, 1989; Thompson & McClintock, 1998). For example, an athletic trainer might offer his services and attend all of the practices and games for a college basketball team in order to observe how the coach's interaction with the players is associated with their risk-taking behavior on the court. In this instance, the trainer would take extensive field notes during each practice and game and use this information to describe the association of interest.

A major advantage of the observation method is that it does not rely on awareness and report of the respondents. The trained observer is present to gather information on each occasion. Added advantages of participant-observation are that the observer has the full experience of being a participant, and the group becomes accustomed to the observer's presence so their behavior is not altered by the presence of an observer. Disadvantages of this method include the fact that the observations made are limited to those of the observer, unless video recordings are made for other observers to validate. Furthermore, it is often difficult for the observer to pay attention to more than one specific event at a time. And as with an interviewer, the cost of providing an observer can become excessive.

Methods may also be mixed in order to obtain needed information. For example, Walter, Bourgois, Loinaz, and Schillinger (2002) used participant-observation, with in-depth interviews to supplement the information, to study the ways in which the social context of undocumented day laborers influenced their risk of occupational injury.

Theory and Qualitative Methods

Until recently, qualitative assessments of injury behavior have been infrequent, and the use of behavioral theory to guide these assessments has been even rarer. This is unfortunate, given the benefits that theory can provide in guiding studies and suggesting targets for intervention. Theory can be incorporated into a qualitative assessment in one of three ways: (1) the information to be collected can be guided by one or more existing behavioral theories, (2) the information can be collected without theoretical guidance and then interpreted from the perspective of an existing theory, and (3) the information can be collected without theoretical guidance and then used to develop a new theory of the injury behavior of interest.

Otis et al. (1992) used the first of these approaches. They conducted a theory-based study of bicycle helmet use, using the theory of reasoned action to guide their data collection. As described in Chapter Two, this theory proposes that the behavior of helmet wearing is determined by the intention to wear a helmet. In turn, the intention to wear a helmet is determined by the individual's attitudes toward wearing a helmet and what the individual believes persons who are important in his or her social network think he or she should do about wearing a helmet. Otis et al. began by asking open-ended questions of children in grades 4 through 6. In order to determine the salient attitudes about helmet use held by students in these grades, they asked the children to list the advantages and disadvantages they perceived to be associated with bicycle helmet use. The attitudes that Otis et al. identified from the children included "makes you look sporty," "makes your feel safe," "would be fun," "would be a bother," "would look ugly," "would look ridiculous," "would make you appear chicken," and "would make you likely to be laughed at." Normative beliefs were explored by asking the children to name people they thought would agree and disagree with wearing a bicycle helmet. Students listed mothers, fathers, and friends.

Addressing the same topic, Loubeau (2000) conducted focus groups to understand failure to wear bicycle helmets among twelve and thirteen year olds in the New York City area. While the design of this study was not specifically theory based, the results can be interpreted in light of three prominent constructs from the health belief model: perceived barriers, perceived severity of an injury, and cues to action. As explained in Chapter Two, the health belief model proposes that the likelihood of taking a preventive action like wearing a helmet is influenced by the perceived benefits of the action minus the perceived barriers. It is also influenced by the perceived threat, which in turn is influenced by perceived susceptibility to the adverse outcome (in this case, injury) and that outcome's perceived severity. The other two influences on perceived threat are cues to action and demographic variables. Barriers reported in Loubeau's study included that helmets were "annoying," "uncomfortable," and "hot," as well as that "they didn't fit," "looked horrible," and "looked stupid." Negative comments from friends were another barrier. In terms of perceived severity, the worst things the youth imagined would happen included "crack your head open," "concussion," and "brain damage," as well as broken bones and a need for surgical intervention. Cues to action reported included parental rules, but most frequently these rules were not enforced. None of the participants recalled guidance from their teachers or doctors, and only one reported intervention by a law enforcement official.

The third approach is to use grounded theory. This entails open coding, a technique that involves closely reviewing the text of interviews, focus groups, or observation field notes to categorize and name the constructs or variables that seem to be mentioned, as well as the relationships among these variables. Chapin and Kewman (2001) used grounded theory to study factors that influenced returning to work after a spinal cord injury. Twelve participants were selected from among those in the University of Michigan Model Spinal Cord Injury Care Systems database. Six of these persons had been continuously employed for the past two years, and six were not employed. Employed and unemployed participants were matched on age, education, race, gender, injury severity, and time since injury. They analyzed their data by having each researcher independently perform open coding and naming the variables. After agreeing on the categories and their meanings, those with strongly related meanings were collapsed. Next, individual categories with related content were grouped and then aggregated into larger concepts. Ultimately the researchers identified a four-step process of employment: job consideration and exploration; job seeking, an offer, and return to work; job maintenance and advancement; and perceived advantages of working. In turn, they found that each of these steps was influenced by four factors: the physical impairment, psychological differences among the individuals, activities and skills, and the environment. The psychological and environmental factors best described the differences between those who were employed and those who were not. Psychologically, those who were employed were more optimistic and had higher self-esteem, greater achievement orientation, and role models. Important contributions from the environment included monetary incentives, disincentives, access, and accommodation.

In Chapter Fifteen, this volume, McDonnell, Burke, Gielen, and O'Campo provide another example of using qualitative methods (in-depth interviews) to examine the utility of the transtheoretical model for understanding women's experience of intimate partner violence.

Collecting Quantitative Information

In this section, the most commonly used methods for collecting quantitative information are reviewed (see Table 8.2).

Introduction to Surveys

A survey is a means of distributing a data collection instrument, usually called a questionnaire, to a selected group of people (Krosnick, 1999; Thompson & McClintock, 1998). Surveys can also be made of observable behaviors, such as observational surveys of home safety practices or car seat use among a selected group of people. Surveys are the most prominent method of collecting quantitative descriptive and correlational information. The survey instrument, or questionnaire, is composed of carefully worded and carefully organized items, or questions (Oppenheim, 1966). This is a benefit in that all respondents answer the same questions in the same order. The instrument may be completed by an observer, an interviewer, or the respondent. Survey instruments can include both close-ended, forced-choice questions providing quantitative data and open-ended items providing qualitative data.

Surveys using observers must be conducted within sight of the person being observed and generally use checklists or other simple data collection instruments to record observations. An advantage of observational surveys is that there is no bias due to the respondent's self-report. Another advantage is the improved data quality resulting from the observer's familiarity with the instrument. A major disadvantage of observation is that the respondent cannot be anonymous. Another disadvantage is the cost of employing and training the observers. If multiple observers are used, quality control and consistency across data collectors are extremely important and best addressed through careful training and supervision.

Surveys using interviewer-completed questionnaires can be administered face-to-face or by telephone. Some advantages of having an interviewer complete a questionnaire are that it does not matter how well the respondent can read, and the interviewer's familiarity with the instrument improves the quality of the information. An additional advantage of telephone surveys is the degree of anonymity added by not being face-to-face. A major disadvantage of interviewer-completed instruments is the cost of employing and training the interviewer. Furthermore, some respondents do not have telephones, do not answer calls from

TABLE 8.2. METHODS OF COLLECTING QUANTITATIVE DATA AT A GLANCE.

Method	Advantages	Disadvantages
Observational surveys	Can access everyone Trained observer ensures better data quality No respondent bias	Costly Time-consuming No anonymity for respondent
Face-to-face surveys	Can access everyone Trained interviewer ensures better data quality Reading level is not a concern	Costly Time-consuming No anonymity for respondent Potential for social desirability may be higher
Telephone surveys	Same as above Fast One supervisor for multiple interviewers Relatively inexpensive	Not everyone has a telephone Easy for respondent to refuse or block call
Distributed surveys	Low cost Anonymity for respondent	Data quality depends on the respondent (for example, literacy) Need incentives for respondents to complete them
Mailed surveys	Anonymity for respondent	Same as above Omit the homeless May require remailing Can be costly
Web-based surveys	Quick Eliminates need for data entry Allows anonymity	Not everyone has equal computer access Respondents are concerned about privacy Respondent can complete more than once Need incentives for respondents to complete them

unfamiliar numbers, or do not open the door to strangers. In addition, as with observational surveys, if multiple interviewers are used, quality control and consistency across data collectors is an important issue that is best addressed through careful training and supervision.

Respondent-completed questionnaires can be distributed by hand, by mail, by e-mail, or on the Web. They have the advantage of anonymity and also allow the respondent to complete them at the most convenient time. Both of these factors contribute to the quality and validity of the responses provided. The key disadvantage of respondent-completed questionnaires is that it can be difficult to get cooperation from the persons to whom they are distributed. Often there is no incentive for completing the questionnaire and returning it on time. This can cause return rates to be very low, limiting their generalizability. Another disadvantage is that self-completed instruments can be difficult or impossible to complete for respondents with a low level of reading ability. Access to the survey can be a problem too. Some people do not have an address to which to mail the questionnaire. Other people do not have access to e-mail or the Web. An additional drawback of Web-based instruments is that it is possible for a respondent to complete the instrument more than one time, which can be a particular problem when incentives are offered.

Observational Surveys

Observational surveys have been a mainstay in injury behavior studies because of the increased validity of not having to rely on self-reported behavior. Observations of seat belt use have been regularly conducted by the National Highway Traffic Safety Administration for decades. In this section, we give three examples of observations.

Weiss (1986) conducted a study in which children were observed arriving at four elementary schools, three junior highs, three senior highs, and one university campus in middle-class neighborhoods of Tucson, Arizona, to determine the frequency of bicycle helmet–wearing behavior. Fewer than 2 percent of the school children and 10 percent of the university students wore helmets in the 1985 data collection period. Subsequently Weiss (1992) reported the results of having an observer return to the same schools in 1990 to observe helmet use. His purpose was to determine whether helmet use had changed in the absence of formal programs designed to increase the use of helmets. There was no change in helmet wearing except among elementary school children. Among these children, the proportion of users increased from 1.9 percent in 1985 to 17.1 percent in 1990.

Eby and Vivoda (2003) conducted an observational study of drivers to assess the frequency of handheld mobile phone use and its association with safety belt use. Observation sites were selected across the state of Michigan so that every intersection in the state had an equal chance of being selected. Day of the week and time of day for observation (between 7:00 A.M. and 7:00 P.M.) were also randomized. Trained observers observed vehicles only in the lane adjacent to the curb, recording the first vehicle they saw and the next one they saw after looking up again. Overall, 2.7 percent of Michigan drivers were using mobile phones at any time, and safety belt use was lower for users of cell phones than for those who were not using.

Face-to-Face Surveys

Rowe, Thorsteinson, and Bota (1995) conducted a roadside survey of consecutive bicyclists traveling past the selected survey locations. This study supplemented observations of behavior with a face-to-face survey to determine the prevalence of helmet wearing, compliance with helmet-wearing recommendations, and attitudes regarding helmet legislation. Survey locations were randomly selected from a list of cycling routes and included both main and residential streets. The thirty-item questionnaire was administered by interviewers in either French or English. The vast majority of the cyclists was students (64 percent), was riding for pleasure (83 percent), and rode every day (72 percent). More than half (57 percent) of the riders over the age of sixteen agreed that there should be a law mandating helmet use for all bicyclists.

Telephone Surveys

Lindsay, Hanks, Hurley, and Dane (1999) conducted a telephone survey of three hundred students at a large, private university to better understand the relationship between sleep and driving among students. Trained student interviewers called participants at least four times on four different days until there were three hundred complete responses. According to the descriptive data, just over three-fourths of the students (76 percent) had their own car on campus. The frequency of motor vehicle trips of more than 150 miles one way ranged from none to one hundred per year, with a median of four per year.

Almost one-third of the respondents (32 percent) said they had experienced an event of dozing while driving. Among those who had dozed while driving, more than half (58 percent) said they had not slept normally before the event, and 56 percent said their schedule during the week before the episode had been irregular, interrupting their normal sleep schedule. Correlational analyses found that almost nine out of ten (89 percent) of the events had occurred when the car was traveling at fifty-five miles per hour or more.

Nelson, Sussman, and Graham (1999) analyzed information from a national telephone survey to assess public knowledge and opinion about the safety of air bags. Respondents were selected using random-digit-dial procedures. Survey administration occurred on the weekend. There were three attempts to call back each telephone number selected at random. A total of 1,005 adults completed the interview, for an overall response rate of 13.4 percent.

The majority of respondents knew about the potential of air bags to harm drivers; that in cars with passenger-side air bags, rear-facing infant seats should not be placed in the front seat; and that air bags are saving the lives of drivers. The majority did not know that air bags can injure belted drivers and that they were involved in more deaths of children than lives saved.

Gielen, Eriksen, Daltroy, and Rost (1984) conducted a statewide telephone survey of 406 parents of children age five and under in Maryland. Guided by the theory of reasoned action, the purpose of the survey was to identify factors that differentiated those who used child safety seats from those who did not. To assess the constructs of Attitude and Perceived Norms, parents were asked their beliefs about the benefits and drawbacks of using safety seats, as well as whose opinions mattered to them in decisions about safety seat use.

Fifty-six parents never used a safety seat for the following reasons: the child's discomfort (27 percent) or resistance (16 percent) or the beliefs that the seat was unnecessary (12 percent), expensive (9 percent), or inconvenient (9 percent). Among safety seat users, most used the seat improperly and inconsistently (38 percent), followed by proper and consistent (28 percent), improper and consistent (23 percent), and proper and inconsistent (10 percent). In a discriminant analysis, parents' attitudes best discriminated between consistent and correct users and all other groups. Approval of spouse also contributed significantly to the discrimination, as did several sociodemographic factors (age of youngest child, family size, and income) and health behavior variables (parents' seat belt use and smoking). The importance of parents' attitudes suggests that this is an important variable to address in interventions to increase safety seat use.

The Behavioral Risk Factor Surveillance System is a prominent telephone survey that includes information on injury behaviors at the state and national level and will be discussed later in this chapter. More information about telephone surveys can be found in Chen (1996).

Distributed Surveys

Kimmel and Nagel (1990) administered a questionnaire in the classroom to three hundred children in grades 4 through 8 in an upper-middle-class suburban school district in Ohio to determine the frequency of bicycle helmet use. The response rate to this survey was 92 percent. Joshi, Beckett, and Macfarlane (1994) conducted a similar survey of secondary school bicycle riders, but the response rate for their survey was not reported. Based on the constructs of the health belief model and the theory of planned behavior, they asked about attitudes, benefits, and barriers of helmet use; conformity to norms; perceived vulnerability; and intention to wear a helmet. Both conformity and perceived vulnerability were significantly associated with intention to wear a helmet.

As noted previously, Otis et al. (1992) conducted a study of bicycle helmet use guided by the theory of reasoned action. For the quantitative portion of the study, they administered a questionnaire to 797 students in grades 4 through 6 to determine factors that influenced their intention to use bicycle helmets. Based on the focus group results, the attitudes measured in the survey included "would be fun," "would be a bother," "would look ugly," "would look ridiculous," "would look sporty," "would make the user feel safe," "would make the user appear chicken," and "would make the user likely to be laughed at." Normative beliefs measured quantitatively were whether the students thought their father, mother, or friends would be supportive of or opposed to the fact that they used a helmet every time they rode a bike.

Results demonstrated that both attitudes and normative beliefs correlated with intention to use a helmet, but attitudes were the stronger correlate, perhaps because this scale had a wider range. Among norms, perceptions regarding friends' beliefs were the strongest influence on intention, followed by perception regarding mothers' beliefs. Perceptions regarding fathers' beliefs did not discriminate those who intended to use helmets from those who did not.

Fullerton and Becker (1991) conducted a survey of students of the University of New Mexico who reported that they rode a bicycle. Students were approached in the vicinity of the student union, asked if they were university students, and then asked if they rode a bicycle in Albuquerque. All of the students who rode bicycles ($N = 100$) agreed to participate. The most frequently reported factor for deciding whether to wear a helmet (34.5 percent) was the length of the bicycle trip. Common reasons for failure to wear a helmet were cost (32.9 percent) and lack of comfort (32.9 percent).

Jones, King, Poteet-Johnson, and Wang (1993) conducted a survey of primary caregivers of children in grades 3 through 6 in Alabama to assess their perceptions regarding bicycle-related head injuries and helmet use. Surveys were distributed to twenty-five hundred children by their homeroom teachers. The children were instructed to take them home and have their caregivers complete them. Using this methodology, fewer than half (40.2 percent) of the caregivers responded.

The Youth Risk Behavior Survey (YRBS), a part of the Youth Risk Behavior Surveillance System, is a national survey distributed to youth in schools that includes information on injury behaviors. The YRBS is discussed later in this chapter.

Mailed Surveys

DiGuiseppi, Rivara, and Koepsell (1988) mailed a questionnaire to the parents of 1,004 third graders attending public schools in Seattle, Washington, who were selected at random. After follow-up of nonrespondents, 48 percent of the parents responded. Comparison of respondents and nonrespondents suggested that the postal codes of responding parents had higher median incomes than those of parents who did not respond.

According to the 482 valid responses, 88 percent of the children owned bicycles, and 77.1 percent of these did not own helmets. Responding parents reported that their children gave the following reasons for failing to wear helmets: "no friends use them" (25.3 percent), "never thought about it" (25.1 percent), and "they are uncomfortable/unattractive" (17.7 percent). When asked, most parents whose children did not own helmets said they "never thought of buying their children a helmet" (57.4 percent), helmets were too costly (28.4 percent), or their children would not wear them (21.6 percent). Parents whose children owned helmets were more likely to know that helmets can prevent head injuries associated with bicycle crashes.

Weiss and Duncan (1986) conducted a survey of pediatricians and family physicians in Tucson, Arizona, to assess their knowledge and behavior regarding bicycle safety and education. Questionnaires were mailed to 161 pediatricians and family physicians listed in the Tucson telephone directory; about two-thirds of them (65.8 percent) completed and returned the questionnaires. The physicians were asked to estimate the percentage of school children who used bicycle helmets, as well as reasons children do not use helmets. Using the scale of "Routinely," "Almost Routinely," "Sometimes," "Almost Never," and "Never," respondents were asked to indicate how often they provided bicycle safety information to their patients.

The vast majority of the respondents (92 percent) correctly estimated the rate of helmet use among children, and most cited lack of parental awareness as the primary reason. In spite of this knowledge, more than one in four (29.2 percent) respondents reported that they never discussed bicycle safety during a well child visit.

Ricker et al. (2002) conducted an anonymous survey of brain injury survivors in New Jersey to determine their interest, familiarity, and skills for using telerehabilitation technology. Questionnaires were mailed through the Brain Injury Association of New Jersey to a random sample of brain injury survivors. Of four hundred surveys mailed in two mailings of two hundred, seventy-one (18 percent) were completed and returned. Among other topics, respondents were asked about their use of e-mail and the Web, their familiarity with computers and the Internet, their access to computers, computer accessibility, and their comfort and interest in using the Internet.

Fifty-nine percent of the respondents currently used a computer. The most frequent uses were for Internet and e-mail (81 percent), followed by games (76 percent) and word processing (71 percent). Almost three-fourths (73 percent) of the computer users responded that they would be comfortable using the Internet for reasons related to health, as long as security of the connection, exchange, and storage was addressed.

Very little injury research using mail surveys has been based in theory. Lee, Jenkins, and Westaby (1997) mailed questionnaires to a representative sample of 1,255 fathers on Wisconsin dairy farms. Based on the theory of planned behavior, the questionnaires elicited information about the fathers' attitudes, subjective norms, and perceived behavioral control related to exposing their children under the age of fourteen to hazards on the farm. Together, attitudes, subjective norms, and perceived behavioral control accounted for a large portion (up to 75 percent) of the fathers' intentions. Attitudes were the strongest predictors.

More information about mailed surveys can be found in Vaux (1996).

Web-Based Surveys

Web-based surveys have been assessed for validity, and found comparable to real-world studies (Eysenbach & Wyatt, 2002). At the same time, Web-based surveys have some limitations. For example, they are not effective for low socioeconomic status populations, who are underrepresented among computer users. Furthermore, as with distributed surveys, Web-based surveys are not likely to be completed without incentives. In addition, studies suggest that respondents worry about the privacy of Web-based surveys (Eysenbach & Wyatt, 2002).

Although Web-based surveys are now being used to describe injury, to date only one article was found in which a Web-based survey was used to describe injury behavior. No articles have used Web-based surveys to study theoretical constructs associated with injury-related behaviors.

Over a period of fifteen months, Attarian (2002) collected data by means of a Web-based questionnaire in order to determine rock climbers' self-perception of their skills in first aid, safety, and rescue. The study was described on the Carolina Climbers' Coalition Web site, and readers were encouraged to participate. It was also announced in the *American Alpine News.*

A total of 241 climbers completed the survey, most of whom were active and experienced climbers and most of whom reported having some first aid training. In terms of behaviors, 82 (34 percent) of respondents reported that they always wore a helmet, and 33 (14 percent) reported that they never did. Only 35 (14 percent) said they always carried a cell phone, while 116 (48 percent) said they never did. Regardless of their beliefs about their rescue capabilities, the vast majority (93 percent) said that if a course was offered in partner and self-rescue techniques, they would take it.

The methodology of several of the Web-based surveys of injury can also provide guidance for future studies of injury-related behaviors. For example, Nathanson and Reinert (1999) combined results of a twenty-four-item questionnaire distributed to a convenience sample of windsurfers on beaches in California, Rhode Island, Massachusetts, Hawaii, and the Dominican Republic with results of a Web-based administration of the same questionnaire. The questionnaire was available online from February through May 1997, and the Web address was posted on a windsurfing news group and distributed to two wind-surfing e-mail distribution lists.

Fifty (78 percent) of the 64 questionnaires distributed on the beaches were returned, and 48 (75 percent) of these had complete responses: 279 questionnaires were completed over the Internet, and 246 (88 percent) of these had complete responses. The authors found no statistically significant differences in type or location of injuries between responses to the questionnaires completed on the Web and those completed on paper.

Nathanson, Haynes, and Galanis (2002) used a Web-based survey alone to collect information from May 1998 to August 1999 on the frequency and mechanisms of surfing injuries. The questionnaire was composed of thirty questions, divided into three sections: demographics, acute injuries, and chronic injuries. Advertisements for the survey were posted in surfing periodicals and on surfing-related Web sites. A total of 1,421 surveys were returned, and 1,348 (95 percent) of these were complete. Lacerations were the most common injury reported (42 percent), and two-thirds (67 percent) of all the injuries were caused by contact with the board.

To assess injury and illness among whitewater paddlers, Schoen and Stano (2002) used a combination of distributed questionnaires and Web-based questionnaires, but they also added a version that was included in club bulletins. The authors described the instrument as long and complex. The purpose of the survey was to assess injury history, compare injuries by type of craft and other variables, and assess reports of diagnosis of giardia infection. They received 319 responses over a six-month period but did not describe the responses by type of survey method used. They did note, however, that 18 percent of their respondents, a larger-than-expected proportion, had paddled for more than fourteen years, suggesting that those with the greatest interest in paddling were the most likely to respond to this long and complex instrument.

In order to determine the incidence of concussion among Division I-A college football players during the 2001 season, Booher, Wisniewski, Smith, and Sigurdsson (2003) conducted an Internet-based survey of head athletic trainers from the Division I-A college football programs. Trainers were first sent letters that explained the purpose of the study. Just over three-fourths (76 percent) of the trainers agreed to participate. Each participating trainer then received, by e-mail, instructions on how to use the data collection Internet site and a unique identification number. Trainers accessed the site weekly and reported the number of practices, number of games, and number of players participating in each and the number of concussions that occurred as well as their grades. Reminder e-mails were sent to the trainers each week, asking them to complete the information on the Web site. Seventy-nine percent (79 percent) of the trainers participated fourteen out of the fifteen weeks and 69 percent all fifteen weeks.

The rate of injury was .74 per 1,000 athlete practice exposures and 5.56 per 1,000 athlete game exposures. The Internet reporting system identified 2.1 times as many game-related injuries and 1.5 times as many practice-related injuries as the National Collegiate Athletic Association (NCAA) reporting system. In part, this is probably due to a difference in the definition used. While the Internet system required reporting of all injuries, the NCAA uses a definition that requires time lost from play beyond the day of the injury.

Theory and Quantitative Methods

A significant benefit of theory-driven studies is that they propose modifiable factors for study. For example, theoretical constructs found to be associated with helmet-wearing behavior, such as attitudes and perceived social norms, can be modified. We can influence attitudes about bicycle helmets, perceptions regarding helmet-wearing social norms, and perceived susceptibility to injury. In contrast, we cannot influence nontheoretical factors such as the age or socioeconomic characteristics of the cyclist or the length of the bicycle trip; although these factors are important for targeting and understanding specific audiences, they are not directly modifiable.

Another advantage of theory-driven studies is that they identify modifiable factors that occur early in the behavioral chain. For example, failure to wear a bicycle helmet can lead to a bicycle-crash-related brain injury. In turn, attitudes about bicycle helmets can lead to a failure to wear a bicycle helmet (see Figure 8.1). From a behavioral perspective, when people fail to wear bicycle helmets, we

FIGURE 8.1. A BEHAVIORAL CHAIN
FOR BICYCLE HELMET BEHAVIOR.

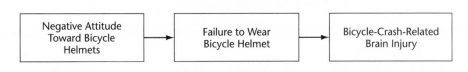

have a public health problem. Thus, true primary prevention requires intervening on the factors that precede the problem behavior, that is, the modifiable behavioral constructs.

Quantitative Measurement and Injury Behavior

An important consideration in collecting quantitative information about any behavior is how the behavior will be measured. We can measure the frequency of the behavior (for example, how often one tests the smoke alarm), the intensity of the behavior (whether a test of the smoke alarm consists of one press of the test button or three), and the quality of the behavior (whether smoke alarm testing includes vacuuming the alarm). Clearly, different measures or definitions produce different results.

When using a theory to guide the study of injury behavior, it is also important to consider how each part of the theory (that is, each theoretical construct) will be measured. For example, one way to measure self-efficacy for child safety seat use is to ask, "How confident are you that you can use a child safety seat correctly?" A more informative way is to ask about the multiple dimensions of using car seats correctly—for example:

- How confident are you that you can:
    Choose the correct car safety seat for your child's age and weight?
    Determine the safest location for your child's safety seat within your vehicle?
    Determine the safest location for your child's safety seat within a vehicle other than your own?
    Correctly position your child within his or her safety seat?
    Correctly install your child's safety seat in your vehicle?
    Correctly install your child's safety seat in a vehicle other than your own?

Because it is difficult to develop sound measures of behaviors and their underlying constructs, it is usually preferable to use existing measures. Such measures can be obtained from other injury control professionals who have already measured the behavior or construct of interest. They can also be obtained from resources such as the Educational Testing Service (n.d.).

Whatever method is used to measure the constructs and behaviors, it is important to determine that the measure is reliable and valid. By reliable, we mean that the measure will produce the same result if used two or more times under the same circumstances. By valid, we mean that the measure actually represents what we think it represents (that our measure of self efficacy actually measures self efficacy). (Further information about measuring reliability and validity can be found in Thompson & McClintock, 1998.)

Using Existing Data

The National Center for Injury Prevention and Control of the Centers for Disease Control and Prevention (CDC) has published an inventory of federal data systems that have data available for use in injury surveillance and prevention programming (Annest, Conn, & James, 1996). A copy of the inventory with Web links to the data sources is provided in the Appendix to this book. There are many benefits of using existing data for describing injury-related behaviors. It almost always takes less time to assess a problem using existing data than it does to gather new information. Less time means less cost. At the same time, there are disadvantages to using existing data. One is that the existing data may not include all the information you would like to obtain. This is particularly true when you want to investigate the relationship of theory-based variables, such as attitudes or self-efficacy, to an injury-related behavior, since most existing data sources are designed to monitor the occurrence of health outcomes rather than their causes. Nonetheless, it is sometimes possible to combine existing sources with other methods to provide the information needed. In addition, existing sources can provide information about where and in whom the behaviors of interest occur.

Death Records

One source of existing information about injury-related behaviors is death records. These records may indicate behaviors such as whether a victim of a motor vehicle crash was using a seat belt or whether a child was restrained in a child safety seat. The Fatality Analysis Reporting System (FARS) of the National Highway Traffic Safety Administration collects data on all motor vehicle crashes on public roadways that involve a fatality. By visiting the FARS Web site (http://www-fars. nhtsa.dot.gov/main.cfm), it is possible to submit queries for data by state that show whether fatal crashes involved the use of restraint systems or alcohol. Information is also available by state for fatal pedal cyclist crashes.

Miles-Doan (1996) investigated whether alcohol use was associated with survival of pedestrians involved in a collision with a car. Data for all pedestrians involved in these collisions were obtained from the Statewide Traffic Accident Management Information System of the Department of Highway Safety and Motor Vehicles of the State of Florida and verified using death certificates. The system also included information on alcohol use.

Hospital Records

Another source of existing data is hospital records, which may include information about behaviors contributing to the injury. For example, Graham, Kittredge, and Stuemky (1992) examined the medical charts of 370 children under the age of two who presented to a pediatric emergency department over a twelve-month period to assess the number of injuries associated with misuse of child safety seats. In order to use these records for this purpose, health care staff had to record not only the nature of the injury but also the cause of the injury in the child's chart.

Tinetti, Doucette, and Claus (1995) investigated the role of situational and behavioral factors in serious fall injuries among a cohort of persons age seventy-two or above. These persons were being followed as a part of a study on fall injuries. The authors supplemented telephone interview data about the events surrounding the fall with a review of hospital records.

Behavioral Risk Factor Surveillance System

Survey data about injury-related behaviors can also be obtained from existing sources. One existing source is the Behavioral Risk Factor Surveillance System (BRFSS) of the CDC. When this system was established in 1984, fifteen states participated in monthly data collection. By 1994, all fifty states, the District of Columbia, and three territories were taking part in the surveillance system. The BRFSS was designed to collect state-level data, but from the beginning, a number of states stratified their samples in such a way that they could estimate prevalence for regions within the state.

The content of the BRFSS questionnaires, which varies slightly from year to year, includes some behavioral data that relate to injury and can be accessed from the CDC Web site (http://www.cdc.gov/brfss/). In recent years, the surveys have included information on firearm use, alcohol use, falls, and seat belt use. Figure 8.2 shows data regarding national seat belt use in 2002, obtained from the CDC Web site. Similar data can be accessed by state.

FIGURE 8.2. FREQUENCY OF SEAT BELT USE NATIONWIDE, 2002.

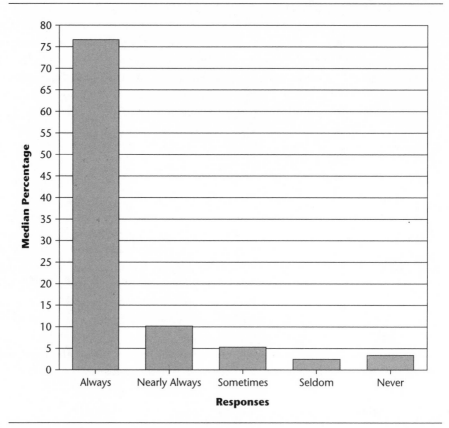

Source: Centers for Disease Control and Prevention.

Chung, Villafuerte, Wood, and Lew (1992) assessed trends in seat belt nonuse and drinking and driving in Hawaii during the five years from 1986 through 1990. During this time, nonuse of seat belts declined an average of 0.9 percent per year, from 8.6 percent in 1986 to 4.8 percent in 1990. This decline was statistically significant ($p < 0.001$). During the same time period, drinking and driving increased from 3.2 percent to 3.9 percent, but this increase was not statistically significant.

Youth Risk Behavior Survey

The Youth Risk Behavior Survey (YRBS) is part of the Youth Risk Behavior Surveillance System (YRBSS). It is also available from the CDC Web site (http://www.cdc.gov/HealthyYouth/yrbs/). The YRBS was created to monitor health risk behaviors that contribute markedly to leading causes of death among youth in the United States. Several behaviors that contribute to unintentional injury and violence are among the behaviors monitored. These include failure to wear a bicycle helmet, failure to wear a seatbelt, drinking and driving as well as riding with a drinking driver, fighting, and carrying a weapon.

The YRBS surveys representative samples of ninth- through twelfth-grade students in schools. These surveys, available at the national, state, and local levels, are conducted every two years. The national survey has representative data for public and private high school students in the United States. The state and local surveys provide representative data for state and local school districts. Figure 8.3 shows data regarding national nonuse of seat belts among youth in 2003, by gender, obtained from the CDC Web site.

In a study by Grunbaum, Lowry, and Kann (2001), behavioral risk data were obtained from students in alternative schools and compared to the data from the 1997 YRBS. Students attending alternative schools had significantly higher rates of failure to wear a seat belt (79 percent versus 67 percent), driving after drinking (24 percent versus 17 percent), carrying a weapon (34 percent versus 18 percent), fighting (62 percent versus 37 percent), and attempting suicide (18 percent versus 8 percent).

FIGURE 8.3. PERCENTAGE OF STUDENTS WHO NEVER OR RARELY WEAR A SEAT BELT WHEN RIDING IN A CAR DRIVEN BY SOMEONE ELSE.

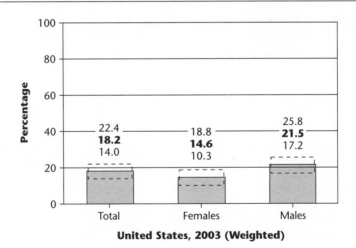

Note: Percentages are displayed in boldface numbers. Ninety-five percent confidence interval boundaries are displayed as the numbers above and below the percentages.

Source: Centers for Disease Control and Prevention.

Current State of Descriptive and Correlational Studies

Descriptive information about injury-related behaviors is increasingly more available, which helps us understand the frequency, timing, and location of specific risk and safety behaviors and the characteristics of the people involved. Unfortunately, there is still little information that allows correlation of theoretical constructs with various injury-related behaviors, although some behaviors, such as bicycle helmet and child safety seat use, have been studied more than others. Thompson, Sleet, and Sacks (2002) have provided a review including theory-based bicycle helmet studies. A similar review of child safety seat studies has also been completed and is under review (Thompson, Rast, Waterman, & Sleet, 2005). There is almost no descriptive information available about the frequency of occurrence of the theoretical constructs themselves. For example, little research has been done to understand the public's general perceptions about risk of injury and violence or the effectiveness of and support for known effective prevention measures. This information would be helpful to framing injury prevention messages. In addition, since longitudinal studies are rare, there is little information to demonstrate the causal association between the theoretical constructs and the behavior. Systematic reviews of the state of knowledge about particularly important injury prevention behaviors would be a welcome addition to the literature. For example, seat belts, car seats, and smoke alarms are prevention measures that have proven effective, yet there are still gaps in their use by segments of the population. A synthesis of what is known about these behaviors and psychosocial correlates would shed light on future behavioral science research needs to facilitate more complete and proper use of these life-saving products. These are important areas for future attention.

References

Annest, J. L., Conn, J. M., & James, S. P. (1996). *Inventory of federal data systems in the United States for injury surveillance, research and prevention activities.* Atlanta: Centers for Disease Control and Prevention.

Attarian, A. (2002). Rock climbers' self-perceptions of first aid, safety, and rescue skills. *Wilderness and Environmental Medicine, 13*(4), 238–244.

Booher, M. A., Wisniewski, J., Smith, B. W., & Sigurdsson, A. (2003). Comparison of reporting systems to determine concussion incidence in NCAA Division I collegiate football. *Clinical Journal of Sport Medicine, 13*(2), 93–95.

Chapin, M. H., & Kewman, D. G. (2001). Factors affecting employment following spinal cord injury: A qualitative study. *Rehabilitation Psychology, 46*(4), 400–416.

Chen, P. Y. (1996). Conducting telephone surveys. In F.T.L. Leong & J. T. Austin (Eds.), *The psychology research handbook: A guide for graduate students and research assistants* (pp. 139–154). Thousand Oaks, CA: Sage.

Chung, C. S., Villafuerte, A., Wood, D. W., & Lew, R. (1992). Trends in prevalences of behavioral risk factors: Recent Hawaiian experience. *American Journal of Public Health, 82*(11), 1544–1546.

Cooper, M. D., Phillips, R. A., Sutherland, V. J., & Makin, P. J. (1994). Reducing accidents using goal setting and feedback: A field study. *Journal of Occupational and Organizational Psychology, 67,* 219–240.

DiGuiseppi, C., Rivara, F. P., & Koepsell, T. (1988). Bicycle helmet ownership and use among schoolage children. *American Journal of Diseases of Children, 142,* 386–387.

Eby, D. W., & Vivoda, J. M. (2003). Driver hand-held mobile phone use and safety belt use. *Accident Analysis and Prevention, 35,* 893–895.

Educational Testing Service. (n.d.). *The ETS test collection.* Retrieved Oct. 17, 2005, from http://www.ets.org/testcoll/index.html.

Eysenbach, G., & Wyatt, J. (2002). Using the Internet for surveys and health research. *Journal of Medical Internet Research, 4*(2), e13.

Fullerton, L., & Becker, T. (1991). Moving targets: Bicycle-related injuries and helmet use among university students. *Journal of American College Health, 39,* 213–217.

Gielen, A. C., Eriksen, M. P., Daltroy, L. H., & Rost, K. (1984). Factors associated with the use of child restraint devices. *Health Education Quarterly, 11*(2), 195–206.

Girasek, D. C. (2003). Public beliefs about the preventability of unintentional injury deaths. *Accident Analysis and Prevention, 33,* 455–465.

Gould, D., Udry, E., Bridges, D., & Beck, L. (1997). Coping with season-ending injuries. *Sports Psychologist, 11*(4), 379–399.

Graham, C. J., Kittredge, D., & Stuemky, J. H. (1992). Injuries associated with child safety seat misuse. *Pediatric Emergency Care, 8*(6), 351–353.

Grunbaum, J. A., Lowry, R., & Kann, L. (2001). Prevalence of health-related behaviors among alternative high school students as compared with students attending regular high schools. *Journal of Adolescent Health, 29,* 337–343.

Haslam, R. A., Sloane, J., Hill, L. D., Brooke-Wavell, K., & Howarth, P. (2002). What do older people know about safety on stairs? *Ageing and Society, 21*(6), 759–776.

Howland, J., Sargent, J., Weitzman, M., Mangione, T., Ebert, R., Mauceri, M., & Bond, M. (1989). Barriers to bicycle helmet use among children. *AJDC, 143,* 741–744.

Jones, C. S., King, W., Poteet-Johnson, D., & Wang, M. Q. (1993). Prevention of bicycle-related injuries in childhood. *Southern Medical Journal, 86*(8), 859–864.

Jorgensen, D. L. (1989). *Participant observation: A methodology for human studie*s. Thousand Oaks, CA: Sage.

Joshi, M. S., Beckett, K., & Macfarlane, A. (1994). Cycle helmet wearing in teenagers— Do health beliefs influence behaviour? *Archives of Disease in Childhood, 71,* 536–539.

Kidd, P., Scharf, T., & Veazie, M. (1996). Linking stress and injury in the farming environment: A secondary analysis of qualitative data. *Health Education Quarterly, 23*(2), 224–237.

Kimmel, S. R., & Nagel, R. W. (1990). Bicycle safety knowledge and behavior in school age children. *Journal of Family Practice, 30*(6), 677–680.

Krosnick, J. A. (1999). Survey research. *Annual Review of Psychology, 50,* 537–567.

Krueger, R. A. (1994). *Focus groups: A practical guide for applied research* (2nd ed.). Thousand Oaks, CA: Sage.

Lee, B. C., Jenkins, L. S., & Westaby, J. D. (1997). Factors influencing exposure of children to major hazards on family farms. *Journal of Rural Health, 13*(3), 206–215.

Lindsay, G. A., Hanks, W. A., Hurley, R. D., & Dane, S. (1999). Descriptive epidemiology of dozing and driving in a college student population. *Journal of American College Health, 47*(4), 157–162.

Loubeau, P. R. (2000). Exploration of the barriers to bicycle helmet use among 12 and 13 year old children. *Accident Analysis and Prevention, 32,* 111–115.

Miles-Doan, R. (1996). Alcohol use among pedestrians and the odds of surviving an injury: Evidence from Florida law enforcement data. *Accident Analysis and Prevention, 28*(1), 23–31.

Nathanson, A., Haynes, P., & Galanis, D. (2002). Surfing injuries. *American Journal of Emergency Medicine, 20*(3), 155–160.

Nathanson, A. T., & Reinert, S. E. (1999). Windsurfing injuries: Results of a paper- and Internet-based survey. *Wilderness and Environmental Medicine, 10*(4), 218–225.

Nelson, T. F., Sussman, D., & Graham, J. D. (1999). Airbags: An exploratory survey of public knowledge and attitudes. *Accident Analysis and Prevention, 31*(4), 371–379.

Oppenheim, A. N. (1966). *Questionnaire design and attitude measurement.* New York: Basic Books.

Otis, J., Lesage, D., Godin, G., Brown, B., Farley, C., & Lambert, J. (1992). Predicting and reinforcing children's intentions to wear protective helmets while bicycling. *Public Health Reports, 107*(3), 283–289.

Peterson, C. (1999). Children's recall for medical emergencies: Two years later. *Developmental Psychology, 35*(6), 1493–1506.

Ricker, J. H., Rosenthal, M., Garay, E., DeLuca, J., Germain, A., Abraham-Fuchs, K., & Schmidt, K. U. (2002). Telerehabilitation needs: A survey of persons with acquired brain injury. *Journal of Head Trauma Rehabilitation, 17*(3), 242–250.

Rowe, B. H., Thorsteinson, K., & Bota, G. W. (1995). Bicycle helmet use and compliance: A northeastern Ontario roadside survey. *Canadian Journal of Public Health, 86*(1), 57–61.

Rubin, H. J., & Rubin, I. S. (1995). *Qualitative interviewing: The art of hearing data.* Thousand Oaks, CA: Sage.

Schoen, R. G., & Stano, M. J. (2002). Year 2000 whitewater injury survey. *Wilderness and Environmental Medicine, 13*(2), 119–124.

Stutts, J. C., & Wilkins, J. W. (2003). On-road driving evaluations: A potential tool for helping older adults drive safely longer. *Journal of Safety Research, 34,* 431–439.

Thompson, N. J., & McClintock, H. O. (1998). *Demonstrating your program's worth: A primer on evaluation for programs to prevent unintentional injury.* Atlanta, GA: Centers for Disease Control and Prevention, National Center for Injury Prevention and Control.

Thompson, N. J., Rast, M. L., Waterman, M. B., & Sleet, D. (2005). *Using behavioral science to increase the effectiveness of child safety seats.* Unpublished manuscript.

Thompson, N. J., Sleet, D., & Sacks, J. (2002). Increasing the use of bicycle helmets: Lessons from behavioral science. *Patient Education and Counseling, 46,* 191–197.

Tinetti, M. E., Doucette, J. T., & Claus, E. B. (1995). The contribution of predisposing and situational risk factors to serious fall injuries. *Journal of the American Geriatrics Society, 43*(11), 1207–1213.

Vaux, A. (1996). Conducting mail surveys. In F.T.L. Leong & J. T. Austin (Eds.), *The psychology research handbook: A guide for graduate students and research assistants* (pp. 127–138). Thousand Oaks, CA: Sage

Walter, N., Bourgois, P., Loinaz, M., & Schillinger, D. (2002). Social context of work injury among undocumented day laborers in San Francisco. *Journal of General Internal Medicine, 17*(3), 221–229.

Weiss, B. D. (1986). Bicycle helmet use by children. *Pediatrics, 77*(5), 677–679.

Weiss, B. D. (1992). Trends in bicycle helmet use by children: 1985 to 1990. *Pediatrics, 89*(1), 78–80.

Weiss, B. D., & Duncan, B. (1986). Bicycle helmet use by children: Knowledge and behavior of physicians. *American Journal of Public Health, 76*(8), 1022–1023.

CHAPTER NINE

INTERVENTION RESEARCH AND PROGRAM EVALUATION

John B. Lowe, Jingzhen Yang, Erin Heiden,
Ralph J. DiClemente

Much of the field of injury prevention and control revolves around the development and implementation of programs designed to influence injury-related behaviors, such as eliminating or reducing risky behaviors and promoting safety behaviors. Programmatic efforts, while critical for injury prevention and control, require rigorous methodological strategies to assess their efficacy. Without appropriate research designs and strategies, it is difficult to evaluate whether injury prevention and control programs are meeting their stated objectives of modifying injury-specific risk and protective behaviors.

The idea of how best to conduct rigorous research to assess programmatic efficacy is not simple and can be confusing or perplexing. However, assessment of programmatic impact is a concept that professionals in the area of injury prevention and control think is critical to identifying evidence-based interventions and advancing the science of injury prevention. While accountability of the project in its effectiveness and direct benefit to society needs to be quantified, the key question is: "What type of evaluation needs to be conducted so individuals outside the program will understand and accept the evaluation results?"

This chapter provides an overview of methods used to evaluate programs in different areas of injury prevention and control. The chapter offers to injury prevention professionals and researchers an understanding of and skills to measure the efficacy and effectiveness of programs and interventions for behavior change and to facilitate an understanding of the array of evaluation research methods and their applicability. Case studies illustrate methods used to assess program efficacy.

Differentiation of Intervention Research and Program Evaluation

Intervention research and program evaluation are different, but the terms are often used similarly in the empirical literature. The type of evaluation conducted may vary greatly by program and be referred to by some to be *program evaluation* and by others *intervention research*. Although there are some commonalities between intervention research and program evaluation, the central one being the assessment of programmatic impact, there are distinct and notable differences as well.

Foremost, intervention research is often referred to as *efficacy trials*. Many are conducted in randomized, controlled trial fashion, where participants are randomized into a treatment or no treatment or minimal treatment control condition. The program in an efficacy trial is usually referred to as an *intervention*. In these trials, intervention research is characterized by a high level of internal validity. Usually researchers control or try to reduce alternate hypotheses that could be viable explanations for why changes in individuals' behavior occurred. Interventions are usually conducted by trained project staff with a high degree of fidelity to the delivery of the intervention.

In comparison, program evaluations are referred to as *effectiveness trials* or *studies*. They are typically characterized by the use of nonrandomized study designs such as case control designs or quasi-experimental designs. Program participants are compared to a similar group that does not receive the program to measure the effect. These studies are characterized by a high level of external validity. The program is delivered in actual situations with staff delivering the program. The researchers impose very little control, and the fidelity of program implementation may or may not be high. For the purposes of this chapter, the terms *intervention* and *program* will be used interchangeably.

Program Planning: The Starting Point for Program Evaluation

Program planning starts with the defining of goals and objectives. These will provide the bases on what the planner believes will be the successes. Without the goals and objectives defined, the program will be successful only in the eye of the beholder.

Program Goals and Objectives

Program goals are an overall status to be reached through continued efforts in the program. Goals are broad statements describing what the program (intervention) is being designed to accomplish (Windsor, Baranowski, Clark, & Cutter, 1994). For example, a program addressing intentional injury may have a goal to reduce the number of deaths due to handguns. Or a program on unintentional injuries may have a goal of limiting or delaying the involvement of youth in motor vehicle crashes.

Program objectives are specific aims needed to accomplish program goals. Objectives should include all of the following: the time period, the specific direction of change that is expected, and how the change will be measured. In addition, objectives must be appropriate for the target population, precise in defining the behavior to be changed, and measurable in terms of health outcomes (Green & Kreuter, 2005). (See also Chapter Seven, this volume.)

Importance of Preparing an Evaluation Plan at the Earliest Phase of Program Planning. In evaluating an intervention, the main purpose is to determine whether the specific goals and stated objectives of the intervention have been met. This typically involves comparing applicable measures before and after the intervention. The programmer must anticipate what needs to be evaluated during program development and needs assessment when data are collected and analyzed to set program objectives. Conversely, the researcher or evaluator looks back during the program evaluation, collecting and analyzing data on what occurred in a program, in accordance with the specified goals and stated objectives of the program. The true impact of a program may not be readily detectable without building in an evaluation during the program planning phase.

Building Evaluation Questions into Program Goals and Objectives. Part of a successful impact or outcome assessment or evaluation is a clear statement of measurable objectives from which meaningful measurements and comparisons can be drawn. Therefore, sound evaluation questions should be developed based on the objectives. For example, with regard to norms of adolescents regarding drunken driving, an objective might be to decrease by 50 percent the proportion of high school students with attitudes favorable to drunken driving. Evaluation questions might include, "Does the target audience think drunken driving is acceptable?" This question could be used to develop specific survey questions in the assessment and evaluation plan, such as, "Do you approve or disapprove of people who drive while drunk?" Similar questions could also be developed for an objective related to a behavioral outcome. If the objective is to increase by 30 percent the number of target high school students who drive a vehicle without the influence of alcohol, the specific survey question used in the evaluation plan might be, "During the past thirty days, how many times did you drive a car or other vehicle when you had been drinking alcohol?"

The Assessment or Evaluation Framework

A sound assessment or evaluation plan needs to have a framework: a plan for evaluating implementation objectives (process evaluation), a plan for evaluating outcome objectives (impact and outcome evaluation), and procedures for managing and monitoring the assessment or evaluation.

An assessment or evaluation framework usually determines what to evaluate, questions to be answered in the evaluation, and the time frame for the evaluation. A plan for evaluating implementation objectives (process evaluation) typically involves the type of information needed, sources of information, time frame for collecting information, and methods for collecting information. A plan for evaluating participant outcome objectives often focuses on the number of participants in the evaluation, data collection points, type of research design (that is, pre-post comparison group design) and specifies a priori applicable methods for data analysis. Procedures for managing and monitoring the assessment or evaluation include training staff to collect data in a reliable and valid manner, conducting quality control checks during the information collection process, and developing a time line for collecting, analyzing and reporting findings.

Types of Evaluation

There are two methods for categorizing evaluations in the literature. The first is based on when an evaluation is conducted (formative versus summative). The second is based on what objectives the evaluation is attempting to measure (process, impact, and outcome). The types of evaluation and temporal relationship between each type of evaluation are displayed in Figure 9.1. As shown, formative evaluation is conducted during program development, and summative evaluation is conducted during the program implementation. While process evaluation can occur in both program development and implementation phases, impact and outcome evaluations occur only in the program implementation phase.

Formative and Summative Evaluation

Formative or assisting in the formation of new information and *summative* or the summing up of the effects of a program are two words used often in the published literature. Although different, both are important to the design and evaluation of a program.

FIGURE 9.1. TYPE OF EVALUATION.

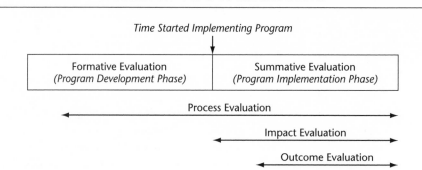

Formative Evaluation

Formative evaluation is designed to produce data and information used to improve an intervention during its developmental phase and document the feasibility of program implementation (Windsor et al., 1994). Although the methods used to conduct a formative evaluation are similar to those used in conducting a needs assessment, the purpose is different. A formative evaluation addresses short-term objectives and is used often in pilot testing or field testing of interventions (Windsor et al., 1994). Formative evaluation is considered a method for judging the worth of an intervention or program while program activities are being developed (Bhola, 1990). Typically, formative evaluation is qualitative in nature and often conducted using small groups of people to pretest various components of the program during its developmental stages. Depending on the goals of the formative evaluation, the methods for formative evaluation can be one or more of the following: observation, in-depth interviews, surveys, focus groups, analysis, reports, and dialogue with participants. In general, formative evaluation can be achieved through one or more of the stages described in Table 9.1 (Dick & Carey, 1990).

Formative evaluation is an important tool for ensuring program success. Although it is challenging to conduct formative evaluations with limited time and tight budgets, it is critical for an injury prevention program to achieve its objectives more effectively.

Summative Evaluation

In contrast to formative evaluation, summative evaluation is designed to produce data and information on the program's efficacy or effectiveness (its ability to do what it was designed to do) during its implementation phase. Summative evalua-

TABLE 9.1. EVALUATION STAGES.

Stages	Contents
Design review	Examining whether intervention goals and objectives match the problem identified
Expert review	Evaluating whether the content of an intervention is accurate, up-to-date, and appropriate to the target population
One-on-one evaluation	Testing specific intervention components with one participant at a time
Small group evaluation	Testing intervention components with a group of participants in an environment similar to the one in which the intervention will be implemented
Field trial	Examining whether the intervention can be used in the context in which it is intended

tion is considered a method of judging the worth of a program after the program is developed and implemented. It is typically quantitative in nature, using numerical scores to assess participants' achievement (for example, behavior change or health status change). Examples of summative evaluations are provided in more detail in a later section.

Process, Impact, and Outcome Evaluation

There are three important areas often referred to in summative evaluation. These three provide a comprehensive approach to measuring what is happening in your program. While the three have different purposes, all three are considered important in evaluating the program.

Process Evaluation

Process evaluation focuses on how a program was implemented and operates. It is designed to document the degree to which the intervention (program) was implemented as intended by assessing how much of the intervention was provided, to whom, when, and by whom. It answers the question, "Was the intervention put into place as planned, and what alterations were required for implementation?" In clinical terms, a process evaluation can be called a *quality assurance review.*

Conducting a Process Evaluation. A process evaluation does not address the question of intervention effectiveness. Typical questions asked in a process evaluation are:

- Is the program (intervention) implemented as planned?
- What aspects of the program are strong? Which ones are weak?
- What can be done to continue to strengthen the program?
- Are there unexpected effects?
- Did problems arise?
- Have remedial actions been developed? Are these being implemented?

Process evaluation does ask the overall question, "Was the intervention delivered as planned?" Process evaluation traditionally includes focus groups, surveys, documentation of dates, processes and participation in activities, and qualitative analysis of intervention materials, such as the content of instructional and training materials.

A number of specific components need to be considered when conducting a process evaluation. Steckler and Linnan (2002) identify seven:

- Context
- Reach
- Dose delivered
- Dose received
- Fidelity
- Implementation
- Recruitment

When developing process measures, it is necessary to consider the larger social, political, or economic factors that may influence the intervention as it is being delivered. These factors can include issues at the program delivery site, such as new organizational policies that could have an impact on the delivery of the intervention. Contextual factors might also include larger social forces, such as war, an increase in the cost of gasoline, or a change of government. Understanding this larger environment and putting it into the context of a process evaluation is important because it has implications for interpreting evaluation results and expectations for how the intervention might perform under different circumstances. The proportion of the intended target audience that participates is critical. Did these intended participants have the opportunity to participate in all aspects of the intervention (dose delivered), and did they receive all the components of the intervention (dose received). Fidelity relates to the quality and integrity of the intervention delivered. Were the components delivered as intended? Finally, re-cruitment is the number of individuals who were invited to participate relative to the number who actually participated in each of the components of the inter-vention. Did the characteristics of those recruited match the intended audience? This helps determine to whom results can be generalized. Process measures should also include the activities conducted and the success of each as measured by num-ber of participants recruited. What worked and what did not work should be the endpoint of a process evaluation.

Importance of Type III Error. Process evaluation provides a measure of the ex-tent to which what was designed to be presented was in truth presented. When an intervention is determined to be effective, process evaluation helps to ensure that it was the intervention and not some other factor that was responsible for suc-cess and provides insights for replicating the program. When an intervention is not effective, good process evaluation measures help to determine whether the in-tervention was in truth ineffective or whether it was not provided to or received by the target audience as intended. This latter lack of fidelity to implementation is often called a type III error. Also of importance, a type III error is unpredictable in that it can result in a type I error (the program or intervention is considered ef-ficacious when, in fact, it is not) or type II error (the program or intervention is considered not efficacious when, in fact, it is). Thus, type III errors can result in invalid results, with the direction of the bias being difficult to gauge or quantify.

An Example of Process Evaluation. To illustrate a process evaluation in the field of injury prevention, we refer to the studies described below. In one study, Cog-gan, Patterson, Brewin, Hooper, and Robinson (2000) conducted a process eval-uation of the community-based Waitakere Community Injury Prevention Project (WCIPP) community-based program implemented in Waitakere City, New Zealand, based on the World Health Organization (WHO) Safe Community model for injury prevention for people of all ages who live in the particular com-munity. The overall goal of this evaluation was to ascertain the process and im-pact of the WCIPP model and the progress toward a reduction in injuries within Waitakere. The evaluation was also designed to provide information relevant to policy development.

The process evaluation occurred over a three-year period during the pilot phase of the project and provided a comprehensive account of the implementa-tion and injury prevention activities of the WCIPP. The evaluation used diverse strategies and methods, including an analysis of project documentation, key in-formant interviews, and participant observation. The evaluation revealed a pri-mary focus on child safety issues but also identified other strategies that targeted the use of smoke alarms and home safety for older adults. Key informant interviews were used to judge the satisfaction of the resources that were developed as a result of the program.

Impact and Outcome Evaluations (Summative Evaluation)

Impact evaluation is designed to assess intervention efficacy or effectiveness in producing midterm (for example, twelve to twenty-four months) cognitive, belief, skill, or behavioral impact (for example, car seat use) for a defined at-risk population (Windsor et al., 1994). Outcome evaluation is designed to assess intervention efficacy or effectiveness in producing long-term changes (for example, one to ten years) in the incidence or prevalence of morbidity rates, mortality rates, or other health status indicators such as injuries among a defined at-risk population (Windsor et al., 1994).

Conducting Impact and Outcome Evaluations. An impact evaluation examines the extent to which desired changes have been achieved immediately after the intervention is complete, and an outcome evaluation focuses on broad and long-term results of program activities. Both evaluations typically compare relevant measures before and after interventions have been implemented. For example, an objective for a program with the goal of reducing motor vehicle crash injuries might be "participants' use of seat belts." An impact evaluation assesses short-term outcomes such as change in knowledge, beliefs, and skills (for example, believing that seat belts are important to wear) or intermediate-term outcomes (for example, seat belt use). An outcome evaluation focuses on long-term outcomes that are related to health outcomes (for example, car crash–related death and injury rates).

Successful impact and outcome evaluations require a clear statement of measurable objectives and an appropriate design for determining if the intervention made a difference. Sometimes impact and outcome evaluations can be hampered by inadequate or incomplete delivery of the intervention, unanticipated events that interrupt its planned flow, or changes made in the message, placement, or timing of media products. These can damage the credibility of an evaluation, leaving the practitioner with few documented results. Therefore, the design and implementation of impact and outcome evaluations are worthy of considerable attention during the development of the program. We illustrate these central evaluation concepts below.

Examples of Impact and Outcome Evaluations. Britt, Silver, and Rivara (1998) conducted a nonrandom, controlled trial to evaluate the effectiveness of a multifaceted bicycle helmet promotion program for low-income children attending preschool enrichment programs throughout Washington State. Eight hundred eighty children from the eighteen intervention sites in the Head Start program were recruited as the intervention group, and two hundred children from the four other sites served as comparison. Intervention activities included classroom activities, education of parents during school meetings and home visits, fitting and distribution of helmets, a bicycle skills and safety "rodeo" event, and helmets required while riding at school. Helmet use was observed at the regularly scheduled home visits before and after the promotion program. The impact of this study was measured by proportion of helmet use among low-income children, comparing proportion between the intervention and comparison groups. The finding showed that use of helmets in the intervention group increased from 43 to 89 percent, while use in the comparison group increased from only 42 to 60 percent ($p < 0.05$ for intervention group changes versus comparison group changes). The outcome evaluation, not reported, would have been the reduction of injuries to low-income children in the intervention groups relative to the comparison groups over the next several years.

In another study, Durkin, Laraque, Lubman, and Barlow (1999) evaluated the impact of the Harlem Hospital Injury Prevention Program (HHIPP) on reducing severe traffic injuries among school-aged children in an urban community. As an outcome measure, the incidence of traffic injuries was compared before and after implementation using hospital discharge and death certificate data on pediatric injuries and census information. The impact evaluation of this study was to measure the change in both knowledge and behavior with respect to traffic safety in school-aged children, while the outcome evaluation focused on a reduction of pediatric injuries resulting in hospital admission or death to persons aged under seventeen years.

There are numerous other examples of intervention evaluations, both programmatic and randomized control trials. Childhood injury prevention has been a topic of particular attention, as has the broader issue of motor vehicle crashes. Detailed reviews of these bodies of literature are beyond the scope of this chapter; however, excellent reviews of evaluated interventions have been previously published. For example, reviews of childhood injury prevention interventions can be found in a special issue of *The Future of Children* (Packard Foundation, 2000) and Harborview Injury Prevention Center's Web site (Harborview Injury Prevention and Research Center, 2005). The *American Journal of Preventive Medicine* published reviews of motor vehicle safety intervention research (Coben & Larkin, 1999; Foss & Evenson, 1999; Grossman & Garcia, 1999; McArthur & Kraus, 1999; Peek-Asa, 1999; Rivara, Thompson, Beahler, & MacKenzie, 1999; Rivara, Thompson, & Cummings, 1999; Segui-Gomez, 1999; Vernick et al., 1999; Zwerling & Jones,

1999). The Task Force on Community Preventive Services makes its CDC-led motor vehicle injury prevention and violence prevention systematic reviews available online (www.TheCommunityGuide.org) and in the Community Guide (Zaza et al., 2005). Work site safety belt interventions have been reviewed by Segui-Gomez (2000), and the Cochrane Collaborations maintain databases synthesizing the intervention literature on a variety of injury prevention topics and can be accessed on the Web. For an instructive injury prevention example of program development and evaluation, readers are also referred to McDonald et al. (2003), who describe quantitative and qualitative results of formative research and process and impact evaluations of a child safety program.

Cost-Effectiveness Analysis and Cost-Benefit Analysis

While rigorous evaluation of injury prevention programs provides a quantitative measure of efficacy or effectiveness with respect to reducing injury-associated risk behaviors among various target populations, a key question is whether these programs, if observed to be efficacious or effective, are also cost-effective. To assess cost-effectiveness, a cost-effectiveness analysis (CEA) can be conducted. A CEA is designed to determine the differences between two programs based on what it costs to deliver them. Stating it another way, cost-effectiveness is a method of evaluation to determine the relationship between intervention or program cost (input) and impact (output). Health economists refer to this as a *ratio of cost per unit of impact*. CEA can only be comparative and has little meaning when feasible alternative interventions or programs do not exist. Unfortunately, this is often the case in the area of injury prevention and control.

A CEA allows the program developers and implementers to answer the question, "How much does this program cost?" For example, assume that a falls prevention program for the elderly has been demonstrated to be effective in reducing the number of falls per participant. The program has a number of components, including changing the physical environment, providing physical exercises, and education to produce the reduction in falls. The program requires direct contact with the participant by a trained nurse. Assume the program has been able to demonstrate a significant difference of a reduction of twenty falls per one hundred individuals participating. Including materials and staff time, it costs the program one hundred dollars for each participant, or five hundred dollars per reduced fall. The previous program the organization was using includes only the presentation of materials to the participant. This type of intervention is able to produce a reduction of one fall per hundred participants, markedly less efficacious. It costs only ten dollars to produce this material; however, it costs a thousand dollars per reduced fall. This example illustrates that the new program is cost-effective in reducing falls as it cost half as much as the current program to produce one less fall.

Cost-benefit analysis (CBA) evaluates the relationship between intervention or program cost (input) and program health outcome. The analysis permits determination of the ratio of cost per unit of economic benefit and net economic benefit (Windsor et al., 1994). Cost-benefit analysis can be used alone when comparable programs do not exist to determine the "value" of the intervention or program. The utility of CBA is that it can yield an absolute economic evaluation. This means the benefit is greater than the cost. CBA also allows the calculation of a standard return on investment (ROI), a calculation used often in non–health care settings.

We illustrate this important analytical strategy using the previous example. The new program was able to achieve twenty fewer falls per hundred participants. If we assume that one fewer fall reduces a disabling injury, we can compute the cost for hospital visit, doctor visits, lost workdays, and quality of life in monetary terms. The program designer can compute the saving to the individual, the company, and society of each fall that is averted through participation in the falls prevention program. This illustrates that the program was not only cost-effective but could be cost-beneficial. Finally, both types of analysis (CEA and CBA) are sensitive to the view of the beholder, typically one of four groups (the individual, provider, insurer or other payer, or society), and are value driven.

Conducting Cost-Effectiveness and Cost-Benefit Analyses

Conducting a cost-effectiveness or cost-benefit analysis can be as straightforward or as complex as you wish to make it. The key to conducting either is the ability to monitor expenditures. Cost expenditures are divided into four groups: (1) developmental cost, (2) production costs, (3) implementation costs, and (4) evaluation costs. The ability to monitor expenditures to determine categorically the different costs requires additional surveillance and data collection systems. These systems need to be structured toward the program and the specific elements of that program. The optimal time to initiate these monitoring systems is during the program development and design stages. Prospective cost assessment yields more precise and valid cost estimates than retrospective cost assessment. Attributing costs to one of these four groups allows the evaluator to have the data needed to compute the cost ratios readily available.

Within the injury prevention literature, there are fewer evaluations of cost-effectiveness and cost-benefit analysis than any other type of evaluation. The majority of cost analysis has been done for policy and environmental interventions, such as seat belts in motor vehicles and changes in roadway design (Miller & Levy, 2000). Analysis of program-based interventions is less frequent. Program-based cost analysis evaluations are useful for broad or single focus injury prevention programs. The HHIPP was evaluated by comparing medical spending pre- and postprogram implementation against a control community and calculating a benefit-cost ratio (Spicer, Miller, Durkin, & Barlow, 2004). In a second example, the cost-effectiveness of a community education campaign to promote the use of rollover protective structures and seat belts on farm tractors was calculated based on a decision analysis of a probability of an injury outcome and the net costs of the intervention (Myers, Cole, & Westneat, 2004).

Haddix, Mallonee, Waxweiler, and Douglas (2001) analyzed the effectiveness of a smoke alarm giveaway program in Oklahoma City. Fatal and nonfatal fire-related injuries from before and after program implementation were compared using surveillance data. Program costs associated with the planning, implementation, and maintenance phases over the five years of the program included expenses related to distributing smoke alarms and batteries, educational materials, program activities, and paid personnel and volunteers. Medical costs and costs associated with productivity loss for fatal and nonfatal injuries were estimated from hospital charges and rates reported previously in the literature. The program was estimated to have prevented twenty fatal and twenty-four nonfatal fire-related injuries and prevented $15 million in productivity loss and $1 million in health care costs.

Use of Cost-Effectiveness and Cost-Benefit Analysis

Robertson et al. (2001) included a cost-effectiveness component in their evaluation of a fall prevention program for women aged eighty years and older living in the community in Dunedin, New Zealand. The costs of implementing the program were used to calculate cost-effectiveness. Measures of program costs included the costs of recruiting participants, time and travel by program personnel to conduct the program, program materials, and overhead costs. Program development cost, a one-time expense, was not included in the total. The cost of a fall occurring was calculated using health care service costs of a fall. The comparison included the total health care costs of all participants in the exercise intervention and control groups. The results indicate that 27 percent of total hospital costs during the trial were related to falls. There were no significant differences in health service costs between the intervention and control groups. Implementing the exercise programs for one and two years, respectively, cost $314 and $265 (1995 New Zealand dollars) per fall prevented and $457 and $426 per fall, resulting in a moderate or serious injury prevented. Cost-effectiveness ratios were lower after two years than after one year of intervention.

Finally, it is also important to reevaluate preprogram estimates of cost-effectiveness and cost benefit after a program has been implemented. When actual costs are not available, estimates are often made based on rates found in the literature or based on certain assumptions when no real-world data exist. Actual benefit and cost estimates may differ, as was the case for estimates of the effectiveness of a standard air bag regulation for motor vehicles between 1984 and 1997 (Thompson, Segui-Gomez, & Graham, 2002).

Research Evaluation Designs

Research evaluation designs have been described in a number of outstanding texts, including the classic Campbell and Stanley (1963) and Cook and Campbell (1979). These books illustrate the advantages and consequences of using different types of research designs. The three types of evaluation designs that have been commonly applied to assess program efficacy or effectiveness in the field of injury prevention are nonexperimental, quasi-experimental, and experimental designs. Nonexperimental designs include case studies, one-group posttest, or one-group pre- and posttest designs. Studies typically using comparison groups such as matched or nonmatched designs and pre- and post-nonrandomized group designs are considered quasi-experimental designs. Randomized designs, or "true" experimental designs, include pretest and posttest control group designs, sometimes referred to as randomized control trials, randomized time series designs, or randomized factorial designs. Randomized designs by definition require that each participant have an equal opportunity to participate in the treatment condition or nontreatment control condition. The ability to scientifically demonstrate the relationship between the intervention or program and the outcome increases along a trajectory from nonexperimental to quasi-experimental to experimental research designs.

According to Campbell and Stanley (1963), by using randomization of subjects, workplaces, and communities, threats to invalidity such as history, maturation, testing, regression to the mean, selection process, mortality, and the interaction of these are eliminated. If the subjects are similar, what happens to one group of subjects is likely to happen to the other group. They will have similar world events affecting them, both groups will learn to the same degree from the instruments used to gather information, and they should have similar characteristics for change. The difference will be the intervention that one group receives. The concerns described above are referred to as threats to internal validity, that is, whether the results are valid to the groups that participated.

How applicable are the results to other groups outside those that participated in the intervention is a question that should be asked. Can you argue that the same effect will occur if a new group participates in the intervention? This is termed *external validity*, that is, how valid the results are to other groups. Unfortunately, randomization does not affect external validity.

Design Utilization Matrix

Studies of programs in the area of injury control and prevention were reviewed regarding their evaluation design (Table 9.2). Electronic search engines were used to collect programs conducted in the United States. Key words used in the primary search included *injury, prevention, intervention, program,* and *evaluation.* Furthermore, search terms used included specific injury mechanism (for example, *fall, fire,*

TABLE 9.2. DESIGN UTILIZATION MATRIX.

Mechanism/Cause	Nonexperimental	Quasi-Experimental	Experimental
Cut/pierce			
Drowning/submersion		Few	
Fall	Few	Some	Some
Fire/burn	Few	Few	Few
Firearm	Some	Some	Few
Machinery			
Motor vehicle traffic	Many	Few	Few
Pedal cyclist	Many	Many	Few
Pedestrian			Few
Transport		Few	Few
Natural/environmental			
Overexertion			
Poisoning	Some	Some	
Struck by, against			
Suffocation			
All injury	Few	Many	Few
All self-inflicted			Few
All assault			Few

Note: None: blank; few: 1–5; some: 6–10; many: 10 or more.

burn, machinery, transportation, and *poisoning*) and the behaviors or populations related to the specific injury mechanism (for example, *young driver, older driver, safety belt use,* and *bicycle helmet use*). Each program was reviewed to determine the method of research evaluation design used to assess program or intervention efficacy or effectiveness. Injury mechanism followed standard injury causes. Articles in each of these areas were classified as incorporating a nonexperimental evaluation design, a quasi-experimental research design, or an experimental research design.

The literature for the period 1995 to 2004 is reviewed in Table 9.2, as only electronic searches of Medline, PsycINFO, and PubMed were used. This review should not be viewed as a comprehensive literature review of research in this area. It should, however, be viewed as reflecting the trends in the choice of evaluation methodology used based on injury mechanism or cause. It is possible that many program evaluations never reach the published literature, which may also be true for intervention research with negative findings. Due to the limitations of our search, the number of studies have been hierarchically categorized into none, a few (one to five), some (six to ten), or many (ten or more).

Examining the design utilization matrix indicates that for road safety, including motor vehicle traffic injuries, pedestrian and bicycle injuries, and firearms and fire injuries, the evaluation methodology used has included nonexperimental, quasi-experimental, and experimental designs to evaluate prevention programs. Other areas such as poisoning and drowning have used less sophisticated evaluation methodologies to determine the effectiveness of prevention programs. One of the most interesting findings relates to the substantial void of cost-effectiveness and cost-benefit analyses conducted in the area of injury prevention programs. Although the search was not comprehensive, the lack of CEA and CBA on any evaluation measuring impact or outcome should be of concern.

Nonexperimental Design Examples

Firearms are frequently purchased with the intent that they will serve as protection against an intruder; as a result, they are often stored unlocked and loaded. In fact, both intentional and unintentional injuries and death by firearm are more likely to occur among family members or acquaintances. Recommended firearm safe storage practices dictate keeping the firearm stored unloaded, in a locked place, separate from ammunition, and secured with an extrinsic safety device.

A media campaign to raise awareness about safe storage practices for firearms and to distribute free gun locks was implemented in an urban county in North Carolina (Coyne-Beasley, Schoenbach, & Johnson, 2001). The "Love your kids, lock your guns" program was held in a Wal-Mart parking lot in October 1998. Preprogram promotions included press conferences, newspaper and television advertisements, radio public service announcements, and targeted announcements to community organizations and gun owners. The program aimed to educate gun owners about the risks of firearm injuries and appropriate gun-safe storage practices, train gun owners how to correctly use a gun lock safety device, and provide gun locks to program participants.

The program was evaluated in a nonexperimental, one-group pre- and posttest design. Participants were recruited on-site at the media event and asked to complete a baseline survey. The survey was adapted from the "Steps to Prevent Firearm Injury in the Home" program by the Center to Prevent Handgun Violence. Evaluation results were based on 112 gun owners who completed the baseline survey. Posttest measures were obtained six months following the program in a telephone interview with study participants. Gun lock use behavior, barriers to gun lock use, and general gun storage practices were assessed at posttest. Trained firearm safety counselors conducted pre- and posttest assessments. Results from baseline and posttest surveys were compared for changes in firearm storage practices. Reported gun storage in a locked compartment increased from 48 percent at baseline to 77 percent at posttest. In addition, 72 percent of participants reported using the gun lock at posttest.

There are only a few strengths when using a one-group pre- and posttest design. The strengths of this evaluation include issues of selection and mortality. The group is compared only to itself. Any selection bias is not an issue in the pre- and posttest comparison. The issue to losing participants will affect the posttest but not differentially. The results are very limited in scope, and there are a number of competitive possible reasons for the outcome of the posttest. These include issues of maturation of participants to learn from other events, historical events including the impact of North Carolina's child access prevention law for firearms, and learning from the pretest. The results are also based on self-reported measures at both baseline and follow-up, making the issue of testing effects an important one. There are a number of possible other reasons for the changes that cannot be attributed to the program. The next major limitation is that it cannot be generalized to any other group that has characteristics different from the test population. The program was implemented and evaluated in a single urban county in the southeast United States, which limits generalizing to other settings.

Quasi-Experimental Designs

A prospective, nonrandomized, controlled community intervention trial was conducted by Ebel, Koepsell, Bennett, and Rivara (2003) to evaluate the intervention implemented in twelve communities, with four communities serving as intervention sites and eight communities serving as control sites. The intervention and control communities were approximately matched on household per capita income and population size. Booster seat use in each community was observed at baseline just before beginning the intervention and again at fifteen months for the follow-up observation. The observations were conducted at eighty-three child care centers and after-school programs. Teams of two or more observers trained to assess the actual restraint use by the driver and all occupants conducted each observation. Information on child's age, weight, height, and distance from home was obtained from the driver's self-report. The difference in prevalence of observed booster seat use was compared between intervention communities and control communities, adjusted for child-level variables such as age and sex, car-level variables such as driver sex and driver seat belt use, and the effect of cluster sampling. Results indicated that fifteen months after the start of the campaign, the adjusted booster seat use had increased to 26.1 percent from 13.3 percent in the intervention communities and to 20.2 percent from 17.3 percent in the control communities ($p = .008$ for the difference in time trends between intervention and control communities).

The strengths of this evaluation design include using a control group and collecting booster seat use for each group at both the baseline and follow-up. This allowed controlling for the main effect of history, maturation, testing, and instrumentation (Campbell & Stanley, 1963). Using intervention and control communities approximately matched on household per capita income and population size also helped to minimize the difference between intervention and control groups at baseline. This evaluation design was theoretically driven. It involved coalition building, used focus groups to guide campaign messages and development, and included an evaluation of campaign effectiveness.

While design strengths are legion, a number of methodological limitations exist as well. The trial was conducted in three Northwest cities and therefore may not be generalizable to other regions of the country. It was a nonrandomized study, so there is the possibility of unmeasured or unidentifiable confounders. The design did not permit determination of which specific intervention components were most effective. Finally, the information on age, weight, and height of child was based on parents' self-report and may have been inaccurate.

Experimental Design

Older adults are disproportionately represented in all suicide deaths and are the most likely to die among all adults who attempt suicide. The majority of older adults who die by suicide have seen their physician within months of their death. Depression is common in later life; the prevalence of major to mild depression has been estimated at between 6 and 40 percent among older patients. Interventions that address depression among older adults in primary care settings may be useful for the prevention of late-life suicide and for suicide's precursor, suicidal ideation. A multisite, randomized trial known as PROSPECT (Prevention of Suicide in Primary Care Elderly: Collaborative Trial) aimed to reduce the risk for suicide in late life was conducted among patients age sixty and older recruited from twenty primary care practices in New York City, Philadelphia, and Pittsburgh regions from May 1999 through August 2001 (Bruce et al., 2004).

Two-stage, age-stratified depression screening of random sampling was used to recruit patients, with selection of primary care practice site at the first stage and selection of patient at the second stage. At the first stage, twenty primary care practices were randomly selected from greater New York City, Philadelphia, and Pittsburgh, with ten practices randomly assigned to intervention and ten to control. At the second stage, an age-stratified (ages sixty to seventy-four and over seventy-five) sample of patients was randomly drawn from an upcoming appointment in twenty selected practices. Patients who were age sixty years or older were able to give informed consent, had a Mini-Mental State Examination score of 18 or higher, were able to communicate in English, and had oral consent were screened for depression using the Centers for Epidemiologic Studies Depression scale (CES-D). Patients with a CES-D score higher than 20 as well as a 5 percent random sample of patients with lower scores were invited to enroll in the research protocol. The purpose of the 5 percent sample included was to assess for false-negative cases of screened depression. To increase the screen's sensitivity, patients scoring 20 or lower and not selected randomly were recruited if they responded positively to supplemental questions about prior depressive episodes or treatment.

Patients in the intervention group received treatment guidelines tailored for the elderly with care management, while patients in the control group received usual care. At baseline, both intervention and control group patients met at the practice with research associates who administered an in-person interview. These patients then received telephone assessments at the fourth and eighth months and an in-person interview at the twelfth month. All assessments were conducted independent of the treating clinicians. Rates of suicidal ideation and depression severity scores were assessed at baseline, as well as three follow-ups. The difference between intervention patients and control patients was compared.

The strengths of this evaluation design include using a randomized control trial and collecting rate of suicidal ideation and depression severity score for each group at baseline, as well as at four-month, eight-month, and twelve-month follow-ups. This evaluation design allowed controlling for the main effects of history, maturation, testing, instrumentation, regression, selection, and mortality. The methodology used in this evaluation also increased the relevance of PROSPECT's findings to real-world practice. Because it was conducted in a variety of practices, the sampling and screening procedures resulted in more heterogeneity than is generally achieved in randomized trials, and the protocol included patients regardless of factors that are typically excluded in most randomized controlled trials, such as mild cognitive impairment, medical comorbidity, concurrent medical treatments, or suicidal ideation. The limitation of this design was that only a small number of patients with minor depression who reported suicidal ideation benefited from the intervention due to the clinical utility that focused on patients with major depression.

Conclusion

This chapter introduced a number of research evaluation concepts related to injury prevention and control. It is important to acknowledge that numerous texts have been written on the topic of program evaluation as well as research design and associated methodology. This chapter was not designed to be comprehensive in addressing the area of evaluation or injury prevention. Rather, the chapter provides a broad overview of issues that researchers and practitioners working in the area of injury prevention and control need to consider when constructing a program evaluation as well as reading and interpreting the findings from empirical articles describing a program evaluation.

Our review found examples of the varying degrees of maturity of evaluations within different causes of injury. Although this was not a systematic review or meta-analysis, the findings, based on a survey of evaluation methods, indicate a continued need to develop evaluation methods specific to injury control. Some conclusions can be suggested for future evaluations. These include the increased need to conduct evaluations using experimental designs. The inclusion of cost-effectiveness and cost benefit studies for most evaluations is critical. The need to continue good formative and summative evaluation is something every practitioner needs to be involved in and comfortable with doing. The importance of being able to demonstrate the worth of a program is pivotal to sustaining efforts in the area of injury prevention and control.

References

Bhola, H. S. (1990). *Evaluating "Literacy for Development" projects, programs and campaigns: Evaluation planning, design and implementation, and utilization of evaluation results.* Hamburg: UNESCO Institute for Education, German Foundation for International Development.

Britt, J., Silver, I., & Rivara, F. P. (1998). Bicycle helmet promotion among low income preschool children. *Injury Prevention, 4,* 280–283.

Bruce, M. L., Ten Have, T. R., Reynolds, C. F., Schulberg, H. C., Mulsant, B. H., Brown, G. K., McAvay, G. J., Pearson, J. L., & Alexopoulos, G. S. (2004). Reducing suicidal ideation and depressive symptoms in depressed older primary care patients—A randomized controlled trial. *JAMA, 291*(9), 1081–1091.

Campbell, D. T., & Stanley, J. C. (1963). *Experimental and quasi-experimental designs for research.* Boston: Houghton Mifflin.

Coben, J. H., & Larkin, G. L. (1999). Effectiveness of ignition interlock devices in reducing drunk driving recidivism. *American Journal of Preventive Medicine, 16*(Suppl. 1), 81–87.

Coggan, C., Patterson, P., Brewin, M., Hooper, R., & Robinson, E. (2000). Evaluation of the Waitakere Community Injury Prevention Project. *Injury Prevention, 6,* 130–134.

Cook, T. D., & Campbell, D. T. (1979). *Quasi-experimentation: Design and analysis issues for field settings.* Skokie, IL: Rand McNally.

Coyne-Beasley, T., Schoenbach, V. J., & Johnson, R. M. (2001). Love our kids, lock your guns: A community-based firearm safety counseling and gun lock distribution program. *Archives of Pediatrics and Adolescent Medicine, 155*(6), 659–664.

Deal, L. W. (2000). Unintentional injuries in childhood. *Future of Children, 10*(1).

Dick, W., & Cary, L. (1990). *The systematic design of instruction* (3rd ed.). New York: HarperCollins.

Durkin, M. S., Laraque, D., Lubman, I., & Barlow, B. (1999). Epidemiology and prevention of traffic injuries in urban children and adolescents [Electronic version]. *Pediatrics, 103*(6). www.pediatrics.org.

Ebel, B. E., Koepsell, T. D., Bennett, E. E., & Rivara, F. P. (2003). Use of child booster seats in motor vehicles following a community campaign: A controlled trial. *JAMA, 289*(7), 879–884.

Foss, R. D., & Evenson, K. R. (1999). Effectiveness of graduated driver licensing in reducing motor vehicle crashes. *American Journal of Preventive Medicine, 16*(1S), 47–56.

Green, L. W., & Kreuter, M. W. (2005). *Health program planning: An educational and ecological approach* (4th ed.). New York: McGraw-Hill.

Grossman, D. C., & Garcia, C. C. (1999). Effectiveness of health promotion programs to increase motor vehicle occupant restraint use among young children. *American Journal of Preventive Medicine, 16*(Suppl. 1), 12–22.

Haddix, A. C., Mallonee, S., Waxweiler, R., & Douglas, M. R. (2001). Cost effectiveness analysis of a smoke alarm giveaway program in Oklahoma City, Oklahoma. *Injury Prevention, 7*(4), 276–281.

Harborview Injury Prevention and Research Center. (2005). *Best practices.* http://depts. washington.edu/hiprc/practices/index.html.

McArthur, D. L., & Kraus, J. F. (1999). The specific deterrence of administrative per se laws in reducing drunk driving recidivism. *American Journal of Preventive Medicine, 16*(1S), 68–75.

McDonald, E. M., Gielen, A. C., Trifiletti, L. B., Andrews, J. S., Serwint, J. R., & Wilson, M. E. (2003). Evaluation activities to strengthen an injury prevention resource center for urban families. *Health Promotion and Practice, 4*(2), 129–137.

Miller, T. R., & Levy, D. T. (2000). Cost-outcome analysis in injury prevention and control: Eighty-four recent estimates for the United States. *Medical Care, 38,* 562–582.

Myers, M. L., Cole, H. P., & Westneat, S. C. (2004). Cost-effectiveness of a ROPS retrofit education campaign. *Journal of Agricultural Safety and Health, 10,* 77–90.

Packard Foundation. (2000). Unintentional injuries in childhood. *The Future of Children, 10.*

Peek-Asa, C. (1999). The effect of random alcohol screening in reducing motor vehicle crash injuries. *American Journal of Preventive Medicine, 16*(Suppl. 1), 57–67.

Rivara, F. P., Thompson, D. C., Beahler, C., & MacKenzie, E. J. (1999). Systematic reviews of strategies to prevent motor vehicle injuries. *American Journal of Preventive Medicine, 16*(Suppl. 1), 1–5.

Rivara, F. R., Thompson, D. C., & Cummings, P. (1999). Effectiveness of primary and secondary enforced seat belt laws. *American Journal of Preventive Medicine, 16*(Suppl. 1), 30–39.

Robertson, M. C., Devlin, N., Scuffham, P., Gardner, M. M., Buchner, D. M., & Campbell, A. J. (2001). Economic evaluation of a community based exercise program to prevent falls. *Journal of Epidemiology and Community Health, 55,* 600–606.

Segui-Gomez, M. (1999). Evaluating interventions that promote the use of rear seats for children. *American Journal of Preventive Medicine, 16*(Suppl. 1), 23–29.

Segui-Gomez, M. (2000). Evaluating worksite-based interventions that promote safety belt use. *American Journal of Preventive Medicine, 18*(Suppl. 4), 11–22.

Spicer, R. S., Miller, T. R., Durkin, M. S., & Barlow, B. (2004). A benefit-cost analysis of the Harlem hospital injury prevention program. *Injury Control and Safety Promotion, 11,* 55–57.

Steckler, A., & Linnan, L. (Eds.). (2002). *Process evaluation for public health interventions and research.* San Francisco: Jossey-Bass.

Thompson, K. M., Segui-Gomez, M., & Graham, J. D. (2002). Validating benefit and cost estimates: The case of airbag regulation. *Risk Analysis, 22*(4), 803–811.

Vernick, J. S., Li, G., Ogaitis, S., MacKenzie, E. J., Baker, B. P., & Gielen, A. C. (1999). Effects of high school driver education on motor vehicle crashes, violations, and licensure. *American Journal of Preventive Medicine, 16*(Suppl. 1), 40–46.

Windsor, R., Baranowski, T., Clark, N., & Cutter, G. (1994). *Evaluation of health promotion, health education, and disease prevention programs.* Mountain View, CA: Mayfield.

Zaza, S., Sleet, D. A., Shults, P. A., Elder, R. W., Dinh-Zarr, T., Nichols, J. L., & Thompson, R. S. (2005). Reducing injuries to motor vehicle occupants. In S. Zaza, P. Briss, & K. Harris (Eds.), *The guide to community preventive services: What works to promote health?* New York: Oxford University Press.

Zwerling, C., & Jones, M. P. (1999). Evaluation of the effectiveness of low blood alcohol concentration laws for younger drivers. *American Journal of Preventive Medicine, 16*(1S), 76–80.

PART THREE

BEHAVIOR CHANGE INTERVENTIONS TO REDUCE INJURY RISK

CHAPTER TEN

BEHAVIOR CHANGE INTERVENTIONS IN ROAD SAFETY

Lawrence P. Lonero, Kathryn M. Clinton, David A. Sleet

What is dangerous driving? I have a tendency to believe that everyone's driving is dangerous, except my own.

—GEORGE BERNARD SHAW

Road safety has always experienced a strategic tension between engineering safer vehicles and roads and trying to influence people to behave more safely. This pattern is paralleled in public health. Passive health measures, such as immunization and water purification, had the greatest early impacts; now the major thrusts in public health are directed toward the promotion of health-related behaviors.

It is clear that efforts to improve safe behaviors on the road have lagged behind vehicle and environment changes as means for reducing injuries. However, crash prevention and safer driver behavior are becoming more critical as we reach the limits of passive protection (Martinez, 2000; Executive Committee of the Transportation Research Board, 2001). More intelligent cars and roads will support driver performance in new ways, but road safety progress is likely to stall unless road users are able to make a more active behavioral contribution themselves. To achieve this requires more effective approaches to influencing the behavior of individual road users, and these approaches in turn will require changes by government leaders and institutions that influence individual behavior (Gielen & Sleet, 2003). In this chapter, we describe the behavior-related tasks associated with driving and review strategies and methods for behavior change that can contribute to reducing motor vehicle deaths and injuries.

Driver Task Demands

Many task demands must be met to operate a motor vehicle safely and efficiently. The widely respected task analysis done by McKnight and colleagues (for example, McKnight & Hundt, 1971) identified as many as fifteen hundred task requirements for a driver behind the wheel. Lonero and colleagues emphasized the central importance of drivers' cognitive skills among a number of distinct traits and skills (Lonero et al., 1995). Seen in slightly modified form in Table 10.1 is a taxonomic

TABLE 10.1. DRIVER TRAIT AND SKILL CATEGORIES.

Category	Definition	Importance
Knowledge	Cognitive/memory: Experiences, facts, rules, principles, and expectations stored in long-term memory	Provides the background against which all perceptual and cognitive functions take place
Attention	Cognitive/perceptual: Controlling, dividing, and switching focus	Real-time management of cognitive resources and perceptual channel capacity, screening out distractions
Detection	Sensory-preattentional: Fixation, formation of images	Identifies changes in the environment that may need identification and evaluation
Perception	Sensory/cognitive: Processing images to extract meaning and produce schemata	Creates awareness and understanding of constantly changing situations
Evaluation	Cognitive/affective: Risk analysis of situation to produce outcome expectations, attributions	Estimates consequences and probabilities of alternative actions in the situation
Decision	Cognitive/affective: Matching options and motives	Selects optimal response: risk acceptance or rejection
Motor skill	Perceptual-motor: Integrating control actions	Execution of intended maneuvers
Imagination	Cognitive: Safety margin, anticipatory responses	Time, speed, and space choices
Motivation	Affective/social: Transient objectives, drives, needs, emotions	Prioritizes and balances a large and often conflicting set of goals and values
Responsibility	Cognitive/affective/cultural: Executive policy skills	Chooses goals and values, directs self-monitoring, consistently controls transient states

model of drivers' sensory, mental, and psychomotor functions. This is intended to indicate the relatively complex set of characteristics that must be considered in improving or changing driver behavior. The model also attempts to account for motivation, a common failure in earlier information-processing driver models (Ranney, 1994).

Lonero and Clinton (1998) pointed out the need to place traditional views of driver safety in a broader behavior change perspective. A first step is recognizing how complex and firmly established the factors that support current behavior are.

Driving behavior is resistant to change. Drivers have both abilities and motives. Perspectives on driver safety usually focus on ability or motives, but rarely both at the same time. Bower (1991) characterized the focus primarily on ability and capacity as "human factors." The human factors perspective sees the driver as an information processor interacting with and responding to the vehicle and environment. He or she is motivated to avoid mistakes but occasionally crashes due to errors of perception or judgment. (The human factors approach to road safety is comprehensively reviewed in Chapter Twenty-One, this volume.)

Changing Individual Behavior

Efforts to change individual behavior have been controversial in injury prevention, and road safety has not escaped this skepticism. While environmental change, rather than individual behavior change, has been seen as the most effective means to prevent injury, the U.S. National Committee for Injury Prevention and Control (1989) agreed that "education/behavior change interventions are less well known within the field of injury prevention. . . . These are interventions that respond to the fact that injuries result from both environmental and behavioral causes. Although 'passive' approaches are usually to be preferred to 'active' ones, it is difficult to envision an environmental change that is without any behavioral component" (p. 11).

We use the term *behavior change* to mean deliberate interventions that are intended to have lasting effects on people's overt actions, beyond some immediate situation, stimulus, or event. Traffic signals, speed bumps, rumble strips, and construction zone signing provide cues and prompts intended to alter drivers' behavior, but only temporarily and in the immediate vicinity. These distinctions cannot be rigid; for instance, behavioral psychologists may use cues and prompts quite effectively as part of broader behavior change programs. In fact, the concept of cues is essential to some behavior change theories, such as the health belief model (see Chapter Two, this volume).

The line between behavioral and engineering methods has become finer still (see Chapter Twenty-One, this volume). For example, nonenforcement speed control can now involve designing roads to produce desired behavior: narrower roads with tighter curves result in more appropriate driver behavior in residential areas. Especially in Europe (European Transport Safety Council, 1997), considerable effort is going into developing road designs that are "self-explaining," so that drivers develop appropriate expectations about what they will encounter (for example, slow-moving traffic, bicyclists) based on road features (Peden et al., 2004).

Behavior is complex and hard to change. Reflecting the challenge of planning effective behavior change programs is Sleet and Gielen's (1998) five-part prescription for effective education leading to behavior change. In order for injury prevention education and behavior change strategies to work, the audience must (1) be exposed to the information; (2) understand and believe the information; (3) have resources and skills to make the change; (4) derive benefit (or perceive a benefit) from the change; and (5) be reinforced to maintain the change. Not only must these factors be considered in planning and executing programs, they should be measured objectively and wherever possible assessed quantitatively, yet this is rarely done.

Both road safety and injury prevention have a common interest in influencing decision making, behavioral choices and protective behaviors, and common factors (if any) that drive them. Factors that might influence safety decisions include Wilde's hypothesized "relative value of future and present time" (2001) or Jessor's "problem behavior" syndrome (1987). These single-factor models suggest that low-risk road use may be strongly linked to other sources of the individual's well-being. At the same time, there are often inconsistencies within the behavior of an individual, with high-risk behaviors in some areas coexisting comfortably with low-risk behaviors in other areas (Wilde, 2001).

In a review of behavior change methods for road safety, Lonero et al. (1994) drew parallels and potential synergies between road safety and injury prevention:

> Both road safety and injury prevention need better understanding of the behavioral dynamics leading to injury in order to refine behavior-change approaches. . . . A number of injury prevention experts emphasized the importance of social norms in determining behaviors and of multifaceted, community-oriented programs for changing them. Similarly, there is emphasis on the need for better means of training risk recognition, of creating "risk literacy." . . . There are useful examples of intensive training and community programs, some of which, such as bicycle helmet use, are directly relevant to and overlap with road safety. The boundary between the two fields will likely continue to blur further. If this leads to planned synergy among programs and further sharing of resources, both fields can benefit [p. 183].

There is little argument that most injuries could have been avoided if different behaviors had preceded the event. Unfortunately, it is much harder to change a behavior than it is to change a technology. Some injury prevention profession-als fear that placing an emphasis on behavior is tantamount to blaming the vic-tim (Baker, 1981; Robertson, 1987), but as Gielen and Sleet (2003) point out, health promotion can often lead to citizen demand for technological and envi-ronmental change. In addition, with many injuries, the critical behaviors may be outside the victim's control. Behavior, technology, and environmental change work best when they work together. Today there is reasonable consensus that a balanced approach should contain behavioral, environmental, and technological change.

Comprehensive Behavior Change Approaches

Aside from drivers, influencing healthier, safer, and more environmentally sus-tainable behaviors has been a major societal challenge. Changing human behav-ior on a large scale is complex, in part because even simple human behaviors are determined by a complex mix of background and context factors: biological, psy-chological, economic, political, and sociocultural. In recent years, however, con-siderable progress in understanding behavior change has occurred, much of it from the field of health promotion. Comprehensive approaches have developed that may influence road safety (Howat, Sleet, Elder, & Maycock, 2004; see also Chapter Two, this volume).

There is a great deal to be learned about efforts to change individual behav-ior from successes in other fields. Sleet (1987) first proposed that road safety could benefit from use of the comprehensive PRECEDE-PROCEED health promotion model (Green & Kreuter, 2005; Green, Kreuter, Deeds, & Partridge, 1980). Green and Kreuter's PRECEDE-PROCEED and other health promotion models and programs (see Chapter Six, this volume) incorporate three broad groupings of fac-tors that are believed to have an impact on behavior:

- *Predisposing* factors—people's or populations' knowledge, attitudes, beliefs, val-ues, perceptions, and motivation for change
- *Enabling* factors—the skills, resources, or barriers that can help or hinder the desired change, be it behavioral or environmental, created mainly by societal forces or systems
- *Reinforcing* factors—the rewards and feedback from others after behavior change, which will support or frustrate the maintenance of the behavior

Individual safety choices are complexly determined. A simple single-factor model will have limited value in predicting behavior or guiding behavior change. More efforts are needed to uncover the critical factors that predispose, enable, and reinforce individual behaviors in road safety and other areas of injury prevention (Sleet & Gielen, 2004).

Using Antecedents and Consequences

Reinforcement was the term used by Lonero et al. (1994) to cover an eclectic variety of incentives and other methods derived from applied behavioral analysis. These were referred to as "nonpunitive" countermeasures by Donelson and Mayhew (1987). These methods represent the behavioral psychologists' technologies applied to road user behavior change (Sleet & Lonero, 2003). The basic theory is that antecedent conditions and consequences control, support, maintain, or influence behavior.

Antecedent influences include the cues, prompts, and other environmental conditions that elicit or trigger a given behavior. Relatively little is known scientifically about the natural antecedents for driver behavior, but carefully designed artificial conditions, such as cues and prompts (reminders), can be effective parts of influence programs for drivers. This has been shown by Van Houten and colleagues in Canada (Malenfant & Van Houten, 1989; Van Houten, Malenfant, & Rolider, 1985), and Geller and colleagues in the United States (Chapter Fourteen, this volume). Effectiveness was shown in a variety of pilot projects addressed to driver behaviors, ranging from seat belt use to yielding to pedestrians. Incentives, which are anticipated rewards, are a particularly powerful antecedent influence on behavior.

Consequences occur after the behavior and include feedback and rewards, as well as punishment. The Lonero et al. (1994) review concluded that behavioral reinforcement techniques are potentially powerful influences, but while widely and effectively used in private fleet management, they are little used in governmental driver programs. Finding practical ways to transfer these technologies to operational programs was seen as a high priority. A carefully designed, systematic series of experiments in California (Harano & Hubert, 1974) explored the use of various reward and incentive schemes with drivers, with mixed results. In one particularly interesting outcome, a poor choice of reward conditions seemed to make drivers worse. It is clear that properly designed incentives can have a positive effect on drivers' safety performance, as has often been demonstrated among employee drivers in industry (Wilde, 2001).

The concept of reinforcing internal controls has significant potential for influencing drivers. It is based on the premise that well-designed behavioral strategies will help build internalized control for long-term self-management and improvement of behavior (see Chapter Fourteen, this volume). A health behavior strategy approach (Elder, Ayala, & Harris, 1999) concluded: "Specifically, individual self-management skills in goal setting, self-monitoring, self-evaluation, and self-reinforcement will translate not only into maintenance of behavior change but also into an ability to generalize that behavior change to novel stimulus conditions and other behaviors. . . . Self-management is critical for long-term behavior change" (p. 280).

In addition to the behavior analysis perspective, there are other ways to look at the effects of outcomes, or expected outcomes, on behavior. Useful perspectives are provided by economic utility, decision theory, and game theory models. These describe the relation between the choices of an individual and the probability of a particular outcome and the value placed on that outcome by the individual. These approaches look at information inputs and outputs with little reference to attitudes or other theoretical processes inside the person (Lonero et al., 1994).

From various theoretical and practical perspectives, behavior-analytic reinforcement techniques may represent a promising future direction for driver improvement program development. Following is a brief overview of some tools for driver behavior change, including the importance of a program mix of law, enforcement, education, and reinforcement.

Legislation and Behavior

Legislation is the most important component of the cultural package that determines how drivers perform on the roads. Shaw and Ogolla (Chapter Twenty, this volume) describe clearly how law and behavior are interconnected. Legislation expresses society's values and expectations and lays down the formal rules for behavior on the public roads. Laws have two main influence functions: the declarative function of law communicates expected standards of behavior, and the deterrent function of law imposes sanctions for those whose behavior violates the standards. Deterrence can work in two ways: special deterrence keeps people who offend the law from doing it again, and general deterrence prevents people from breaking the law in the first place.

Bonnie (1986) quoted B. F. Skinner, who observed that rules sometimes derive from hazards and are part of society's way of telling its citizens to learn from the mistakes of others. This is necessary because people do not directly experience the outcomes of the risks others have taken (Rumar, 1988).

While it is clear that law can have a major impact on behavior, and thus crashes and injuries, desirable effects are by no means automatic. This was made clear by the Organisation for Economic Cooperation and Development's paper (OECD Scientific Expert Group, 1990) on behavioral adaptation to safety countermeasures, which points out that there are often negative, perverse effects from law as drivers "adapt" to change. Informal rules in driving culture often predominate and may bear limited resemblance to the formal rules (for example, posted speed limits versus average driving speeds). Research and theory on behavioral adaptation to safety measures has continued (Jiang, Underwood, & Howarth, 1992; Traynor, 1993), although the concept remains controversial (Wilde, 2001).

Licensing and Behavior

Most licensing-related actions take place within the framework of administrative law. Less relevant is civil law, especially given the widespread movement to no-fault insurance. The incentive effects of the threat of civil liability have probably been diminished by no-fault insurance (Cummins & Weiss, 1999). Reviews of studies from California and internationally (McKnight & Voas, 1991; Peck, 1991; Ross, 1991b) concluded that license actions have succeeded better than any other to change drinking and driving behavior. While most drivers with suspended licenses continue to drive (Peck, 1991; Ross, 1991a) and they have higher-than-average crash risk (Griffin & DeLaZerda, 2000), suspended drivers (apparently) drive more carefully than they would otherwise because of their suspended status (Hurst, 1980). According to Hurst's hypothesis, the longer the license is suspended, the more practice drivers have with careful, inconspicuous driving. This would explain why longer suspensions for driving-while-intoxicated drivers are more effective for reducing subsequent collisions, while longer jail sentences are not (Mann, Vingilis, Gavin, Adlaf, & Anglin, 1991; Voas, 1986).

Many jurisdictions have adopted administrative license revocation (ALR) for drinking drivers (Williams, Weinberg, & Fields, 1991), and there is ample evidence it works (Chapter Eleven, this volume; McArthur & Kraus, 1999). The immediacy of these actions (suspension on the spot) is likely responsible for their effectiveness and contrasts with other measures with long delays between infraction and punishment. Unfortunately, many locations offer education or treatment in lieu of license suspensions, which removes the infraction from the driving record. The Presidential Commission on Drunk Driving recommended that such diversionary programs be eliminated (Nichols, 1990).

Enforcement and Behavior

Enforcement threat is the sharp end of the legal stick. Visible enforcement on the roads has long been considered basic support for road safety (Lonero et al., 1994). Evaluations have suggested that enforcement on its own may not have as much impact as has been traditionally assumed, at least over the short term (Hauer, Ahlin, & Bowser, 1982; Shinar & McKnight, 1985; Shinar & Stiebel, 1986). Over the long term, it seems plausible that enforcement threat may have influenced the informal driving norms and drivers' habits that form current driving cultures. In their overview of the enforcement evaluation literature, Bjornskau and Elvik (1992) concluded that the effects of enforcement are local and transient in nature and that no studies show that traditional enforcement alone produces a permanent change in violation rates.

By itself, traffic enforcement suffers from many limitations. First, it is almost exclusively connected with punishment, and punishment is a relatively weak behavior modifier (Friedland, Trebilcock, & Roach, 1990; Geller et al., 1990; Mann et al., 1991; Moskowitz, 1989). Second, there are severe limits to the intensity of surveillance that can be maintained (Ross, 1985) to support enforcement-influenced behavior, at least by conventional, nonautomated means (Rothengatter, 1991). Heavy enforcement pressure, such as random breath testing programs, and selective traffic enforcement programs have shown significant impacts on driving while impaired (Canadian Council of Motor Transport Administrators, 1990; Hingson, Swahn, & Sleet, 2006; Elder et al., 2004; Dussault, 1990). Low levels of enforcement have long been seen as a problem, as Peck (1992) suggested: "All things being equal, the accuracy of risk assessments and the net impact of the countermeasures will increase as a function of the volume of traffic citations (or accidents) that are issued or reported to DMV [Department of Motor Vehicles]. The traffic enforcement level of many states is very poor, resulting in low volumes of traffic citations and minimal investigations and reporting of accidents" (p. 20).

Rothengatter (1997) reflected the concern for weak enforcement levels in Europe by noting that below a certain level, enforcement is inconsequential; increases or decreases will not affect driver behavior, and in Europe "normal levels of police enforcement are indeed below that level" (p. 230).

Bjornskau and Elvik's meta-analysis (1992) of speed enforcement and Engel's analyses (1980) concluded that by simply increasing enforcement, little effect was seen on violations, and the public did not notice the changes in patrol intensity. Perhaps a three to five times increase in enforcement is the minimum that drivers will notice, at least without heavy publicity (Lonero et al., 1995).

There may be a number of reasons for decreases in enforcement seen recently in North America. Rippey (1999) identified the following concerns regarding Ontario traffic policing and enforcement:

- Fragmentation and lack of coordination of traffic enforcement
- The subordination of traffic safety in the mandates of the police community
- Possible deprofessionalizing or privatizing traffic policing
- Poor training and morale in traffic police
- Loss of specialist expertise
- Lack of standards for traffic policing and accident investigation

- Loss of crash data quality and quantity due to reduced police collision reporting
- Inappropriate and inconsistent fines
- Resistance to automated enforcement technology

Programs to Improve Driver Behavior

Many specific measures are implemented within the framework of driver improvement, including warning letters, individual interviews, group classes or educational remediation, and driving ability retests. License suspension and the threat of it are at the core of traditional driver improvement programs. A recent review by Lonero et al. (in press) provides an update of recent evaluation research and program practice. Evaluations of administrative driver improvement (ADI) actions other than suspension are inconsistent, but some have shown surprisingly strong effects from modest measures, such as warning letters and home study packages.

For a number of years, California ran ongoing evaluation experiments with a rotating control group continuously being shielded for comparison purposes from driver improvement actions that were being evaluated. California dropped the continuous evaluation structure in 1995 as a result of political and liability concerns. It seems to be acceptable to not know whether a program is effective but not acceptable to withhold the program from a small group of randomly chosen drivers. Of course, most jurisdictions do no empirical evaluation of their programs. Relatively little progress has been made in innovative application of behavior change to driver improvement programs in the past two decades. In fact, driver improvement as a behavior change strategy may have moved backward.

Most research in driver improvement took place in the 1960s and 1970s. Support for the utility of warning letters was found in California and Oregon, but other states found them ineffective. Studies confirmed that individual hearings could result in lower subsequent conviction rates, and California found reductions in crashes. One study found that drivers most amenable to treatment were collision-involved drivers with a minimum of convictions, which suggests matching drivers with different, tailored programs (Donelson & Mayhew, 1987).

Donelson and Mayhew (1987) also identified differences in results of different types of group meetings. The defensive driving course reduced violations but not crashes. Other driver reeducation courses have generally failed to improve driver performance. Group meetings that emphasized attitude change were shown to have positive effects on subsequent violations and crashes.

The once-optimistic driver improvement movement has slowed. In fact, the impact of ADI programs has actually diminished due to lack of evaluation, reductions in enforcement, and the diversion of offenders from modestly effective ADI programs into clearly ineffective private violator schools. (Lonero et al., in press). There is little reason to think that current driver behavior change programs are effective in reducing crashes or injuries.

Education and Behavior

Education provides an important avenue to influence behavior. It can provide a supplement to laws and policies or be used to reinforce desirable behaviors. It can also be used to teach and improve skills. The aspects of education most relevant to road safety are driver education, on-road driver skill acquisition and training, school-based safety training, and public education programs. What makes educational techniques effective is well known in theory, but rarely is it put into practice in road safety (Cirillo, Council, Griffith, Hauer, & Paniati, 2000; Elder et al., 2004).

While education appears to be a popular prescription for improving safety, demonstrated effectiveness in improving drivers' safety through education alone is rare. Aside from relevant knowledge and skills, safe road user behavior needs community support, social norms and models, environmental cues and prompts, and external incentives and disincentives. Knowledge and skills are necessary but not sufficient for safe behavior, and without motivation and social support, people do not always choose safer behaviors (Orleans, Gruman, Ulmer, Emont, & Hollendonner, 1999).

Driver Education and Training

After a number of years of relative obscurity, driver education and training seems to be developing rapidly. Graduated licensing implies multistage training and has shown positive effects in reducing teen driver crashes (Lonero et al., 1995; Simons-Morton & Hartos, 2002). It combines controlled exposure and on-road practice with education and training.

Technology changes, such as computer-based instruction and simulation, are also changing driver education and training (Brock, 1997). More individualized and self-paced instruction, with active involvement of peers and parents, is seen as promising (see Chapter Three, this volume). Especially in the United States, traditional driver education in high schools is being replaced by private driving schools, some associated with motor vehicle manufacturers or insurance companies. Integration of driver education with other motoring services and establishment of ongoing relationships with drivers may permit a version of lifelong learning for drivers (Smiley, Lonero & Chipman, 2004).

The impact of advanced driver training suffers from the fact that increased skill does not automatically lead to safer driving. In a review of fourteen evaluations of the Defensive Driving Course in the United States, Lund and Williams (1985) pointed out that the better-controlled studies were the ones that showed no effect on collisions. The course did impart knowledge, and there was a moderate effect on violations (a decline of 10 percent). Numerous evaluations of specialized car handling training suggest the counterintuitive conclusion that raising levels of these skills may lead to a *higher* crash risk (Jones, 1993; OECD Scientific Expert Group, 1990; Siegrist & Ramseier, 1992).

Not all advanced skill training actually increases the targeted skill, let alone some consequent measure of safety. Gregersen's slippery road training with young drivers showed increases in confidence without any increase in skill (Gregersen & Bjurulf, 1996). Unfortunately, most training evaluations have not looked at intermediate effects, such as changes in skill or confidence.

The current trend in technology suggests that vehicle usability may get worse before it gets better (Sharfman & Lonero, 1999; Smiley, 2000). For example, the rapid penetration of antilock braking systems (ABS) into the vehicle fleet reduced the need for a key driver skill component, threshold braking, while adding a new skill, continuous braking pressure, and it required drivers to "unlearn" pumping the brakes to achieve braking control.

People may also adapt to changes in technology in unexpected ways. For instance, navigation systems intended to improve travel time appear to navigate drivers onto residential roads to avoid congestion on main roads, posing greater risks for pedestrians (Smiley, 2000). Better brakes have led drivers to follow too close (Sagberg, Fosser, & Saetermo, 1997). Aids such as adaptive cruise control and collision warning devices may cause drivers to engage in more distracting tasks while driving. The societal context for driver improvement is changing rapidly, and driver education and training must develop as rapidly as vehicle technology.

School-Based Education

Evaluations of school-based road safety education for young children have been primarily focused on pedestrian skills and behavior, with some attention being given to bicycling, bicycle helmet use, and seat belt use. A review by Michon (1981) concluded that (1) effective programs are those limited to traffic tasks that are performed frequently and are relatively most dangerous; (2) traffic education for young children should aim at skill development rather than knowledge acquisition; (3) realistic training environments are essential; (4) positive reinforcement is important to the effectiveness of training; and (5) parent participation is a major requirement for an effective program. Ampofo-Boateng and Thomson (1989) also concluded that simulations and participative skill training are "by far the most promising approach to road safety training" (p. 267), with realistic simulation being extremely effective with younger children (those five to six years old).

Cross and Pitkethly (1991) tried an unusual approach to improving road safety abilities in young children. They hypothesized that children's concept of speed led to erratic road crossing behavior. A teaching unit on speed was incorporated into the primary science curriculum in two schools in Melbourne, Australia. In real-life situations, significantly more trained children correctly judged the speed of oncoming vehicles. The authors suggested that educational programs should target children's conceptual frameworks in developmentally appropriate ways.

Preusser and colleagues (Preusser & Blomberg, 1984; Preusser & Lund, 1988) succeeded in conducting a landmark series of pilot education programs to change road crossing behavior in children. These programs were constructed according to a clear set of educational and behavior change principles and were found to change crossing behavior and pedestrian crashes. Despite successful pilot results, the program was never implemented.

Educational programs are an important part of developing a safer road culture, but there still exists a noticeable gap between educational theory and the practice of road safety education. Routine programs need to be examined, evaluated, and improved to take advantage of theory and established principles of effective school-based education.

Mass Communications

Driving behavior may be influenced by the media and by the driving culture—that is, the common practices, expectations, and informal rules that drivers learn by observation from others in their communities. Driving-related information in the media comes through:

- Explicit advertising messages, whether paid or public service
- Deliberately placed public relations by commercial businesses, trade and lobbying groups, and nonprofit public service organizations
- Multimedia campaigns
- News coverage of collisions, technical developments, legislative and regulatory mandates, litigation, and political matters

Mass media often encompass interactive features of the local environments and media advocacy "as a means of mobilizing social and political support for policy and regulatory changes" (Green & Kreuter, 1999, p. 78; see also Chapter Five, this volume).

Much effort and many resources have been dedicated to influence drivers' behavior through paid or public service advertising. Lonero et al. (1994) concluded that public education and advertising promotions have limited demonstrable effect on their own, but that they have a strong role to play in supporting broader behavior change efforts.

Communications researchers have identified critical factors affecting message effectiveness. Four principal elements in mass media communication that determine effectiveness have been identified by Wilde (1993) and others:

- *Source*—Credibility, expertise, trustworthiness, and similarity to the recipient
- *Content*—Close to recipient's views, positive message presented first, concrete effectiveness, personally relevant, modeling and imitation, arousing attention, motivating appeals, not humor or fear
- *Channel of communication*—Selection of medium, rates of exposure, immediacy to targeted behavior
- *Recipient*—Self-selected exposure to medium, opinion leaders and followers, conspicuous target behavior, multistage communication through personal influence, persuadability, reactance

Rather than telling us what to think, media communications can establish agendas, telling us what to think about. Wilde (1993) conceives of the media audience as "active decision makers" rather than "passive message absorbers."

Yanovitzky and Bennett (1999) confirmed a strong (but indirect) effect of communication campaigns on driver behavior: "Public communication campaigns aimed at regulating people's behavior may be more successful in meeting their goals if they focus on promoting actions by social institutions rather than targeting at risk individuals with persuasive messages. . . . In doing so, it is also important to recognize that human behavior change is likely to be slow and gradual rather than rapid and substantial" (p. 447).

In addition to targeted communications in the media, news reporting may affect public perception and lead to behavior change. Wilde and Ackersviller (1981) experimentally altered the newspaper treatment of local collisions in Kingston, Ontario. The human interest context of the crash was highlighted, along with general safety information. Surveys before and after showed that the public in Kingston had changed their perception of road safety. No change was seen in a control community. Lonero et al. (1994) suggested finding approaches to the recruitment and training of local, regional, and national media on how to cover road safety more effectively.

News reporting may engender support for legal and policy actions to support road safety. Tyler and Cook (1984) showed that even conventional media coverage influenced risk-related judgments at the societal but not personal level. This may help explain findings that information programs can change attitudes toward legislation without changing compliance with the targeted behavior (Lonero et al., 1994).

A more recent example of mass communications efforts in Victoria, Australia, demonstrates the need to "market traffic safety as a consumer product." The program developers concluded: "All the evidence suggests that when the ads are off-air, the road toll goes up. And when the ads are back on-air, the road toll goes down. We are beginning to conclude that road safety is not a rational considered-purchase decision. Road safety is an impulse decision that requires constant, high, top-of-mind product promotion" (Forsyth & Ogden, 1993, p. 1440).

Social marketing approaches can be understood from a behavioral psychology perspective, where the ads act as cues and prompts, reminding drivers frequently about the choices they have to drive more safely.

New Perspectives

Changing behavior does not necessarily require understanding every detail of the reasons and causes for the behavior in every individual. However, a reasonably comprehensive and detailed understanding of the influences that support current behavior is necessary. One such approach, context theory, has been used to explain how minor and superficial changes in local communities in New York City altered behavioral expectations and, it is argued, contributed to the reduction of crime rates (Gladwell, 2000). Could such subtle changes in context alter the driving behavior of drivers? We may not yet know all of the potential interventions that could leverage drivers' behavior change. The trend to larger, quieter, more powerful vehicles may influence driving actions. A context or driving culture in which there are increasing numbers of unpunished violations such as red light running could induce additional drivers to commit similar violations, making stepped-up (or automated) enforcement critical in the future.

The practical purpose of a theory, model, or philosophy is to provide a set of assumptions and rules that lead to better decisions. We can base intervention programs on either explicit theory (behavioral, economic, or educational) or common sense. Common sense, as a framework for changing behavior, has not succeeded (Haight, 1985), and "feel good" programs (Waller, 1992) are no longer acceptable alternatives to evidence-based approaches (Task Force on Community Preventive Services, 2005; Zaza et al., 2001). The use of a social-psychological approaches to predicting and influencing injury prevention behavior (see Chapter Two, this volume) holds promise for the future of driver improvement (Lonero et al., 1994). However, most programs have not been given a fair chance to succeed and have not been designed using the best behavior change techniques. The practice of designing road safety programs for administrative convenience rather than for safety impact must be discontinued (Donelson & Mayhew, 1987).

Conclusions

Both unhealthy and unsafe behaviors are established by many strong, and perhaps redundant, influences. Cross-fertilization of theories and practical ideas from different fields may help drivers change unsafe habits and tendencies. Effective driver improvement and behavior change tools must develop congruently with the contemporary changes in vehicle technology, roads, and driving environments. As driver attitudes and demographics shift, so must the use of behavioral strategies. There is an apparently widespread belief that changing the way that people drive is simply a matter of increasing awareness and that it therefore should be relatively easy (Haight, 1985). This belief unfortunately is not correct, and it has greatly hindered road safety progress.

As the global impact of road traffic injury becomes better known, the demand for more effective interventions will increase (Sleet & Branche, 2004). Significant time and resources have been spent worldwide in search of effective behavior change strategies for traffic safety, yet no single behavior change initiative, or even class of them, has emerged as a panacea. Of course, theory must be at the heart of any behavior change program affecting driver performance. Moreover, what is needed is a varied portfolio of program components that takes advantage of the additive contributions that legislation, enforcement, education, behavior change, and communications make to safer road travel. Driver improvement programs need to be revamped rather than simply withdrawn or diverted. Mashaw and Harfst (1990) suggested that there might be new market-driven strategies to advance road safety, such as incentives, which are less abrasive to personal freedom. In the longer term, it will be necessary to raise the level of safety coordination and restructure organizational incentives to achieve such improvements. A new model must also consider various definitions of safety improvement. Important intermediate outcomes, including changes in infrastructure, cultural norms, driver and pedestrian knowledge, attitudes, intentions, and motivations, as well as specific behaviors, will enhance safety practices of drivers, passengers, and pedestrians.

References

Ampofo-Boateng, K., & Thomson, J. A. (1989). Child pedestrian accidents: A case for preventive medicine. *Health Education Research, 5*(2), 265–274.

Baker, S. P. (1981, Sept.). Childhood injuries: The community approach to prevention. *Journal of Public Health Policy,* 236–246.

Bjornskau, T., & Elvik, R. (1992). Can road traffic law enforcement permanently reduce the number of accidents? *Accident Analysis and Prevention, 24*(5), 507–520.

Bonnie, R. (1986). The efficacy of law as a paternalistic instrument. In G. Melton (Ed.), *Nebraska symposium on human motivation, 1985: The law as a behavioral instrument* (pp. 131–211). Lincoln: University of Nebraska Press.

Bower, G. H. (1991). Incentive programs for promoting safer driving. In M. J. Koornstra & J. Christensen (Eds.), *Enforcement and rewarding: Strategies and effects. Proceedings of the International Road Safety Symposium in Copenhagen, Denmark, Sept. 19–21, 1990.* Leidschendam, The Netherlands: SWOV Institute for Road Safety Research.

Brock, J. (1997). Computer-based instruction. In G. Salvendy (Ed.), *Handbook of human factors and ergonomics* (2nd ed.). New York: John Wiley.

Canadian Council of Motor Transport Administrators. (1990). *National Occupant Restraint Program.* Ottawa, Ontario: Ministers Responsible for Transportation and Highway Safety.

Cirillo, J. A., Council, F. M., Griffith, M. S., Hauer, E., & Paniati, J. F. (2000). *Making safety management knowledge based.* Washington, DC: Transportation Research Board, Committee on Safety Data, Analysis, and Evaluation.

Cross, R. T., & Pitkethly, A. (1991). Concept modification approach to pedestrian safety: A strategy for modifying young children's existing conceptual framework of speed. *Research in Science and Technological Education, 9*(1), 93–106.

Cummins, J. D., & Weiss, M. A. (1999). The incentive effects of no fault automobile insurance. In G. Dionne & C. Laberge-Nadeau (Eds.), *Automobile insurance: Road safety, new drivers, risks, insurance fraud and regulation* (pp. 283–308). Norwell, MA: Kluwer.

Donelson, A. C., & Mayhew, D. R. (1987). *Driver improvement as post-licensing control: The state of knowledge.* Toronto: Ontario Ministry of Transportation and Communications.

Dussault, C. (1990). Effectiveness of a selective traffic enforcement program combined with incentives for seat belt use in Quebec. *Health Education Research, 5*(2), 217–223.

Elder, J. P., Ayala, G. X., & Harris, S. (1999). Theories and interventions approaches to health-behavior change in primary care. *American Journal of Preventive Medicine, 17*(4), 275–284.

Elder, R. E., Shults, R., Sleet, D. A., Nichols, J., Zaza, S., Thompson, R. S., & Compton, R. (2002). Effectiveness of sobriety checkpoints for reducing alcohol-involved crashes. *Traffic Injury Prevention, 3*, 266–274.

Elder, R. W., Shults, R. A., Sleet, D. A., Nichols, J. L., Thompson, R. S., & Rajab, W. (2004). Task Force on Community Preventive Services. Effectiveness of mass media campaigns for reducing drinking and driving and alcohol involved crashes: A systematic review. *American Journal of Preventive Medicine, 27*(1), 57–65.

Engel, R. (1980). *Summary of traffic enforcement literature.* Ottawa: Solicitor General of Canada.

European Transport Safety Council. (1997). *A strategic road safety plan for the European Union.* Brussels: European Transport Safety Council.

Executive Committee of the Transportation Research Board. (2001). Critical issues in transportation 2002. *TR News, 217*, 3–11.

Forsyth, I., & Ogden, E.J.D. (1993). Marketing traffic safety as a consumer product in Victoria, Australia. In H. D. Utzelmann, G. Berghaus, & G. Kroj (Eds.), *Alcohol, drugs and traffic safety–T'92: Proceedings of the 12th International Conference* (pp. 1437–1442). Cologne, Germany: Verlag TUV Rheinland.

Friedland, M. L., Trebilcock, M., & Roach, K. (1990). Regulating traffic safety. In M. L. Friedland (Ed.), *Securing compliance: Seven case studies* (pp. 165–324). Toronto, Ontario: University of Toronto Press.

Geller, E. S., Berry, T. D., Ludwig, T. D., Evans, R. E., Gilmore, M. R., & Clarke, S. W. (1990). A conceptual framework for developing and evaluating behavior change interventions for injury control. *Health Education Research, 5*(2), 125–137.

Gielen, A. C., & Sleet, D. (2003). Application of behavior change theories and methods to injury prevention. *Epidemiologic Reviews, 25,* 65–76.

Gladwell, M. (2000). *The tipping point. How little things can make a big difference.* Boston: Little, Brown.

Green, L. W., & Kreuter, M. W. (1999). *Health promotion planning: An educational and ecological approach* (3rd ed.). Mountain View, CA: Mayfield.

Green, L. W., & Kreuter, M. W. (2005). *Health program planning: An educational and ecological approach* (4th ed.). New York: McGraw-Hill.

Green, L. W., Kreuter, M. W., Deeds, S. G., & Partridge, K. B. (1980). *Health education planning: A diagnostic approach.* Mountain View, CA: Mayfield.

Gregersen, N. P., & Bjurulf, P. (1996). Young novice drivers: Towards a model of their accident involvement. *Accident Analysis and Prevention, 28*(2), 229–241.

Griffin, L. I., & DeLaZerda, S. (2000). *Unlicensed to kill.* Washington, DC: AAA Foundation for Traffic Safety.

Haight, F. A. (1985). Road safety: A perspective and a new strategy. *Journal of Safety Research, 16*(3), 91–98.

Harano, R. M., & Hubert, D. E. (1974). *An evaluation of California's "Good Driver" Incentive Program* (Rep. No. 6). Sacramento: California Department of Motor Vehicles.

Hauer, E., Ahlin, F. J., & Bowser, J. S. (1982). Speed enforcement and speed choice. *Accident Analysis and Prevention, 14*(4), 267–278.

Howat, P., Sleet, D. A., Elder, R., & Maycock, B. (2004). Preventing alcohol-related traffic injury: A health promotion approach. *Traffic Injury Prevention, 5*(3), 208–219.

Hingson, R., Swahn, M., & Sleet, D. A. (2006). Alcohol and injuries. In L. Doll, J. Mercy, S. Bonzo, & D. Sleet (Eds.), *Handbook for injury and violence prevention.* New York: Kluwer.

Hurst, P. M. (1980). Can anyone reward safe driving? *Accident Analysis and Prevention, 12,* 217–220.

Jessor, R. (1987). Risky driving and adolescent problem behavior: An extension of problem-behavior theory. *Alcohol, Drugs and Driving, 3*(3–4), 1–11.

Jiang, C., Underwood, G., & Howarth, C. I. (1992). Towards a theoretical model for behavioural adaptations to changes in the road transport system. *Transport Reviews, 12*(3), 253–264.

Jones, B. (1993). *The effectiveness of skid-car training for teenage novice drivers in Oregon.* Salem: Oregon Department of Motor Vehicles.

Nansel, T. R., Weaver, N., Donlin, M., Jacobsen, H., Kreuter, M. W., & Simons-Morton, B. (2002). Baby, be safe: The effect of tailored communications for pediatric injury prevention provided in primary care setting. *Patient Education and Counseling, 46*(3), 175–190.

Lonero, L., & Clinton, K. (1998). *Changing road user behavior: What works and what doesn't.* Toronto: PDE Publications,

Lonero, L., Clinton, K., Brock, J., Wilde, G., Laurie, I., & Black, D. (1995). *Novice driver education model curriculum outline.* Washington, DC: AAA Foundation for Traffic Safety.

Lonero, L. P., Clinton, K., Mayhew, D. R., Peck, R. C., Smiley, A. M., & Black, D. R. (in press). *Driver improvement programs, state of knowledge and trends: Report 1: Review and Jurisdiction Survey.* Ottawa, Transport Canada, Société de L'Assurance Automobile du Québec.

Lonero, L. P., Clinton, K. M., Wilde, G.J.S., Roach, K., McKnight, A. J., MacLean, H., Guastello, S. J., & Lamble, R. (1994). *The roles of legislation, education, and reinforcement in changing road user behaviour.* Toronto: Ontario Ministry of Transportation.

Lund, A. K., & Williams, A. F. (1985). A review of the literature evaluating the defensive driving course. *Accident Analysis and Prevention, 17*(6), 449–460.

Malenfant, L., & Van Houten, R. (1989). Increasing the percentage of drivers yielding to pedestrians in three Canadian cities with a multifaceted safety program. *Health Education Research, 5*(2), 275–279.

Mann, R. E., Vingilis, E. R., Gavin, D., Adlaf, E., & Anglin, L. (1991). Sentence severity and the drinking driver: Relationships with traffic safety outcome. *Accident Analysis and Prevention, 23*(6), 483–491.

Martinez, R. (2000). The status of traffic safety in the United States. In H. von Holst, A. Nygren, & A. E. Andersson (Eds.), *Transportation, traffic safety and health—Human behavior. Fourth International Conference, Tokyo, Japan, 1998* (pp. 7–13). New York: Springer.

Mashaw, J. L., & Harfst, D. L. (1990). *The struggle for auto safety.* Cambridge, MA: Harvard University Press.

McArthur, D. L., & Kraus, J. F. (1999). The specific deterrence of administrative per se laws in reducing drunk driving recidivism. *American Journal of Preventive Medicine, 16*(Suppl. 1), 68–75.

McKnight, A. J., & Hundt, A. G. (1971). *Driver education task analysis: Instructional objectives.* Washington, DC: U.S. Department of Transportation, National Highway Traffic Safety Administration.

McKnight, A. J., & Voas, R. B. (1991). The effect of license suspension upon DWI recidivism. *Alcohol, Drugs and Driving, 7*(1), 43–54.

Michon, J. A. (1981). Traffic education for young pedestrians: An introduction. *Accident Analysis and Prevention, 13*(3), 163–167.

Moskowitz, J. M. (1989). The primary prevention of alcohol problems: A critical review of the research literature. *Journal of Studies on Alcohol, 50*(1), 54–88.

Nichols, J. L. (1990). Treatment versus deterrence. *Alcohol Health Research World, 14*(1), 44–51.

OECD Scientific Expert Group. (1990). *Behavioural adaptations to changes in the road transport system.* Paris: Organisation for Economic Cooperation and Development, Road Transport Research.

Orleans, C. T., Gruman, J., Ulmer, C., Emont, S. L., & Hollendonner, J. K. (1999). Rating our progress in population health promotion: Report card on six behaviors. *American Journal of Health Promotion, 14*(2), 75–82.

Parker, D., & Manstead, A.S.R. (1996). The social psychology of driver behaviour. In G. R. Semin & K. Fielder (Eds.), *Applied social psychology* (pp. 198–224). Thousand Oaks, CA: Sage.

Peck, R. C. (1991). The general and specific deterrent effects of DUI sanctions: A review of California's experience. *Alcohol, Drugs and Driving, 7*(1), 13–42.

Peck, R. C. (1992). *The identification of high-risk target groups.* Sacramento: California Department of Motor Vehicles.

Peden, M., Scurfield, R., Sleet, D. A., Mohan, D., Hyder, A., Jarawan, E., & Mathers, C. (Eds). (2004). *World report on road traffic injury prevention.* Geneva: World Health Organization.

Preusser, D. F., & Blomberg, R. D. (1984). Reducing child pedestrian accidents through public education. *Journal of Safety Research 15*(2), 47–56.

Preusser, D. F., & Lund, A. K. (1988). And keep on looking: A film to reduce pedestrian crashes among 9 to 12 year olds. *Journal of Safety Research, 19*(4), 177–185.

Ranney, T. A. (1994). Models of driving behavior: A review of their evolution. *Accident Analysis and Prevention, 26*(6), 733–750.

Rippey, K. (1999). *Road safety and the police: Who can coordinate the road safety policy community?* Unpublished M.P.A. thesis, Queen's University, Kingston.

Robertson, L. S. (1987). Injury prevention: Limits to self-protective behavior. In N. D. Weinstein (Ed.), *Taking care: Understanding and encouraging self protective behavior* (pp. 280–297). Cambridge, MA: Cambridge University Press.

Ross, H. L. (1985). Deterring drunken driving: An analysis of current efforts. *Journal of Studies on Alcohol, 10,* 122–128.

Ross, H. L. (1991a). License deprivation as a drunk-driver sanction. *Alcohol, Drugs and Driving, 7*(1), 63–68.

Ross, H. L. (1991b, Dec.). *Punishment as a factor in preventing alcohol-related accidents.* Paper presented at the International Symposium: Alcohol-Related Accidents and Injuries, Yverdon-les-Bains, Switzerland.

Rothengatter, T. (1991). Automatic policing and information systems for increasing traffic law compliance. *Journal of Applied Behavior Analysis, 24*(1), 85–87.

Rothengatter, T. (1997). Psychological aspects of road user behaviour. *Applied Psychology: An International Review, 46*(3), 223–234.

Rumar, K. (1988). Collective risk but individual safety. *Ergonomics, 31*(4), 507–518.

Sagberg, F., Fosser, S., & Saetermo, I.-A. F. (1997). An investigation of behavioral adaptation to airbags and antilock brakes among taxi drivers. *Accident Analysis and Prevention, 29*(3), 293–302.

Siegrist, S., & Ramseier, E. (1992). *Evaluation of advanced driving courses.* Bern, Switzerland: BFU.

Sharfman, W. L., & Lonero, L. P. (1999, Aug. 23). Smarter cars need smarter drivers. *Automotive News,* 16.

Shinar, D., & McKnight, A. J. (1985). The effects of enforcement and public information on compliance. In L. Evans & R. C. Schwing (Eds.), *Human behavior and traffic safety* (pp. 385–414). New York: Plenum Press.

Shinar, D., & Stiebel, J. (1986). The effectiveness of stationary versus moving police vehicles on compliance with speed limit. *Human Factors, 28*(3), 365–371.

Simons-Morton, B., & Hartos, J. (Eds). (2002). Reducing young driver crash risk: Proceedings of an expert conference on young drivers. *Injury Prevention, 8*(Suppl II), ii1–ii38.

Sleet, D. A. (1987). Health education approaches to motor vehicle injury prevention. *Public Health Reports, 102*(6), 607–608.

Sleet, D. A., & Branche, C. (2004). Road safety is no accident. *Journal of Safety Research, 35*(2), 173–174.

Sleet, D. A., & Gielen, A. C. (1998). Injury prevention. In S. Sheinfeld Gorin & J. Arnold (Eds.), *Health promotion handbook* (pp. 247–275). St. Louis: Mosby.

Sleet, D. A., & Gielen, A. C. (2004). Developing injury interventions: The role of behavioural science In R. McClure, M. Stevenson, & S. McEvoy (Eds.), *The scientific bases of injury prevention and Control.* Melbourne, Australia: IP Communications.

Sleet, D. A., & Lonero, L. (2003). Behavioral approaches to traffic safety. In L. Breslow, J. Last, L. Green, & M. McGinnis (Eds.), *Encyclopedia of public health* (pp. 105–107). St. Louis: Mosby.

Smiley, A. (2000). Behavioral adaptation, safety and ITS. *Transportation Research Record, 1724,* 47–51.

Smiley, A., Lonero, L., & Chipman, M. (2004). *Final report: A review of the effectiveness of driver training and licensing programs in reducing road crashes.* Paris: MAIF Foundation.

Task Force on Community Preventive Services. (2005). *Guide to community preventive services: What works to promote health?* New York: Oxford University Press.

Traynor, T. L. (1993). The Peltzman hypothesis revisited: An isolated evaluation of offsetting driver behavior. *Journal of Risk and Uncertainty, 7*(7), 237–247.

Tyler, T. R., & Cook, F. L. (1984). The mass media and judgments of risk: Distinguishing impact on personal and societal level judgments. *Journal of Personality and Social Psychology, 47*(4), 693–708.

U.S. National Committee for Injury Prevention and Control. (1989). *Injury prevention: Meeting the challenge.* New York: Oxford University Press.

Van Houten, R., Malenfant, L., & Rolider, A. (1985). Increasing driver yielding and pedestrian signalling with prompting, feedback and enforcement. *Journal of Applied Behaviour Analysis, 18*(2), 103–110.

Voas, R. B. (1986). Evaluation of jail as a penalty for drunk driving. *Alcohol, Drugs and Driving, 2*(2), 47–70.

Waller, P. F. (1992). New evaluation horizons: Transportation issues for the 21st century. *Evaluation Practice, 13*(2), 103–115.

Wilde, G.J.S. (1993). Effects of mass media communications on health and safety habits: An overview of issues and evidence. *Addiction, 88,* 983–996.

Wilde, G.J.S. (2001). *Target risk 2. A new psychology of safety and health.* Toronto: PDE Publications.

Wilde, G.J.S., & Ackersviller, M. J. (1981). *Accident journalism and traffic safety education: A three-phase investigation of accident reporting in the Canadian daily press.* Ottawa: Transport Canada.

Williams, A. F., Weinberg, K., & Fields, M. (1991). The effectiveness of administrative license suspension laws. *Alcohol, Drugs and Driving, 7*(1), 55–62.

Yanovitzky, I., & Bennett, C. (1999). Media attention, institutional response, and health behavior change. The case of drunk driving, 1978–1996. *Communication Research, 26*(4), 429–453.

Zaza, S., Carande-Kulis, V. G., Sleet, D. A., Sosin, D. M., Elder, R. W., Shults, R. A., Dinh-Zarr, T. B., Nichols, J. L., & Thompson, R. S. (2001). Task Force on Community Preventive Services: Methods for conducting systematic reviews of the evidence of effectiveness and economic efficiency of interventions to reduce injuries to motor vehicle occupants. *American Journal of Preventive Medicine, 21*(Suppl. 4), 23–30.

CHAPTER ELEVEN

MODIFYING ALCOHOL USE TO REDUCE MOTOR VEHICLE INJURY

Ralph Hingson, David A. Sleet

Traffic crashes are the leading cause of death in the United States for people ages one to thirty-four (Centers for Disease Control and Prevention, 2005). According to the National Highway Traffic Safety Administration (2003b), 41 percent of traffic crash fatalities are alcohol related (those in which a driver or pedestrian had a blood alcohol concentration [BAC] greater than zero), and 35 percent involve someone with a BAC of 0.08 percent or higher. Nine percent of all traffic crashes (225,000 out of 2,926,000) result in alcohol-related injury.

Traffic crashes are more likely to result in death or injury if alcohol is involved. In 2002, 4 percent of all alcohol-related crashes resulted in a death, and 42 percent resulted in an injury. By contrast, 0.6 percent of crashes where alcohol was not a factor resulted in a death, and 31 percent resulted in an injury.

An alcohol-impaired driver (AID) has the capacity to injure or kill not only himself or herself, but many others. Overall in 2002, 44 percent of those who died in traffic crashes involving a drinking driver with a BAC of 0.01 percent or higher were people other than the drinking driver. From 1985 to 1996, nearly two-thirds of the 5,555 children under the age of fifteen who died in drinking-driver-related crashes were riding in the same car as the drinking driver (Quinlan, Brewer, Sleet, & Dellinger, 2000).

Impaired driving is the leading cause of police arrests in the United States. Over 10 percent of all police arrests are for AID (1.4 million annually). The National

Highway Traffic Safety Administration (NHTSA) estimates that alcohol-related crashes cost society $45 billion annually in medical costs and lost productivity.

Blood Alcohol Concentration and Fatal Crash Involvement

A person's BAC is determined by a combination of behavioral and physiological factors, including his or her drinking rate and the body's absorption, distribution, and metabolism of the alcohol. Within a few seconds after ingestion, alcohol reaches the liver, which begins to break it down, or metabolize it. Any BAC measurement therefore reflects not only a person's drinking rate but also his or her rate of metabolism. The human body metabolizes alcohol much more slowly than it absorbs alcohol, so the concentration in the body increases when the person consumes additional drinks before earlier drinks have been metabolized. Physiological and biological factors that influence BAC during and after drinking alcohol include age, gender, the proportion of body mass made up by fatty tissue, and whether food is eaten with the alcoholic beverage. Although individual rates can vary, a 170-pound man who has four drinks in an hour on an empty stomach or a 135-pound woman who has three drinks under similar conditions would reach a BAC of 0.08 percent (National Highway Traffic Safety Administration, 1992), the legal blood alcohol limit in all U.S. states. A number of reports have concluded that safe driving is impaired at very low BACs (Howat, Sleet, & Smith, 1991). Experimental laboratory studies (Moskowitz & Fiorentino, 2000) have reported clear behavioral and psychomotor deficits at a 0.08 percent BAC:

- Reduced peripheral vision
- Poorer recovery from glare
- Poor performance in complex visual tracking
- Reduced divided attention performance (the simultaneous performance of two or more tasks such as tracking, visual search, number monitoring, and detection of auditory stimuli)

Driver simulation and road course studies have revealed poorer parking performance, poorer driver performance at slow speeds, and steering inaccuracy at BACs of 0.05 percent (Finnigan & Hammersley, 1992; Hindmarch et al., 1992; Starmer, 1989).

Finally, in a comparison of alcohol test results, Zador (1991) found that each 0.02 increase in a driver's BAC nearly doubled his or her risk of being in a single-vehicle fatal crash. The study found that for all age and gender groupings, the likelihood of being a fatally injured driver was at least nine times greater at BACs of 0.05 to 0.09 percent than at zero BAC. For each 0.02 percent increase in BAC, the fatal crash risk increased even more for drivers under age twenty-one and for female drivers.

In an update of this study, Zador, Krawchuk, and Voas (2000) found that drivers in all age and gender groups examined who had BACs between 0.08 percent and 0.099 percent had at least an eleven times greater risk of dying in a single-vehicle crash than nondrinking drivers. Male drivers age sixteen to twenty with 0.08 percent BAC had fifty-two times greater risk of death than zero-BAC drivers of the same age.

In addition, a review of 112 studies provided strong evidence that impairment in driving skills begins with any departure from zero BAC (Moskowitz & Fiorentino, 2000). The majority of studies reported impairment by 0.05 percent BAC. The authors concluded that virtually all drivers tested in the studies reviewed exhibited impairment on some critical driving measure by the time they reached a BAC of 0.08 percent.

Characteristics of Alcohol-Related Fatalities and Fatal Crashes

Data from the Fatality Analysis Reporting System (FARS) (National Highway Traffic Safety Administration, 2003a) reveal that alcohol involvement in fatal crashes varies considerably by gender, age, race/ethnicity, type of vehicle driven, time of day, day of the week, and whether the person involved was a driver, motor vehicle passenger, or pedestrian. Behaviors associated with increased risk of AID include previous drinking while intoxicated (DWI) convictions and license suspensions, amount of alcohol consumed and BAC, speeding, and nonuse of safety belts.

Alcohol-related traffic crashes are more likely to occur from driving at night and on weekends. Seventy-seven percent of fatal alcohol-related traffic crashes occurred between 6:00 P.M. and 6:00 A.M., compared with 33 percent of non-alcohol-related fatal crashes (National Highway Traffic Safety Administration 2003a). More alcohol-related fatal crashes occur on Saturday (24 percent) than any other day, followed by Sunday (twenty-one percent) and Friday (16 percent).

Age and Gender

Drivers between the ages of sixteen and twenty, and especially those ages twenty-one to forty-five, are disproportionately likely to be involved in alcohol-related fatal crashes. Although 14 percent of drivers in alcohol-related fatal crashes in 2002 were between the ages of sixteen and twenty, this age group represents only 7 percent of the population. Most drivers in alcohol-related fatal crashes are male: 73 percent (National Highway Traffic Safety Administration, 2003a).

Race/Ethnicity

Voas and Tippetts (1999) found that between 1990 and 1994, 72 percent of people killed in alcohol-related fatal crashes were white, 12.1 percent were African American, 2.4 percent were Native American, 1.2 percent were Asian Americans and Pacific Islanders (AAPIs), and 12.7 percent were Hispanic (Mexican Americans, 8.7 percent; Puerto Ricans, 0.6 percent; Cubans, 0.3 percent; Central and South Americans, 1.1 percent; and people of other Hispanic origins, 2.0 percent).

Native Americans had the highest percentage of traffic deaths that were alcohol related (68 percent). Whites and African Americans had similar proportions (38 percent and 39 percent, respectively). Alcohol was involved in 50 percent of traffic deaths among Mexican Americans, 42 percent among Central and South Americans, 36 percent among Puerto Ricans, and 24 percent among Cubans. AAPIs had the lowest percentage of alcohol-related traffic deaths of any ethnic group (19 percent).

License Suspension and Convictions

Drivers in fatal crashes who had positive BACs were more likely than other drivers in fatal crashes to have had their driver's license suspended. Eight percent of drivers in fatal crashes who had BACs of zero had a suspended license, compared with 19 percent of drivers with BACs between 0.01 and 0.07 percent, twenty-one percent of drivers with BACs between 0.08 and 14 percent, and 24 percent of drivers with BACs of 0.15 percent or greater.

Driver BAC

The higher the BAC of a driver in a fatal crash, the greater the likelihood was that the crash involved only one vehicle. Thirty percent of zero BAC drivers in fatal crashes were involved in single-vehicle crashes, compared with 68 percent of drivers with BACs of 0.15 percent or higher.

Speeding

In 2002, 42 percent of intoxicated drivers (those with BACs of 0.08 percent or higher) in fatal crashes were speeding, as were 43 percent of drivers with BACs of 0.15 percent or higher. In contrast, 15 percent of zero BAC drivers in fatal crashes were speeding (National Highway Traffic Safety Administration, 2003a, 2003c). Alcohol interferes with sensorimotor coordination and reaction time, making drinking drivers more dangerous as their speeding behavior increases.

Non–Safety Belt Use

Drivers who drink are less likely to wear seat belts. The higher the driver's BAC, the less likely drivers are to wear a safety belt (National Highway Traffic Safety Administration, 2003a; Quinlan et al., 2000). People who wear safety belts reduce their risk of injury or death in traffic crashes by one-half (National Highway Traffic Safety Administration, 2002). We estimate that if all states adopted primary enforcement of safety belt laws, six hundred fewer alcohol-related traffic deaths would occur each year and over one thousand non-alcohol-related traffic deaths would be prevented annually.

Interventions to Reduce Alcohol-Related Crashes

During the past two decades, alcohol-related traffic deaths have declined 35 percent, from 26,173 in 1982 to 17,013 in 2003 (Figure 11.1). During the same time period, the U.S. population has grown and the amount of travel has increased. Alcohol-related traffic deaths have declined 48 percent per 100,000 population and 63 percent per 100 million vehicle miles of travel. The age group fifteen to twenty years had the greatest proportional decline in alcohol-related traffic deaths: alcohol-related deaths declined 56 percent from 5,504 in 1982 to 2,395 in 2003 (National Highway Traffic Safety Administration, 2005).

The behavior of driving while intoxicated or under the influence of alcohol is not only shaped by individual choice and motivation, but also strongly associated with organizational, economic, environmental, and social factors. Approaches that use one approach alone to bring about change in AID are likely to have limited success. Each preventive intervention builds on the strength of every other one. The long-term view of change favors the cumulative effects of interventions over time (Sleet, Wagenaar, & Waller, 1989; Howat, Sleet, Elder, & Maycock, 2004).

Three types of interventions have been shown to reduce alcohol-impaired driving behaviors and alcohol-related traffic crashes: (1) individually oriented interventions to change knowledge attitudes and drinking and driving behaviors, (2) environmental interventions to reduce alcohol availability and deter drinking and driving behaviors, and (3) comprehensive community interventions designed to reduce alcohol availability and drinking driving behaviors.

Individually Oriented Interventions

Evidence is available that many, if not most, drinking drivers involved in alcohol-related fatal crashes are alcohol dependent or abusers. Baker, Braver, Chen, and

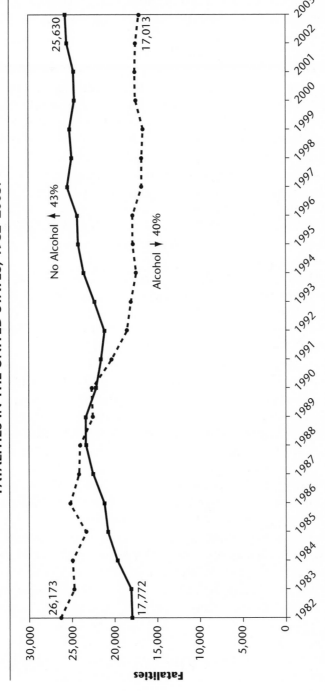

FIGURE 11.1. ALCOHOL AND NON-ALCOHOL-RELATED TRAFFIC FATALITIES IN THE UNITED STATES, 1982–2003.

Source: National Highway Traffic Safety Administration Fatality Analysis Reporting System.

Williams (2002) explored the issue of alcohol dependence and involvement in fatal crashes. Researchers contacted informants—usually a spouse, parents, children, or siblings of drivers killed in alcohol-related traffic crashes. These data were matched with data on previous drinking and driving convictions for 818 of the fatally injured drivers in the study. Fatally injured drivers with BAC of 0.15 percent or higher relative to zero BAC drivers were much more likely to have been classified (by informants) as problem drinkers: 31 percent versus 1 percent. Fatally injured drivers with BAC of 0.15 percent or higher were more likely than those with no BAC to reportedly have had five or more drinks at a time at least once per week (43 percent versus 5 percent) and to usually consume five or more drinks before driving (26 percent versus 2 percent). This relationship between increases in AID behavior and binge drinking has recently been confirmed by the CDC (Quinlan et al., 2005). Finally fatally injured drivers with BACs of 0.15 percent or higher were much more likely than those with no BAC to be driving from bars (28 percent versus 0 percent) or from restaurants or other people's homes (34 percent versus 22 percent).

Evidence about the relationship between alcohol dependence and alcohol-related crashes also comes from Hingson and Winter (2003), who found that people who are alcohol dependent are disproportionately involved in alcohol-related crashes, accounting for approximately two-thirds of motor vehicle crashes involving alcohol.

Currently, thirty-two states have laws requiring people convicted of drinking and driving to be assessed for alcohol abuse or dependence and to attend an alcohol treatment program (Mothers Against Drunk Driving, 2002). A meta-analysis (Wells-Parker, Bangert-Drowns, McMillen, & Williams, 1995) of 215 independent evaluations of mandated treatment of convicted drinking and driving offenders revealed that alcohol treatment programs reduce the behaviors leading to recidivism by up to 9 percent more than standard sanctions such as license suspension, revocations, or fines. The average recidivism rate for those who did not receive treatment over a two-year period was 19 percent. Treatment strategies that combined behavioral change strategies such as punishment, education, and individual and group therapy (with follow-up mandating after-care) were more effective than any single approach for first-time and repeat offenders (Wells-Parker et al., 1995).

Because most drivers in alcohol-related fatal crashes have not been convicted for driving while intoxicated, efforts to screen, diagnose, and treat alcohol problems (outside the criminal justice system) are also needed. A systematic review of randomized controlled trials to reduce alcohol dependence and abuse among the general population (Dinh-Zarr, Diguiseppi, Heitman, & Roberts, 1999) has found beneficial effects in reducing alcohol consumption, as well as drinking and driving offenses.

Trauma center and emergency department experimental studies of screening and brief intervention counseling for alcohol problems among people who experienced alcohol-related injuries have also shown reductions in drinking and driving offenses and alcohol-related injuries (Gentilello et al., 1999; Monti et al., 1999; Longabaugh et al., 2001). The reductions are often greater than those found in primary care or general internal medicine settings.

Larimer and Cronce (2002) and D'Amico and Fromme (2000) specifically identified interventions that reduced driving after drinking (and riding with an intoxicated driver) among college students. But a major unresolved issue is how to involve college students in screening that can refer those at risk to counseling programs. Even the most successful programs to date have linked fewer than 50 percent of eligible freshman to screening and potential counseling (Marlatt et al., 1998).

Reducing Alcohol Availability

Efforts to reduce alcohol availability include raising the legal drinking age, increasing the price of alcohol, reducing alcohol outlet density, and measures to reduce hours and days of sale. Availability of alcohol can also be reduced by beer keg registration, responsible beverage service, social host and dram shop liability, and server training programs. These interventions reduce the likelihood of consuming alcohol before driving.

Minimum Drinking Age. In 1984 only twenty-five states had a legal drinking age of age twenty-one. By 1988, all states had adopted this law. A review of forty-nine studies of legal drinking age changes concluded that in the 1970s and 1980s, when many states lowered the legal drinking age, alcohol-related traffic crashes increased 10 percent. In contrast, when states increased the drinking age to twenty-one, alcohol-related crashes among people under age twenty-one decreased 16 percent on average (Shults et al., 2001). Wagenaar and Toomey (2002) concluded that increases in the age of legal sales of alcohol have been the most successful intervention to date in reducing drinking and alcohol-related crashes among persons under age twenty-one. One national study of laws raising the drinking age to twenty-one indicated that persons who grew up in states with a drinking age of twenty-one not only drank less when they were twenty-one but also when they were twenty-five (O'Malley & Wagenaar, 1991). NHTSA (2005) estimates that a legal drinking age of twenty-one saves seven hundred to one thousand lives annually and that more than twenty-two thousand traffic deaths have been prevented by such laws since 1976.

Zero-tolerance laws, which make it illegal for persons under age twenty-one to drive after any drinking, have also contributed to declines in alcohol-related traffic deaths. A comparison of the first eight states to adopt zero-tolerance laws with nearby states without such laws revealed a 21 percent greater decline in single-vehicle fatal crashes in zero-tolerance-law states, the type of crash most likely to involve alcohol. Wagenaar, O'Malley, and LaFond (2001) found that in the first thirty states to adopt zero-tolerance laws, relative to the rest of the nation, there was a 19 percent decline in the proportion of people younger than age twenty-one who drove after any drinking and a 23 percent decline in the proportion who drove after five or more drinks. Most recently, an analysis of states with and without a minimum legal drinking age of twenty-one and zero-tolerance laws from 1982 to 1997, controlling analytically for per capita driving exposure per capita, beer consumption per se laws (which makes driving above the legal BAC limit a criminal offense and BAC test results sufficient evidence for conviction) at 0.10 percent and 0.08 percent, administrative license revocation, and safety belt laws, found the minimum legal drinking age zero tolerance associated with independent declines of 19 percent and 24 percent in the proportions of underage drinking drivers in fatal crashes (Voas, Tippetts, & Fell, 2003).

Stepped-up enforcement of alcohol purchase laws aimed at sellers and buyers can reduce sales and consumption and driving after drinking (Preusser, Ulmer, & Preusser, 1992; Wagenaar, Murray, & Toomey, 2000; Wagenaar et al., 2000) if resources are made available. In some states, zero-tolerance laws are not enforced independent of DWI. In New Mexico, for example, where this situation exists, most teenagers are unaware that there is a zero-tolerance law (Ferguson & Williams 2002), which can hamper efforts to change behavior.

Modifying the Price of Alcohol. With rare exceptions (Chaloupka & Wechsler, 1996; Dee, 1999), research since the early 1980s has concluded that increases in the price of alcoholic beverages lead to reductions in drinking, heavy drinking, and alcohol-related problems (Chaloupka, Grossman, & Saffer, 2002; National Academy of Sciences, 2003). Higher alcohol prices have been found to reduce motor vehicle deaths (Dee, 2001; Kenkel, 1993; Saffer & Grossman 1987), robberies, rapes, and cirrhosis deaths (Cook & Moore, 1993a, 1993b; Cook & Tauchen, 1982; Ruhn, 1996). Among moderate drinkers, a 1 percent price increase has been associated with a 1.19 percent decrease in consumption (Manning, Blumberg, & Moulton 1995). Younger drinkers tend to be more affected by price than older drinkers are (Chaloupka, Saffer, & Grossman, 1993a, 1993b; Godfrey, 1997; Kenkel, 1993; Sutton & Godfrey, 1995) perhaps because younger drinkers have less discretionary income. For example, Kenkel (1993) found a 10 percent increase in the price of alcohol would be enough to reduce DWI by 7 percent among men and 8 percent among women over age twenty-one. For those under age twenty-one, a 13 percent decrease among men and a twenty-one percent decrease among women could be realized.

Reducing Alcohol Outlet Density. High alcohol outlet density has been associated with alcohol-related problems (Gruenwald, Ponicki, & Holder, 1993) and traffic crashes. However, in six prospective studies of changes in outlet density, results were small and inconsistent.

Hours of Sale. Grube and Stewart (2004) report that studies of reducing hours of sale and its effects on drinking and driving behavior are mixed. Graham, McLeod, and Steedman (1998) in the U.K. found no significant changes in alcohol-related or assault hospital admissions as a result of restriction on hours of sales. A temporary extension of sale hours in Australia was not associated with increases in maximum consumption (McLaughlin & Harrison-Stewart, 1992). In contrast Smith (1988) found a 12 percent increase in traffic injury crashes after pub closing hours were extended from 6:00 P.M. to 10:00 P.M., Monday through Saturday in Victoria, Australia. Howat et al. (2004) found that closing bars earlier in Australia would have a positive effect on reducing drinking-and-driving behavior.

Dram Shop Laws. Dram shop laws enable individuals injured by those under legal drinking age who are under the influence to recover damages from (or sue) the alcohol retailer who sold alcohol to the persons causing the injury (Grube & Stewart, 2004). Overall dram shop liability has been estimated to reduce traffic fatalities among underage drinkers 3 percent to 4 percent (Chaloupka et al., 1993a, 1993b). In their review of this law, Grube and Stewart identified numerous studies that found these laws were associated with reduction in traffic crashes (Sloan, Reilly, & Schenzler, 1994, Sloan, Stout, Whetten-Goldstein, & Liang, 2000; Young & Likens, 2000; Benson, Rasmussen, & Mast 1999; Wagenaar & Holder, 1991).

Keg Registration. Cohen, Mason, and Scribner (2001) reported that keg registration is negatively correlated with traffic fatality rates, and Howat et al. (2004) in Australia support this finding. However, no other studies of this intervention have been reported (Grube & Stewart, 2004).

Responsible Behavior on the Part of Beverage Servers. Purchase surveys indicate from 40 to 90 percent of outlets sell alcohol to underage persons. Forster et al. (1994), Pruesser and Williams (1992), Grube (1997), and Holder and Wagenaar (1994) found that responsible beverage service (RBS) can reduce car crashes. RBS requires all servers to be above age twenty-one and not selling to persons under age twenty-one, checking identification for anyone appearing under the age of thirty-five, training managers and checks in identifying false identification, and monitoring drinks consumed by patrons. Lang, Stockwell, Rydon, and Beel (1998) and Saltz and Stanghetta (1997) found little impact of RBS on car crashes. Server training, however, which provides education and training to servers with the goal of altering their serving practices to prevent patron intoxication, can be effective. Shults et al. (2001) in a review of server training behavior found evidence of effectiveness under conditions of face-to-face instruction and strong management support. Wagenaar and Holder (1991) reported a 23 percent decrease in single-vehicle nighttime injury crashes associated with a statewide mandatory server training behavior change program.

Social Host Liability. Grube and Stewart (2004) identified only one study (Whetten-Goldstein, Sloan, Stout, & Liang, 2000) that found social host liability laws (where hosts whose serving behavior contribute to AID) were associated with lower alcohol-related motor vehicle crash deaths. This effect was found among adults but not among minors.

Alcohol Licensing. There is strong evidence that monopoly systems that control liquor licensing limit both the levels of alcohol consumption and alcohol-related problems like drinking and driving behavior. Total consumption generally increases when government-owned off-premise outlets are replaced by privately owned ones (Howat et al., 2004).

Laws to Deter Drinking and Driving Behavior

Deterrence theory suggests that if there is swift, certain, and severe punishment for an undesired behavior, people will be less likely to engage in that behavior (Ross, 1992). Specific deterrence laws target persons already convicted of DWI.

General Deterrence Laws. There are three types of general deterrence laws:

- *Administrative license revocation.* Enactment and enforcement of administrative license revocation laws, in place in forty states, allow police to immediately seize the driver's license of anyone operating a motor vehicle above the legal blood limit. Although this action might not reduce alcohol consumption, it has a general deterrence effect by reducing or eliminating the behavior of driving while impaired, since the driver no longer holds a valid driver's license. Although this practice does not eliminate all AID behavior (some people continue to drink and drive without a valid license), these laws have been associated with 6 to 12 percent declines in alcohol-related traffic deaths (Zador, Lund, Fields, & Weinberg, 1989; Voas, Tippetts, & Fell, 2000; Tippetts, Voas, Fell, & Nichols, 2005).
- *Criminal per se laws.* Criminal per se laws make the behavior of driving above the legal blood alcohol limit a criminal offense. These laws, in place in all U.S. states, have been shown to reduce traffic deaths (Voas et al., 2000).

- *0.08 per se legal blood alcohol limits.* In 2000, the U.S. Congress passed legislation that would withhold federal highway construction funds from states unless they lowered the legal limit from 0.10 percent to 0.08 percent. By 2004 all states had done so. Ten analyses of enactment of 0.08 percent laws in multiple states have all found that 0.08 laws are a general behavioral deterrent associated with significant declines in alcohol-related fatal crash and fatality measures (Johnson & Fell, 1995; Hingson, Heeren, & Winter, 1996, 2000; Voas et al., 2000; Shults et al., 2001; Eisenberg, 2003; Bernat, Dunsmuir, & Wagenaar, 2004; Tippetts et al., 2005). Proportional declines in alcohol-related fatalities in the United States ranged from 3 to 10 percent, and the estimate of annual lives saved ranged from five hundred to a thousand.

Specific Deterrence Laws. There are two specific types of deterrence laws:

- *Lower limits for convicted DWI offenders.* In 1988 Maine lowered its illegal BAC limit for persons with prior DWI convictions from 0.10 to 0.05 percent. A comparison of the effects of the six years before the law to the six years after showed a 25 percent reduction in the proportion of fatal crashes involving drivers with prior convictions and a 35 percent decline in the proportions with prior convictions and very high blood alcohol levels of 0.15 percent or higher (Hingson, Heeren, & Winter, 1998). This specific deterrent targeting the behavior of convicted DWI offenders seemed to work, since no changes were observed in the rest of the U.S. population during the same time period. Jones and Rodriguez-Iglesias (2005) reported that both Maine's lowering of the limit to 0.05 percent for prior convictions and the subsequent zero-tolerance law for them each produced significant behavior change with alcohol-related fatal crash declining among the targeted drivers.
- *Other laws targeting convicted offenders.* Impounding vehicles or license plates of previously convicted DWI offenders to prevent drinkers from driving (Voas, Tippetts, & Lange, 1997; Voas, Tippetts, & Taylor, 1997, 1998) and mandated use of ignition interlocks, which prevents an intoxicated person from driving (Beck, Rooch, & Baker, 1999), have been found to significantly reduce AID recidivism. The ignition interlock method of behavior change is effective only when it is in use and loses its behavioral deterrence effect when removed.

The Role of Enforcement and Education

Passage of a law does not by itself ensure behavior change (see Chapter Twenty, this volume). The extent to which drunk driving laws are enforced will influence their impact on impaired driving. Awareness of the law is vital. Publicity about the law and about efforts to enforce the law can strengthen its impact (Elder et al., 2004). A process of informing the public about new laws, their rationale, and how these will be enforced is critical to achieving behavior change. This educational function can also inoculate the public against efforts to overturn or repeal the law.

Sobriety Checkpoints. Publicizing the presence of sobriety checkpoints is a highly effective strategy for motivating changes in drinking and driving behavior (Castle et al., 1995; Lacey, Jones, & Smith, 1999; Shults et al., 2001). Some statewide efforts have yielded declines up to 20 percent in alcohol-related fatal crashes (Lacey et al., 1999). Fell, Lacey, and Voas (2004) recently reviewed the literature on sobriety checkpoint effectiveness in the United States and reported alcohol-related fatal crash declines ranging from 18 to 24 percent. The effectiveness of checkpoint programs is linked to their deterring drinking and driving behavior, not the likelihood that many driving under the influence offenders will be caught and removed from the highway. Fell et al. (2004) reported that despite demonstrated effectiveness and efforts of the NHTSA to promote checkpoint use, only about a dozen of thirty-seven states that conduct checkpoints do so on a weekly basis. A new key finding is that checkpoints conducted by as few as three to five officers can be just as effective as checkpoints conducted by fifteen or more officers. Clearly the behaviors of police officers in enforcing the law and the behaviors related to publicizing checkpoint programs have a positive effect on public perception and behavior related to drinking and driving.

Mass Media Campaigns. Elder et al. (2004) conducted a systematic review of the effectiveness of mass media campaigns to reduce alcohol-related traffic crashes. Among five studies that estimated the effects of mass media campaigns on traffic crashes, the median decrease in injury-producing crashes was 10 percent. Two studies used roadside BAC tests and found net decreases of 15 percent and 30 percent in the proportion of drivers with BAC levels of 0.05 percent and 0.08 percent and higher. The effects were similar whether the messages focused on the legal consequences or the health consequences of drinking and driving. They concluded that media campaigns that are carefully planned, well executed, attain adequate audience exposure, and are implemented in conjunction with other ongoing prevention activities such as enhancing alcohol-impaired law enforcement are effective in reducing alcohol-impaired driving behavior and alcohol-related crashes.

Comprehensive Community Programs. Community-based initiatives have succeeded in reducing drinking and related alcohol problems among young people (Hingson & Howland, 2002). These programs typically coordinate efforts of city officials from multiple departments of city government, school, health, police, alcohol beverage control, alcohol sellers, and others. Often multiple intervention strategies are used, including school-based programs involving students, peer leaders, and parents; media advocacy; community organizing and mobilization; environmental policy change to reduce alcohol availability to youth; and heightened enforcement of laws regulating sales and distribution of alcohol and laws to reduce alcohol-related traffic injuries and deaths.

Illustrative examples of comprehensive community programs include the Communities Mobilizing for Change Program (Wagenaar, Murray, & Toomey, 2000; Wagenaar et al., 2000), the Community Trials Program (Holder et al., 2000), the Saving Lives Program (Hingson et al., 1996), the Matter of Degree Program (Weitzman, Nelon, Lee, & Wechsler, 2004), the Fighting Back Program (Hingson et al., 2005), and a college community intervention (Clapp et al., 2005). Two programs (Holder et al., 2000; Wagenaar, Murray, & Toomey, 2000; Wagenaar et al., 2000) concentrated efforts on underage alcohol purchase attempt surveys with feedback to alcohol sales merchants and the community about the proportion of attempts that resulted in sales and penalties for continued violations. Three programs (Holder et al., 2000; Hingson et al., 1996; Clapp et al., 2005) focused on publicized police enforcement of drinking and driving laws, and one program targeted risky motorist behaviors disproportionately engaged in by drinking drivers, such as speeding, running red lights, and failure to wear safety belts and yield to pedestrians in crosswalks. Another combined strategies to reduce alcohol availability with increased substance abuse treatment participation (Hingson et al. 2005).

Relative to the comparison communities, the Communities Mobilizing for Change communities achieved a 17 percent increase in outlets checking the age identification of youthful-appearing alcohol purchasers, a 24 percent decline in sales by bars and restaurants to potential underage purchasers, a 25 percent decrease in the proportion of those eighteen to twenty years old seeking to buy alcohol, a 17 percent decline in the proportion of older teens who provided alcohol to younger teens, and a 7 percent decrease in the percentage of respondents younger than age twenty-one who drank in the previous thirty days (Wagenaar, Murray, & Toomey, 2000). Furthermore, arrests for drinking and driving declined significantly among those eighteen to twenty years old, and arrests for disorderly conduct declined among those fifteen to seventeen years old (Wagenaar et al., 2000).

In the Community Trials Program, single-vehicle crashes at night declined 11 percent more in program than in comparison communities. Alcohol-related trauma visits to emergency departments declined 43 percent (Holder et al., 2000).

The Saving Lives Program focused on reducing impaired alcohol driving and risky driving behaviors common among drinking drivers (Hingson et al., 1996).

During the five years of the program, the proportion of drivers younger than age twenty who reported driving after drinking declined from 19 to 9 percent over the course of the program. The proportion of vehicles observed speeding through use of radar was cut in half, and there was a 7 percent increase in safety belt use. Minimal change in these outcomes occurred in comparison areas. Fatal crashes declined from 178 to 120 during the five program years, a 25 percent greater reduction than in the rest of Massachusetts. Fatal crashes involving alcohol declined 42 percent, and the number of fatally injured drivers with positive blood alcohol levels declined 47 percent relative to the rest of Massachusetts. Visible injuries per one hundred crashes declined 5 percent more in Saving Lives cities than in the rest of the state during the program period.

Weitzman et al. (2004) recently evaluated the impact of college-community partnerships implementing environmentally based interventions to reduce drinking and related problem behaviors among college students. Interventions included keg registration, mandatory responsible beverage service, increased enforcement of community police collaboration or wild party enforcement, substance-free residence halls, and a variety of media efforts. Significant reductions were achieved in binge and frequent binge drinking, frequent intoxication, driving after drinking, alcohol-related injury, and a variety of other alcohol-related problems.

Five Fighting Back communities that combined environmental interventions to reduce availability of alcohol with interventions to increase substance abuse treatment use observed over a 20 percent decline in alcohol-related fatal crashes during ten program years related to the ten preprogram years and relative to companion comparison community drawn from the same states (Hingson et al., 2005).

Efforts to reduce alcohol availability included compliance check surveys to monitor underage access to alcohol over time, responsible beverage training, ordinances to prohibit public consumption or beverage sales, closing of liquor stores, and monitoring problematic outlets and advertising. Initiatives to expand treatment included increasing publicly funded treatment, establishment of referral or expanded treatment and after-care programs, initiating hospital emergency department screening and referral establishing drug courts, and opening of new treatment and after-care facilities. Communities varied somewhat in the initiatives that they pursued, but most of the five communities pursued most of the activities described above.

All of the community studies cited above indicate that community organizing can have an impact on reducing alcohol-related traffic deaths and injury. However, these community programs may not be sufficient to reduce alcohol-related problems unless they specifically identify and implement interventions that have previously had demonstrable benefits or have a plausible rationale for reducing alcohol-related problems (Hingson et al., 2005). Ecological and health promotion approaches in the community that focus on using a multidisciplinary and multi-sector strategies for prevention have the greatest potential for preventing alcohol-impaired driving (Sleet et al., 1989; Howat et al, 2004; Chapter Six, this volume).

Conclusion

Research has identified a variety of behavioral, environmental, and comprehensive community-based interventions strategies to reduce alcohol-impaired driving behavior and reduce alcohol-related traffic injury and death. Important progress has been made over the past two decades in reducing alcohol-related traffic crash deaths in high-income countries such as the United States, but there is still a long way to go in reducing the influence of alcohol on deaths and injuries in low- and middle-income countries elsewhere in the world (Peden et al., 2004).

Ecological strategies emphasizing changing behaviors, environments, policies, and practices exhibit the strongest impacts on reducing drinking and have also been associated with the greatest reductions in traffic injuries and deaths. For example, raising the drinking age to twenty-one has had its greatest effects on alcohol consumption and traffic deaths among persons under age twenty-one, but it is also associated with consumption declines for persons twenty-one to twenty-four and clearly reduces deaths of people injured by drivers under age twenty-one. Price increases also tend to disproportionately affect young people because they have less discretionary income. The onset of drinking is related to alcohol-related injuries and motor vehicle crashes not only during adolescence but also in adult years (Hingson et al., 2000; Hingson, Heeren, Zakocs, Kopstein, & Wechsler, 2002). Whether interventions that reduce drinking during adolescence will also reduce these behaviors that increase risk of alcohol-related injury during adulthood also warrants investigation.

The interventions that have produced the greatest declines in alcohol-related traffic deaths are raising the legal drinking age to twenty-one and general and specific deterrence laws that discourage behavior, such as criminal per se laws, administrative license revocation, lowering of legal blood alcohol limits for adult drivers, zero-tolerance laws for drivers under age twenty-one, and mandatory screening and treatment programs to modify behaviors of drivers convicted of driving while intoxicated.

Undoubtedly, the behaviors of grassroots activist organizations such as Mothers Against Drunk Driving (MADD) have played a pivotal role in motivating change. MADD, which has an organized chapter in every state, has helped to stimulate passage of over two thousand state-level laws and has played a key role in persuading legislators to pass key legislation to reduce AID. Other partners in this effort, such as the Centers for Disease Control and Prevention, American Medical Association, American Public Health Association, American Academy of Pediatrics, American Association of Emergency Room Physicians, Encare Nurses, National Safety Council, and Advocates for Highway Safety illustrate that not all behavior change is individual; collective action can stimulate change as well.

This chapter illustrates that alcohol and driving are complex behaviors, and the prevention of alcohol-impaired driving has no simple solution. Public policy, education, law, enforcement, alcohol outlets and servers, industry, the media, and the health care industry are all necessary partners to prevent alcohol-impaired driving behavior. At the community level, a growing number of evaluations of comprehensive community interventions indicate that education, reducing alcohol availability, enforcement of alcohol control, and drinking and driving laws, particularly using sobriety checkpoints at the community level and expansion of substance abuse treatment, can further reduce behaviors related to alcohol and traffic injuries and death. Changing behavior and societal practices with regard to alcohol and driving will require actions by legislators, employers, citizen groups, schools, taverns, and others. Individual and community actions, fostered by education, stimulated by social norms, and encouraged through public policy, ought to be our goal in efforts to prevent alcohol-impaired driving.

References

Baker, S. P., Braver, E. R., Chen, L. H., & Williams, A. (2002). Drinking histories of fatally injured drivers. *Injury Prevention, 8,* 221–226.

Beck, K., Rooch, W. J., & Baker, E. (1999). Effects of ignition interlock license restrictions on drivers with multiple alcohol offenses: A randomized trial in Maryland. *American Journal of Public Health, 89*(11), 1646–1700.

Benson, B. L., Rasmussen, D. W., & Mast, B. D. (1999). Deterring drunk driving fatalities: An economics of crime perspective. *International Review of Law Economics, 19,* 205–225.

Bernat, D. H., Dunsmuir, W. T., & Wagenaar, A. (2004). Effects of lowering the legal BAC to 0.08 on single-vehicle-nighttime fatal traffic crashes in 19 jurisdictions. *Accident Analysis and Prevention, 36,* 1089–1097.

Castle, S. P., Thompson, J. D., Spataro, J. A., Sewell, C. M., Flint, S., Scirmer, J., Justice, M., & Lacey, J. (1995). Early evaluation of a statewide sobriety checkpoint program. In *Proceedings of the Thirty-Ninth Annual AAAM* (pp. 65–78). Des Plaines, IL: Association for the Advancement of Automotive Medicine.

Centers for Disease Control and Prevention. (2005). Web-based injury statistics query and reporting system (Wisqars) [database]. Retrieved June 5, 2005, from http://www.cdc.ncipc/wisqars.

Chaloupka, F., Grossman, M., & Saffer, H. (2002). The effects of price on alcohol consumption on alcohol related problems. *Alcohol Research and Health, 26*(1), 22–33.

Chaloupka, F. J., Saffer, H., & Grossman, M. (1993a). Alcohol control policies and motor vehicle fatalities. *Journal of Law and Economics, 22,* 161–186.

Chaloupka, F. J., Saffer, H., & Grossman, M. (1993b). Effects of price on the consequences of
alcohol use and abuse. In M. Galanter (Ed.), *Recent developments in alcoholism. The consequences
of alcoholism* (pp. 331–346). New York: Plenum Press.

Chaloupka, F. J., & Wechsler, H. (1996). Binge drinking in college: The impact of price, availability, and alcohol control policies. *Contemporary Economic Policy, 14*(4), 112–124.

Clapp, J. D., Johnson, M., Voas, R. B., Lange, J. E., Shillington, A., & Russell, C. (2005).
Reducing DUI among US college students: Results of an environmental prevention trial.
Addiction, 100, 327–334.

Cohen, D. A., Mason, K., & Scribner, R. A. (2001). The population consumption model,
alcohol control practices, and alcohol-related traffic fatalities. *Preventive Medicine, 34,*
187–197.

Cook, P. J., & Moore, M. J. (1993a). *Economic perspectives on reducing alcohol-related violence. Alcohol
and interpersonal violence: Fostering multidisciplinary perspectives.* Washington, DC: Department
of Transportation.

Cook, P. J., & Moore, M. J. (1993b). Taxation on alcoholic beverages. In M. E. Hilton &
G. Bloss (Eds.), *Economics and the prevention of alcohol-related problems* (pp. 33–58). Rockville,
MD: National Institute on Alcohol Abuse and Alcoholism.

Cook, P. J., & Tauchen, G. (1982). The effect of liquor taxes on heavy drinking. *Bell Journal
of Economics, 13*(2), 379–390.

D'Amico, E. J., & Fromme, K. (2000). Implementation of the Risk Skills Training Program:
A brief intervention targeting adolescent participation in risk behaviors. *Cognitive and Behavioral Practice, 7,* 101–117.

Dee, T. S. (1999). State alcohol policies, teen drinking and traffic accidents. *Journal of Public
Economics, 72*(2), 289–215.

Dee, T. S. (2001). Does setting limits save lives? The case of 0.08 BAC laws. *Journal of Policy
Analysis and Management, 20*(1), 113–130.

Dinh-Zarr, T., Diguiseppi, C., Heitman, E., & Roberts, I. (1999). Preventing injuries through
interventions for problem drinking: A systematic review of randomized controlled trials.
Alcohol and Alcoholism, 34, 609–621.

Eisenberg, D. (2003). Evaluating the effectiveness of policies related to drunk driving. *Journal
of Policy Analysis and Management, 22*(2), 249–274.

Elder, R., Shults, R., Sleet, D., Nichols, J. L., Thompson, R., & Rajab, W. (2004). Effectiveness of mass media campaigns for reducing drinking and driving and alcohol involved
crashes. *American Journal of Preventive Medicine, 27*(1), 57–65.

Fell, S., Lacey, J., & Voas, R. (2004). Sobriety checkpoints: Evidence of effectiveness is strong,
but use is limited. *Traffic Injury Prevention, 5*(3), 220–227.

Ferguson, S. A., & Williams, A. F. (2002). Awareness of zero tolerance laws in three states.
Journal of Safety Research, 33, 293–299.

Finnegan, F., & Hammersley, R. (1992). The effects of alcohol on performance. In
A. P. Smith & D. M. Jones (Eds.), *Handbook of human performance, Vol. 2: Health and performance* (pp. 73–126). Orlando, FL: Academic Press.

Forster, J. L., McGovern, P. G., Wagenaar, A. C., Wolfson, M., Perry, C. L., & Anstine, P. S.
(1994). The ability of young people to purchase alcohol without age identification in
northeastern Minnesota, USA. *Addiction, 89,* 699–705.

Gentilello, L. M., Rivara, F. P., Donovan, D. M., Jurkovich, G. J., Daranciang, E., Dunn, C. W., Villaveces, A., Copass, M., & Ries, R. R. (1999). Alcohol intervention in a trauma center as a means of reducing the risk of injury recurrence. *Annals of Surgery, 230*(4), 473–483.

Godfrey, C. (1997). Can tax be used to minimize harm? A health economist's perspective. In M. Plant, E. Single, & T. Stockwell (Eds.), *Alcohol: Minimizing the harm: What works?* London: Free Association Books.

Graham, C. A., McLeod, L. S., & Steedman, D. J. (1998). Restriction extensions to permitted licensing hours does not influence the numbers of alcohol or assault-related attendances at an inner city accident and emergency department. *Journal of Accident and Emergency Medicine, 15,* 23–25.

Grube, J. W. (1997). Preventing sales of alcohol to minors: Results from a community trial. *Addiction, 92*(Suppl. 2), S251–S260.

Grube, J., & Stewart, K. (2004). Preventing impaired driving using alcohol policy traffic. *Injury Prevention, 5*(4), 199–207.

Gruenwald, P. J., Ponicki, W. R., & Holder, H. D. (1993). The relationship of outlet densities to alcohol consumption: A time series cross-sectional analysis. *Alcoholism: Clinical and Experimental Research, 17*(1), 38–47.

Hindmarch, I., Bhatti, J. Z., Starmer, G. A., Mascord, D. J., Kerr, J. S., & Sherwood, N. (1992). The effects of alcohol on the cognitive function of males and females and on skills relating to car driving. *Human Pharmacology, 7*(2), 105–114.

Hingson, R., Heeren, T., & Winter, M. (1996). Lowering state legal blood alcohol limits to 0.08 percent: The effect on fatal motor crashes. *American Journal of Public Health, 86*(9), 1297–1299.

Hingson, R., Heeren, T., & Winter, M. (1998). Effects of Maine's 0.05 percent legal blood alcohol level for drivers with DWI convictions. *Public Health Reports, 113,* 440–446.

Hingson, R., Heeren, T., & Winter, M. (2000). Effects of recent 0.08 percent legal blood alcohol limits on fatal crash involvement. *Injury Prevention, 6,* 109–114.

Hingson, R., Heeren, T., Zakocs, R., Kopstein, A., & Wechsler, H. (2002). Magnitude of alcohol-related mortality and morbidity among U.S. college students. *Journal of Studies on Alcohol, 63,* 136–144.

Hingson, R., & Howland, J. (2002, Mar.). Comprehensive community interventions to promote health: Implications for college-age drinking problems. *Journal of Studies on Alcohol, 14*(Suppl.), 226–240.

Hingson, R., & Winter, M. (2003). Epidemiology and consequences of drinking and driving. *Alcohol Research and Health, 27*(1), 63–78.

Hingson, R., Zakocs, R., Heeren, T., Winter, M., Rosenbloom, D., & DeJong, W. (2005). Effects on alcohol related fatal crashes of a community based initiative to increase substance abuse treatment and reduce alcohol availability. *Injury Prevention, 11,* 84–90.

Holder, H., Gruenewald, P. J., Ponicki, W. R., Treno, A. J., Grube, J. W., Saltz, R. F, Voas, R. B., Reynolds, R., Davis, J., Sanchez, L., Gaumont, G., & Roeper, P. (2000). Effects of community-based interventions on high risk driving and alcohol-related injuries. *JAMA, 284*(18), 2341–2347.

Holder, H. D., & Wagenaar, A. C. (1994). Mandated server training and reduced alcohol-involved traffic crashes: A time series analysis of the Oregon experience. *Accident Analysis and Prevention, 26,* 89–97.

Howat, P., Sleet, D., Elder, R., & Maycock, B. (2004). Preventing alcohol related traffic injury: A health promotion approach. *Traffic Injury Prevention, 5*(3), 199–208.

Howat, P., Sleet, D. A., & Smith, D. I. (1991). Alcohol and driving: Is the 0.05 percent blood alcohol concentration limit justified? *Drug and Alcohol Review* (Australia), *10*(1), 151–166.

Johnson, D., & Fell, J. (1995, Oct.). The impact of lowering the illegal BAC limit in five states in the US. In *Thirty-Ninth Annual Proceedings of the Association for the Advancement of Automotive Medicine*. Washington, DC: National Highway Traffic Safety Administration.

Jones, R. K., & Rodriguez-Iglesias, C. (2005, Dec.). *Evaluation of lower BAC limits for convicted OUI offenders in Maine*. DOT HS 809-827. Washington, DC: National Highway Traffic Safety Administration.

Kenkel, D. S. (1993). Drinking, driving and deterrence: The effectiveness and social costs of alternative policies. *Journal of Law and Economics, 36*(2), 877–814.

Lacey, J. H., Jones, R. K., & Smith, R. G. (1999). *Evaluation of Checkpoint Tennessee: Tennessee's state sobriety checkpoint program*. DOT HS 808-841. Washington, DC: National Highway Traffic Safety Administration.

Lang, E., Stockwell, T., Rydon, P., & Beel, A. (1998). Can training bar staff in responsible serving practices reduce alcohol-related harm? *Drug and Alcohol Review, 17*, 39–50.

Larimer, M., & Cronce, J. (2002, Mar.). Identification prevention treatment: A review of individually focused strategies to reduce problematic alcohol consumption by college students. *Journal of Studies on Alcohol, 14*(Suppl.), 148–163.

Longabaugh, R., Woolard, R., Nirenberg, T., Minugh, A. P., Becker, B., Clifford, P. R., Carty, K., Sparadeo, F., & Gogineni, A. (2001). Evaluating the effects of a brief motivational intervention for injured drinkers in the emergency department. *Journal of Studies on Alcohol, 62*, 806–816.

Manning, W. G., Blumberg, L., & Moulton, L. H. (1995). The demand for alcohol: The differential response to price. *Journal of Health Economics, 14*(2), 123–148.

Marlatt, G. A., Baer, J. S., Kivlahan, D. R., Dimeff, L. A., Larimer, M. E., Quigley, L. A., Somers, J. M., & Williams, F. (1998). Screening and brief intervention for high risk college student drinkers. Results from a 2 year follow up assessment. *Journal of Consulting and Clinical Psychology, 66*, 604–615.

McLaughlin, K. L., & Harrison-Stewart, A. J. (1992). The effect of temporary period of relaxing licensing laws on the alcohol consumption of young male drinkers. *International Journal of the Addictions, 27*, 409–423.

Monti, P., Colby, S., Barnett, P., Spirito, A., Rohsenow, D. J., Myers, M., Woolard, R., & Lewander, W. (1999). Brief intervention for harm reduction with alcohol-positive older adolescents in a hospital emergency department. *Journal of Consulting and Clinical Psychology, 67*, 989–994.

Moskowitz, H., & Fiorentino, D. (2000). *Review of the literature on the effects of doses of alcohol on driving related skills*. DOT HS 809-028. Springfield, VA: U.S. Department of Transportation, National Highway Safety Administration.

Mothers Against Drunk Driving. (2002). *Rating the states: An assessment of the nation's attention to the problem of drunk driving and underage drinking*. Irving, TX: Author.

National Academy of Sciences. (2003). *Reducing underage drinking: A collective responsibility*. Washington, DC: Author.

National Highway Traffic Safety Administration. (1992). *BAC Estimation* (computer program). Springfield, VA: National Technical Information Service.

National Highway Traffic Safety Administration. (2002). *Traffic Safety facts 2001: Occupant protection.* DOT 809-474. Washington, DC: U.S. Department of Transportation.

National Highway Traffic Safety Administration. (2003a). *2002 Annual assessment of motor vehicle crashes based on the Fatality Analysis Reporting System, the National Accident Sampling System and the General Estimates System.* Washington, DC: U.S. Department of Transportation.

National Highway Traffic Safety Administration. (2003b). *Traffic safety facts 2002: Alcohol.* DOT HS 809-606. Washington, DC: U.S. Department of Transportation.

National Highway Traffic Safety Administration. (2003c). *Traffic safety facts 2002: Overview.* DOT HS 809-612. Washington, DC: U.S. Department of Transportation.

National Highway Traffic Safety Administration. (2005). *Traffic safety facts 2003.* DOT HS 809-775. Washington, DC: U.S. Department of Transportation.

O'Malley, P., & Wagenaar, A. C. (1991). Effects of minimum drinking age laws on alcohol use, related behavior and traffic crash involvement among American youth. *Journal of Studies on Alcohol, 52,* 478–491.

Peden, M., Scurfield, R., Sleet, D., Mohan, D., Hyder, A., Jarawan, E., & Mathers, C. (Eds.). (2004). *World report on road traffic injury prevention.* Geneva: World Health Organization.

Preusser, D. F., Ulmer, R. B., & Preusser, C. W. (1992). *Obstacles to enforcement of youthful (under twenty-one) impaired driving.* DOT HS 807-878. Washington, DC: National Highway Traffic Safety Administration.

Preusser, D. F., & Williams, A. F. (1992). Sales of alcohol to underage purchasers in three New York counties and Washington DC. *Journal of Public Health Policy, 13,* 306–317.

Quinlan, K. P., Brewer, R. D., Siegel, P., Sleet, D. A., Mokdad, A. H., Shults, R. A., & Flowers, N. (2005). Alcohol-impaired driving among U.S. adults, 1993–2002. *American Journal of Preventive Medicine, 28*(4), 346–350.

Quinlan, K. P., Brewer, R. D., Sleet, D. A., & Dellinger, A. M. (2000, May 3). Characteristics of child passenger deaths and injuries involving drinking drivers. *JAMA,* 2249–2252.

Ross, H. L. (1992). *Confronting drunk driving: Social policy for saving lives.* New Haven, CT: Yale University Press.

Ruhn, C. J. (1996). Alcohol policies and highway vehicle fatalities. *Journal of Health Economics, 15*(4), 435–454.

Saffer, H., & Grossman, M. (1987). Beer taxes, the legal drinking age, and youth motor vehicle fatalities. *Journal of Legal Studies, 16*(2), 351–374.

Saltz, R. F., & Stanghetta, P. (1997). A community-wide responsible beverage service program in three communities: Early findings. *Addiction, 92*(Suppl. 2), S237–S249.

Shults, R. A., Elder, R. W., Sleet, D. A., Nichols, J. L., Alao, M. O., Carande-Kulis, V. G., Zaza, S., Sosin, D. M., & Thompson, R. S. (2001). Reviews of evidence regarding interventions to reduce alcohol-impaired driving. *American Journal of Preventive Medicine, 21*(Suppl. 4), 66–88.

Sleet, D. A., Wagenaar, A., & Waller, P. (1989). Introduction: Drinking, driving and health promotion. *Health Education Quarterly, 16*(3), 329–333.

Sloan, F. A., Reilly, B. A., & Schenzler, C. (1994). Effects of prices, civil and criminal sanctions, and law enforcement on alcohol-related mortality. *Journal of Studies on Alcohol, 55,* 454–465.

Sloan, F. A., Stout, E. M., Whetten-Goldstein, K., & Liang, L. (2000). *Drinkers, drivers and bartenders: Balancing private choices and public accountability.* Chicago: University of Chicago Press.

Smith, D. I. (1988). Effect of casualty traffic accidents of the introduction of 10 P.M. Monday to Saturday hotel closing in Victoria. *Australian Drug and Alcohol Review, 7,* 163–166.

Starmer, G. A. (1989). Effects of low to moderate doses of ethanol on human driving-related performance. In K. E. Crow & R. D. Batt (Eds.), *Human metabolism of alcohol, Vol. 1: Pharmacokinetics, mediocolegal aspects, and general interests* (pp. 101–130). Boca Raton, FL: CRC Press.

Sutton, M., & Godfrey, C. (1995). A grouped data regression approach to estimating economic and social influences on individual drinking behavior. *Health Economics, 4,* 237–247.

Tippetts, A. S., Voas, R. B., Fell, J. C., & Nichols, J. L. (2005). A meta-analysis of 0.08 BAC laws in 19 jurisdictions in the U.S. *Accident Analysis and Prevention, 37,* 149–161.

Voas, R. B., & Tippetts, A. (1999). *Ethnicity and alcohol-related fatalities, 1990–1994.* Washington, DC: National Highway Traffic Safety Administration.

Voas, R. B., Tippetts, A., & Fell, J. (2000). The relationship of alcohol safety laws to drinking drivers in fatal crashes. *Accident Analysis and Prevention, 32,* 483–492.

Voas, R. B., Tippetts, A., & Fell, J. (2003). Assessing the effectiveness of minimum legal drinking age and zero tolerance laws in the United States. *Accident Analysis and Prevention, 35*(4), 579–587.

Voas, R. B., Tippetts, A., & Lange, J. (1997). Evaluation of a method for reducing unlicensed driving: The Washington and Oregon license plate sticker laws. *Accident Analysis and Prevention, 29*(5), 627–634.

Voas, R. B., Tippetts, A., & Taylor, E. (1997). Temporary vehicle immobilization: Evaluation of a program in Ohio. *Accident Analysis and Prevention, 29*(5), 635–642.

Voas, R. B., Tippetts, A., & Taylor, E. (1998). Temporary vehicle impoundment in Ohio: A replication and confirmation. *Accident Analysis and Prevention, 30*(5), 651–656.

Wagenaar, A. C., & Holder, H. D. (1991). Effects of alcohol beverage server liability law on traffic crash injuries. *Alcoholism: Clinical and Experimental Research, 15,* 942–947.

Wagenaar, A. C., Murray, D. M., Gehan, J. P., Wolfson, M., Forster, J., Toomey, T., Perry, C. L., & Jones-Webb, R. (2000). Communities mobilizing for change: Outcomes from a randomized community trial. *Journal of Studies on Alcohol, 161*(1), 85–94.

Wagenaar, A. C., Murray, D. M., & Toomey, T., (2000). Communities mobilized for change on alcohol effects of a randomized trail on arrests and traffic crashes. *Addiction, 95,* 209–217b.

Wagenaar, A. C., O'Malley, P. M., & LaFond, C. (2001). Lowered legal blood alcohol limits for young drivers: Effects on drinking, driving and driving after drinking behaviors in 30 states. *American Journal of Public Health, 91,* 801–804.

Wagenaar, A. C., & Toomey, T. L. (2002). Effects of minimum drinking age laws: Review and analysis of the literature from 1960–2000. *Journal of Studies on Alcohol* (Suppl. 14), 206–226.

Weitzman, E. R., Nelon, T. F., Lee, H., & Wechsler, H. (2004). Reducing drinking and related harms in college: Evaluation of the Matter of Degree Program. *American Journal of Preventive Medicine, 27,* 187–196.

Wells-Parker, E., Bangert-Drowns, R., McMillen, R., & Williams, M. (1995). Final results from a meta-analysis of remedial intervention with drink/drive offenders. *Addiction, 90,* 907–926.

Whetten-Goldstein, K., Sloan, F. A., Stout, E., & Liang, L. (2000). Civil liability, criminal law, and other policies and alcohol-related motor vehicle fatalities in the United States: 1984–1995. *Accident Analysis and Prevention, 32*(6), 723–733.

Young, D. J., & Likens, T. W. (2000). Alcohol regulation and auto fatalities. *International Review of Law and Economics, 20,* 107–126.

Zador, P. L. (1991). Alcohol-related relative risk of fatal driver injuries in the relation to driver age and sex. *Journal of Studies on Alcohol, 52*(4), 302–310.

Zador, P., Krawchuk, S., & Voas, R. (2000). Alcohol related relative risk of driving fatalities and driver impairment in fatal crashes in relation to driver age and gender: An update using 1996 data. *Journal of Studies on Alcohol, 61*, 387–395.

Zador, P., Lund, A., Fields, M., & Weinberg, K. (1989). Fatal crash involvement and laws against alcohol-impaired driving. *Journal of Public Health Policies, 10*(4), 467–485.

CHAPTER TWELVE

BEHAVIORAL CONSIDERATIONS FOR SPORTS AND RECREATIONAL INJURIES IN CHILDREN AND YOUTH

Morag MacKay, Karen Liller

Children and youth spend a considerable amount of time participating in sports and recreational activities, which society views as beneficial to their physical, social, and emotional development. On average, Canadian children between the ages of five and twelve spend eighteen hours engaged in physical activity every week, while those between thirteen and seventeen years spend fifteen hours (Canadian Fitness and Lifestyle Research Institute, 1998). In the United States, it is estimated that over 30 million children and youth participate in organized sports annually (Centers for Disease Control, 2002b; Micheli, 1995; Patel & Nelson, 2000). As a result, it is perhaps not surprising that sport and recreational activities account for a large number and substantial proportion of all injuries to children and youth (Bijur et al., 1995; Health Canada, 1997). With children and youth being encouraged to participate in sports and recreational activities in record numbers, protective behaviors in sport and understanding and preventing injuries are becoming increasingly important (Danmore, Metzl, Ramundo,

Portions of this chapter were excerpted with permission from MacKay, M., Scanlan, A., Olsen, L. N., Reid, D., Clark, M., McKim, K., & Raina, P. (2004). Looking for the evidence: A systematic review of prevention strategies addressing sport and recreational injury among children and youth. *Journal of Science & Medicine in Sport, 7*(1), 58–73.

Pan, & van Amerongen, 2003; Flynn, Lou, & Ganley, 2002; Jones, Lyons, Sibert, Evans, & Palmer, 2001; Marshall & Guskiewicz, 2003; Shephard, 2003).

The prevention of sport and recreational injuries among children and youth has merit on several fronts. First, increasing physical activity through participation in sport and recreational activities has numerous benefits, including reducing the risk of obesity and its associated health-related conditions (Bar-Or, 2000; Epstein & Goldfield, 1999; Ewart, Young, & Hagberg, 1998; Gutin, Cucuzzo, Islam, Smith, & Stachura, 1996), increasing motor skills (American College of Sports Medicine, 2001; Hoover Wilson, Baker, Teret, Shock, & Garbarino, 1991), and self-esteem (Myers, Raynor, & Epstein, 2001). According to the National Center for Injury Prevention and Control (2002), injuries are a leading reason that people stop participating in potentially beneficial physical activity (Centers for Disease Control, 2002b). Limiting the risk of injury during sport and recreational activities through the application of effective preventive strategies increases the likelihood of continued benefit.

Second, although the majority of sport and recreational injuries among children and youth are not severe enough to require hospitalization and current injury classification systems make it difficult to accurately capture the economic impact of these injuries alone, they occur frequently enough to collectively have a significant impact in terms of direct costs of medical care and indirect costs (Danseco, Miller, & Spicer, 2000; Miller, Lestina, & Galbraith, 1995; Miller, Romano, & Spicer, 2000; SMARTRISK, 1998). When injuries are catastrophic, the costs to society can be even higher if they result in litigious activities (Posner, 2000).

In this chapter, we review the epidemiology of sports and recreational injuries and preventive interventions, and we discuss the role of behavior change theory in better understanding these types of injury and their prevention.

Epidemiology of Sports and Recreational Injuries in Children and Youth

To be effective, the practice of injury prevention needs to be evidence based. However, the prevention of sports and recreational injuries is hampered by several factors. First is the challenge of definitions. What makes a sport a sport and a recreational activity a recreational activity? There are no internationally agreed-on definitions for sport or sport injury (Chalmers, 2002). Furthermore, within sport itself, there are various levels of play and organization, which have implications for funding, training, coaching, and refereeing and, thus, injury potential and prevention options. A related issue is the difficulty in obtaining true exposure data, which affects the determination of injury rates. Another challenge is on what level or severity of injury to focus prevention efforts. As a result, understanding the epidemiology and prevention of sports and recreational injuries is a challenge, and it becomes problematic to design, implement, and evaluate effective prevention programs.

Nevertheless, data on sports and recreational injuries have been compiled so that we do have some information on the scope of the problem and some risk and protective factors. According to the Centers for Disease Control and Prevention (2002b), for example, data from the National Electronic Injury Surveillance System showed that from July 2000 to June 2001, approximately 4 million nonfatal sports and recreation injuries were treated in U.S. hospital emergency departments (EDs). Rates were highest for boys ages ten to fourteen. Sports and recreation injuries were 16 percent of all unintentional injury-related ED visits.

The types of sports and injury visits varied. For ages zero to nine years, for example, the leading types of injury were playground and bicycle-related injuries. Football, basketball, and bicycle-related injuries were most common for older males (ages ten to nineteen). Basketball produced the most injuries for females ages ten to nineteen. Approximately 715,000 sports and recreation injuries occur each year in school settings alone. Exercise injuries were most common among older individuals, and the most frequent injury diagnosis across the board was strains and sprains. Injuries were reported to be a leading reason that people stop participating in potentially beneficial physical activity.

According to the CDC data, participant age is crucial. Children younger than age fifteen account for about 40 percent of all sports- and recreation-related ED visits. Adolescents and young adults under age twenty-five participate in many such activities and experience almost one-third of these injuries. Although not the focus of this chapter, it is interesting to point out that there also has been a 54 percent increase in sports and recreational injuries among people sixty-five and older since 1990. These numbers do not include injuries that are treated in primary care settings, sports medicine clinics, orthopedic clinics, and chiropractic clinics. Therefore, these data clearly underestimate the burden of these injuries, which includes not only monetary costs but major quality-of-life costs as well.

Risk factors for exercise- and sports-related injuries can be intrinsic or extrinsic to the participant. Extrinsic factors include duration, frequency, and intensity of exercise; environmental conditions; and equipment. Intrinsic factors include age, sex, anatomic and musculoskeletal factors, and behavioral factors, such as previous physical activity and lifestyle, smoking and alcohol use, and current levels of fitness (Gilchrist, Jones, Sleet, & Kimsey, 2000). How these factors act singly or in combination to influence injury risk is not well understood, but behavioral factors likely play an important role.

Preventing Sports and Recreational Injuries Among Children and Youth

To date, the majority of research in the area of sports and recreational injury has been descriptive, with too few studies examining prevention strategies in any rigorous manner. This is particularly true when one examines sports and recreational injuries in children and youth. In 1999, a team of researchers in Canada undertook a systematic review of interventions to address sports and recreational injuries in children and youth to assess what had been done to date and provide direction for future research (MacKay et al., 2004). Much of what follows is drawn from that study.

The specific objectives of the study were to (1) examine existing evidence on the effectiveness of current prevention strategies in twenty-five selected sport and recreational activities; (2) determine the applicability of this evidence to children and youth; and (3) make recommendations related to best practice (policy and programming) and future research needs in this area. The detailed study methods and limitations and sport and recreational activity specific results are reported elsewhere (MacKay et al., 2004; Olsen et al., 2004; Scanlan & MacKay, 2001). The study examined alpine skiing, baseball, basketball, cycling, football, golf, gymnastics, hockey, horseback riding, ice skating, in-line skating, martial arts, ringette,[1] rugby, sledding, skateboarding, snowboarding, soccer, swimming, track and field, trampolining, volleyball, wrestling, and a mixed category called general sport. The study excluded biomechanical interventions evaluated in laboratory settings, instead focusing on interventions in actual sports and recreational settings.

Electronic searches identified 21,499 articles, and a review of abstracts and titles reduced this to 740 potentially relevant articles. Hand searching identified 124 additional potentially relevant articles. Only 117 (13.5 percent) of the 864 potentially relevant articles were evaluations of the effectiveness of a prevention measure using a control group and including children and youth in the study population. All 117 of these were published in English and came from many countries, with the majority from the United States (72 percent). Relevant articles were found for only sixteen of the original twenty-six activities, and only eight activities had three or more relevant articles and were included in the final review: alpine skiing, baseball, basketball, cycling, football, ice hockey, rugby, and soccer. The 93 articles that related to those eight activities represented 89 percent of relevant articles found.

Study designs varied from randomized controlled trials to simple one-group pretest-posttest designs (Table 12.1). The most frequently used design was the prospective cohort (30 percent), followed by simple one-group pretest-posttest designs (20 percent) and randomized controlled trials (16 percent). The most common

TABLE 12.1. STUDY DESIGN AND QUALITY RATING BY SPORT OR RECREATIONAL ACTIVITY.

	Study Design							Quality Rating		
	Randomized Control Trial	Nonequivalent Control Group	Prospective Cohort	Retrospective Cohort	Case Control	Time Series	One-Group Pretest-Posttest	Poor	Moderate	Good
Baseball (n = 4)	—	—	4	—	—	—	—	1	3	0
Basketball (n = 3)	3	—	—	—	—	—	—	2	1	0
Cycling (n = 12)	3	4	1	—	1	—	3	5	7	0
Football (n = 47)	6	2	21	4	—	4	10	23	23	1
Hockey (n = 8)	—	2	1	—	—	—	5	4	4	0
Rugby (n = 5)	—	2	1	1	—	—	1	1	4	0
Alpine skiing (n = 10)	2	1	—	—	7	—	—	8	2	0
Soccer (n = 4)	1	1	—	—	—	2	—	1	3	0
Total (n = 93)	15	12	28	5	8	6	19	45	47	1

Source: MacKay et al. (2004). Reproduced with permission.

interventions evaluated were those examining the effectiveness of environmental or equipment modifications (72 percent) (Figure 12.1). These examined equipment design, such as shoe and cleat design in soccer and football, equipment maintenance such as correct adjustment of ski bindings, and playing surfaces such as the impact of playing on artificial turf (Scanlan & MacKay, 2001).

Educational and behavior change interventions were most common for cycling, skiing, and soccer, whereas regulatory interventions (such as policy requiring certain equipment and game rules) were most common for cycling, football, and hockey. Examples of the educational and behavior change interventions in-

FIGURE 12.1. TYPE OF INTERVENTION BEING EVALUATED.

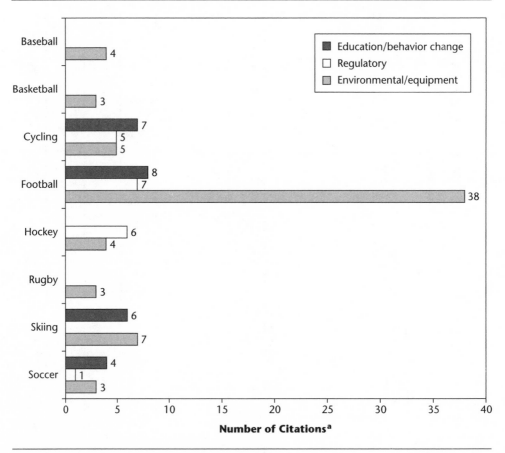

aA citation might include more than one intervention type.

Source: MacKay et al. (2004). Reproduced with permission.

cluded multifaceted educational campaigns aimed at increasing skills and encouraging equipment modification (skiing and cycling) and the introduction of preseason training and conditioning and warm-up stretching (soccer and football), behaviors designed to reduce the risk of injury. Regulatory interventions included introduction of rules to reduce unsafe actions (for example, disallowing spearing in football) and introduction of legislation to increase protection (for example, bicycle helmets). It is important to note that although the regulatory interventions focused on policy change, they all still include behavioral aspects, such as wearing equipment and following rules, so that participant, coach, and referee behavior all still play an important role in achieving injury reductions. Given this, it is somewhat surprising that none of the ninety-three studies reviewed made reference to a theoretical framework, including behavior change theory, as the basis for their intervention design. Overall, the quality of the relevant studies was found to be low, with approximately 48 percent rated as poor, 51 percent as moderate, and only 1 percent as good (Table 12.1). Children and youth were identified as the specific target group in forty-two studies (45 percent), while eleven additional studies (12 percent) included children in their sample (Figure 12.2).

The purpose of conducting the systematic review was to examine evidence-based practice. It highlighted the lack of evidence in relation to effectiveness of interventions, with very few evaluative studies found for the sport and recreational activities. In fact, relevant evaluations were found for less than two-thirds of the targeted sport and recreational activities. For many of the most popular activities, no studies were found at all. Although the review is now several years old, there have been few articles since to suggest that this situation is improving. This raises the following question: What is the basis for current best practice with respect to injury prevention for these sports and recreational activities? It is clear that many strategies perceived to be preventive and in common practice on playing fields across the globe have not been evaluated, particularly among children and youth. This is not to say they are not effective, just that there is no empirical evidence. Obvious starting points for future research would be these common practices.

Theory and Behavioral Considerations in Sports and Recreational Injury Prevention

Several approaches for organizing sports injury prevention have been proposed. In their discussion of these models, Weaver, Moore, and Howe (1996) propose a schema that integrates nicely with Haddon's matrix to examine host, agent, and

FIGURE 12.2. EVALUATIONS TARGETING
CHILD AND YOUTH PARTICIPANTS (*n* = 93).

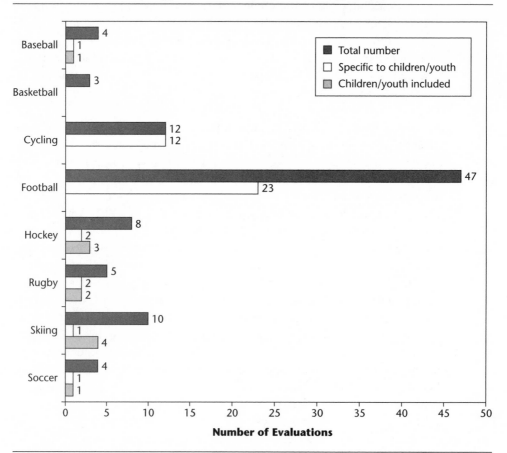

Source: MacKay et al. (2004). Reproduced with permission.

environment. Using the three E's of injury prevention—engineering, education/
behavior change, and enforcement—the schema suggests that sport and recreational injuries should be preventable by:

- Ensuring that design, development, and maintenance of sport and recreational
  equipment and facilities meet safety standards
- Influencing attitudes toward, and promoting uptake of, protective behaviors or
  equipment (for example, wearing protective equipment and physical conditioning)
- Adapting playing rules to the participants with respect to age and other characteristics and ensuring their enforcement

Effective engineering-based interventions do not ensure reduction of injury in and of themselves. Often educational and promotional activities to encourage uptake and policy or regulation requiring safety product use are necessary. Without such efforts, people can still behave unsafely despite good evidence to support the safety practice in question. For example, the use of bicycle helmets illustrates how a known, effective engineering-based intervention is practiced most often when a combination of both education and legislation is in place (Klassen, MacKay, Moher, Walker, & Jones, 2000). Preventing sport and recreational injuries requires an understanding of the factors that contribute to both the occurrence of injury and the uptake of, or compliance with, potential preventive strategies (Meeuwisse, 1991). Challenges for current prevention efforts include poor knowledge regarding both intrinsic and extrinsic contributing factors, their interaction to increase susceptibility, and a gap between what is known and what is used in developing and implementing prevention strategies (Meeuwisse, 1994).

The *Injury Research Agenda* of the Centers for Disease Control and Prevention (2002a) has set priorities for the prevention of sports, recreation, and exercise-related injuries. Several of these priorities focus on behavior factors and determinants, as well as effective interventions and dissemination strategies. In addition, a priority on collecting exposure data must be addressed before true sports injury rates can be determined and used comparatively. Better statistical study designs must be used and careful implementation of effective strategies carried out to improve the chances of better utilization of future research findings (Shephard, 2005).

While the history of injury prevention and control efforts has clearly included behavioral factors (Lett, Kobusingye, & Sethi, 2002), these factors have not been fully investigated with regard to the prevention of injuries in sports and recreation activities. But the issue is more than simply including behavior change efforts when injury prevention initiatives are developed. The incorporation of behavior change strategies needs to be based on tested theories and models that allow us not only to understand why people change their behavior but also the mechanisms of those changes, the determination of why some programs succeed or fail, and how to build stronger and better programs (Gielen & Sleet, 2003). According to Glanz, Rimer, and Lewis (2002), the theories and models can be based on individual health behavior (such as in the health belief model, theory of reasoned action and planned behavior, and the transtheoretical model); models of interpersonal health behavior that include interaction with the environment, including the social environment (for example, social cognitive theory, social networks, and social support); and community and group models that involve community organization and community building, diffusion of innovations, and communication. (These theories are discussed in detail in Chapters Two and Three, this volume.)

While the field of injury prevention and control has used the study of behavior and the incorporation of models and theories in some areas such as parental supervision to prevent injuries, motor vehicle injuries (including pedestrian injuries and bicycle helmet use), falls, fires, and others, very few studies have focused on these concepts in the prevention of sports and recreation injuries. Reviews of literature produce little to no results, and although best practice documents include promoting the wearing of protective gear in sports (Centers for Disease Control and Prevention, 1995), there are no examples or guidelines of how to accomplish this using theories and models to build behavioral interventions (Scanlan & MacKay, 2001).

More can be learned from the psychological literature and from behavioral research (Sleet & Hopkins, 2004). Division 47 of the American Psychological Association (APA) is dedicated to exercise and sport psychology. APA scientists and practitioners in Division 47, founded in 1986, study motivation in sport and psychological and behavioral considerations in sport injury and rehabilitation.

More can also be gleaned from recent studies. For example, a publication of safety attitudes and beliefs of junior Australian football players used the theory of reasoned action to determine the attitudes toward safety behaviors and perceived outcomes of these behaviors, subjective norms, and perceived behavioral control. The results showed that certain environments were perceived to be more dangerous than others, and negative beliefs needed to be addressed in a more comprehensive injury prevention strategy (Finch, Donohue, & Granham, 2002).

Psychosocial constructs from behavioral sciences have been the focus of some research in sports-related injuries. Andersen and Williams (1988) posited a model of stress and injury, which has been widely used in studies of athletes and their injuries. According to this model, stress responsivity increases injury risk in athletes, and the degree of stress responsivity is influenced by one's history of stressors (for example, major life events), personality characteristics (for example, "hardiness"), and coping resources (for example, social support). This model has been used by a number of researchers seeking to understand the complex relationships between such intra- and interpersonal factors and injury risk; which variables moderate or mediate the stress and injury connection remain the subject of debate (Andersen & Williams, 1999; Ford, Eklund, & Gordon, 2000; Rider & Hicks, 1995; Smith, Smoll, & Ptacek, 1990).

The incorporation and testing of behavioral theories and constructs can be carefully designed within health education and health promotion interventions (Gielen & McDonald, 2002). What are needed are more systematic studies so that appropriate theoretically based behavioral interventions can be developed, implemented, and evaluated. Evaluations of engineering or environmental interventions should also include an analysis of their reciprocal effects on behavior to more fully understand the role of behavior and behavior change in prevention.

Furthermore, most of the studies that met inclusion criteria for the review of sports and recreational activities described previously did not specifically address children and youth. This is troubling because of the physical, behavioral, and developmental differences between children and adults, especially because most of the interventions involved the modification of either the environment or a piece of protective equipment. Is it safe to assume that what works for an elite twenty-six-year-old athlete is reasonable for a sixteen year old or a nine year old? Accounting for developmental differences in allowable sport behaviors (such as matching for size and skill rather than age), environments (such as surfaces and playing fields selected), and agents of injury (such as the type of equipment allowed) can profoundly affect injury risk and injury prevention (Sleet, 1994). In the field of transportation safety, effective strategies have taken into account the fact that physiological and psychological differences between children, youth, and adults require child- and youth-specific preventive strategies such as child passenger restraints and graduated licensing (Hoover Wilson et al., 1991; Mayhew, Simpson, Williams, & Desmond, 2002). It is not clear why similar attention to age and developmental differences that have been noted in the area of sports and recreation safety has not been acted on (Maffuli & Baxter-Jones, 1995; Macgregor, 2003; Mercy, Sleet, & Doll, 2003; Outerbridge & Micheli, 1995; Posner, 2000; van Mechelen, 1997). It is clear that the development of evidence-based best practices for children and youth will be accomplished only through significant research and evaluation that addresses these physical and psychosocial differences. The need for this approach has been recognized for nearly three decades (Smoll et al., 1979).

Conclusions

Despite the magnitude of the injury problem in sports and recreation, there has been little rigorous study to understand and address the behavioral causes and prevention of these injuries. A systematic review of the sport and recreational literature retrieved revealed surprisingly few well-designed and controlled studies investigating strategies to prevent injuries, particularly those focusing on behavioral approaches. An even smaller number of publications evaluated strategies to reduce injury in children and youth. Even where studies and evidence were found, too little existed to specify best practices. For the activities where evaluative studies were found, few employed a randomized control group design (Barrett et al., 1993; Ekstrand & Gillquist, 1983; Garrick & Requa, 1973; Hauser, 1989; Hendrickson & Becker, 1998; Jorgensen, Fredensborg, Haraszuk, & Crone, 1998; Kaufman & Kaufman, 1984; Kim, Rivara, & Koepsell, 1997; Kraus, Anderson, & Mueller, 1970a, 1970b; Macarthur, Parkin, Sidky, & Wallace, 1998; Quillian, Simms, & Cooper, 1987; Sitler et al., 1990, 1994; Stevenson & Anderson, 1981). Only one study was judged to have good quality of reporting, a nonequivalent control group design (Grace et al., 1988). Future studies should employ more rigorous study protocols, where possible applying a randomized control group design (Caine, Caine, & Lindner, 1996; Walter & Hart, 1990). In circumstances where randomization is not possible, studies should attempt to control for factors including, age, gender, size, playing position, and experience, through either design or analysis (Meeuwisse, 1994; Caine et al., 1996). Furthermore, while a consistent definition of injury is essential to allow a comparison of results across studies, stronger measures of exposure will better elucidate the true magnitude of the issue (Caine et al., 1996; van Mechelen, Hlobil, & Kemper, 1992; Walter & Hart, 1990). Many of the studies included in this review failed to apply these basic research standards. This situation does not seem to have changed much in the past decade (Caine et al., 1996; Walter & Hart, 1990). The consequence of methodological and reporting weaknesses is that the validity of results is called into question and cannot be generalized to other populations (Hart & Meeuwisse, 1994; Walter & Hart, 1990).

Perhaps of more concern is the lack of studies examining preventive strategies for the majority of sport and recreational activities. As governments in developed countries continue to focus on increasing physical activity among children and youth, thought must be given to the issue of risk of injury and the relative lack of evidence regarding effective preventive measures. Behavior change theory provides a basis on which researchers may investigate potential causes and preventive strategies for reducing sport and recreational injuries. Stronger linkages between those working in the fields of injury prevention and health promotion and behavior change should be encouraged so that this potential can be maximized.

Future Needs

The lack of good evidence to support preventive strategies is both surprising and concerning given the burden of sport and recreational injuries among children and youth. Further research is required to ascertain the scope of sport and recreational injuries in children and youth and intrinsic and extrinsic factors related to this population; evaluate existing prevention strategies among this age group; and develop interventions specific to the population where none exist. Despite a lack of studies, the synthesis of existing research provides some direction for current practice, although the majority of our recommendations are for further research. In the absence of strong evidence to the contrary, the cessation of existing practices not previously tested among children and youth cannot be recommended, unless they can be linked with specific harms. Rather, rigorous evaluation of existing practices is strongly recommended, thereby allowing the development of evidence-based practice recommendations.

It is perhaps at this point that behavior change theory offers a relatively new opportunity. Although rare, there are some examples where theory has been used to assist in the design of an intervention, for example in relation to helmet use during bicycling (Thompson, Sleet, & Sacks, 2002). However, to our knowledge, no one has yet tested behavior change theories in the context of trying to reduce sport and recreational injuries (Trifiletti, Gielen, Sleet, & Hopkins, 2005). Engineering and environmental changes and enforcement of policies and legislation all have the potential to benefit from the application of behavior change theory, and this connection should be systematically explored.

Note

1. Ringette is an international sport, developed in Canada, which was first introduced in 1963 in North Bay, Ontario. Developed originally for girls, ringette is a fast-paced team sport on ice in which players use a straight stick to pass, carry, and shoot a rubber ring to score goals. Ringette is played on a rink and there are five players plus a goalie on the ice at the same time from each team. Ringette is fun and fast, it has no body contact, and there is a need to cooperate to be able to move from one side to another.

References

American College of Sports Medicine. (2001, Dec.). Plyometric training for children and adolescents. *Current Comments, 1.*

Andersen, M. B., & Williams, J. M. (1988). A model of stress and athletic injury: Prediction and prevention. *Journal of Sport and Exercise Psychology, 10,* 294–306.

Andersen, M. B., & Williams, J. M. (1999). Athletic injury, psychosocial factors and perceptual changes during stress. *Journal of Sports Sciences, 17,* 735–741.

Bar-Or, O. (2000). Juvenile obesity, physical activity, and lifestyle changes: Cornerstones for prevention and management. *Physician and Sports Medicine, 28*(11), 51–58.

Barrett, J. R., Tanji, J. L., Drake, C., Fuller, D., Kawasaki, R. T., & Fenton, R. M. (1993). High- versus low-top shoes for the prevention of ankle sprains in basketball players: A prospective randomized study. *American Journal of Sports Medicine, 21*(4), 582–585.

Bijur, P. E., Trumble, A., Harel, Y., Overpeck, M. D., Jones, D., & Scheidt, P. C. (1995). Sports and recreation injuries in US children and adolescents. *Archives of Pediatrics & Adolescent Medicine, 149*(9), 1009–1016.

Caine C. G., Caine D. J., & Lindner, K. J. (1996). *The epidemiologic approach to sports injuries.* In C. G. Caine, D. J. Caine, & K. J. Lindner (Eds.), *Epidemiology of sports injuries.* Champaign, IL: Human Kinetics Publishers.

Canadian Fitness and Lifestyle Research Institute. (1998). *1998 physical activity monitor.* Retrieved from http://www.cflri.ca/cflri/pa/surveys/98survey/98survey.html.

Centers for Disease Control and Prevention. (1995). Injury control recommendations for bicycle helmets. *Journal of School Health, 65*(4), 133–139.

Centers for Disease Control and Prevention. (2002a). *CDC injury research agenda.* Atlanta, GA: Centers for Disease Control and Prevention. http://www.cdc.gov/ncipc/pub-res/research_agenda/Research percent20Agenda.pdf.

Centers for Disease Control and Prevention. (2002b). Nonfatal sports- and recreation-related injuries treated in emergency departments—United States, July 2000–June 2001. *Morbidity and Mortality Weekly Report, 51,* 736–740.

Chalmers, D. J. (2002). Injury prevention in sport: Not yet part of the game? *Injury Prevention, 8,* 22–25.

Danmore, D. T., Metzl, J. D., Ramundo, M., Pan, S., & van Amerongen, R. (2003). Patterns in childhood sports injury. *Pediatric Emergency Care, 19*(2), 65–67.

Danseco, E. R., Miller, T. R., & Spicer, R. S. (2000). Incidence and costs of 1987–1994 childhood injuries: Demographic breakdowns. *Pediatrics, 105*(2), E27.

Ekstrand, J., & Gillquist, J. (1983). Soccer injuries and their mechanisms: A prospective study. *Medicine & Science in Sports & Exercise, 15*(3), 267–270.

Epstein, L. H., & Goldfield, G. S. (1999). Physical activity in the treatment of childhood overweight and obesity: Current evidence and research issues. *Medicine & Science in Sports & Exercise, 31*(Suppl. 11), S553–S559.

Ewart, C. K., Young, D. R., & Hagberg, J. M. (1998). Effects of school-based aerobic exercise on blood pressure in adolescent girls at risk for hypertension. *American Journal of Public Health, 88,* 949–951.

Finch, C., Donohue, S., & Granham, A. (2002). Safety attitudes and beliefs of junior Australian football players. *Injury Prevention, 8,* 151–154.

Flynn J. M., Lou, J. E., & Ganley, T. J. (2002). Prevention of sports injuries in children. *Current Opinion in Pediatrics 14*(6), 719–722.

Ford, I. W., Eklund, R. C., & Gordon, S. (2000). An examination of psychosocial variables moderating the relationship between life stress and injury time-loss among athletes of a high standard. *Journal of Sports Sciences, 18,* 301–312.

Garrick, J. G., & Requa, R. K. (1973). Role of external support in the prevention of ankle sprains. *Medicine & Science in Sports, 5*(3), 200–203.

Gielen, A. C., & McDonald, E. M. (2002). Using the PRECEDE/PROCEED planning model to apply health behavior theories. In K. Glanz, B. K. Rimer, & F. M. Lewis. (Eds.), *Health behavior and health education* (3rd ed.). San Francisco: Jossey-Bass.

Gielen, A. C., & Sleet, D. (2003). Application of behavior-change theories and methods to injury prevention. *Epidemiologic Reviews, 25,* 65–76.

Gilchrist, J., Jones, B. H., Sleet, D. A., & Kimsey, C. D. (2000, Mar. 31). Exercise-related injuries among women: Strategies for prevention from civilian and military studies. *MMWR Recommendations and Reports, 49*(RR-2), 15–33.

Glanz, K., Rimer, B. K., & Lewis, F. M. (Eds.). (2002). *Health behavior and health education* (3rd ed.). San Francisco: Jossey-Bass.

Grace, T. G., Skipper, B. J., Newberry, J. C., Nelson, M. A., Sweetser, E. R., & Rothman, M. L. (1988). Prophylactic knee braces and injury to the lower extremity. *Journal of Bone & Joint Surgery—American Volume, 70*(3), 422–427.

Gutin, B., Cucuzzo, N., Islam, S., Smith, C., & Stachura, M. E. (1996). Physical training, lifestyle education, and coronary risk factors in obese girls. *Medicine & Science in Sports & Exercise, 28,* 19–23.

Hart, L. E., & Meeuwisse, W. H. (1994). Evaluating methodology in the sport medicine literature. *Clinical Journal of Sport Medicine, 4(1),* 64.

Hauser, W. (1989). Experimental prospective skiing injury study. In R. J. Johnson, C. D. Mote Jr., & M. H. Binet (Eds.), *Skiing trauma and safety: Seventh International Symposium.* Philadelphia: American Society for Testing and Materials.

Health Canada. (1997). *For the safety of Canadian children and youth: From injury data to preventive measures.* Ottawa: Minister of Public Works and Government Services Canada.

Hendrickson, S. G., & Becker, H. (1998). Impact of a theory based intervention to increase helmet use in low income children. *Injury Prevention, 4,* 126–131.

Hoover Wilson, M., Baker, S. P., Teret, S. P., Shock, S., & Garbarino, J. (1991). *Saving children: A guide to injury prevention.* New York: Oxford University Press.

Jones, S. J., Lyons, R. A., Sibert, J., Evans, R., & Palmer, S. R. (2001). Changes in sports injuries to children between 1983 and 1998: Comparison of case series. *Journal of Public Health Medicine, 23,* 268–271.

Jorgensen, U., Fredensborg, T., Haraszuk, J. P., & Crone, K. L. (1998). Reduction of injuries in downhill skiing by use of an instructional ski-video: A prospective randomized intervention study. *Knee Surgery, Sports Traumatology, Arthroscopy, 6*(3), 194–200.

Kaufman, R. S., & Kaufman, A. (1984). An experimental study on the effects of the MORA on football players. *Basal Facts, 6*(4), 119–126.

Kim, A. N., Rivara, F. P., & Koepsell, T. D. (1997). Does sharing the cost of a bicycle helmet help promote helmet use? *Injury Prevention, 3,* 38–42.

Klassen, T. P., MacKay, J. M., Moher, D., Walker, A., & Jones, A. L. (2000). Community-based injury prevention interventions. *Future of Children, 10*(1), 83–110.

Kraus, J. F., Anderson, B. D., & Mueller, C. E. (1970a). The effectiveness of a new touch football helmet to reduce head injuries. *Journal of School Health, 40*(9), 496–500.

Kraus, J. F., Anderson, B. D., & Mueller, C. E. (1970b). The quality of officiating as an injury prevention factor in intramural touch football. *Medicine & Science in Sport, 3*(3), 143–147.

Lett, R., Kobusingye, O., & Sethi, D. (2002). A unified framework for injury control: The public health approach and Haddon's matrix combined. *Injury Control and Safety Promotion, 9,* 199–205.

Macarthur, C., Parkin, P. C., Sidky, M., & Wallace, W. (1998). Evaluation of a bicycle skills training program for young children: A randomized controlled trial. *Injury Prevention, 4,* 116–121.

Macgregor, D. M. (2003). Don't save the ball! *British Journal of Sports Medicine, 37,* 351–353.

MacKay, M., Scanlan, A., Olsen, L. N., Reid, D., Clark, M., McKim, K., & Raina, P. (2004). Looking for the evidence: A systematic review of prevention strategies addressing sport and recreational injury among children and youth. *Journal of Science & Medicine in Sport, 7*(1), 58–73.

Maffuli, N., & Baxter-Jones, A. (1995). Common skeletal injuries in young athletes. *Sports Medicine, 19,* 137–149.

Marshall, S. W., & Guskiewicz, K. M. (2003). Sports and recreational injury: The hidden cost of a healthy lifestyle. *Injury Prevention, 9,* 100–102.

Mayhew, D. R., Simpson, H. M., Williams, A. F., & Desmond, K. (2002). *Specific and long-term effects of Nova Scotia's graduated licensing program.* Arlington, VA: Insurance Institute for Highway Safety.

Meeuwisse, W. H. (1991). Predictability of sports injuries. What is the epidemiologic evidence? *Sports Medicine, 12*(1), 8–15.

Meeuwisse, W. H. (1994). Assessing causation in sport injury: A multifactorial model. *Clinical Journal of Sport Medicine, 4,* 166–170.

Mercy, J. A., Sleet, D. A., & Doll, L. S. (2003). Applying a developmental approach to injury prevention. *American Journal of Health Education, 34*(5), S6–S12.

Micheli, L. J. (1995). Sports injuries in children and adolescents: Questions and controversies. *Clinics in Sports Medicine, 14*(3), 727–745.

Miller, T. R., Lestina, D. C., & Galbraith, M. S. (1995). Patterns of childhood medical spending. *Archives of Pediatrics & Adolescent Medicine, 149*(4), 369–373.

Miller, T. R., Romano, E. O., & Spicer, R. S. (2000). The cost of childhood unintentional injuries and the value of prevention. *Future of Children, 10*(1), 137–163.

Myers, M. D., Raynor, H. A., & Epstein, L. H. (2001). Predictors of child psychological changes during family-based treatment for obesity. *Archives of Pediatrics & Adolescent Medicine, 152*, 855–861.

National Center for Injury Prevention and Control. (2002). *CDC Injury Research Agenda.* Atlanta, GA: Centers for Disease Control and Prevention, Department of Health and Human Services.

Olsen, L., Scanlan, A., MacKay, M., Babul, S., Reid, D., Clark, M., & Raina, P. (2004). Soccer-related injury prevention strategies: A systematic review. *British Journal of Sports Medicine, 38*, 89–94.

Outerbridge, A. R., & Micheli, L. J. (1995). Overuse injuries in the young athlete. *Clinics in Sports Medicine, 14(3)*, 503–516.

Patel, D., & Nelson, T. L. (2000). Sports injuries in adolescents. *Medical Clinics of North America, 844*, 983–1007.

Posner, M. (2000). *Preventing school injuries: A comprehensive guide for school administrators, teachers and staff.* New Brunswick, NJ: Rutgers University Press.

Quillian, W. W., Simms, R. T., & Cooper, J. S. (1987). Knee-bracing in preventing injuries in high school football. *International Pediatrics, 2*, 255–256.

Rider, S. P., & Hicks, R. A. (1995). Stress, coping, and injuries in male and female high school basketball players. *Perceptual and Motor Skills, 81*, 499–503.

Scanlan, A., & MacKay, M. (2001). *Sports and recreation injury prevention strategies: Systematic review and best practices: Executive summary.* Vancouver: British Columbia Injury Research and Prevention Unit, Vancouver, and Plan-It Safe, Children's Hospital of Eastern Ontario, Ottawa. www.injuryresearch.bc.ca/publicns.html.

Shephard, R. J. (2003). Can we afford to exercise, given current injury rates? *Injury Prevention, 9*, 99–100.

Shephard, R. J. (2005). Towards an evidence based prevention of sports injuries. *Injury Prevention, 11*, 65–66.

Sitler, M., Ryan, J., Hopkinson, W., Wheeler, J., Santomier, J., Kolb, R., & Polley, D. (1990). The efficacy of a prophylactic knee brace to reduce knee injuries in football: A prospective, randomized study at West Point. *American Journal of Sports Medicine, 18*(3), 310–315.

Sitler, M., Ryan, J., Wheeler, B., McBride, J., Arciero, R., Anderson, J., & Horodyski, B. (1994). The efficacy of a semi-rigid ankle stabilizer to reduce acute ankle injuries in basketball: A randomized clinical study at West Point. *American Journal of Sports Medicine, 22(4)*, 454–461.

Sleet, D. A. (1994). Injury prevention. In K. Middleton & P. Cortese (Eds.), *The comprehensive school health challenge* (pp. 443–489). Santa Cruz, CA: ETR Associates.

Sleet, D. A., & Hopkins, K. (2004). *Bibliography of behavioral science research in unintentional injury prevention.* Atlanta, GA: Division of Unintentional Injury Prevention, Centers for Disease Control and Prevention. www.cdc.gov/pub-res/behavioral.

SMARTRISK. (1998). *The economic burden of unintentional injury in Canada.* Toronto, Ontario: SMARTRISK. www.smartrisk.ca/PDF/main_study_canada.pdf.

Smith, R. E., Smoll, F. L., & Ptacek, J. T. (1990). Conjunctive moderator variables in vulnerability and resiliency research: Life stress, social support and coping skills, and adolescent sport injuries. *Journal of Personality and Social Psychology, 58*(2), 360–370.

Smoll, F. L., Lefebvre, L. M., Fujita, A., Ismail, A. H., Pauwels, J., Pilz, G. A., & Sleet, D. A. (1979). Psychology of children in sport. *International Journal of Sports Psychology, 10*(3), 173–176.

Stevenson, M. J., & Anderson, B. D. (1981, May). The effects of playing surfaces on injuries in college intramural touch football. *Journal of National Intramural Recreational Sports Association*, 59–64.

Thompson, N., Sleet, D. A., & Sacks, J. (2002). Increasing the use of bicycle helmets: Lessons from behavioral science. *Patient Education and Counseling, 46*(3), 191–197.

Trifiletti, L. B., Gielen, A. C., Sleet, D. A., & Hopkins, K. (2005). Behavioral and social sciences theories and unintentional injury. *Health Education Research, 20*(3), 298–307.

van Mechelen, W. (1997). The severity of sports injuries. *Sports Medicine, 243*, 176–180.

van Mechelen, W., Hlobil, H., & Kemper, H. C. (1992). Incidence, severity, aetiology and prevention of sports injuries: A review of concepts. *Sports Medicine, 14*(2), 82–89.

Walter, S. D., & Hart, L. E. (1990). Application of epidemiological methodology to sports and exercise science research. *Exercise and Sport Sciences Reviews, 18*, 417–448.

Weaver, J., Moore, C. K., & Howe, W. B. (1996). In C. G. Caine, D. J. Caine, & K. J. Lindner (Eds.), *Injury prevention in epidemiology of sports injuries*. Champaign, IL: Human Kinetics Publishers.

CHAPTER THIRTEEN

HOUSE FIRES AND OTHER UNINTENTIONAL HOME INJURIES

Eileen M. McDonald, Andrea Carlson Gielen

Mid pleasures and palaces though we may roam,
Be it ever so humble, there's no place like home.

—JOHN HOWARD PAYNE, U.S. ACTOR AND DRAMATIST (1791–1852)

Home conjures up feelings of warmth, belonging, respite, and rejuvenation. Home rarely evokes concerns about injury. But hazards are common in and around the home and result in injuries to people across the life span. Until recently, details about injuries that occurred in the home were scarce. A recent report by the Home Safety Council (Runyan & Casteel, 2004) sheds new light on the variety of injuries that occur within (for example, falls on stairs, burns from stove) and around (falls from trees, cut injury occurring in the garage) the home. Other sources are also available to help describe specific household injuries to children and adults in or around the home (O'Donnell & Mickalide, 1998; National Center for Injury Prevention and Control, 2001).

Despite the recent work of the Home Safety Council, the profile of home-based injuries provided in this chapter is at best an underrepresentation of the problem. Information about the location of injuries is still difficult to obtain and remains problematic. Consider the standardized death certificate used as the basis of the National Vital Statistics System, where information about fatal injuries is recorded (National Center for Health Statistics, 2005c). When a death results from an injury, among the information requested on the death certificate is date, time,

---

The authors would like to thank Dr. Deborah C. Girasek for her review and comments to this chapter.

and location of the injury. In the Home Safety Council study, location of injury was available for only about one-third of all fatal unintentional injuries: 20 percent home and 13 percent location other than home (Runyan et al., 2005b). The picture is even further compromised when examining nonfatal injuries. Several sources are available to potentially determine the magnitude and scope of morbidity associated with unintentional home injuries, including the National Health Interview Survey (National Center for Health Statistics, 2005a), the National Ambulatory Medical Care Survey, and the National Hospital Ambulatory Medical Care Surveys for Outpatient and Emergency Departments (National Center for Health Statistics, 2005b). Investigators who have used these data sources report "differences with respect to the definition of the home environment, the definition of populations used for rates, and the presence of systematically missing data" (Runyan et al., 2005a, p. 81).

Another challenge rests in defining the term *home*. The U.S. Census Bureau (2005) defines *housing unit* as any house, apartment, mobile home or trailer, group of rooms, or single room that is occupied or intended for use as a separate living quarters. Excluded from this definition are institutional (for example, nursing homes and hospitals) and noninstitutional (for example, college dormitories and military barracks) group facilities. However, some of the data sources listed above include some group facilities in their definition of housing unit.

In 2003, the Census Bureau estimated the number of housing units at 120,879,390 (U.S. Census Bureau, 2005). When one considers the amount of time (exposure) that the more than 280 million Americans spend in their residences, it is not surprising that injuries in the home are common. This chapter describes the major contributors to the household injury problem, including falls, poisonings, and fires and burns, and their impact on the U.S. population. The chapter also highlights the myriad other ways in which children and adults get injured or killed in and around the home. (Intentional injury events that may occur in the home, such as intimate partner violence and suicide, are addressed in Chapters Fourteen and Fifteen, this volume.) To address the specific issue of behavior and injury, we have chosen to focus on the home injury topic of fire prevention behaviors: smoke detector behaviors to illustrate behavior change theories, methods, and applications. The chapter concludes with a brief discussion of future research implications for home injuries.

Incidence and Mechanisms of Home Injury

Usually considered a place of respite and relief, the home is too frequently the location of injuries. The extent to which injuries occur in the home varies by age, gender, and type of injury as well as other factors.

Fatal Home Injury

The Home Safety Council estimated more than 18,000 injury deaths each year between 1992 and 1999, yielding an overall death rate from home injuries of 6.83 deaths per 100,000 persons (Runyan & Casteel, 2004). While all ages are at risk of death from household injuries, individuals at either end of the life span are among the high-risk groups (see Table 13.1). The highest rate of death from unintentional household injury is among people eighty years and older (47.91 per 100,000). Males and females between the ages of seventy and seventy-nine follow a distant second (14.57 per 100,000), and children under the age of one rank third, with an injury death rate of 12.19 deaths per 100,000 persons. Rates of home injury death for those between the ages of five and thirty-nine are below 6 deaths per 100,000 persons. Males across the life span have higher rates of death overall from home injury compared to females (8.78 versus 4.97 deaths per 100,000).

TABLE 13.1. UNINTENTIONAL HOME INJURY DEATHS: AVERAGE ANNUAL NUMBER AND RATE (PER 100,000 PERSONS), BY AGE GROUP AND SEX, UNITED STATES, 1992–1999.

	Male		Female		Total	
Age Group	Number	Rate	Number	Rate	Number	Rate
Below 1	286	12.34	201	9.81	469	12.19
1–4	616	7.48	382	5.23	998	6.42
5–9	215	2.17	139	1.58	354	1.85
10–14	194	1.99	81	.095	275	1.47
15–19	327	3.40	81	0.96	408	2.22
20–29	1,010	6.00	302	2.08	1,312	3.53
30–39	1,896	9.93	657	3.88	2,553	5.88
40–49	1,965	10.98	672	3.98	2,637	6.85
50–59	941	7.63	428	3.55	1,369	5.32
60–69	931	9.94	513	5.25	1,444	7.21
70–79	1,253	18.07	1,017	11.94	2,270	14.57
80 and over	1,715	57.37	2,245	39.80	39,602	47.91
Total	11,331	8.78	6,718	4.97	18,048	6.83

Source: Runyan and Casteel (2004). Reproduced with permission of the Home Safety Council, Washington, DC.

Nonfatal Home Injury

The National Health Interview Survey (NHIS) is the principal source of information on the health of the civilian, noninstitutionalized population of the United States (National Center for Health Statistics, 2005a). The household survey is conducted every year among adults seventeen years of age and older. NHIS data are used to monitor trends in illness, injury, and disability and to track progress toward achieving national health objectives, such as Healthy People 2010. NHIS data from 1997 to 2001 were used to estimate that more than 12 million nonfatal, unintentional home injuries occurred and required either medical attention or lost time from work or school (Casteel & Runyan, 2004b).

As holds true for other injury causes, most home injuries do not result in death. For every 1 home injury death, more than 650 nonfatal injury events occur in or around the home (Casteel & Runyan, 2004b). As displayed in Table 13.2,

TABLE 13.2. NONFATAL UNINTENTIONAL HOME INJURIES: AVERAGE NUMBER AND RATE (PER 100,000 PERSONS), BY AGE GROUP AND SEX, UNITED STATES, 1997–2001.

Age Group	Male		Female		Total	
	Number	Rate	Number	Rate	Number	Rate
Under 1	71,412	3,451	45,120	2,343	116,531	3,459
1–4	715,857	8,957	545,057	7,042	1,260,914	9,995
5–9	619,030	5,905	423,988	4,259	1,043,018	5,933
10–14	539,266	5,272	356,557	3,640	895,822	5,119
15–19	387,178	3,851	271,274	2,763	658,452	4,065
20–29	539,034	2,999	671,706	3,649	1,210,740	3,921
30–39	858,876	4,162	761,856	3,553	1,620,732	4,460
40–49	718,661	3,518	873,703	4,139	1,592,364	4,516
50–59	510,166	3,651	720,303	4,817	1,230,469	5,085
60–69	371,171	4,022	581,896	5,545	953,066	5,568
70–79	304,308	4,522	716,844	8,183	1,021,152	7,641
80 and over	176,440	6,503	616,164	12,787	792,604	11,547
Total	5,811,398	4,389	6,584,466	4,733	12,395,864	4,410

Source: Runyan and Casteel (2004). Reproduced with permission of the Home Safety Council, Washington, DC.

the highest rate of nonfatal home injuries is among individuals eighty years of age and older. Children ages one to four rank second, and older adults ages seventy to seventy-nine rank third in their rate of injury morbidity due to home injuries.

When comparing injury morbidity (nonfatal) and mortality (fatal), the landscape of home injuries yields both similarities and differences. Similarities include consistently higher mortality and morbidity risks at either end of the life span as well as for young males (see Tables 13.1 and 13.2). Beginning at age forty, however, gender differences begin to emerge. Whereas males have consistently higher mortality rates, females over age forty experience consistently higher nonfatal injury rates. The nonfatal injury rate for women eighty and older is almost double that of males in the same age group (12,787 versus 6,503 injuries per 100,000 persons). Investigators hypothesize that these higher nonfatal rates for women may be a reflection of their spending more time at home compared to males, differences in what females would seek care for or would report as an injury compared to males, and contributions from specific injury mechanisms such as falls, which affect women more than men (Casteel & Runyan, 2004a).

Leading Causes of Fatal and Nonfatal Home Injury

Falls, poisonings, and fires and burns are the top three leading causes of unintentional home injury deaths (see Table 13.3) and account for 78.6 percent of all home injury deaths. Ten other injury mechanisms account for the remaining 21.4 percent of deaths and include, in addition to those listed in Table 13.3, machinery (0.7 percent), a cut or pierce (0.3 percent), and overexertion (less than 0.1 percent).

The top three mechanisms for nonfatal home injuries are fall, struck by/against, and cut/pierce events (Table 13.3). These three causes represent 64.3 percent of all nonfatal home injuries. The remaining 35.7 percent of nonfatal injuries are caused by, in addition to those listed in Table 13.3, transport, other (1.1 percent), machinery (1.0 percent), motor vehicle (0.7 percent), pedestrian, other (0.2 percent), choking/suffocation (0.1 percent), firearm (0.1 percent), and near-drowning/submersion (less than 0.1 percent).

Each of the three leading mechanisms of fatal injury will be explored in more detail in the following sections.

Falls. A fall is an event that results in a person coming to rest inadvertently on the ground or floor or other lower level (World Health Organization, 2004). Falls can occur on the same level, as when an older adult trips or loses balance. Falls also can occur from one level to another, as when a child falls from a window or an infant rolls off a bed. Risk of death or permanent impairment is strongly related to the height of the fall and the protective nature of the material struck. Serious injury or

TABLE 13.3. TOP CAUSES OF FATAL AND NONFATAL HOME INJURIES: AVERAGE ANNUAL NUMBER, PERCENTAGE, AND RATE (PER 100,000 PERSONS), UNITED STATES, 1992–1999.

Injury Event	Fatal, 1992–1999			Nonfatal, 1997–2001		
	Number	Percentage (Rank)	Rate	Number	Percentage (Rank)	Rate
Fall	5,961	33.0 (1)	2.25	5,105,558	41.2 (1)	1,884.0
Poisoning	4,833	26.8 (2)	1.83	726,296	5.9 (5)	263.9
Fire/burn	3,402	18.8 (3)	1.29	261,326	2.1 (9)	96.4
Choking/suffocation	1,092	6.1 (4)	0.41			
Drowning/submersion	823	4.6 (5)	0.31			
Firearm	590	3.3 (6)	0.22			
Natural/environmental	427	2.4 (7)	0.16	580,343	4.7 (6)	213.4
Struck by/against	285	1.6 (8)	0.11	1,467,203	11.8 (2)	541.4
Miscellaneous	230	1.3 (9)	0.09	560,903	4.5 (7)	206.0
Unspecified	215	1.2 (10)	0.08	464,922	3.8 (8)	171.9
Cut/pierce				1,398,434	11.3 (3)	515.5
Overexertion				1,262,619	10.2 (4)	466.2
Pedal cyclist, other				169,530	1.4 (10)	62.5
Total	18,048	100.0	6.63	12,395,864	100.0	4,410.0

Source: Runyan and Casteel (2004). Reproduced with permission of the Home Safety Council, Washington, DC.

death is more likely to occur when falls occur at significant heights and when the victim falls on an unforgiving surface. A direct fall on the head, regardless of the height of the fall, may be fatal (Chiaviello, Cristof, & Bond, 1994; Wilson, Baker, Teret, Shock, & Garbarino, 1991; American Academy of Pediatrics, 2001).

The Home Safety Council (Runyan & Casteel, 2004) study revealed that the cause of most fatal falls (63.0 percent) that occurred in the home was "unspecified." When the location was reported, falls on or from stairs accounted for 17.4 percent of fatal falls, and falls on the same level (tripping, slipping, stumbling) described another 5.8 percent. Falls from or out of a building (3.7 percent), falls from a ladder (3.2 percent), and falls from a chair or bed (3.2 percent) explained an additional 10 percent of fatal falls. The rate of fall deaths increases dramatically with age, with relatively few deaths occurring among those under sixty years of age but rising rapidly for those above the age of sixty.

Recommended safety behaviors and effective devices exist for preventing falls. Parents of young children are counseled to use safety gates on stairs, use nonslip surfaces on their tubs, and avoid the use of baby walkers (Committee on Injury Prevention, 1994). The use of window bars in high-rise buildings has been shown to be effective in reducing falls among young children (Spiegel & Lindaman, 1977). To protect older adults, modifications to the home environment are recommended and include improved lighting, the use of grab bars in the bathroom or near the bed, and railings on stairs (American Geriatric Society, 2001). Marshall and colleagues (2005) surveyed more than one thousand U.S. households to determine the use of such devices and found low use of grab bars in bathrooms overall (25 percent) and low use of window guards (34 percent) among households with children under the age of seven. About half of those surveyed (53 percent) with children under the age of seven reported use of safety gates (Marshall et al., 2005). Rates of safety practices may be lower depending on the community and the method of data collection. For example, in an observational study, we found only about one-quarter of families in a low-income, urban neighborhood were using stair gates (Gielen et al., 2002).

Poisonings. A poison exposure is defined as an ingestion of or contact with a substance that can produce toxic effects (National Center for Injury Prevention and Control, 2001). While there is no universally agreed-on definition of a poisoning from either a clinical or epidemiological perspective (Institute of Medicine, 2004), the Home Safety Council defined it as "the ingestion, inhalation, absorption through the skin, or injection of so much of a drug, toxin or other chemical that a harmful effect results" (Runyan & Casteel, 2004, p. 133). Such harmful effects can range in severity from mild to fatal, and the physical effects of nonfatal injuries caused by poisonings can be temporary in nature or can result in lifelong disability.

Every thirteen seconds, a poison control center in the United States fields a call about a poison exposure; more than 90 percent of them are exposures that occur in the home (Watson et al., 2004). More than half of these 2,395,582 incidents occur among children under the age of six. Their most common ingestions are household products such as cosmetics, cleaning supplies, and pain relievers. Under the age of thirteen, more males are the victims of poison exposures, but among teenagers and adults, more females are likely to be involved in poison exposures. The substances most commonly involved in poison exposures among adults were pain relievers, sedatives, cleaning products, and antidepressants.

Most calls to poison control centers do not result in a hospital or emergency department visit. In fact, three-quarters of all such calls are managed at the site of the exposure (Watson et al., 2004; National Safe Kids Campaign, 2004b).

Nevertheless, one-fourth of all home injury deaths are caused by poisoning. Unlike other injury causes, fatal poisoning rates are highest among adults between twenty and fifty-nine years of age. While fatal poisoning rates stayed relatively stable between 1992 and 1999 for all other age groups (fewer than 1 per 100,000), fatal poisoning among those twenty to fifty-nine years old rose to a rate greater than 4 per 100,000 in 1999 (Runyan & Casteel, 2004). Many fatal poisonings occurring at home have been attributed to unintentional overdoses of prescription, over-the-counter, and illegal substances, including heroin, appetite suppressants, caffeine, antidepressants, and alcohol. Less than 3 percent of unintentional poisoning deaths were the result of motor vehicle exhaust (Casteel & Runyan, 2004a).

Poisoning fatalities differ from exposures in several ways according to the Toxic Exposure Surveillance System of the American Association of Poison Control Centers. First, while children younger than six years of age are responsible for the majority of poisoning reports but only 3 percent of fatalities, adults twenty to forty-nine years old make up 58 percent of poisoning fatalities (Watson et al., 2004). Second, more than 90 percent of poisoning exposures involve a single substance. In contrast, 49 percent of fatal cases involved two or more drugs or products. Finally, almost 92 percent of exposures are acute compared to 54 percent of chronic poisonings, which are fatal.

The costs related to poisoning deaths and injury are staggering: nearly $21.8 billion for children under the age of fifteen alone (National Safe Kids Campaign, 2004b). The Children's Safety Network (2005) reports poisoning fatality costs in excess of $150 billion, including $102 billion for quality-of-life costs and $48 billion for work-lost costs. Poisoning injuries not resulting in death add to these costs, with $1.5 billion in work-lost costs and $2.3 billion in medical costs.

A variety of safety products and behaviors are recommended to prevent unintentional poisoning, mostly aimed at preventing child poisonings. Many countermeasures require action and vigilance on the part of adult caretakers of children. For instance, installing cabinet and drawer latches or locks along with lock boxes are consistently recommended countermeasures by safety advocacy groups (National Safe Kids Campaign, 2004b). However, a recent survey of homes where children younger than age six live or visit found that few adults practice these behaviors or use the recommended safety products. The study found that adults keep medicines out in the open (33 percent), in an unlocked drawer or cabinet (82 percent), and in their purse (42 percent) (Coyne-Beasley, Runyan, Baccadlini, Perkis, & Johnson, 2005). In our study of low-income urban families, we observed cabinet locks in use in only 11 percent of households (Gielen et al., 2002).

Using child-resistant containers on all prescription medications is another recommended behavior for adults. Numerous studies indicate that the Poison Prevention Packaging Act of 1970 and child-resistant packaging significantly reduce the morbidity and mortality of childhood poisonings (Walton, 1982; Dole, Czajka, & Rivara, 1986; Hingley, 1997) but require the caps to be replaced properly on medicines after every use. Similarly, adults bringing any hazardous products into the home, such as household cleaners or over-the-counter preparations, should consider carefully the toxicity and packaging of the products. One aspect of packaging that is less clear in its protective abilities is warning labels, commonly referred to as "Mr. Yuk." First created by the National Poison Control Center in Pittsburgh, Mr. Yuk is a bright green picture of a scowling face with a protruding tongue designed to be placed onto containers of harmful substances. Mr. Yuk stickers are well known among many parents and are frequently perceived as a sufficient countermeasure to protecting children from hazardous substances. However, a study of two year olds showed no effect in reducing poisonings with the use of Mr. Yuk stickers (Fergusson, Harwood, Beautrais, & Shannon, 1982). A second study of children age twelve to thirty months showed an actual increase in the children's handling of medicines labeled with Mr. Yuk stickers (Vernberg, Culver-Dickinson, & Spyker, 1984). Children may be attracted to these substances due to the colorful stickers on the medicine container.

Once previously recommended by pediatric and poison control groups, syrup of ipecac, a pharmaceutical agent that induces vomiting, is now contraindicated for home use (Committee on Injury, Violence and Poison Prevention, 2003). This change in policy and practice was brought about by several factors, including the dramatic decrease in childhood poisonings over the past forty years and recent research evidence that failed to show a benefit for children who were treated with it (Bond, 2003).

Our review of PubMed and Internet sources found no mention of interventions aimed at reducing accidental poisoning among older people. The literature does identify common causes for unintentional poisoning among the elderly, including senility and confusion, improper use or storage of chemical products, and mistakes in identifying nonfood items or therapeutic agents (Klein-Schwartz, Oderda, & Booze, 1983).

Fires and Burns. Different types of energy can be implicated in burn injuries and include thermal (heat), electrical, and chemical energy. When thermal energy is in the form of a liquid or steam and results in an injury, this is usually referred to as a scald burn. Burn injuries can be classified by either the percentage of body surface involved or the depth of the skin involved (first-degree through fourth-degree burns). The depth of the burn depends on the temperature and duration of the heat applied, as well as on characteristics of the skin. In the case of house fires, death or injury can be caused by burns from the fire or inhaling the toxic gases produced as fires develop and spread (National Safe Kids, 2004a).

More than twenty-six hundred people died as a result of a home fire in 2002, the latest year for which national mortality data are available (Centers for Disease Control and Prevention, 2004). Mortality rates are highest among adults over the age of sixty-five (2.04 per 100,000) and children under the age of five (1.22 per 100,000). Age-related morbidity rates reveal a different picture. The highest rate of injury from house fires is among children zero to four years (355 per 100,000), followed by those twenty to twenty-four years old (217 per 100,000) and those fifteen to nineteen years old (216 per 100,000). Seniors eighty to eighty-four years of age have the lowest morbidity rates from house fires: 39.52 per 100,000. Others known to be at increased risk for house fire deaths are individuals who are impaired by alcohol or other drugs, have physical or cognitive disability, have low socioeconomic status, and live in substandard housing or mobile homes (Runyan, Bangdiwala, Linzer, Sacks, & Butts, 1992; Marshall et al., 1998).

According to the U.S. Fire Administration (2005), more than 500,000 structure fires occurred in 2001; 76 percent of the structures burned were residences. For both single-family homes and apartments, fires most often start in the kitchen, bedroom, or living room. Cooking is the leading cause of home fire injuries, while cigarette smoking causes the most home fire deaths. The cause of death due to home fires is more likely to be from smoke, fumes, or carbon monoxide compared to burn injuries: 69 percent versus 15 percent, respectively (Casteel & Runyan, 2004a).

Smoke alarms have been called the "residential fire safety success story of the past quarter century" by the National Fire Protection Association (NFPA; 2004). Smoke detectors have been repeatedly found to be effective, reliable, and inexpensive early warning devices that prompt evacuation behavior (Runyan et al., 1992; Marshall et al., 1998; Istre, McCoy, Osborn, Barnard, & Bolton, 2001). It has been estimated that if a home fire occurs, a working smoke detector can reduce the risk of death by as much as 50 percent (Ahrens, 2003). About 70 percent of residential fire deaths occur in homes without a working smoke alarm. As such, support for smoke alarm use is encouraged by a wide variety of professional and advocacy groups including the National Fire Protection Association (2004), the American Academy of Pediatrics (Committee on Injury and Poison Prevention, 2000), the American Association of Retired Persons (2005), and the National Safe Kids Campaign (2004a). The presence of smoke alarms is reported in 95 percent of homes in the United States, and recommendations call for at least one working smoke alarm on each level and in each sleeping area (NFPA, 2004). However, reported rates of working smoke alarms may be an overestimate. In our research with low-income urban families, we found that 96 percent of families reported having working smoke alarms, but only about half were actually functional when tested by home observers (Chen, Gielen, & McDonald,

2003). Thus, there continues to be a need for behavioral interventions promoting their proper and consistent use and maintenance.

Behavioral Interventions to Reduce Home Fires and Their Related Injuries

This section highlights the potential and actual role of behavioral interventions in reducing the problem of home fires and their related injuries. A growing area of research and attention relates to the intersection of human behavior and the built environment, not addressed in this chapter. Readers interested in this topic are directed to conference proceedings of three international symposia on this topic (www.intercomm.dial.pipex.com).

Conceptualizing Prevention Strategies

A variety of primary, secondary, and tertiary prevention initiatives to reduce residential fire deaths and injuries have been implemented in communities around the world. Primary prevention consists of strategies to prevent or minimize the likelihood that the injury event (home fires) will occur. For example, because cigarette smoking is implicated as the leading cause of home fire deaths, considerable efforts have been aimed at reducing their ability to initiate fires. The use of less porous cigarette paper, which slows the burn rate of a cigarette, allows it to self-extinguish if left unattended, thereby reducing the likelihood of starting a fire (Children's Safety Network, 2005). Secondary prevention includes strategies that prevent death or injury in the event of a home fire. Perhaps the most widely recognized secondary prevention strategy is the use of residential smoke alarms to cue evacuation behaviors of residents in the event of a fire. Tertiary prevention comprises those efforts to minimize the extent of damage to individuals injured during the event (home fire). One such example is the development of comprehensive trauma systems designed to efficiently and effectively care for, in this case, burn victims.

As with all other injury control strategies, fire prevention strategies can be placed on an active-passive continuum as determined by their dependence on modifying human behavior. Passive strategies attempt to remove human factors from the equation and rely instead on changing environments or products to reduce injury. Self-extinguishing cigarettes, residential sprinkler systems, and smoke alarms are all examples of more passive fire prevention strategies. Active strategies rely on individuals to be active, that is, engaged in behavior to protect or promote their own safety. Injury control professionals may prefer passive strategies, but as Gielen and Sleet (2003, p. 65) argue, "[i]t is rarely feasible to achieve injury reduction without some element of behavior change." For example, although a smoke alarm offers passive protection that does not rely on human behavior (it alerts individuals rather than relying on them to detect a fire on their own), it must be installed and properly maintained and residents must perform evacuation behaviors. The same could be said for self-extinguishing cigarettes and residential sprinkler systems, both of which require consumer action (purchasing behavior). Behavior and social change theories have a largely untapped potential to improve our understanding of the active strategies necessary for preventing injuries in general and in fire safety in particular (Thompson, Waterman, & Sleet, 2004).

A Historical Perspective

A number of authors have noted the historical lack of scholarship in the application of social and behavior change theories to injuries (Sleet & Hopkins, 2004; Trifiletti, Gielen, Sleet, & Hopkins, 2005). Trifiletti and colleagues (2005) conducted a systematic review of the literature published between 1980 and 2001 on behavioral and social sciences theory applications to all unintentional injuries and found an underuse of such theories applied to injury, especially for the purpose of testing theory. In the review, home fires were included with other household injuries in a few studies, but there were no studies that dealt exclusively with home fires and theory-based approaches to understanding fire safety behaviors. Warda, Tenenbein, and Moffatt (1999) reviewed forty-three studies published between 1983 and 1997 that focused on home fire injury prevention interventions. DiGuiseppi and Higgins (2000) reviewed twenty-six trials from 1970 to 1998 that addressed interventions specific to promoting residential smoke alarms. In an update to the last two reviews, Ta, Frattaroli, Bergen, and Gielen (2005) reviewed an additional twelve new studies of fire prevention interventions. This body of literature is also not theory based, with none of the studies explicitly mentioning the use of theory in guiding their interventions. The general conclusions that can be drawn from these reviews are that smoke alarm distribution programs that use the canvassing method of going to homes are an effective and efficient means of getting smoke alarms into people's homes but that smoke alarm functionality over time remains a problem.

From a behavioral perspective, we can note that distribution programs address barriers to behavior change, an important construct in many behavior change theories. Also, the reduced functionality over time (mostly from missing batteries) is a behavioral challenge that has yet to be addressed. There is an important opportunity here to use behavioral theory to better understand and address this unsafe behavior. We conclude that despite the lack of explicit use of behavioral theory to guide home fire safety intervention research, many studies have used constructs that cut across a variety of behavioral theories, which will be described in more detail in the following sections.

A Contemporary Perspective

Contemporary health promotion and injury prevention practice supports the notion that behavior is affected by and affects multiple levels of influence. This ecological perspective organizes these multiple levels of influence into ever larger spheres of social influence (see also Chapter Seven, this volume). Glanz and Rimer (1995) organize and identify these levels of influence as intrapersonal factors, interpersonal factors, institutional factors, community factors, and public policy. Kaplan, Everson, and Lynch (2000) offer a more refined delineation of levels to examine the distribution of diseases within populations by preceding the individual level with pathophysiological pathways and genetic factors and following it with social relationships and living conditions. The exact manner in which levels of influence are divided and organized is not as important as the consideration given to multiple levels of influence.

In this chapter, we organize our discussion around two main levels of influence: individual-level and community-level influences on our specific behavior of interest, smoke alarm use. Individual-level theories, such as the health belief model and the theory of planned behavior, more broadly applied to injury prevention, are reviewed in detail in Chapter Two, this volume. Community-level models, such as community organization and diffusion of innovations, represent the combined elements of institutional factors, community factors, and public policy approaches and are covered in Chapter Four, this volume. Chapter Three in this volume includes a detailed description of social cognitive theory, which acknowledges the importance of reciprocal determinism, that is, the bidirectional nature of how individuals influence and are influenced by their environments, as well as their behavior (Green & Kreuter, 2005). In this chapter, we highlight examples of this reciprocity where appropriate.

Individual-Level Influences. Individual characteristics that influence behavior include factors such as knowledge, attitudes, beliefs, and personality traits. Among the individual-level factors that affect the use of smoke alarms are knowledge about their efficacy, attitudes about the seriousness and likelihood of a house fire, and beliefs about one's ability to obtain and install a smoke alarm. Research has focused primarily on describing the frequency and correctness of smoke alarm behaviors in populations and the demographic factors associated with specific fire safety practices (Sleet et al., 2004; Trifiletti, Gielen, Sleet, & Hopkins, 2005; Warda et al., 1999; DiGuiseppi & Higgins, 2000).

Knowledge, skills, and attitudes are individual-level factors addressed by the constructs of a number of social and behavior theories and are often the target of educational interventions. However, while educational campaigns have been effective in increasing knowledge of burn prevention, there is little evidence that educational approaches alone achieve reductions in burn rates (Towner, Dowswell, Mackereth, & Jarvis, 2001). Azeredo and Stephens-Stidham (2003) found knowledge gains among elementary school children who received a multifaceted injury prevention curriculum that included smoke alarm giveaways and installations. In terms of attitude change, research has demonstrated that it is more effective to enhance people's positive beliefs than to refute their negative beliefs and that fear-based communication is not effective, although we could find no examples of research that has tested this specifically with regard to fire safety beliefs (Wilde, 1993).

DiGuiseppi and Roberts (2000) conducted a systematic review of individual-level injury prevention interventions in clinical (medical) settings. As related to smoke alarms, the authors found that educational interventions such as counseling, especially when linked with free or low-cost safety devices, did increase smoke alarm ownership (Kelly, Sein, & McCarthy, 1987; Barone, 1988; Thomas, Hassanein, & Christophersen, 1984; Clamp & Kendrick, 1998). In our randomized controlled trials of home safety interventions delivered in pediatric well-child-care settings, we were unable to demonstrate changes in smoke alarm use using either self-report or observed outcomes (Gielen et al., 2001, 2002). These negative results may be due to several factors: we did not give away smoke alarms, we addressed multiple home safety topics rather than focusing exclusively on smoke alarms, and there were high rates of smoke alarm use among our families at baseline, perhaps due to the city fire department's giveaway program.

Community-Level Influences. Here, community-level influences are defined broadly to encompass institutional factors (policies and rules that affect behavior), community factors (social networks and norms among groups or organizations), and public policy (local, state, and federal laws or policies that effect behavior). In essence, this level of influence encompasses aspects related to the larger social structures in which individuals live. Requiring smoke alarms in all new residential construction and making landlords responsible for ensuring working alarms in rental properties are examples of community-level interventions. We could find no studies evaluating the effectiveness of these types of policy-related interventions.

Another type of community-level intervention is the broad-scale campaign that includes distribution (or installation) of smoke alarms in communities, often selected because they have high rates of fires or fire-related injuries. This type of intervention seeks to get the product into the homes of those in need and educate the residents about fire safety, and in doing so may also facilitate changing social norms and strengthening social networks. In their work distributing free smoke alarms to low-income, urban homes in the U.K., DiGuiseppi and colleagues (2002) found that giving out free smoke alarms in an economically deprived urban community resulted in few alarms actually being installed (only 8 percent were installed by program staff), few alarms working at the time of follow-up (9 percent of the intervention group), and little effect on reducing fire-related injuries. Douglas, Mallonee, and Istre (1998) tested different distribution techniques and found that canvassing resulted in significantly more alarms being distributed and at cheaper cost compared to three other distribution methods tested. Mallonee (2000) implemented a smoke alarm giveaway program targeted to neighborhoods with the highest rates of burn injuries. This highly successful program found an 81 percent reduction in residential fire-related injuries in the targeted communities (compared to 7 percent in the comparison communities) and a five-year cost savings of $15 million. Harvey et al. (2004) evaluated two methods of promoting smoke alarms in five U.S. cities: direct distribution or redeemable vouchers. High-risk households randomized to the direct distribution group were more likely to have a working smoke alarm at follow-up compared to those randomized to the voucher group.

Additional examples of individual- and community-level interventions can be found in the review articles cited previously (Sleet et al., 2004; Trifiletti, Gielen, Sleet, & Hopkins, 2005; Warda et al., 1999; DiGuiseppi & Higgins, 2000; Ta et al., 2005). Now we turn our attention to a specific example of how theory is currently being applied to the issue of smoke alarm behaviors.

Applying Behavioral Science and Theory to Smoke Alarm Behaviors: Implications for Practitioners

In his review of health behavior models for the Behavioral Approaches to Injury Control Conference, Fishbein (2005) identified defining the behavior of interest as one of the most important tasks in developing and using behavioral theory. The work reviewed above defines smoke alarm behavior quite broadly and therefore may fail to intervene at the correct or necessary point to bring about change. Recent novel applications of theory to injury behaviors are shedding light on this issue.

A New Behavioral Science Model for Smoke Alarm Use

Recent work by Thompson, Waterman, and Sleet (2004) offers an example of an effective way to apply behavioral science not only to define behavior better but also to push our understanding of prevention behaviors. Building on the realization by McKnight, Struttmann, and Mays (1995) that smoke alarm use is a composite of several distinct behaviors, Thompson and colleagues defined smoke alarm use not only in terms of acquiring and installing the alarm but also in reacting appropriately to it in the event of activation. They identified seven behavioral aspects of smoke alarm use in their model: (1) acquiring the alarm, (2) installing the alarm, (3) testing the alarm, (4) maintaining the alarm, (5) formulating an escape plan, (6) practicing an escape plan, and (7) implementing the escape plan. A panel of experts was then convened to confirm that these were the most important target behaviors related to smoke alarms and to develop a model to influence them. By separating out each behavior, it was then possible to consider legislative, engineering, and behavioral solutions for each. Eventually a model was developed that could be used by injury program personnel to improve the array of target behaviors and advance future research on how best to influence smoke alarm behaviors. In this model, behavioral solutions had the most significant role in bringing about change related to formulating, practicing, and implementing the plan, while legislative and engineering solutions play a more significant role in acquiring and installing the alarm (Thompson et al., 2004).

Application of the Precaution Adoption Process Model to Smoke Alarm Use

To better understand the practical utility afforded by the use of behavioral theories, what follows is the application of one specific theory, the precaution adoption process model (Weinstein, 1988), to one particular behavior: smoke alarm use. The precaution adoption process model (PAPM) provides the theoretical basis for understanding the adoption of specific health behaviors. As previously described (see Chapter Two, this volume), the PAPM has a sequence of seven stages: stage 1, unaware of precaution; stage 2, not engaged; stage 3, undecided; stage 4, not planning; stage 5, planning; stage 6, acting; and stage 7, maintenance (see Figure 13.1). The stages proposed by the model can be assessed by a series of questions for a behavior that identify a person's position in the adoption process. This simple and direct method for evaluating a person's stage makes this model highly desirable for both researchers and practitioners. By recognizing that behavior change occurs as a staged process, rather than a static one, this model helps target communication messages and educational methods to an individual's or a group's stage of readiness. The PAPM shares the stage-based approach with the Transtheoretical Model (see Chapter Two, this volume), but differs in the number and definition of the stages, and in the inclusion of the notion of both a hazard (house fires) and a precaution (smoke alarm).

Trifiletti (2005) was the first to apply the PAPM to research on parents' readiness to adopt home safety behaviors (see also Chapter Two, this volume). Based on

FIGURE 13.1. PRECAUTION ADOPTION PROCESS MODEL.

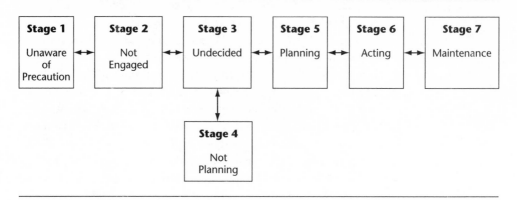

her results and in consultation with Neil Weinstein, the creator of the PAPM, the model has been adapted for use with injury behaviors, including smoke alarm use, in a currently funded National Institute for Child Health and Human Development (NICHD) trial being conducted by the authors (McDonald and Gielen). Although the trial is still in the field, we offer this adaptation as an illustration of how theory can have practical utility for designing and evaluating interventions. Answers to the question of this particular application's utility to smoke alarm behaviors await the trial results.

In the new adaptation, behaviors are better specified, much along the lines suggested by Thompson's model described for smoke alarms. Specifically, profiles have been added to more fully define and stage components of a safety behavior. For example, the safety behavior of "smoke alarm use" is made up of several complex behaviors or "profiles," including (1) not having a working smoke alarm, (2) having one but not changing the batteries in the past six months, (3) having a working smoke alarm but not on all levels of the home, and (4) having a working smoke alarm on every level and changing batteries at correct intervals. More fully articulating smoke alarm behaviors through the use of these profiles offers benefit to defining the problem, directing the interventions, and evaluating its impact. Figure 13.2 shows a person in profile 2, stage 3 for smoke alarms (the person has an alarm but has not changed batteries and has not made a decision about changing the batteries).

Problem definition is enhanced by the application of this theory because it allows a more precise and complete snapshot of the intended target audience's smoke alarm behavior. Compared to the dichotomous response evoked from the question, "Do you have a smoke alarm?" responses to the PAPM staging questions illustrated in Figure 13.2 reveal much more information. A clearer picture of the problem in turn promotes better interventions. Consider the differential

FIGURE 13.2. STAGING SAFETY PROFILES
USING THE PAPM: SMOKE ALARM USE.

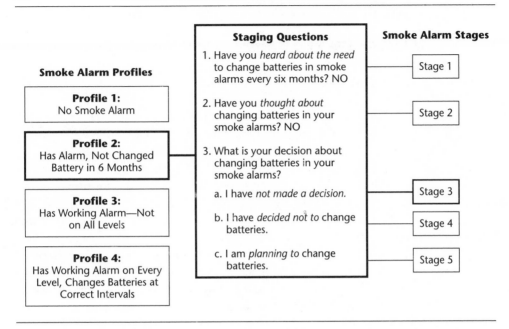

impact of a communication campaign or a counseling message that promoted smoke alarm use in general compared to one that could, through the application of PAPM, hone in on a message that communicated the need for a smoke alarm on every level of the home (if that was determined to be the priority message needed based on a group's or individual's responses to the staging items). The final benefit of using a stage-based model such as the PAPM is its utility for evaluating an intervention. Because behavior change is a process that occurs in stages over time, success can be measured as progress through these stages. This creates the potential for evaluations that allow both static outcomes (absolute number of safety practices) and dynamic outcomes (stage movement).

Conclusion

Home injuries remain all too common, and the most vulnerable among us—young children and older adults—are hardest hit by unintentional home injury. The home injury problem has recently come into more focus, in large part due to the efforts of the Home Safety Council. However, many aspects of the home injury problem remain blurred because of inadequate data sources. While the work of the Home Safety Council has shed light on the problem of injuries in the home, still too little is known to guide much-needed intervention and evaluation studies. The Home Safety Council's work was hampered by poor injury reporting, which limited the ability to provide a complete picture of the home injury problem.

Because of the large number of types of home injuries, it was beyond the scope of this chapter to review all of the intervention literature to determine how theory has been used. However, based on the findings of the Trifiletti and colleagues (2005) review of multiple types of unintentional injuries and the three reviews of smoke alarms (Warda et al., 1999; DiGuiseppi & Higgins, 2000; Ta et al., 2005), it seems reasonable to conclude that behavior change theories have not been widely used in constructing prevention programs for unintentional home injuries or for developing a solid understanding of the determinants of specific safety behaviors. In the review of the smoke alarm literature, we found that many incorporated constructs commonly found in behavior change theories, such as reducing barriers to adopting a behavior and influencing social norms. We hope this review will encourage additional behavioral science explorations into safety behaviors and how best to influence them. Glanz and Rimer (1995, p. 12) wrote, "Effective practice depends on marshaling the most appropriate theory or theories and practice strategies for a given situation." Better integration and application of social and behavioral sciences theories could result in more carefully designed intervention trials and more rigorous standards for professional practice.

References

Ahrens, M. (2003). *US experience with smoke alarms and other alarms.* Quincy, MA: National Fire Protection Agency.

American Academy of Pediatrics Committee on Injury and Poison Prevention. (2001). Falls from heights: Windows, roofs, and balconies. *Pediatrics, 107*(5), 1188–1191.

American Association of Retired Persons. (2005, June). *Smoke detectors.* http://www.aarp.org/families/home_design/safety_lighting/a2004–03–02-s-smokedetectors.html.

American Geriatric Society. (2001). Guidelines for the prevention of falls in older persons. *Journal of the American Geriatric Society, 49,* 664–672.

Azeredo, R., & Stephens-Stidham, S. (2003). Design and implementation of injury prevention curricula for elementary schools: Lessons learned. *Injury Prevention, 9*(3), 274–278.

Barone, V. J. (1988). *An analysis of well-child parenting classes: The extent of parent compliance with healthcare recommendations to decrease potential injury of their toddlers.* Unpublished doctoral dissertation, University of Kansas.

Bond, G. R. (2003). Home syrup of ipecac use does not reduce emergency department use or improve outcome. *Pediatrics, 112*(5), 1061–1064.

Casteel, C., & Runyan, C. W. (2004a). Leading causes of unintentional home injury death. In C. W. Runyan & C. Casteel (Eds.), *The state of home safety in America: Facts about unintentional injuries in the home* (2nd ed.). Washington, DC: Home Safety Council.

Casteel, C., & Runyan, C. W. (2004b). Nonfatal unintentional home injury. In C. W. Runyan & C. Casteel (Eds.), *The state of home safety in America: Facts about unintentional injuries in the home* (2nd ed.). Washington, DC: Home Safety Council.

Centers for Disease Control and Prevention. (2004, Mar.). Web-based Injury Statistics Query and Reporting System (WISQARS), Unintentional residential fire/flame deaths and rates per 100,000, 2002. http://www.cdc.gov/ncipc/wisqars.

Chen, L. H., Gielen, A. C., & McDonald, E. M. (2003). Validity of home safety practices. *Injury Prevention, 9*(1), 73–75.

Chiaviello, C. T., Christof, R. A., & Bond, G. R. (1994). Infant walker-related injuries: A prospective study of severity and incidence. *Pediatrics, 93*(6), 974–976.

Children's Safety Network. (2005). *Injury prevention: What works? Cost-outcome analysis of injury prevention programs.* Calverton, MD: CSN Economics and Data Analysis Resource Center, Pacific Institute for Research and Evaluation.

Clamp, M., & Kendrick, D. (1998). A randomized controlled trial of general practitioner safety advice for families with children under 5 years. *British Medical Journal, 16,* 1576–1579.

Committee on Injury and Poison Prevention. (2000). Reducing the number of deaths and injuries from residential fires. *Pediatrics, 105*(6), 1355–1357.

Committee on Injury Prevention. (1994). *The Injury Prevention Program (TIPP).* Chicago: American Academy of Pediatrics.

Committee on Injury, Violence and Poison Prevention. (2003). Poison treatment in the home. *Pediatrics, 112*(5), 1182–1185.

Coyne-Beasley, T., Runyan, C. W., Baccadlini, L., Perkis, D., & Johnson, R. M. (2005). Storage of poisonous substances and firearms in homes with young children visitors and older adults. *American Journal of Preventive Medicine, 28,* 109–115.

DiGuiseppi, C., & Higgins, J.P.T. (2000). Systematic review of controlled trails of interventions to promote smoke alarms. *Archives of Diseases of Children, 82,* 341–348.

DiGuiseppi, C., & Roberts, I. G. (2000). Individual level injury prevention strategies in the clinical setting. *Future of Children, 10*(1), 53–82.

DiGuiseppi, C., Roberts, I., Wade, A., Sculper, M., Edwards, P., Godward, C., Pan, H., & Slater, S. (2002). Incidence of fires and related injuries after giving out free smoke alarms: Cluster randomized controlled trial. *British Medical Journal, 325,* 995–998.

Dole, E. J., Czajka, P. A., & Rivara, F. P. (1986). Evaluation of pharmacists' compliance with the Poison Prevention Packaging Act. *American Journal of Public Health, 76*(11), 1335–1336.

Douglas, M. R., Mallonee, S., & Istre, G. R. (1998). Comparison of community based smoke detector distribution methods in an urban community. *Injury Prevention, 4,* 28–32.

Fergusson, D. M., Harwood, L. J., Beautrais, A. L., & Shannon, F. T. (1982). A controlled trial of a poisoning prevention method. *Pediatrics, 69*(5), 515–520.

Fishbein, M. (2005, May). Models of health behavior. In *Behavioral approaches to injury control: Conference proceedings.* www.hiprc.org. Seattle: Harborview Injury Prevention and Research Center.

Gielen, A. C., & Sleet, D. (2003). Application of behavior-change theories and methods to injury prevention. *Epidemiologic Reviews, 25,* 65–76.

Gielen, A. C., Wilson, M.E.H., McDonald, E. M., Serwint, J. R., Andrews, J. A., Hwang, W., & Wang, M. (2001). Randomized trial of enhanced anticipatory guidance for injury prevention. *Archives of Pediatrics and Adolescent Medicine, 155*(1), 42–44.

Gielen, A. C., McDonald, E. M., Wilson, M.E.H., Hwang, W., Serwint, J. R., Andrews, J. A., & Wang, M. (2002). Effects of improved access to safety counseling, products, and home visits on parents' safety practices: Results of a randomized trial. *Archives of Pediatrics and Adolescent Medicine, 156*(1), 33–40.

Glanz, K., & Rimer, B. K. (1995, July). *Theory at a glance: A guide for health promotion practice.* Rockville, MD: National Cancer Institute.

Green, L., & Kreuter, M. W. (2005). *Health program planning: An educational and environmental approach.* (4th ed.). New York: McGraw-Hill.

Harvey, P. A., Aitken, M., Ryan, G. W., Demeter, L. A., Givens, J., Sundararaman, R., & Goulette, S. (2004). Strategies to increase smoke alarm use in high-risk households. *Journal of Community Health, 29*(5), 375–385.

Hingley, A. T. (1997). Preventing childhood poisoning. *FDA Consumer Magazine, 30*(2), 1–7.

Institute of Medicine. (2004). *Forging a poison prevention and control system.* Washington, DC: National Academy of Sciences.

Istre, G. R., McCoy, M. A., Osborn, L., Barnard, J. J., & Bolton, A. (2001). Deaths and injuries from house fires. *New England Journal of Medicine, 344,* 1911–1016.

Kaplan, G. A., Everson, S. A., & Lynch, J. W. (2000). The contribution of social and behavioral research to an understanding of the distribution of disease: A multi-level approach. In B. D. Smedley & S. L. Syme (Eds.), *Promoting health: Intervention strategies from social and behavioral research* (pp. 37–80). Washington, DC: National Academy Press.

Kelly, B., Sein, C., & McCarthy, P. L. (1987). Safety education in a pediatric primary care setting. *Pediatrics, 79,* 818–824.

Klein-Schwartz, W., Oderda, G. M., & Booze, L. (1983). Poisoning in the elderly. *Journal of the American Geriatric Society, 31*(4), 195–199.

Mallonee, S. (2000). Evaluating injury prevention programs: The Oklahoma City Smoke Alarm Project. *Future of Children, 10*(1), 164–74.

Marshall, S. W., Runyan, C. W., Bangdiwala, S. I., Linzer, M. A., Sacks, J. J., & Butts, J. D. (1998). Fatal residential fires: Who dies and who survives? *Journal of the American Medical Association, 279,* 1633–1637.

Marshall, S. W., Runyan, C. W., Yang, J., Coyne-Beasley, T., Waller, A. E., Johnson, R. M., & Perkis, D. (2005). Prevalence of selected risk and protective factors for falls in the home. *American Journal of Preventive Medicine, 28*(1), 95–101.

McKnight, R., Struttmann, T., & Mays, J. (1995). Finding homes without smoke detectors: One step in planning burn prevention programs. *Journal of Burn Care and Rehabilitation, 16,* 548–556.

National Center for Health Statistics, Centers for Disease Control and Prevention. (2005a, Feb.). National Health Interview Survey description. http://www.cdc.gov/nchs/about/major/nhis/hisdesc.htm.

National Center for Health Statistics, Centers for Disease Control and Prevention. (2005b, Feb.). National Hospital Ambulatory Medical Care Surveys for Outpatient and Emergency Department. http://www.cdc.gov/nchs/about/major/ahcd/namcsdes.htm.

National Center for Health Statistics, Centers for Disease Control and Prevention. (2005c, Feb.). U.S. Standard Death Certificate. http://www.cdc.gov/nchs/data/dvs/DEATH11–03final-ACC.pdf.

National Center for Injury Prevention and Control. (2001). *Injury fact book, 2001–2002.* Atlanta, GA: Centers for Disease Control and Prevention.

National Fire Protection Association. (2004, Aug.). *NFPA fact sheets: Smoke alarms: Make them work for your safety.* http://www.nfpa.org/Research/NFPAFactSheets/Alarms/Alarms.asp.

National Safe Kids Campaign. (2004a.). *Residential fire injury fact sheet*. Washington, DC: National Safe Kids Campaign.

National Safe Kids Campaign. (2004b, Sept.). *Injury facts: Poisoning*. http://www.safekids.org/tier3_printable.cfm?content_item_id=1152&folder_id+540.

O'Donnell, G. W., & Mickalide, A. D. (1998, May). *SAFE KIDS at home, at play and on the way: A report to the nation on unintentional childhood injury*. Washington, DC: National Safe Kids Campaign.

Runyan, C. W., Bangdiwala, S. I., Linzer, M. A., Sacks, J. J., & Butts, J. (1992). Risk factors for fatal residential fires. *New England Journal of Medicine, 37*(12), 859–863.

Runyan, C. W., & Casteel, C. (2004). *The state of home safety in America: Facts about unintentional injury in the home* (2nd ed.). Washington, DC: Home Safety Council.

Runyan, C. W., Perkis, D., Marshall, S. W., Johnson, R. M., Coyne-Beasely, T., Waller, A. E., Black, C., & Baccaglini, L. (2005a). Unintentional injuries in the home in the United States. Part II: Morbidity. *American Journal of Preventive Medicine, 28*(1), 80–87.

Runyan, C. W., Casteel, C., Perkis, D., Black, C., Marshall, S. W., Johnson, R. M., Coyne-Beasley, T., Waller, A. E., & Viswanathan, S. (2005b). Unintentional injuries in the home in the United States. Part I: Mortality. *American Journal of Preventive Medicine, 28*(1), 73–79.

Sleet, D. A., & Hopkins, K. (2004). *Bibliography of behavioral science research in unintentional injuries*. Atlanta, GA: National Center for Injury Prevention and Control.

Spiegel, C., & Lindaman, F. (1977). Children can't fly: A program to prevent childhood morbidity and mortality from window falls. *American Journal of Public Health, 67*, 1143–1146.

Ta, V., Frattaroli, S., Bergen, G., & Gielen, A. C. (2005). *Community fire safety interventions: A review of the current literature*. Unpublished manuscript, Johns Hopkins Bloomberg School of Public Health, Baltimore, MD.

Thomas, K. A., Hassanein, R. S., & Christophersen, E. R. (1984). Evaluation of group well-child care for improving burn prevention practices in the home. *Pediatrics, 74*, 879–882.

Thompson, N. J., Waterman, M. B., & Sleet, D. A. (2004). Using behavioral science to improve fire escape behaviors in response to a smoke alarm. *Journal of Burn Care and Rehabilitation, 45*, 179–188.

Towner, E., Dowswell, T., Mackereth, C., & Jarvis, S. (2001). *What works in preventing unintentional injuries in children and young adolescents? An updated systematic review*. London: Health Development Agency.

Trifiletti, L. B. (2005). *The utility of the precaution adoption process model for understanding car safety seat use*. Unpublished manuscript.

Trifiletti, L. B., Gielen, A. C., Sleet, D. A., & Hopkins, K. (2005). Behavioral and social sciences theories and models: Are they used in unintentional injury prevention research? *Health Education Research, 20*(3), 298–307.

U.S. Census Bureau. (2005, Feb.). *American community survey, 2003 data profile: Table 4, Selected Household Characteristics*. http://www.census.gov/acs/www/Products/Profiles/Single/2003/ACS/Tabular/010/01000US4.htm.

U.S. Fire Administration. (2005, Feb.). *Home fire safety fact sheet*. http://www.usfa.fema/gov/public/factsheets/facts.shtm.

Vernberg, K., Culver-Dickinson, P., & Spyker, D. A. (1984). The deterrent effect of poison warning stickers. *American Journal of Diseases of Children, 138*(11), 1018–1020.

Walton, W. W. (1982). An evaluation of the Poison Prevention Packaging Act. *Pediatrics, 69*(3), 363–370.

Warda, L., Tenenbein, M., & Moffatt, M. E. (1999). House fire injury prevention update. Part II. A review of the effectiveness of preventive interventions. *Injury Prevention, 5*, 217–225.

Watson, W. A., Litovitz, T. L., Klein-Schwartz, W., Rodgers, G. C., Jr., Reid, N., Rouse, W. G., Rembert, R. S., & Borys, D. (2004). 2003 annual report of the American Association of Poison Control Centers Toxic Exposures Surveillance System. *American Journal of Emergency Medicine, 22*(5), 335–404.

Weinstein, N. D. (1988). The precaution adoption process. *Health Psychology, 7*(4), 355–386.

Wilde, G.J.S. (1993). Effects of mass media communications on health and safety habits: An overview of issues and evidence. *Addiction, 88*, 983–996.

Wilson, M.E.H., Baker, S. P., Teret, S. P., Shock, S., & Garbarino, J. (1991). *Saving children: A guide to injury prevention*. New York: Oxford University Press.

World Health Organization. (2004, Sept.). *Injuries and violence prevention*. http://www.who.int/violence_injury_prevention/unintentional_injuries/falls/falls1/en/.

CHAPTER FOURTEEN

OCCUPATIONAL INJURY PREVENTION AND APPLIED BEHAVIOR ANALYSIS

E. Scott Geller

Occupational injuries have been vastly reduced during the twentieth century. There were approximately eighteen thousand to twenty-three thousand workplace fatalities per year in the early 1900s compared to fewer than six thousand in 2000 (Stout & Linn, 2002). Much of the early success in reducing occupational fatalities has been attributed to intervention by the safety sciences—safety engineering, industrial hygiene, and safety managements—and legislative and regulatory reforms in response to horrific mining disasters (Stout & Linn, 2002).

Unfortunately, the rate of decline is not uniform across types of industries or causes of death. According to Stout and Linn (2002), the rates are dropping more rapidly for motor vehicles, machine-related deaths, and electrocutions than for homicides and falls. And rates of fatal and nonfatal workplace injuries remain unacceptably high when considering the existence of effective prevention measures.

On average, nearly eleven thousand workers are treated in emergency departments each day in the United States, and approximately two hundred of these workers are hospitalized daily (Centers for Disease Control and Prevention, 2005). Injuries and diseases account for nearly 73 billion dollars in workers' compensation (National Academy of Social Insurance, 2002). According to the National Occupational Research Agenda Report (National Institute for Occupational Safety and Health, 1998), an estimated sixteen U.S. workers are killed and thirty-six thousand U.S. workers are injured every day. On an annual basis, about 3.6 million occupational injuries result in hospital emergency room treatment. International and national prevention practices during the preceding three decades have reduced these losses, but morbidity and mortality from occupational hazards are still a major social and economic burden (Centers for Disease Control and Prevention, 2005).

The ongoing problem of occupational injuries requires collaboration among public health scientists, safety scientists, and social and behavioral scientists (Stout & Linn, 2002). The identification and widespread implementation of effective prevention strategies remain challenges for the field of occupational injury. While engineering changes and regulatory interventions remain critical to protecting workers, how workers behave in environments that are more or less safe can greatly influence their risk for injury. For example, motor vehicle travel is by far the greatest single cause of occupational injury death in the United States, yet strategies to prevent it are often ignored (Sleet & Lonero, 2002; Peden et al., 2004).

Thus, it is vitally important to study individual behavior in the workplace and determine how to influence it. Applied behavior analysis attempts to reduce workplace injury by discovering environmental determinants of injury risk and ways to reduce that risk through behavior change. This chapter offers a detailed review of applied behavior analysis (or behavior-based safety) as used effectively to prevent occupational injuries.

Overview of Behavior-Based Safety

For more than two decades, applied behavior analysis has been used to improve occupational safety in industrial settings. The popular label for this approach to injury prevention is *behavior-based safety* (BBS). Several books detail the principles and procedures of BBS and provide empirical evidence for its success (Geller, 1996a, 1998c, 2001g, 2001h; 2005; Geller & Williams, 2001; Krause, 1995; Krause, Hidley, & Hodson, 1996; McSween, 2003; Petersen, 1989; Sulzer-Azaroff, 1998). Moreover, a number of reviews of the literature provide solid evidence for the success of this approach to injury prevention (Geller, 1998a; Grindle, Dickinson, & Boettcher, 2000; McAfee & Winn, 1989; Petersen, 1989; Sulzer-Azaroff & Austin, 2000).

Principles of Behavior-Based Safety

The effective applications of BBS generally follow seven key principles described below. Each principle is broad enough to include a wide range of practical applications but narrow enough to guide the applied behavior analysis approach to improving safety and health. These principles can guide the development and implementation of interventions to improve safety-related behaviors and attitudes in the workplace as well as in homes and neighborhoods, and throughout the community (Elder, Geller, Hovell, & Mayer, 1994; Geller, 1997b, 1998b, 1998c, 2001b, 2001c; Geller & Williams, 2001; Geller, Elder, Hovell, & Sleet, 1991).

Principle 1: Target Observable Behavior

The BBS approach is grounded in empirical behavioral research as conceptualized and described by B. F. Skinner (1938/1991, 1953, 1974). Experimental behavior analysis and, later, applied behavior analysis emerged from Skinner's research and laid the groundwork for numerous therapies and interventions to improve the quality of life among individuals, groups, and entire communities (Goldstein & Krasner, 1987; Greene, Winett, Van Houten, Geller, & Iwata, 1987). Whether working one-on-one in a clinical setting or with work teams throughout an organization, the intervention procedures always target specific behaviors in order to produce constructive change. In other words, applied behavior analysis focuses on what people do, analyzes why they do it, and then applies a research-supported intervention strategy to improve what people do.

The focus of BBS is on changing behaviors or actions rather than changing internal awareness, intentions, attitudes, cognitions, or emotions. This latter approach is often used successfully in clinical psychology but is considered too labor and time intensive for use in a group, organizational, or communitywide setting.

Principle 2: Focus on External Factors to Explain and Improve Behavior

Skinner did not deny the existence of internal determinants of behavior (such as personality characteristics, feelings, perceptions, attitudes, and values), but considered them unobservable for scientific study. Given the difficulty in objectively defining internal traits or states, Skinner believed it is more cost-effective to identify environmental conditions that influence behavior and to change these factors as a means to improve behavior.

A behavior analysis of risky work practices can pinpoint many determinants of risky behavior, including inadequate management systems or supervisor behaviors that promote or inadvertently encourage at-risk work practices. Without the objective problem-solving perspective fostered by BBS principles, these inadequacies that shape and maintain undesirable behaviors may never be identified.

Examining external factors that explain or control behavior is a primary focus of BBS and organizational behavior management (Austin, 2000; Austin, Carr, & Agnew, 1999; Bailey & Austin, 1996; Gilbert, 1978). In occupational safety, this approach has been termed *behavioral safety analysis* (Geller, 2000, 2001b, 2001c, 2001f). It involves a search for answers to the following questions in the sequence given in Figure 14.1.

FIGURE 14.1. SAMPLE OF TEN SEQUENTIAL QUESTIONS ASKED IN A BEHAVIORAL SAFETY ANALYSIS.

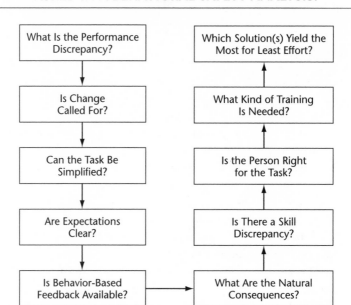

Source: Adapted from Geller, E. S. (2000). Behavioral safety analysis: A necessary precursor to corrective action. *Professional Safety, 45*(3), 32.

Can the Task Be Simplified? Before designing an intervention program to improve behavior, it is critical to implement all possible engineering controls to simplify the task or reduce the likelihood of injury. Consider the many ways an environment could be changed to reduce physical effort, reach, and repetition. This is the rationale behind ergonomics and the search for engineering solutions to occupational safety and health (Kroemer, 1991).

Sometimes behavior facilitators can be added, such as control designs with different shapes to aid discrimination by touch or sight, clear instructions placed at the point of application, color codes to aid memory and task differentiation (Norman, 1988), or convenient machine lifts or conveyor rollers to help with physical jobs. In addition, complex assignments might be redesigned to involve fewer steps or more people. To reduce boredom or repetition, simple tasks might allow job swapping. At the start of a behavioral safety analysis, ask these questions:

- Can an engineering intervention make the job more user friendly?
- Can the task be redesigned to reduce physical demands?

- Can a behavior facilitator be added to improve response differentiation, reduce memory load, or increase reliability?
- Can the challenges of a complex task be shared?
- Can boring, repetitive jobs be cross-trained and swapped?

Is a Quick Fix Available? From their more than sixty combined years of analyzing and solving human performance problems, Mager and Pipe (1997) concluded that many discrepancies between real and ideal behavior can be eliminated with relatively little effort. More specifically, behavioral risks might be present because expectations are unclear, resources are inadequate, or feedback is unavailable. In these cases, behavior-based instruction or demonstration can overcome informal expectations, and behavior-based feedback can enable continuous improvement. When conducting such an analysis, behavioral scientists consider these questions:

- Does the individual know what safety precautions are expected?
- Are there environmental barriers to safe work practices?
- Is the equipment safe to operate for most people?
- Is protective equipment readily available and as comfortable as possible?
- Do employees receive frequent behavior-based feedback related to their safety?

Is Safe Behavior Punished? In some work cultures, there are consequences for reporting an environmental hazard or minor injury. These can range from a reprimand for sullying the company safety record to negative social consequences by coworkers. In some work cultures, it might be considered "cool" or "macho" to work unprotected and take risks. Mager and Pipe (1997) refer to these situations as "upside-down consequences" and suggest they are the cause of many, if not most, of the undesirable behaviors occurring in the workplace. Ask these questions during a behavioral safety analysis:

- What are the consequences for desired behavior?
- Are there more negative than positive consequences for safe behavior?
- What negative consequences for safe behavior can be reduced or removed?

Is Risky Behavior Rewarded? At-risk behavior is often followed by natural positive consequences, including comfort, convenience, and efficiency. Risky short-cuts are usually taken to save time and are perceived to lead to higher performance output. Therefore, taking risky short cuts may be considered "efficient" behavior. People take calculated risks because they expect to gain something positive or avoid something negative. Behavioral safety analysis asks:

- What are the immediate, certain, and positive consequences for risky behavior?
- Does a worker receive more attention, prestige, or status from coworkers for at-risk than safe behavior?
- How can rewards for risky behaviors be reduced or removed?

Are Extra Consequences Used Effectively? Since the natural consequences of comfort, convenience, or efficiency usually support risky over safe behavior, it is often necessary to add extra consequences. These usually take the form of incentive and reward or disincentive and penalty programs. Unfortunately, many of these programs do more harm than good because they are implemented ineffectively (Geller, 1996b, 2001g, 2001h). Disincentives are often ineffective because they are used incorrectly and tend to motivate avoidance behavior rather than positive change. BBS asks these questions when analyzing the impact of using extra consequences to motivate improved safety performance:

- How can punishing consequences be implemented consistently and fairly?
- Can safety incentives stifle the reporting of injuries and close calls?
- Do the safety incentives motivate the achievement of safety process goals?
- Are workers recognized individually and as teams for completing process activities related to safety improvement?

Is There a Skill Discrepancy? What about those times when the individual really does not know how to do the prescribed safe behavior? The person is "knowingly at risk." This situation might call for training, a relatively expensive approach to corrective action. Mager and Pipe (1997) claim that undesirable work behavior is most often not caused by lack of knowledge or skill. People can usually perform the recommended safe behavior if the conditions and the consequences are right. So training should be used relatively infrequently for corrective action. Ask these questions to determine whether the behavioral discrepancy is caused by a lack of knowledge or skill:

- Could the person perform the task safely if his or her life depended on it?
- Are the person's current skills adequate for the task?
- Did the person ever know how to perform the job safely?
- Has the person forgotten the safest way to perform the task?

What Kind of Training Is Needed? Answers to the previous two questions can help pinpoint the kind of intervention needed to eliminate a skill discrepancy. More specifically, a yes answer to these questions implies the need for a skill maintenance program. Skill maintenance might be needed to help a person stay skilled, as when police officers practice regularly on a pistol range to stay ready to use their guns effectively in the rare situation when they need it. This is the rationale behind periodic emergency training. People need to practice the behaviors that could prevent injury or save a life during an emergency. Fortunately, emergencies do not occur very often, and since they do not, people need to go through the motions to stay in practice so that if the infrequent event does occur, they will be prepared.

A very different kind of situation also calls for skill maintenance training. This is when certain behaviors occur regularly but discrepancies still exist. Contrary to circumstances requiring emergency training, this problem is not lack of practice. Rather, the person gets plenty of practice doing the behavior ineffectively or unsafely. In this case, practice does not make perfect but rather serves to entrench a bad (or at-risk) habit.

Vehicle driving behavior is perhaps the most common and relevant example of this second kind of situation in need of skill maintenance training. Most experienced drivers know how to drive a vehicle safely and at one time performed most of their driving behaviors safely, as prescribed by teachers, parents, driving instructors, or peers. For many drivers, however, safe driving practices can decrease over time, especially with the onset of aging, and drivers require retraining or skill modification for the behaviors to remain adaptive in traffic.

Practice with appropriate behavior-based feedback is critical for solving both types of skill discrepancies. However, if the skill is already used frequently but has deteriorated (as in the driving example), it is often necessary to add an extra feedback intervention to overpower the natural consequences that have caused the behavior to drift from the ideal. Later in this chapter, this critical component of the BBS approach to injury prevention is explained. Ask these questions to determine whether the cause of the apparent skill discrepancy is due to lack of practice or lack of feedback:

- How often is the desired skill performed?
- Does the performer receive regular feedback relevant to skill maintenance?
- How does the performer find out how well he or she is doing?

Is the Person Right for the Task? A skill discrepancy can be handled in one of two ways: change the job or change the behavior. The first approach is exemplified by simplifying the task, and the second is reflected in practice with behavior-based feedback. But what if a person's interests, skills, or prior experiences are incompatible with the job? Before investing in skill training for a particular individual, it is a good idea to assess whether the person is right for the task. If the person does not have the motivation or the physical and mental capabilities for a particular job assignment, including risky tasks such as driving, the cost-effective solution is to replace the performer. Not doing this reduces productive work and increases the risk for personal injury. Ask these questions to determine whether the individual has the potential to handle the job safely and effectively:

- Does the person have the physical capability to perform as desired?
- Does the person have the mental capability to handle the complexities of the task?
- Is the person overqualified for the job and thus prone to boredom or dissatisfaction?
- Can the person learn how to do the job as desired?

Summary. Before deciding on an intervention approach, conduct a careful analysis of the situation, the behavior, and the individuals involved in any observed discrepancy between desired and actual behavior. Do not impulsively assume that corrective action to improve behavior requires training or "discipline." A behavioral safety analysis as summarized here and outlined previously in Figure 14.1 will likely give priority to a number of alternative intervention approaches.

Principle 3: Direct with Activators and Motivate with Consequences

This principle enables understanding of why behavior occurs and guides the design of interventions to improve behavior. We do what we do because of the consequences we expect to get for doing it. As Carnegie (1936) put it, "Every act you have ever performed since the day you were born was performed because you wanted something" (p. 62). It is noteworthy that Carnegie cited the research and scholarship of B. F. Skinner as the foundation of this motivation principle.

The important point here is that activators (or signals preceding behavior) are only as powerful as the consequences supporting them. In other words, activators tell us what to do in order to receive a consequence, from the ringing of a telephone or doorbell to the instructions from a training seminar or one-on-one coaching session. We follow through with the particular behavior activated (from answering a telephone or door to following a trainer's instructions) to the extent we expect doing so will give us a pleasant consequence or enable us to avoid an unpleasant consequence.

This principle is typically referred to as the ABC model or three-term contingency, with A for activator (or antecedent), B for behavior, and C for consequence. Proponents of the BBS approach use this ABC principle to design interventions for improving behavior at individual, group, and organizational levels. More than forty years of behavioral science research have demonstrated the efficacy of this general approach to directing and motivating behavior change (Geller, 2001g; McSween, 2003).

Principle 4: Focus on Positive Consequences to Motivate Behavior

B. F. Skinner's concern for people's feelings and attitudes is reflected in his antipathy toward the use of punishment (or negative consequences) to motivate behavior: "The problem is to free men, not from control, but from certain kinds of control" (Skinner, 1971, p. 41). He goes on to explain why control by negative consequences must be reduced in order to increase perceptions of personal freedom.

Years ago, Atkinson and his associates (for example, Atkinson, 1957, 1964; Atkinson & Litwin, 1960) compared the decision making of individuals with a high need to avoid failure and those with a high need to achieve success, and found dramatic differences. While those motivated to achieve positive consequences set challenging but attainable goals, participants with a high need to avoid failure were likely to set goals that were either overly easy or overly difficult.

Easy goal setting ensures avoidance of failure, while setting unrealistic goals provides a readily available excuse for failure, termed *self-handicapping* by later researchers (for example, Berglas & Jones, 1978; Rhodewalt, 1994; Rhodewalt & Fairfield, 1991). Thus, a substantial amount of behavioral research and motivational theory justifies the advocacy of positive reinforcement over punishment contingencies, whether contrived to improve someone else's behavior or imagined to motivate personal rule-governed behavior (see the review by Wiegand & Geller, 2004/2005).

Punishment contingencies are relatively easy to implement on a large scale. That is why the government often selects this approach to behavior management through legislation and enforcement. And when monetary fines are paid for transgressions, the controlling agency obtains financial support for continuing their enforcement efforts.

In many areas of large-scale behavior management, including transportation management, control by negative consequences is seemingly the only feasible approach. Classic research in experimental behavior analysis taught us to expect only temporary suppression of a punished behavior (Azrin & Holz, 1966) and to predict that some drivers in their "Skinner box on wheels" will drive faster to compensate for the time they lost when slowing down in an "enforcement zone" (Estes & Skinner, 1941).

Practical ways to apply positive reinforcement contingencies to driving are available (for example, Everett, Haywood, & Meyers, 1974; Geller, Kalsher, Rudd, & Lehman, 1989; Kalsher, Geller, Clarke, & Lehman, 1989; Hagenzieker, 1991; Rudd & Geller, 1985), but much more long-term research is needed in this domain. Various positive reinforcement contingencies need to be applied and evaluated with regard to their ability to offset the negative side effects of the existing negative reinforcement contingencies (Geller, 2001e).

Regarding industrial safety, we can often intervene to increase people's perceptions that they are working to achieve success rather than working to avoid failure. Even verbal behavior directed toward another person, perhaps as a statement of genuine approval or appreciation for a task well done (Geller, 1997a), can influence motivation in ways that increase perceptions of personal freedom and empowerment. Of course, we cannot be sure the intervention will have the effect intended. Therefore, we need to measure objectively the impact of our intervention procedures, as implicated in the next basic principle of BBS.

Principle 5: Apply the Scientific Method to Improve Intervention

Safety professionals frequently suggest that dealing with the human aspects of safety requires only "good common sense" (Eckenfelder, 1996). This premise is unsupportable because common sense is based on people's selective listening and interpretation and is usually founded on what sounds good to the individual listener, not necessarily on what works (Daniels, 2000, 2001). In contrast, systematic and scientific observation enables the kind of objective feedback needed to know what works and what does not work to improve behavior.

The occurrence of specific behaviors can be objectively observed and measured before and after the implementation of an intervention process. This application of the scientific method provides feedback by which behavioral improvement can be shaped. The acronym DO IT (define, observe, intervene, test; Figure 14.2) is used to teach the principles of BBS to employees and can help empower them to intervene on behalf of others. The DO IT process can put people in control of improving safety-related behaviors and thereby preventing injuries. It represents the scientific method behavior analysts have used for decades to demonstrate the impact of a particular behavior change intervention (Geller, 1996b, 1998a, 2001g).

"D" for Define. The process begins by defining specific behaviors to target. These are at-risk behaviors that need to decrease in frequency or safe behaviors that need to occur more often. Avoiding at-risk behaviors often requires certain safe behaviors, and therefore safe targets might be behaviors to substitute for particular at-risk behaviors. A safe target behavior can also be defined independently of an associated at-risk behavior. The definition of a safe target might be as basic as using certain personal protective equipment or "walking within pedestrian walkways." Or the safe target could be a process requiring a particular sequence of safe behaviors, as when lifting or locking out energy sources.

Deriving a precise definition of a DO IT target is facilitated with the development of a behavioral checklist to evaluate objectively whether a certain target

FIGURE 14.2. THE DO IT MODEL.

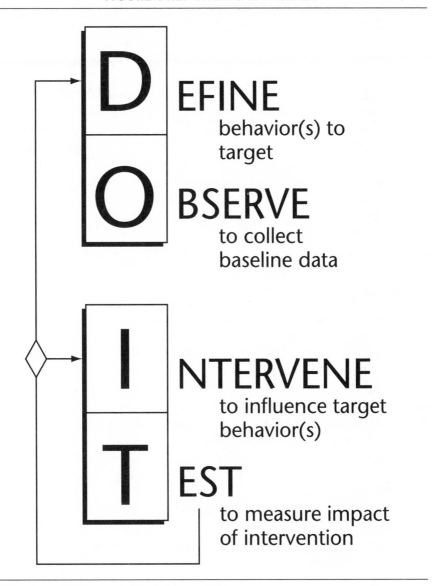

Source: Geller (1996a). Reproduced with permission.

behavior or process is being performed safely. The development of such behavioral definitions enables an invaluable learning experience. When people are involved in deriving a behavioral checklist, they own a training process that can improve human dynamics on both the outside (behaviors) and the inside (feelings and attitudes) of people.

"O" for Observe. When people observe each other for certain safe or at-risk behaviors, they realize everyone performs at-risk behavior, sometimes without even realizing it. The observation stage is not a fault-finding procedure but a fact-finding learning process to facilitate the discovery of behaviors and conditions that need to be changed or continued in order to prevent injuries. Thus, no behavioral observation is made without awareness and explicit permission from the person being observed. Observers should be open to learning as much (if not more) from the postobservation feedback conversation as they expect to teach from completing the behavioral checklist.

Regarding an observation process, teams of workers answer the following critical questions:

- What kind of behavioral checklist should be used during one-on-one observations?
- Who will conduct the behavioral observations?
- How often will the observations be conducted?
- How will data from the checklist be summarized and interpreted?
- How will people be informed of the results from an observation process?

There is not one generic observation procedure for every situation, and the customization and refinement of a process for a particular setting never stops. It is often beneficial to begin with a limited number of behaviors and a relatively simple checklist. This reduces the possibility of people feeling overwhelmed in the beginning. Starting small also enables the broadest range of voluntary participation and provides numerous opportunities to successively improve the process by expanding coverage of both behaviors and work areas. Details on how to design and use a critical behaviorial checklist for constructive observation and feedback are given elsewhere (Geller, 1998c, 2001g, 2001h; Krause et al., 1996; McSween, 2003; Geller & Williams, 2001).

"I" for Intervene. During this stage, interventions are designed and implemented in an attempt to increase safe behavior or decrease at-risk behavior. As reflected in principle 2, intervention means changing the external conditions of the behavioral context or system in order to make safe behavior more likely than at-risk behavior. When designing interventions, principles 3 and 4 are critical. Specifically, the most motivating consequences are soon, certain, and sizable (principle 3), and positive consequences are preferable to negative consequences (principle 4).

The process of observing and recording the frequency of safe and at-risk behavior on a checklist provides an opportunity to give individuals and groups valuable behavior-based feedback. When the results of a behavioral observation are shown to individuals or groups, they receive the kind of information that enables practice to improve performance. Considerable research has shown that providing workers with feedback regarding their ongoing behavior is a highly cost-effective intervention approach. (See, for example, the important analysis of the Hawthorne effect by Parsons, 1974, and comprehensive reviews by Alvero, Bucklin, & Austin, 2001, and Balcazar, Hopkins, & Suarez, 1986.) Furthermore, occupational safety has significantly improved following the feedback display of workers' percentages of safe versus at-risk behavior (Austin, Kessler, Riccobono, & Bailey, 1996; Sulzer-Azaroff & de Santamaria, 1980; Williams & Geller, 2000; Zohar, Cohen, & Azar, 1980).

In addition to behavioral feedback, researchers have found a number of other intervention strategies to be effective at increasing safe work practices. These include worker-designed safety slogans, "near miss" and corrective action reporting, safe behavior promise cards, individual and group goal setting, actively caring thank-you cards, safety coaching, and incentive and reward programs for individuals or groups. (These are detailed in Geller, 1998c, 2001g, 2001h; McSween, 2003; and Petersen, 1989.)

"T" for Test. The test phase of DO IT provides work teams with the information they need to refine or replace a behavior change intervention and thereby improve the process. If observations indicate that significant improvement in the target behavior has not occurred, the work team analyzes and discusses the situation and refines the intervention or chooses another intervention approach. If the target has reached the desired frequency level, the participants can turn their attention to another set of behaviors. They might add new critical behaviors to their checklist, thus expanding the domain of their behavioral observations. Alternatively, they might design a new intervention procedure to focus on only the new behaviors.

Summary. Every time the participants evaluate an intervention approach, they learn more about how to improve safety performance. They have essentially become behavioral scientists, using the DO IT process to diagnose a human factors problem, monitor the impact of a behavior change intervention, and refine interventions for continuous improvement. The results from such testing provide motivating consequences to support this learning process and keep the participants involved. The systematic evaluation of a number of DO IT processes can lead to a body of knowledge worthy of integration into a theory or reflected in the next principle.

Principle 6: Use Theory to Integrate Information, Not to Limit Possibilities

While much, if not most, research is theory driven, Skinner (1950) was critical of designing research projects to test theory. Theory-driven research can narrow the perspective of the investigator and limit the extent of findings from the scientific method. In other words, applying the DO IT process to merely test a theory can be like putting blinders on a horse. It can limit the amount of information gained from systematic observation.

This is an important perspective for safety and health professionals, especially when applying the DO IT process. It is often better to be open to many possibilities for improving safety performance than to be motivated to support a certain process. Numerous intervention procedures are consistent with a BBS approach, and an intervention process that works well in one situation will not necessarily be effective in another setting. Thus, my colleagues and I teach safety leaders to make an educated guess about what intervention procedures to use at the start of a BBS process, but to be open to results from a DO IT process and refine procedures accordingly. Of course, principles 1 to 4 should always be used as guides when designing intervention procedures.

After many systematic applications of the DO IT process, distinct consistencies will be observed. Certain procedures will work better in some situations than others, with some individuals than others, or with some behaviors than others. Summarizing functional relationships between intervention impact and specific situational or interpersonal characteristics can lead to the development of a research-based theory of what works best under particular circumstances. This implies the use of theory to integrate information gained from systematic behavioral observation. Skinner (1950) approved of this use of theory, but cautioned that premature theory development can lead to premature theory testing and limited profound knowledge.

Principle 7: Design Interventions with Consideration of Internal Feelings

That Skinner was concerned about unobservable attitudes or feeling states is evidenced by his criticism of punishment because of its impact on people's feelings or perceptions. This perspective also reflects a realization that intervention procedures influence feeling states, and these can be pleasant or unpleasant, desirable or undesirable. The rationale for using more positive than negative consequences to motivate behavior is based on the differential feeling states provoked by positive reinforcement versus punishment procedures (for example, Wiegand & Geller, 2004/2005). Similarly, the way we implement an intervention process can increase or decrease feelings of empowerment, build or destroy trust, or cultivate or inhibit a sense of teamwork or belonging (Geller, 2001g, 2001h, 2002b, 2005). It is important to assess feeling states or perceptions that occur concomitantly with an intervention process. This can be accomplished informally through one-on-one interviews and group discussions or formally with a perception survey (O'Brien, 2000; Petersen, 2001). Thus, decisions regarding which intervention to implement and how to refine existing intervention procedures should be based on both objective behavioral observations and subjective evaluations of feeling states.

The Challenge of Sustaining Behavior Change

The intervention approaches can change behavior, but will the target behavior continue when the intervention is removed? Some behavior analysts consider this primarily a challenge of institutionalizing the ABC contingencies of the intervention process (Malott, 2001; McSween & Matthews, 2001). In other words, the external and extrinsic activators and consequences need to be transferred from the behavior analyst or intervention agent to the indigenous personnel of the organizational setting in which the target behavior occurs. Hence, the intervention is not actually removed; rather, those who deliver the intervention contingencies are changed. McSween and Mathews (2001) concluded that five factors are critical for developing institutionalization: training and education, employee involvement in intervention design, a monitoring or accountability system, a formal data system, and supportive consequences.

Other behavior analysts talk about this maintenance challenge in terms of the behavior continuing in the absence of the external and extrinsic intervention process (Baer, 2001; Boyce & Geller, 2001; Geller, 2001d; Stokes & Baer, 1977). Some presume the objectives of the intervention are internalized, and people act themselves into thought processes consistent with the new behavior (Geller, 2001f). As such, personal change is viewed as a continuous spiral of behavior causing thinking, thinking inducing more behavior, and then this additional behavior influencing more thinking consistent with the behavior, and so on. However, programmatic research indicates that some interventions do not facilitate an attendant change in thinking. This is reflected profoundly in Bem's classic behavior-based theory of self-perception (1972).

Behavioral Self-Perception

Bem (1972) prefaced his behavioral presentation of self-perception theory in this way: "Individuals come to 'know' their own attitudes, emotions, and other internal states by inferring them from observations of their own overt behavior and/or the circumstances in which this behavior occurs" (p. 2). Consistent with this theory, children who had the excuse of a severe threat for not playing with a "forbidden toy" did not internalize a rule, and therefore played with the forbidden toy when the threat contingency was removed (Lepper & Greene, 1978). Analogously, college students paid twenty dollars for telling other students a boring task was fun did not develop a personal view that the task was enjoyable (Festinger & Carlsmith, 1959). The reinforcement contingency made their behavior incredible as a reflection of their personal belief or self-perception. In contrast, participants who received a mild threat or low compensation (only one dollar) to motivate their behavior developed a self-perception consistent with their behavior. The children avoided playing with the forbidden toy in a subsequent situation with no threat, and the college students who lied for low compensation decided they must have liked the boring task. In theory, these participants viewed their behavior as a valid guide for inferring their private views, since their behavior was not under strong contingency control.

The More Outside Control, the Less Self-Persuasion

Much additional research supports the notion that self-persuasion is more likely when the extrinsic control is less obvious or perhaps indirect. In other words, when there are sufficient external consequences to justify the amount of effort required for a particular behavior, the performer does not develop an internal justification for the behavior. There is no self-persuasion (Aronson, 1999), and performing the behavior does not alter self-perception (Bem, 1972). Under these circumstances, the maintenance of the behavior is unlikely, unless it is possible to keep a sufficient accountability system (such as incentives or disincentives) in place over the long term, as was the case for a thirteen-year incentive process that successfully reduced injuries in an open pit mine (Fox, Hopkins, & Anger, 1987).

Direct Persuasion. Advertisers use direct persuasion to change consumer behaviors. Advertisements for products and services show people enjoying positive consequences or avoiding negative consequences by taking action. As such, advertisers apply the three-term contingency or ABC paradigm to sell their goods and services. The activator (the "A" of the ABC contingency) announces the availability of a reinforcing consequence (the "C" of the ABC contingency) if the purchasing behavior is performed (the "B" of the ABC contingency). Safety-related behaviors, in contrast, are usually more inconvenient and require more effort than switching brands at a supermarket. In other words, long-term participation in a safety-related work process is far more cumbersome and lifestyle changing than the consumer behavior targeted by advertisers. The direct approach can give the impression that the target behavior is accomplished for someone else's benefit. This can cause a disconnection between the behavior and self-perception.

Indirect Persuasion. Self-persuasion is more likely to occur when the motivational strategy is less obvious. For example, compliments regarding a person's performance are often more powerful when they are more indirect than direct (Allen, 1990; Geller, 1997a). This is because the direct approach is tainted by the possibility the flattery is given for an ulterior motive. Indirect persuasion deviates significantly from the standard command-and-control method of promoting compliance with safety regulations. Both approaches might be equally effective at motivating behavior change, but an indirect approach will be far more successful at enhancing the kind of internal dialogue needed to maintain behavior in the absence of an external motivator or accountability system.

Defining intervention conditions that can make this happen is not easy but starts by asking, "Does the situation promote individual choice, ownership, and personal accountability?" "Does the context in which injury prevention participation is desired contribute to connecting or disconnecting the link between what people do and what they think of themselves?" "Are the safety-related activities only behaviors, or do they stimulate supportive cognitive activity or self-persuasion?"

These questions reflect the role of psychological states, or expectancies in facilitating safety-related behavior. Indeed, if certain feelings or beliefs affect people's participation in safety-related activities, then enhancing these states could be a powerful indirect way to improve safety performance. This is reflected in another theoretical perspective relevant to the large-scale prevention of unintentional injuries and fatalities: the actively caring model. For over a decade, research on actively caring has proposed that certain psychological states or expectancies affect the propensity for individuals to actively care for the environment (Geller, 1995, 2002a) and for the safety or health of others (Geller, 1991a, 1996a, 2001a, 2001g, 2001h). Furthermore, it is theorized that certain conditions (including behavioral antecedents and consequences) can influence these psychological states and thereby enhance the probability an individual will emit caring-related behavior, thus contributing to long-term maintenance of behavior change.

Future Research Directions

This chapter offers many examples of the need for systematic research on applied behavior analysis for injury prevention. A critical issue in need of empirical study is how to design an incentive and reward or disincentive and penalty program that is sufficient to increase desired safety-related behavior or decrease undesired at-risk behavior but does not detract from the development of self-accountability or personal responsibility. When people are self-directed and feel responsible for injury prevention, they are likely to also engage in other safety-relevant behaviors than the one targeted for change. This raises the need to assess the issue of response generalization as well as test the validity of the actively caring model and examine critical issues related to intrinsic versus extrinsic motivation.

Response Generalization Versus Risk Compensation

A shortcoming of most behavioral intervention research is that it often focuses on a single target response, failing to consider that a variety of responses may covary as a function of similar response classes and reinforcement histories (Geller, 1991b, 2001b; Ludwig & Geller, 1991, 1997, 2001). Thus, safety behaviors can be considered as groups of functionally related behaviors (for example, the response class of safe-driving practices). If safety practices covary in a consistent fashion, then intervening to increase one desired behavior can have indirect effects on other desired safety behaviors within the same response class. This behavioral covariation can occur in one of two ways, resulting in either an increase in safety-related behaviors (response generalization; Bandura, 1969; Carr, 1988) or a decrease in safety-related behaviors (risk compensation; Peltzman, 1975).

Response generalization occurs when multiple behaviors clustered in a functional response class such as safe driving increase as a result of intervening on one of the behaviors within the response class (Russo, Cataldo, & Cushing, 1981). Risk compensation occurs when an increase in the targeted behavior results in a decrease in other behaviors within the same functional response class.

Ludwig and Geller (1991) demonstrated that an intervention that targeted only safety belt use among pizza delivery drivers influenced a significant increase in the use of both safety belts and turn signals, thus indicating response generalization. In a subsequent study, Ludwig and Geller (1997) found a similar effect when targeting complete intersection stops among pizza deliverers.

Risk compensation is based on risk homeostasis theory (Wilde, 1982), which purports that at any point in time, individuals perceive (and are willing to accept) a certain level of risk. When perceived and accepted levels of risk are not in equilibrium, the individual presumably alters his or her behavior in order to bring the perceived and accepted levels of risk into homeostatic balance. Thus, efforts to increase the frequency of one safe behavior can have the undesirable side effect of decreasing other safe behaviors within the same response class. Girasek (Chapter Five, this volume) has reviewed this literature and its relevance to risk communications and injury prevention.

Although some experiments have been conducted to assess this phenomenon among driving behaviors (McKenna, 1985; O'Neill, Lund, & Ashton, 1985; Streff & Geller, 1988) and in the laboratory (Wilde, Claxton-Oldfield, & Platenius, 1985), the findings have been mixed and inconclusive. Research is needed to evaluate the circumstances under which response generalization versus risk compensation occurs when interventions target certain behaviors, while other nontargeted safety-related behaviors are also observed and evaluated.

Intrinsic Versus Extrinsic Motivation

Some investigators (Deci, 1971; Deci & Ryan, 1987; Kohn, 1993; Lepper, Greene, & Nisbett, 1973) have reported that external control of behavior through either punishment or reinforcement will undermine an individual's natural desire to engage in a particular behavior. Although proponents of intrinsic motivation theory believe all external consequences are perceived as controlling, applied behavior analysts disagree, claiming behaviors are shaped and maintained by the consequences that follow them. Some behaviors are followed by natural consequences (inherent to the task). For example, at-risk behaviors are supported by consequences of comfort, convenience, or faster performance.

Safe behaviors are often inconvenient and uncomfortable and can require support by some type of extrinsic (or external) intervention. This could include participative or mandated goal setting (Ludwig & Geller, 1997), commitment strategies (Geller & Lehman, 1991; Streff, Kalsher, & Geller, 1993), or consequence procedures, including both reward and punishment techniques (Geller, 1988). In a comprehensive review of twenty-eight employer-based programs to motivate safety belt use, Geller, Rudd, Kalsher, Streff, and Lehman (1987) found reward strategies to be more effective than punishment strategies and more effective in the short term than commitment strategies. However, commitment strategies were most effective in maintaining long-term behavior change.

Streff et al. (1993) used a promise card commitment strategy to increase the use of personal protective equipment. After a group meeting where line employees discussed the importance of using this equipment, they were asked to make a voluntary personal commitment to use safety glasses, gloves, and earplugs (the target behaviors) on the job for two months by signing a promise card. The voluntary commitment presumably empowered employees and was effective in increasing the target behaviors over the pledge period. In addition, these investigators reported response generalization to safety belt use. Specifically, safety belt use by the employees who signed promise cards to use safety glasses, gloves, and earplugs increased from 12.8 percent on 654 occasions before the intervention to 35.1 percent on 166 occasions after the promise card intervention.

The results of these studies, however, leave an important question: Under what circumstances will response generalization occur? Few injury prevention studies have evaluated changes in more than the behaviors targeted by the intervention. Obviously interventions that facilitate response generalization will be especially effective in reducing work-related injuries and will be ecologically valid (Willems, 1974, 1977). A key component of achieving response generalization may be personal choice or empowerment as discussed above, an issue worthy of further research.

Conclusion

Occupational safety remains an important public health problem in the United States and one for which behaviorally focused interventions offer promise. This chapter reviewed the applied behavior analysis approach or behavior-based safety (BBS) and its application to reducing occupational injury. The appeal of the applied behavior analysis approach to injury control can be attributed to a number of advantages over other approaches:

- Behaviorally focused interventions can be administered by individuals with minimal professional training.
- The intervention can reach people in the setting where behavior change is needed (for example, the workplace, school, or community at large).
- The indigenous staff can be taught the straightforward behavior change techniques most likely to work under given circumstances.
- An objective and ongoing evaluation process can be readily conducted by the local change agents, who are likely to be motivated by the learning opportunities available from behavioral data.

The applied behavior analysis approach is not a panacea. While it may be relatively easy to empower change agents to initiate and evaluate this approach, and even to institutionalize it, there are some disadvantages. Particularly, there is often little maintenance of the targeted behavior after the intervention is withdrawn. This implies a need to institutionalize the BBS approach in a wide variety of occupational settings with managers and supervisors. An ongoing BBS system requires observers (for example, supervisors or trained coworkers) to administer the program and manage an accountability system. Although straightforward, this program can be quite time-consuming. Furthermore, there are many situations where external accountability is impossible, as when people drive or work alone.

Research reviewed in this chapter suggests that an external motivational or accountability system can detract from the development of internal control or self-accountability—a disposition needed for the lone worker and most occupational drivers. And when the external control or enforcement is too strong or obvious, some workers may resist accepting personal responsibility and even engage in risky behavior to assert personal freedom. These and other issues raised in this chapter should activate future intervention research to enhance BBS approaches to occupational safety. More research using the tenets of applied behavior analysis in other areas of injury prevention is needed for BBS to reach its practical long-term and large-scale potential.

References

Allen, J. (1990). *I saw what you did and I know who you are: Bloopers, blunders and success stories in giving and receiving recognition.* Tucker, GA: Performance Management Publications.

Alvero, A. M., Bucklin, B. R., & Austin, J. (2001). An objective review of the effectiveness and characteristics of performance feedback in organizational settings (1985–1998). *Journal of Organizational Behavior Management, 21*(1), 3–29.

Aronson, E. (1999). The power of self-persuasion. *American Psychologist, 54,* 875–884.

Atkinson, J. W. (1957). Motivational determinants of risk-taking behavior. *Psychological Review, 64,* 359–372.

Atkinson, J. W. (1964). *An introduction to motivation.* Princeton, NJ: Van Nostrand.

Atkinson, J. W., & Litwin, G. F. (1960). Achievement motive and test anxiety conceived as motive to approach success and motive to avoid failure. *Journal of Abnormal and Social Psychology, 60,* 52–63.

Austin, J. (2000). Performance analysis and performance diagnostics. In J. Austin & J. E. Carr (Eds.), *Handbook of applied behavior analysis* (pp. 321–349). Reno, NV: Context Press.

Austin, J., Carr, J. E., & Agnew, J. (1999). The need for assessing maintaining variables in OBM. *Journal of Organizational Behavior Management, 19*(2), 59–87.

Austin, J., Kessler, M. L., Riccobono, J. E., & Bailey, J. S. (1996). Using feedback and reinforcement to improve the performance and safety of a roofing crew. *Journal of Organizational Behavior Management, 16*(2), 49–75.

Azrin, N. H., & Holz, W. C. (1996). *Punishment.* In W. K. Honig (Ed.), *Operant behavior: Areas of research and application.* New York: Appleton-Century-Crofts.

Baer, D. M. (2001). Since safety maintains our lives, we need to maintain maintaining. *Journal of Organizational Behavior Management, 21*(1), 61–64.

Bailey, J. S., & Austin, J. (1996). Evaluating and improving productivity in the workplace. In B. Thyer & M. Mattaini (Eds.), *Behavior analysis and social work* (pp. 179–200). Washington, DC: American Psychological Association.

Balcazar, F., Hopkins, B. L., & Suarez, I. (1986). A critical, objective review of performance feedback. *Journal of Organizational Behavior Management, 7*(3/4), 65–89.

Bandura, A. (1969). *Principles of behavior modification.* New York: Holt, Rinehart & Winston.

Bem, D. J. (1972). *Self-perception theory.* In L. Berkowitz (Ed.), *Advances in experimental social psychology* (Vol. 6, pp. 1–60). Orlando, FL: Academic Press.

Berglas, S., & Jones, E. E. (1978). Drug choice as a self-handicapping strategy in response to noncontingent success. *Journal of Personality and Social Psychology, 36,* 405–417.

Boyce, T. E., & Geller, E. S. (2001). Applied behavior analysis and occupational safety: The challenge of response maintenance. *Journal of Organizational Behavior Management, 21*(1), 31–60.

Bureau of Labor Statistics. (2003a). *Workplace injuries and illness in 2003.* http://www.bls.gov/news.realease/pdf/osh.pdf.

Bureau of Labor Statistics. (2003b). National census of fatal occupational injuries in 2003. http://www.bls.gov/news.realease/pdf/cfoi.pdf.

Carnegie, D. (1936). *How to win friends and influence people.* New York: Simon & Schuster.

Carr, E. G. (1988). Functional equivalence as a mechanism of response generalization. In R. H. Horner, G. Dunlap, & R. L. Koegel (Eds.), *Generalization and maintenance* (pp. 221–241). Baltimore, MD: Paul H. Brookes.

Centers for Disease Control and Prevention. (2005, Apr. 29). Workers' Memorial Day. *MMWR,* 1.

Daniels, A. C. (2000). *Bringing out the best in people: How to apply the astonishing power of positive reinforcement* (2nd ed.). New York: McGraw-Hill.

Daniels, A. C. (2001). *Other people's habits: How to use positive reinforcement to bring out the best in people around you.* New York: McGraw-Hill.

Deci, E. L. (1971). Effects of externally mediated rewards on intrinsic motivation. *Journal of Personality and Social Psychology, 18*(1), 105–115.

Deci, E. L., & Ryan, R. M. (1987). The support of autonomy and the control of behavior. *Journal of Personality and Social Psychology, 53,* 1024–1037.

Eckenfelder, D. J. (1996). *Values-driven safety.* Rockville, MD: Government Institutes.

Elder, J. P., Geller, E. S., Hovell, M. F., & Mayer, J. A. (1994). *Motivating health behavior.* Clifton Park, NY: Delmar.

Estes, W. K., & Skinner, B. F. (1941). Some quantitative properties of anxiety. *Journal of Experimental Psychology, 29,* 390–400.

Everett, P. B., Haywood, S. C., & Meyers, A. W. (1974). Effects of a token reinforcement procedure on bus ridership. *Journal of Applied Behavior Analysis, 7,* 1–9.

Festinger, L., & Carlsmith, J. M. (1959). Cognitive consequences of forced compliance. *Journal of Abnormal and Social Psychology, 58,* 203–210.

Fox, D. K., Hopkins, B. L., & Anger, W. K. (1987). The long-term effects of a token economy on safety performance in open-pit mining. *Journal of Applied Behavior Analysis, 20,* 215–224.

Geller, E. S. (1988). A behavioral science approach to transportation safety. *Bulletin of the New York Academy of Medicine, 64*(7), 632–661.

Geller, E. S. (1991a). If only more would actively care. *Journal of Applied Behavior Analysis, 24,* 607–612.

Geller, E. S. (1991b). Where's the validity in social validity? In E. S. Geller (Ed.), *Social validity: Multiple perspectives.* Lawrence, KS: Society for the Experimental Analysis of Behavior.

Geller, E. S. (1995). Integrating behaviorism and humanism for environmental protection. *Journal of Social Issues, 51,* 179–195.

Geller, E. S. (1996a). *The psychology of safety: How to improve behaviors and attitudes on the job.* Radnor, PA: Chilton.

Geller, E. S. (1996b). The truth about safety incentives. *Professional Safety, 41*(10), 34–39.

Geller, E. S. (1997a). Key processes for continuous safety improvement: Behavior-based recognition and celebration. *Professional Safety, 42*(10), 40–44.

Geller, E. S. (1997b). What is behavior-based safety, anyway? *Occupational Health and Safety, 66*(1), 25–35.

Geller, E. S. (1998a). *Applications of behavior analysis to prevent injury from vehicle crashes* (2nd ed.). Cambridge, MA: Cambridge Center for Behavioral Studies.

Geller, E. S. (1998b). Light up safety in the new millennium. In *Principles of behavior-based safety: Proceedings of the ASSE Behavioral Safety Symposium* (pp. 13–24). Orlando, FL, Des Plaines, IL: American Society of Safety Engineers.

Geller, E. S. (1998c). *Understanding behavior-based safety: Step-by-step methods to improve your workplace* (2nd ed.). Neenah, WI: J. J. Keller & Associates.

Geller, E. S. (2000). Behavioral safety analysis: A necessary precursor to corrective action. *Professional Safety, 45*(3), 29–32.

Geller, E. S. (2001a). Actively caring for occupational safety: Extending the performance management paradigm. In C. M. Johnson, W. K. Redmon, & T. C. Mawhinney (Eds.), *Organizational performance: Behavior analysis and management* (pp. 303–326). Binghamton, NY: The Haworth Press.

Geller, E. S. (2001b). *Beyond safety accountability.* Rockville, MD: Government Institutes.

Geller, E. S. (2001c). *Building successful safety teams.* Rockville, MD: Government Institutes.

Geller, E. S. (2001d). Dream—operationalize—intervene—test: If you want to make a difference—just DO IT. *Journal of Organizational Behavior Management, 21*(1), 109–121.

Geller, E. S. (2001e). From ecological behaviorism to response generalization: Where should we make discriminations? *Journal of Organizational Behavior Management, 21*(4), 55–73.

Geller, E. S. (2001f). Sustaining participation in a safety improvement process: Ten relevant principles from behavioral science. *Professional Safety, 46*(9), 24–29.

Geller, E. S. (2001g). *The psychology of safety handbook.* Boca Raton, FL: CRC Press.

Geller, E. S. (2001h). *Working safe: How to help people actively care for health and safety* (2nd ed.). New York: Lewis Publishers.

Geller, E. S. (2002a). The challenge of increasing pro-environmental behavior. In R. B. Bechtel & A. Churchman (Eds.), *The new environmental psychology handbook* (pp. 525–540). Hoboken, NJ: Wiley.

Geller, E. S. (2002b). *The participation factor: How to get more people involved in occupational safety.* Des Plaines, IL: American Society of Safety Engineers.

Geller, E. S. (2005). *People-based safety: The source.* Virginia Beach, VA: Coastal Training and Technologies Corporation.

Geller, E. S., Elder, J., Hovell, M., & Sleet, D. (1991). Behavioral approaches to drinking-driving interventions. In W. Ward & F. Lewis (Eds.), *Advances in health education and promotion* (Vol. 3, pp. 45–68). London: Jessica Kingsley Press.

Geller, E. S., Kalsher, M. J., Rudd, J. R., & Lehman, G. (1989). Promoting safety belt use on a university campus: An integration of commitment and incentive strategies. *Journal of Applied Social Psychology, 19,* 3–19.

Geller, E. S., & Lehman, G. R. (1991). The buckle-up promise card: A versatile intervention for large-scale behavior change. *Journal of Applied Behavior Analysis, 24,* 91–94.

Geller, E. S., Rudd, J. R., Kalsher, M. J., Streff, F. M., & Lehman, G. R. (1987). Employer-based programs to motivate safety belt use: A review of short-term and long-term effects. *Journal of Safety Research, 18*, 1–17.

Geller, E. S., & Williams, J. (Eds.). (2001). *Keys to behavior-based safety from Safety Performance Solutions*. Rockville, MD: Government Institutes.

Gilbert, T. F. (1978). *Human competence: Engineering worthy performance*. New York: McGraw-Hill.

Goldstein, A. P., & Krasner, L. (1987). *Modern applied psychology*. New York: Pergamon Press.

Greene, B. F., Winett, R. A., Van Houten, R., Geller, E. S., & Iwata, B. A. (Eds.). (1987). *Behavior analysis in the community: Readings from the* Journal of Applied Behavior Analysis. Lawrence: University of Kansas.

Grindle, A. C., Dickinson, A. M., & Boettcher, W. (2000). Behavioral safety research in manufacturing settings: A review of the literature. *Journal of Organizational Behavior Management, 20*(1), 29–68.

Hagenzieker, M. P. (1991). Enforcement or incentive? Promoting safety belt use among military personnel in the Netherlands. *Journal of Applied Behavior Analysis, 24*, 23–30.

Kalsher, M. J., Geller, E. S., Clarke, S. W., & Lehman, G. R. (1989). Safety-belt promotion on a naval base: A comparison of incentives vs. disincentives. *Journal of Safety Research, 20*, 103–113.

Kohn, A. (1993). *Punished by rewards: The trouble with gold stars, incentive plans, A's, praise, and other bribes*. Boston: Houghton Mifflin.

Krause, T. R. (1995). *Employee-driven systems for safe behavior: Integrating behavioral and statistical methodologies*. New York: Van Nostrand Reinhold.

Krause, T. R., Hidley, J. H., & Hodson, S. J. (1996). *The behavior-based safety process: Managing improvement for an injury-free culture* (2nd ed.). New York: Van Nostrand Reinhold.

Kroemer, K. H. (1991). Ergonomics. In R. Dulbecco (Ed.), *Encyclopedia of human biology* (Vol. 3, pp. 473–480). San Diego: Academic Press.

Lepper, M., & Greene, D. (1978). *The hidden cost of reward*. Mahwah, NJ: Erlbaum.

Lepper, M. R., Greene, D., & Nisbett, R. E. (1973). Undermining children's intrinsic interest with extrinsic rewards: A test of the overjustification hypothesis. *Journal of Personality and Social Psychology, 28*, 129–137.

Ludwig, T. D., & Geller, E. S. (1991). Improving the driving practices of pizza deliverers: Response generalization and moderating effects of driving history. *Journal of Applied Behavior Analysis, 24*, 31–44.

Ludwig, T. D., & Geller, E. S. (1997). Managing injury control among professional pizza deliverers: Effects of goal setting and response generalization. *Journal of Applied Psychology, 82*, 253–261.

Ludwig, T. D., & Geller, E. S. (2001). *Intervening to improve the safety of occupational driving*. New York: Hawthorn Press.,

Mager, R. F., & Pipe, P. (1997). *Analyzing performance problems or you really oughta wanna* (3rd ed.). Atlanta, GA: Center for Effective Performance.

Malott, R. W. (1992). A theory of rule-governed behavior and organizational behavior management. *Journal of Organizational Behavior Management, 12*(2), 45–65.

Malott, R. W. (2001). Occupational safety and response maintenance: An alternative view. *Journal of Organizational Behavior Management, 21*(1), 85–102.

McAfee, R. B., & Winn, A. R. (1989). The use of incentives/feedback to enhance workplace safety: A critique of the literature. *Journal of Safety Research, 20*(1), 7–19.

McKenna, F. P. (1985). Do safety measures really work? An examination of risk homeostasis theory. *Ergonomics, 28*(2), 489–498.

McSween, T. E. (2003). *The values-based safety process: Improving your safety culture with a behavioral approach* (2nd ed.). New York: Van Nostrand Reinhold.

McSween, T., & Matthews, G. A. (2001). Maintenance in organizational safety management. *Journal of Organizational Behavior Management, 21*(1), 75–83.

National Academy of Social Insurance. (2002). *Workers' compensation: Benefits, coverages, and costs.* http://www.nasi.org/usr_doc/workers_comp_2002.pdf.

National Institute for Occupational Safety and Health. (1998). *National occupational research agenda, Traumatic occupational injury research needs and priorities.* DHHS(NIOSH). Publication No. 98-134. Available at http://www.cdc.gov/niosh/traumado.html.

Norman, D. A. (1988). *The psychology of everyday things.* New York: Basic Books.

O'Brien, D. P. (2000). *Business measurements for safety performance.* New York: Lewis Publishers.

O'Neill, B., Lund, A. K., & Ashton, S. (1985). Mandatory belt use and driver risk taking: An empirical evaluation of the risk compensation hypothesis. In L. Evans & R. Schwing (Eds.), *Human behavior and traffic safety* (pp. 93–107). New York: Plenum Press.

Peden, M., Scurfield, R., Sleet, D., Mohan, D., Hyder, A., Jarawan, E., & Mathers, C. (Eds.). (2004). *World report on road traffic injury prevention.* Geneva: World Health Organization.

Parsons, H. M. (1974). What happened at Hawthorne? *Science, 183,* 922–932.

Peltzman, S. (1975). The effects of automobile safety regulation. *Journal of Political Economics, 83,* 677–725.

Petersen, D. (1989). *Safe behavior reinforcement.* Goshen, NY: Aloray.

Petersen, D. (2001). *Authentic involvement.* Itasca, IL: National Safety Council.

Rhodewalt, F. (1994). Conceptions of ability achievement goals, and individual differences in self-handicapping behavior: On the application of implicit theories. *Journal of Personality, 62,* 67–85.

Rhodewalt, F., & Fairfield, M. (1991). Claimed self-handicaps and the self-handicapper: The relations of reduction in intended effort to performance. *Journal of Research in Personality, 25,* 402–417.

Rudd, J. R., & Geller, E. S. (1985). A university-based incentive program to increase safety-belt use: Toward cost-effective institutionalization. *Journal of Applied Behavior Analysis, 18,* 215–226.

Russo, D. C., Cataldo, M. F., & Cushing, P. J. (1981). Compliance training and behavioral covariation in the treatment of multiple behavior problems. *Journal of Applied Behavior Analysis, 14,* 209–222.

Skinner, B. F. (1950). Are theories of learning necessary? *Psychological Review, 57,* 193–216.

Skinner, B. F. (1953). *Science and human behavior.* New York: Macmillan.

Skinner, B. F. (1971). *Beyond freedom and dignity.* New York: Knopf.

Skinner, B. F. (1974). *About behaviorism.* New York: Knopf.

Skinner, B. F. (1991). *The behavior of organisms: An experimental analysis.* Acton, MA: Copley Publishing Group. (Originally published in 1938)

Sleet, D., & Lonero, L. (2002). Behavioral approaches to preventing motor vehicle crashes. In L. Breslow, J. Last, L. Green, & M. McGinnis (Eds.), *Encyclopedia of public health* (pp. 105–107). St. Louis, MO: Mosby.

Stokes, T. F., & Baer, D. M. (1977). An implicit technology of generalization. *Journal of Applied Behavior Analysis, 10,* 349–367.

Stout, N. A., & Lin, H. I. (2002). Occupational injury prevention research: Progress and priorities. *Injury Prevention, 8*(Suppl. 4), iv9–iv14.

Streff, F. M., & Geller, E. S. (1988). An experimental test of risk compensation: Between-subject versus within-subject analyses. *Accident Analysis and Prevention, 20*(4), 277–287.

Streff, F. M., Kalsher, M. J., & Geller, E. S. (1993). Developing efficient workplace safety programs: Observations of response covariation. *Journal of Organizational Behavior Management, 13*(2), 3–15.

Sulzer-Azaroff, B. (1998). *Who killed my daddy? A behavioral safety fable.* Cambridge, MA: Cambridge Center for Behavioral Studies.

Sulzer-Azaroff, B., & Austin, J. (2000). Does BBS work? Behavior-based safety and injury reduction: A survey of the evidence. *Professional Safety, 45*(7), 19–24.

Sulzer-Azaroff, B., & de Santamaria, M. C. (1980). Industrial safety hazard reduction through performance feedback. *Journal of Applied Behavior Analysis, 13*, 287–295.

Wiegand, D. M., & Geller, E. S. (2004/2005). Connecting positive psychology and organizational behavior management: Achievement motivation and the power of positive reinforcement. *Journal of Organizational Behavior Management, 24*(1/2), 3–25.

Wilde, G.J.S. (1982). The theory of risk homeostasis: Implications for safety and health. *Risk Analysis, 2*(4), 209–225.

Wilde, G.J.S., Claxton-Oldfield, S. P., & Platenius, P. H. (1985). Risk homeostasis in an experimental context. In L. Evans & R. Schwing (Eds.), *Human behavior and traffic safety* (pp. 119–149). New York: Plenum Press.

Willems, E. P. (1974). Behavioral technology and behavioral ecology. *Journal of Applied Behavior Analysis, 7*, 151–165.

Willems, E. P. (1977). Steps toward an ecobehavioral technology. In A. Rogers-Warren & S. F. Warren (Eds.), *Ecological perspectives in behavior analysis.* Baltimore, MD: University Park Press.

Williams, J. H., & Geller, E. S. (2000). Behavior-based intervention for occupational safety: Critical impact of social comparison feedback. *Journal of Safety Research, 31*, 135–142.

Zohar, D., Cohen, A., & Azar, N. (1980). Promoting increased use of ear protectors in noise through information feedback. *Human Factors, 22*, 69–79.

CHAPTER FIFTEEN

INTIMATE PARTNER VIOLENCE

Karen A. McDonnell, Jessica G. Burke,
Andrea Carlson Gielen, Patricia J. O'Campo

Intimate partner violence is an important public health problem that demands increased intervention attention. Despite a wealth of research illustrating the profound negative consequences that intimate partner violence has on women's physical and psychological health (Campbell, 2002; Heise, Ellsburg, & Gottemoeller, 1999; McCauley et al., 1995; McDonnell, Gielen, & O'Campo, 2003; McDonnell, Gielen, O'Campo, & Burke, 2005), little is known regarding the effectiveness of existing intimate partner violence intervention programs. The field of intimate partner violence program development could be greatly strengthened with the integration of behavior change theories to develop innovative and responsive intimate partner violence programs. This chapter provides an overview of intimate partner violence and the injury implications of this public health issue, examines the state of intimate partner violence interventions within the health care setting, and outlines additional research needs with regard to the application of behavioral theory to intimate partner violence.

Intimate partner violence, also referred to as domestic violence, is a form of violence against women that has gained increased recognition over the past two decades. Intimate partner violence is violence perpetrated by one intimate partner (a husband, boyfriend, or female partner) against another and includes psychological aggression, physical assault, and sexual coercion (Straus, Hamby, Boney-McCoy, & Sugarman, 1996). According to the National Institute of Mental Health's Committee on Family Violence (Crowell & Burgess, 1996), "intimate [partner] violence may include acts that are physically and emotionally harmful or that carry the potential to cause physical harm. Abuse of adult partners may include sexual coercion or assaults, physical intimidation, threats to kill or harm, restraint of normal activities or freedom, and the denial of access to resources" (p. 10).

Epidemiology of Intimate Partner Violence

Recognition of the magnitude of intimate partner violence in the United States has occurred only within the past two decades as there were no studies on its prevalence, determinants, and consequences prior to that time. Although estimates suggest that 3 to 4 million women may be affected by intimate partner violence each year in the United States (Tjaden & Thoennes, 1998), methodological challenges in determining prevalence and incidence have precluded an accurate assessment of the extent of the problem. Estimates of the magnitude of intimate partner violence vary by population sampled and instruments used to measure the problem. Comparisons of annual and lifetime (adult) prevalence of domestic violence were found to differ for two types of U.S. samples: health clinic samples (excluding prenatal clinics) and population-based surveys. Lifetime prevalence rates of intimate partner violence from women in both types of samples range from 21 to 55 percent, and annual prevalence rates range from 4 to 47 percent (Jones et al., 1999; Commonwealth Fund, 1998; Tjaden & Thoennes, 1998; Coker, Smith, McKeown, & King, 2000; McDonnell et al., 2003; Gielen, O'Campo, & McDonnell, 2002). Even if we omit the extreme values, we still end up with a wide range of estimates. Population-based surveys yielded lower lifetime prevalence rates than clinical studies. This is partially due to the fact that women who experience intimate partner violence are not only seeking medical assistance for their injuries but also use other clinical services at a higher rate than women who do not have a history of intimate partner violence (Campbell & Soeken, 1999; Eby, Campbell, & Sullivan, 1995; Plichta, 1996; Plichta & Falik, 2001; Coker et al., 2000; Commonwealth Fund, 1998). Despite the wide range of prevalence estimates, intimate partner violence remains an important public health problem.

More than a decade of research on battered women has made it clear that women have significant physical and mental health effects as a result of being abused (Campbell, 2002; Koss, Ingram, & Pepper, 2000; Gielen, McDonnell, O'Campo, & Burke, 2005). Intimate partner violence is the largest single cause of injury to women requiring emergency medical treatment, accounting for up to half of all injuries to women who seek care at emergency care sites (Stark et al., 1981). Women who are physically or sexually abused by a male partner present to health care services with multiple injuries to various parts of the body, especially the face, neck, head, throat, breast, chest, or abdomen; defensive injuries to the forearms; bruises in various stages of healing; neurological symptoms; chronic pelvic pain; and gastrointestinal disorders, including any type of injury caused by sexual assault (Stark et al., 1981; Campbell et al., 2002). Injuries that abused women experience can be as a direct result of the abuse, such as bodily bruises or lacerations, or an indirect result of the chronic heightened stress response and psychosocial distress (McCauley et al., 1995; Koss et al., 2001; McDonnell et al., 2003). Female victims of homicide are more likely than men to be killed by a spouse, intimate acquaintance, or family member (Wyatt, 1992). Data from 1996 show that almost 30 percent of homicide deaths in women are at the hands of these intimate partner perpetrators (Federal Bureau of Investigation, 1996). Homicide, clearly the most serious and tragic outcome, represents only the tip of the iceberg with regard to violence against women. A majority of domestic homicides are preceded by episodes of physical abuse (U.S. Department of Health and Human Services 2000). Healthy People 2010 (U.S Department of Health and Human Services, 2000) recently concluded that although there has been a decline in the homicide of intimates, including spouses, partners, boyfriends, and girlfriends, over the past decade, this problem remains significant and deserves research attention.

Research on intimate partner violence reveals that women experience significant poorer quality of life as a function of the physical and mental health consequences of abuse (Leserman, Drossman, & Hu, 1998; Peterson, Saltzman, Goodwin, & Spitz, 1997; Pitzner & Drummond, 1997; Wingood, DiClemente, & Raj, 2000; McDonnell, Gielen, O'Campo, & Burke, 2005). The Commonwealth Fund survey of women's health found that abused women were significantly more likely than nonabused women to rate their health as fair to poor and to say that although they were in need of medical care, they never sought such assistance (Plichta, 1996). Although physical injury is the most visible effect of abuse, battered women often also suffer from a range of more hidden psychological injuries.

Much of the work with battered women has made it clear that abused women experience a range of emotional effects, among which depression and anxiety predominate (Rath & Jarratt, 1990). In general population surveys, depression has been estimated to affect 10 to 20 percent of abused women and may affect as many as one-third when anxiety disorders are included (Kessler et al., 1994; Weissman & Kleman, 1992). Although the dynamics of depression in abused women are not clearly understood, coercive control through emotional abuse, fear engendered through frequency and severity of physical abuse, demoralization through undermining of self-esteem, and physical sequelae of abuse may foster depressive states (McCauley et al., 1995; Bergman & Brismar, 1991; Campbell, Kub, & Rose, 1996; Campbell, Kub, Belknap, & Templin, 1997; Campbell &

Humphreys, 1993; Cascadi & O'Leary, 1992). That depression results from long-standing abuse by intimate partners is supported by evidence that indicators of physical and mental health improve when women cease to be abused, although women often continue to suffer long-term sequelae (Campbell, 2002; McDonnell, Gielen, O'Campo, & Burke, 2005; McDonnell et al., 2003). Women who have experienced abuse are at an increased risk of suicide ideation as well as attempts (Stark & Flitcraft, 1991; Thakker, Gutierrez, Kuczen, & McCanne, 2000; Gielen et al., 2005). Stark and Flitcraft (1991) report that approximately 10 percent of abused women attempt suicide at least once, and among those who attempt suicide, 50 percent do so multiple times.

Mitchell and Hodson (1983) propose that the impact of violence on a woman's psychological health (self-esteem) is a function of her level of social support, her repertoire of coping skills, her personal resources (education, income, employment), and the extent to which appropriate institutions (criminal justice, legal, mental health) have been used or are responsive to her needs. Social isolation, self-esteem, and depression are often mentioned in the literature as characteristics of abused women (Gelles & Cornell, 1990; Coley & Beckett, 1998; Sackett & Saunders, 1999; Wise, Zierler, Krieger, & Harlow, 2001; Abraham, 2000; National Committee for Injury Prevention and Control, 1989; Bassuk, Dawson, Perloff, & Weinreb, 2000). Social isolation may in fact be a significant component of the abuse, being forced on the woman by her abuser (Abraham, 2000).

Intimate Partner Violence Interventions

Intimate partner violence, by its very definition, is a problem that involves two intimate partners and has several associated health behaviors: the abusive behaviors and acts of the perpetrator and the safety-enhancing or help-seeking behaviors of victim. While intervention programs addressing male perpetration of intimate partner violence are an important approach for addressing the problem, this chapter focuses on intervention programs to address women's experiences of intimate partner violence.

Although men and women may be victims or perpetrators of intimate partner violence, most perpetrators are men and most victims are women. Compared with interventions for women who experience intimate partner violence, more evaluation data exist on programs for perpetrators. This lack of evaluation data on programs for victims is particularly troubling for practitioners in the health care system who are being asked or required to screen their female patients for intimate partner violence (for a review, see Rhodes & Levinson, 2003). Currently health care providers have limited information available on how to address the needs of women who, when asked, screen positive for intimate partner violence.

Research suggests a number of actions that victims can take to address violence perpetrated by an intimate partner. Empirical evidence on women's help-seeking behaviors from our team's research on intimate partner violence among a sample of low-income women found that 64 percent of women who had ever been abused by an intimate partner reported that they could predict violent episodes (O'Campo, McDonnell, Gielen, Burke, & Chen, 2002). What women actually did when experiencing intimate partner violence included nothing, fighting back, leaving the partner, calling law enforcement, and talking with family and friends. A study by Goodman, Dutton, Weinfurt, and Cook (2003) found that among a sample of 406 battered women recruited from a shelter or district court rated informal (family and friends, for example), legal, and safety planning strategies as most helpful. Although resistance and placating strategies were used more often, they were less likely to be rated as helpful.

The focus of interventions for women experiencing intimate partner violence has been on safety enhancement, helping women develop a plan that addresses her safety, and can help women deal with and end the abuse. Recommended safety behaviors, enumerated by McFarlane and Parker (1994) and used in their subsequent intervention work (McFarlane et al., 2002; Parker, McFarlane, Soeken, Silva, & Reel, 1999), include the following items:

- Hide money.
- Hide an extra set of house and car keys.
- Establish a safety or assistance code with family or friends.
- Ask neighbors to call police if violence begins.
- Remove weapons.
- Have social security number.
- Have rent and utility receipts.
- Have birth certificates for self and children.
- Have identification or driver's license for self and children.
- Have bank account numbers.
- Have insurance policies and numbers.
- Have marriage license.
- Have valuable jewelry.
- Have important telephone numbers.
- Hide bag with extra clothing.

Among the studies that support women's development of safety planning is Sullivan and Bybee's shelter-based intervention (1999), designed to help women devise safety plans and provide needed advocacy services. Women in this ten-week intervention experienced less physical violence and increased quality of life over time. Parker and colleagues (1999) used a quasi-experimental design in a prenatal clinic study to compare giving women community resource cards to a three-session counseling intervention delivered by nurses. Both study groups improved over the twelve-month postdelivery follow-up period, as indicated by improved scores on measures of physical and nonphysical abuse, although the intervention group scores were lower than the comparison group at both six months and twelve months postdelivery. In another intervention, McFarlane, Soeken, and Wiist (2000) attempted to enhance abused pregnant women's safety by providing referrals, support, safety planning education, and help accessing community resources (such as housing and legal services). Women seen in a prenatal clinic were randomized to receive a list of community resources (Brief), unlimited access to a clinic-based professional counselor (Counseling), or a peer "mentor mother," who was a paraprofessional peer advocate (Outreach), in addition to the counseling. These women were followed up at the two-, six-, twelve-, and eighteen-months postdelivery. The group that received the mentor mother had lower physical violence scores than the other two groups at a two-month follow-up, but these findings did not persist at the later follow-up points.

Despite the identification of these types of safety strategies and the growing public interest in domestic violence, there remains much more to learn about the effectiveness of interventions to facilitate and support women as they consider and undertake these safety-enhancing behaviors (Chalk & King, 1998b; Hadley, Short, Lezin, & Zook, 1995; Janinksi & Willimas, 1998). The Committee on the Assessment of Family Violence Interventions identified only thirty-four intimate partner violence intervention studies from 1980 to 1996 that were sufficiently rigorous to inform the discussion of how best to help women end the abuse (Chalk & King, 1998b). Of these, nineteen were legal, eight were health care, and seven were social service interventions. In addition, in a more recent assessment that systematically reviewed all available evidence on interventions aimed at preventing abuse or reabuse, twenty-two articles were found to meet minimal inclusion criteria, eleven of which described four interventions for primary care physician or shelter referral mechanisms and eleven for batterer and couple programs (Wathen & MacMillan, 2003). None of the interventions aimed at women achieved an evaluation of good by the authors, and four were rated as fair, with the remaining being viewed as poor in quality. Clearly there is a need for the development, implementation, and evaluation of rigorous, behaviorally based interventions aimed at assisting women with intimate partner violence.

Stark and Flitcraft (1996) noted that while domestic violence has been the subject of extensive descriptive research, there is a "dearth of systematic theorizing (or theory testing)" (p. 130). The authors describe three major theoretical models for understanding domestic violence. First is the interpersonal violence model, in which individuals or families are considered to have underlying psychiatric or behavioral problems. Second, in the family violence model, individuals are thought to learn violence in childhood, have it reinforced by the family and cultural institutions, and have it provoked by stresses, such as poverty. Third, in the gender politics model, domestic violence is seen as caused by male dominance that extends from dating relationships, through marriage and parenting, to economic life. In addition, the descriptive research in intimate partner violence has integrated the use of the cycle of abuse theory, which posits that there are three distinct phases that most couples in intimate partner violence experience (Walker, 1979): the tension-building phase, the acute battering phase, and the loving or calm phase. Each phase may vary in duration and intensity between couples. Although these models suggest reasons for or the context within which violence occurs, they do not offer guidance in how or when to intervene. These models need to be integrated with behavior change theories so that we can understand the process by which women are eventually successful in ending the abuse, and we can design interventions to facilitate that process. In the context of intimate partner violence (IPV) interventions for women and for the purposes of this chapter, behavior change refers to women's safety-enhancing behaviors.

Although no behavior change theory has been used in its entirety or explicitly with the terminology that is used in the behavioral sciences (for example, cues to action or normative behavior), some interventions have incorporated components of widely used theories. Of the interventions described in the literature, the majority engage women in the intervention at the point where they are ready to seek or are seeking assistance (shelter populations, seeking protective services). A handful of interventions have engaged women at the point of screening in the health care setting (McFarlane, Soeken, Reel, Parker, & Silva, 1997; Parker et al., 1999; McFarlane et al., 2000). Therefore, these women's cues to action may predate the intervention itself or may be the screening tool used in the intervention. These interventions tend to use a one-on-one or group advocate or advocacy approach, and the intention to instill skills in the women to maintain her safety is evident. The intervention literature discusses the necessity of working with women to gain the knowledge of and positive attitude toward existing environmental resources and to become competent in safety planning. In this way, interventions may assist in changing women's perception of a social norm to one that supports the implementation of safety-enhancing behaviors and the belief that the abusive behaviors are destructive and need to cease. The skill building, social norms, and beliefs that the advantages of taking action outweigh the disadvantages of inaction are all components that can enhance a woman's self-efficacy to perform the safety-enhancing behaviors.

Furthermore, while the nomenclature of behavior change theory and processes may not have been used in the intervention literature, neither have the intervention components and process outcomes been operationalized or systematically measured. Interventions that exist do not necessarily present process outcomes such as changes in women's knowledge of services, enhancement in self-efficacy, or social norms, but rather concentrate on outcomes that may not be under the control of women. Therefore, while women may engage in the components of the intervention and be successful in increasing their awareness of safety resources, self-efficacy, or their intention to end the abuse, their intervention success is determined by the frequency or intensity of abuse experienced—outcomes that are not necessarily under the women's control. Ultimately, then, women may be labeled an intervention failure even though they may have taken some steps to try to improve their situations. Interventions that use behavior change theories will see behavior change as a process by which women engage in the intervention and achieve positive gains in the precursors to behavior change, such as intention, beliefs, and knowledge. These theory-based precursors, outcomes in and of themselves, are not restricted to actions that the women may not have direct control over. The use of theory will allow intervention designers to efficiently evaluate their programs and determine what components were most successful in promoting women's behavior change. While an intervention's impact on women's actual experience of violence is important to measure as well, the integration of behavior change theory will allow a more refined assessment of what helps women adopt safety-enhancing behaviors.

Theories of behavior change that are widely available and rigorously evaluated can be usefully applied to investigate and intervene in the complex problem of intimate partner violence. Behavioral theories have been used in two ways: for behavioral prediction and for understanding mechanisms of change. Models of behavioral prediction are designed to determine factors that predict the performance or nonperformance of a behavior, whereas behavior change theories focus on the phases, states, or stages that people go through in their attempt at successful behavior change. While this distinction is important to make in dealing with intimate partner violence, it is not to say that these two ideas are not complementary. What is identified as a predictor of behavior could be used as a mechanism for promoting change in a behavior change intervention. Although understanding the process or stage-based process of behavior change is important, it is equally important to be able to explain why people behave the way they do. Also important to recognize is the need to have available interventions to assist abused women once they recognize the behaviors of their partner as abusive. Women may not recognize their partner's behavior as abusive for many reasons, including lack of awareness or their cultural patterns that permit men to abuse women. Therefore, it is imperative that the choice of a behavior change theory in the design of an intervention take into account that even though women may screen positive for experiencing abuse by an intimate partner, they may not be ready to actively engage in the intervention as they may not see themselves as abused and in need of assistance. We describe in the next section an example of how a behavior change theory can be used to design a responsive and effective intervention to assist women experiencing intimate partner violence.

An Application of the Transtheoretical Model to Intervention Development and Evaluation

Relationships are ever changing in their existence, content, and intensity. Campbell, Rose, Kub, and Nedd (1998) interviewed women in abusive relationships three times over a three-year period. Their study demonstrated that intimate partner relationships are fluid with regard to their abuse status, and success in ending abuse is a process that occurs over time, with women using different strategies to facilitate the process (Anderson & Saunders, 2003). Campbell, Rose, Kub, and Nedd (1998), Brown (1997), and Burke, Gielen, McDonnell, O'Campo, and Maman (2001) suggest that a promising conceptual framework for understanding such a process is the transtheoretical model (TM; Prochaska & DiClemente, 1983). The transtheoretical model, also known as the stages of change model, addresses an individual's readiness to change behavior and has been successfully applied to a range of health behaviors in diverse settings (Polacsek, Celentano, O'Campo, & Santelli, 1999; Cabral, Pulley, Artz, Brill, & Macaluso, 1998; Prochaska, 1994; Kelly et al., 1994; Carey et al., 2000; Perz, DiClemente, & Carbonari, 1996; Rossi et al., 1994; Belding, Iguchi, Lamb, Lakin, & Terry, 1995; Keefe et al., 2000; Fogarty et al., 2001; Gielen et al., 2001; Grimley, DiClemente, Prochaska, & Prochaska, 1995; Lauby et al., 1998; Milstein, Lockaby, Fogarty, Cohen, & Cotton, 1998; O'Campo et al., 1999; Prochaska & DiClemente, 1983; Prochaska, Redding, Harlow, Rossi, & Velicer, 1994).

The TM, which originated in the early 1980s from an examination of psychotherapy and behavior change theories, conceptualizes behavior change as a process that occurs in five stages: precontemplation, contemplation, preparation, action, and maintenance (Prochaska & DiClemente, 1982; see also Chapter Two, this volume). Behavior change is seen as often being cyclical, with individuals progressing and relapsing between stages before achieving the success of maintenance.

The TM also incorporates ten processes of change to describe how an individual moves from one stage of change to the next (Prochaska, 1994; Prochaska, DiClemente, & Norcross, 1992). These processes can be categorized into two groups; cognitive processes and behavioral processes. According to Prochaska et al. (1994), these processes of change "provide important guides for intervention programs, since the processes are like the independent variables that people need to apply to move from stage to stage" (p. 39). Thus, understanding how each process is used for a particular behavior change is a critical element in the design of effective stage-tailored interventions. By first determining an individual's stage of change, those who are using intervention programs can apply stage-specific processes that will facilitate movement toward the desired behavior.

Using TM for Intimate Partner Violence Research

Some work has been done examining the application of the TM to male batterers and their abusive behaviors (Daniels & Murphy, 1997; Murphy & Baxter, 1997) and there is great promise in the application of the TM to women's experiences of intimate partner violence. To our knowledge, our work (described below) was some of the first to examine the TM stages, processes, and constructs of behavior change for women's experiences of ending abuse within intimate relationships (Burke et al., 2001; Burke, Denison, Gielen, McDonnell, & O'Campo, 2004). We recognize that some would argue that a TM approach to women's experiences of intimate partner violence is inherently victim blaming because the abusive behavior belongs to the perpetrator. However, women in abusive relationships do take action to survive, cope with, and eventually find ways to have the abuse end (Anderson & Saunders, 2003; Campbell, Miller, Cardwell, & Belknap, 1994; Jacobson, Gottman, Berns, & Shortt, 1996; Okun, 1986). Those who provide health care or other services to women in abusive relationships recognize their responsibility to help these women keep themselves safe.

Interventions based on the TM are tailored to an individual's stage of readiness to change and thus should be effective. For example, early in the change process, individuals may respond better to cognitive and emotional appeals to promote awareness and motivation, whereas later in the process, individuals may need more social and behavioral, action-oriented approaches (Prochaska, 1994).

In addition to helping to build more effective interventions, the TM has been shown to have utility for program evaluation. Evaluation of domestic violence interventions typically focuses on outcome measures such as the type and frequency of abuse experienced by women as measured by instruments such as the Conflict Tactics Scale (Straus, Hamby, Boney-McCoy, & Sugarman, 1996) and the Abusive Behavior Inventory (Shepard & Campbell, 1992). These scales and other frequently used dichotomous questions about current abuse status shed little light on the complexity of the situation. According to Brown (1997), "we must go beyond outcome measures looking at instances of violence and leaving the abusers and examine the incremental and measurable processes of change" (p. 7). Measuring progress toward ending the abuse should be possible with the TM, as suggested by studies evaluating interventions for other health-related behaviors (Prochaska, 1994; Kelly et al., 1994; Carey et al., 2000; Perz et al., 1996; Rossi et al., 1994; Belding et al., 1995; Keefe et al., 2000; Grimley et al., 1995; Milstein et al., 1998; Prochaska et al., 1994).

Qualitative Research to Explore the TM

As a first step in the process of applying the TM to intimate partner violence, we used qualitative research methods to explore how abused women describe their experiences trying to end the abuse (Burke et al., 2001, 2004). Our talking at length with currently or recently abused women recruited from health service settings in a low-income urban area provided a greater understanding of their experiences. These results support the application of the TM to women's descriptions of the stages and processes they go through when ending abuse in their intimate relationships.

Our qualitative analysis suggests that women talk about five stages: (1) not recognizing the abuse and safety as a problem (precontemplation), (2) acknowledging the problem (contemplation), (3) considering their options (preparation), (4) selecting an option and deciding to take an action toward ending the abuse/safety enhancement (action), and (5) keeping themselves safe using various strategies (maintenance) (Table 15.1). For example, one woman in the initial phase of precontemplation stated, "I still haven't accepted [that it's abuse]. No way—it hasn't come down on me yet." Another woman poignantly described how "flower-colored glasses" contributed to her denial of the abuse as a problem: "Well, basically, you

TABLE 15.1. STAGES OF CHANGE FOR INTIMATE PARTNER VIOLENCE.

Stage of Change	Definition
Precontemplation	The woman does not recognize the abusive behavior as a problem and is not interested in change.
Contemplation	The woman recognizes the abusive behavior as a problem and has an increasing awareness of the pros and cons of change.
Preparation	The woman recognizes the abusive behavior as a problem, intends to change, and has developed a plan.
Action	The woman is actively engaged in making changes related to ending the abusive behavior.
Maintenance	The abusive behavior has ended, and the woman is taking steps to prevent relapse.

Source: Burke, Gielen, McDonnell, O'Campo, & Maman (2001). Reproduced with permission.

know, when we first started seein' each other I didn't, I won't say I didn't detect some obsessiveness, but I kinda wore the flower-colored glasses. Then I was like, 'Oh well, you know, he just cares about me' kinda thing." Women were able to pinpoint the exact moment in which they recognized their partners' abusive behavior. One woman, while in the contemplation stage, reported that she started to recognize her safety and the abuse as a problem when "the hits got more harder. . . . It wasn't just a slap or something."

For women in the preparation stage who had begun to consider their options, several factors, including concerns about personal safety and financial stability, affected their decisions about how to move forward: "I think that if someone had said you can come and stay, or provided me with a place to stay [I would have left]. Because I did try to get into the Y a couple times, but no beds were available. I was afraid to leave and I was afraid to stay. I was afraid to leave because I felt as though he may find me and kill me." The women used several strategies for ending their abusive situations. This phase of selecting an option and deciding to take an action toward ending the abuse incorporated a range of behaviors. Some women chose to handle the situation themselves, and others sought help from outside sources such as family, friends, and law enforcement. Finally, women in the maintenance phase talked about their experiences since ending the abuse and how they have kept themselves safe. Although these women were able to end the abusive relationships, the experiences left some of them emotionally fragile. According to one woman, "I wouldn't have never took him back. Never look back. I see myself now as just struggling and taking it day by day [after having left him]. Doing the right thing."

Results from our research also show that women attempting to end abuse within intimate relationships use processes of change to facilitate movement from one stage to the next (Burke et al., 2004). Out of the ten processes of change defined by Prochaska (1994), abused women were found to use seven in their movement through the stages of change (consciousness raising, self-reevaluation, environmental reevaluation, self-liberation, social liberation, helping relationships, and stimulus control). Support for the use of the counterconditioning, dramatic relief, and reinforcement management processes was not apparent. Data from abused women show that women in the early stages of behavior change (precontemplation, contemplation, and preparation) tend to use the more cognitive processes (for example, consciousness raising, self-reevaluation, environmental reevaluation), while women in the action or maintenance stage use more behavioral processes (for example, stimulus control and self-liberation) In the case of abused women, we found that consciousness raising was important in both the earlier and later stages of change, and helping relationships were important throughout. (Figure 15.1).

In addition to the processes of change, the two constructs of decisional balance and self-efficacy also related to women's ability to end abuse within intimate partner relationships. Several of the women in this sample reported remaining in con-

FIGURE 15.1. STAGES, PROCESSES, AND CONSTRUCTS
OF CHANGE FOR ENDING INTIMATE PARTNER VIOLENCE.

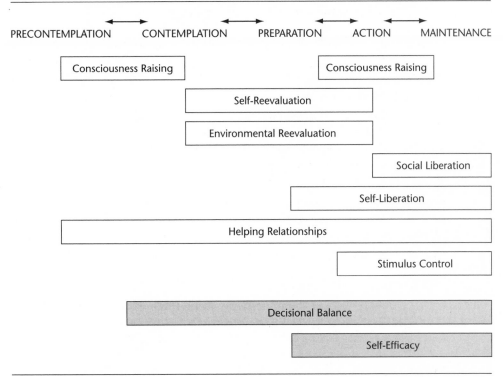

Note: The processes of change are represented by the white boxes and the constructs of change are represented by the darker shaded boxes.

Source: Burke, Denison, Gielen, McDonnell, & O'Campo (2004). Reproduced with permission.

templation about the abuse for a prolonged period of time during which they felt the disadvantages outweighed the advantages of taking action. According to Prochaska et al.'s review of the transtheoretical model (1994), individuals in the contemplation stage are "acutely aware of the cons. This balance between the costs and benefits of changing can produce profound ambivalence that can keep people stuck in this stage for long periods of time" (p. 39). Conversely, as women moved toward action and ultimately maintenance, the pros of the behavior change outweighed the cons.

Implications for Interventions

The results from our research and that of others (Anderson & Saunders, 2003; Campbell, Rose, Kub, & Nedd, 1998; Brown, 1997) support the application of the TM model to understanding women's experiences ending abuse, implementing safety behaviors, and designing, implementing, and evaluating a stage-tailored intervention for women experiencing abuse. Practitioners could use specific questions to determine a woman's stage of change and then identify which influencing processes and constructs of change would be most beneficial for the woman. For example, based on our findings, a woman staged in precontemplation should receive a consciousness-raising intervention activity such as receiving information about what constitutes abuse (Table 15.2). Table 15.2 provides an example of what a tailored intervention using the stages of change and corresponding processes of change would entail with specific examples of counseling activities.

When designing an intervention that would be responsive to abused women, an initial screening, using widely used and evaluated tools, could be conducted to identify women who have experienced intimate partner violence (Straus et al., 1996; Tolman, 1999; Hudson & Mcintosh, 1981; Feldhaus et al., 1997; McFarlane et al., 1997). A woman classified as abused would be assessed to determine what stage she was in for readiness to engage in the intervention. The intervention components would then follow the TM: tailoring the intervention to accommodate women's stages of readiness by using stage-specific processes of change, self-efficacy,

TABLE 15.2. STAGE OF CHANGE AND SAMPLE PROCESSES OF CHANGE AND COUNSELING ACTIVITIES FOR INTIMATE PARTNER VIOLENCE.

Stage of Change and Sample Processes of Change	Sample Counseling Activity
Precontemplation: Consciousness raising	Fact or fiction: The advocate reads a list of statements about intimate partner violence to the client and asks her which are true and which are false.
Contemplation: Self-reevaluation	Relationship reflection: The advocate helps the client explore her ideas of a healthy relationship, including discussion of beliefs about her current intimate partner relationship.
Preparation: Self-liberation	Safety planning: The advocate shares key safety planning steps with client, such as identifying a safe place and practicing getting there when safe and not under stress, and keeping an extra set of house and car keys, cash or credit card, emergency telephone numbers, copies of important documents, and spare clothing where they can be gotten to quickly.
Action: Helping relationships	Who can I turn to? The advocate asks the client to list and talk about the people whom she trusts and could rely on.
Maintenance: Social liberation	Becoming involved: The advocate encourages the client to become involved in organizations that assist abused women or promote other healthy behaviors.

and decisional balance mechanisms. Components of the intervention activities and goals that correspond to TM would need to be operationalized and measured to ensure adequate evaluation of the intervention before, during, and after administration of the program. Outcomes and goals of the program would include such aspects described below, as well as an assessment of women's stage of change to ascertain if they had progressed a stage as a result of the intervention efforts. This approach seems most appropriate for clinical or social service settings in which women are screened for other issues already, although it may be possible to implement in other settings as well, as long as the screening and stage assessments could be done privately and safely.

Ecological Approaches to Intimate Partner Violence

Researchers such as Heise (1998; Heise et al., 1999) and Dutton (1996) have advocated for the adoption of an integrated, ecological framework for a fuller understanding of the multiple levels of factors influencing women's experiences of abuse. Ecological models, based on the premise that multiple factors influence health and that those factors are interrelated (Sallis & Owen, 1997), can "help [intimate partner violence] activists and researchers grapple with the complexity of real life" (Heise, 1998, p. 285; see also Chapter Six, this volume).

Ecological models of health behavior focus on the relationship and connections between people and their environments. Such models propose that behaviors are influenced by the characteristics of individuals and their social and physical environments (Sallis & Owen, 1997). Accordingly, ecological models are multilevel in nature and permit the identification of multiple levels for intervention. For example, McLeroy, Bibeau, Steckler, and Glanz's ecological model of health behavior (1988) identifies five levels of influence: intrapersonal factors, interpersonal processes, institutional factors, community factors, and public policy. A growing consensus suggests that multilevel interventions derived from ecological models and targeting individuals and their environments are a promising approach for addressing improvements in health (Sallis & Owen, 2002).

The use of ecological models is a promising approach for intervening to address intimate partner violence. However, work remains to be done regarding the operationalization and application of ecological frameworks. Although there is a growing wealth of research on the intra- and interpersonal characteristic associated with intimate partner violence experiences and help seeking (O'Campo, Burke, Peak, McDonnell, & Gielen, 2005; Burke et al., 2005), additional work is needed to identify the broader macrolevel determinants. Neighborhood context is one such area that has received increased attention in the past decade. For example, O'Campo et al.'s multilevel study (1995) of violence by male partners against women during the childbearing years found that women residing in neighborhoods characterized by low per capita income, high unemployment rates, and a high versus low ratio of renters to home owners were at increased risk of intimate partner violence. Cunradi, Caetano, Clark, and Schafer (2000) found that couples who lived in impoverished neighborhoods were at an increased risk of intimate partner violence compared to couples who did not reside in impoverished neighborhoods. And Browning's recent work (2002) found that neighborhoods characterized as having high social cohesion (for example, a willingness of neighbors to help other neighbors) and high informal social control (for example, the likelihood that neighbors would intervene to address issues such as child delinquency) had a decreased likelihood of intimate partner homicide and increased likelihood that an abused woman would disclose her situation.

Recent work by O'Campo and colleagues contributes to our understanding of the relationship between neighborhood factors and intimate partner violence outcomes (O'Campo et al., 2005; Burke et al., 2005). Results from our work applying the innovative methodology of concept mapping (Trochim, 1989) uncovered a range of neighborhood characteristics that far exceeded the handful of factors that have been examined in the research literature in relation to perpetration of partner violence.

In response to a focal question asking women about all the neighborhood-level characteristics that could in any way, good or bad, affect intimate partner violence experiences, participants generated a range of neighborhood items, including descriptions of physical attributes (for example, lots of trash, abandoned houses), economic characteristics (for example, poverty, unemployment, income and wealth), attributes of residents (for example, people who do not care, public drunkenness, people who take a stand), resources (for example, community centers, emergency assistance programs), and beliefs or attitudes of residents (for example, macho attitudes about control). Rating information captured participants' perceptions regarding the strength of the relationship between neighborhood characteristics and four intimate partner violence outcomes: prevalence, severity, perpetration, and cessation. In general, the severity and perpetration ratings are virtually identical. That is, the items were rated as being similarly important for these two outcomes. The prevalence ratings were also similar to those for severity and perpetration. However, for cessation, the ratings were almost reversed compared to severity or perpetration. That is, items that received a high rating for severity and perpetration received a low rating for cessation. While neighborhood characteristics related to violence attitudes and behaviors and negative social attributes were felt to be strongly related to prevalence, severity, and perpetration, neighborhood characteristics such as community enrichment resources and community networks were felt to be most strongly related to cessation of intimate partner violence.

As part of the concept mapping activities, participants were asked to and were able to articulate the relationship between neighborhood characteristics and intimate partner violence experiences. Results from these discussions provided valuable information regarding the perceived pathways through which neighborhood context influences intimate partner violence outcomes. For example, several noted that with high levels of home ownership, there would be a greater likelihood that residents would take a stand and would be more alert. This in turn would increase the likelihood of intimate partner violence cessation. Participants also noted that low levels of home ownership might negatively affect job availability, which might lead to stress, which leads to increased prevalence of intimate partner violence in the neighborhood.

Explorative research such as that described previously assists in the determination of how neighborhood context is related to intimate partner violence and begins to highlight areas for intervention at the neighborhood level. Results from this line of neighborhood effects research can be coupled with data regarding intrapersonal and interpersonal factors associated with intimate partner violence experiences to develop multilevel, ecologically oriented approaches to intimate partner violence interventions.

Conclusions and Future Directions

Intimate partner violence interventions for women thus far have focused on either health care delivery systems or legal advocacy. The interventions have been secondary prevention using active approaches focusing on the victim and perpetrator and have been largely devoid of behavior change theory. Components of theories have been used or concentrated within social justice and cycle of violence frameworks. Few interventions focused on women's safety behaviors have been rigorously evaluated. Rather, evaluations have concentrated on increases in knowledge or those behaviors that the woman has no control over.

Recommendations for enhancing IPV programs and their evaluation include using comprehensive theoretical frameworks that incorporate a stage-based approach that sees behavior as a process of change that occurs progressively through phases and individualized to take into account the person's state of readiness to institute a behavioral change. In this way, proximal, intermediate, and distal goals can be established, and behavior change can be seen as a progressive process and not necessarily an all-or-none phenomenon. Theory-based interventions and evaluations are critically important to advance both the theory and practice of reducing intimate partner violence. Ecological approaches that incorporate an under-standing of neighborhood and other social-contextual factors with individual-level factors represent an important new frontier in intimate partner violence research.

References

Abraham, M. (2000). Isolation as a form of marital violence. *Journal of Social Distress and the Homeless, 9*(3), 221–236.

Anderson, D. K., & Saunders D. G. (2003). Leaving an abusive partner: An empirical review of predictors, the process of leaving, and psychological well-being. *Trauma, Violence and Abuse, 4,* 163–191.

Bassuk, E. L., Dawson, R., Perloff, J., & Weinreb, L. (2001). Post-traumatic stress disorder in extremely poor women: Implications for health care clinicians. *Journal of American Medical Women's Association, 56*(2), 79–85.

Belding, M. A., Iguchi, M. Y., Lamb, R. J., Lakin, M., & Terry, R. (1995). Stages and processes of change among polydrug users in methadone maintenance treatment. *Drug and Alcohol Dependence, 39,* 45–53.

Bergman, B., & Brismar, B. (1991). A five-year follow-up study of 117 battered women. *American Journal of Public Health, 81*(11), 1486–1488.

Brown, J. (1997). Working toward freedom from violence: The process of change in battered women. *Violence Against Women, 3*(1), 5–26.

Browning, C. (2002). The span of collective efficacy: Extending social disorganization theory to partner violence. *Journal of Marriage and Family, 64,* 833–850.

Burke, J. G., Denison, J., Gielen, A. C., McDonnell, K., & O'Campo, P. (2004). What helps women end abuse in intimate relationships? An application of the transtheoretical model. *American Journal of Health Behavior, 28*(2), 122–133.

Burke, J. G., Gielen, A. C., McDonnell, K. A., O'Campo, P., & Maman, S. (2001). The process of ending abusive relationships: A qualitative exploration of the transtheoretical model. *Violence Against Women, 7*(10), 1144–1163.

Burke, J. G., O'Campo, P., Peak, G., Gielen, A., McDonnell, K., & Trochim, W. (2005). *An introduction to concept mapping as a participatory public health research methodology.* Unpublished manuscript.

Cabral, R., Pulley, L., Artz, L., Brill, I., & Macaluso, M. (1998). Women at risk of HIV/STD: The importance of male partners as barriers to condom use. *AIDS and Behavior, 2,* 75–85.

Campbell, J. C. (2002). Health consequences of intimate partner violence. *Lancet, 359,* 1331–1336.

Campbell, J. C., & Humphreys, J. (1993). *Nursing care of survivors of family violence.* St. Louis, MO: Mosby.

Campbell, J., Jones-Snow, A., Dienemann, J., Kub, J., Schollenberger, J., O'Campo, J., Gielen, A. C., & Wynne, C. (2002). Intimate partner violence and physical health consequences. *Archives of Internal Medicine, 162,* 1157–1163.

Campbell, J. C., Kub, J., Belknap, R. A., & Templin, T. (1997). Predictors of depression in battered women. *Violence Against Women, 3,* 276–293.

Campbell, J. C., Kub, J., & Rose, L. (1996). Depression in battered women, *Journal of the American Women's Association, 51*(3), 106–110.

Campbell, J. C., Miller, P., Cardwell, M., & Belknap, R. A. (1994). Relationship status of battered women over time. *Journal of Family Violence, 9,* 99–111.

Campbell, J. C., Rose, L., Kub, J., & Nedd, D. (1998). Voices of strength and resistance: A contextual and longitudinal analysis of women's responses to battering. *Journal of Interpersonal Violence, 13*(6), 743–762.

Campbell, J. C., & Soeken, K. L. (1999). Forced sex and intimate partner violence: Effects on women's risk and women's health. *Violence Against Women, 5*(9), 1017–1035.

Carey, M. P., Bratten, L. S., Maisto, S. A., Gleason, J. R., Forsyth, A. D., Durant, L. E., & Jaworski, B. C. (2000). Using information, motivational enhancement, and skills training to reduce the risk of HIV infection for low-income urban women: A second randomized clinical trial. *Health Psychology, 19*(1), 3–11.

Cascadi, M., & O'Leary, K. D. (1992). Depressive symptomatology, self-esteem, and self-blame women, *Journal of Family Violence, 7*(4), 249–256.

Chalk, R., & King, P. (1998a). Assessing family violence interventions. *American Journal of Preventive Medicine, 14,* 289–292.

Chalk, R., & King, P. A. (Eds.). (1998b). *Violence in families.* Washington, DC: National Academy Press.

Coker, A., Smith, P. H., McKeown, R. E., & King, M. J. (2000). Frequency and correlates of intimate partner violence by type: Physical, sexual, and psychological battering. *American Journal of Public Health, 90*(4), 553–559.

Coley, S. M., & Beckett, J. O. (1988). Black battered women: A review of empirical literature. *Journal of Counseling and Development, 66,* 266–270.

Commonwealth Fund. (1998). *Addressing domestic violence and its consequences: Policy report on the Commonwealth Fund Commission on Women's Health.* New York: Commonwealth Fund.

Crowell, N. A., & Burgess, A. W. (1996). *Understanding violence against women.* Washington, DC: National Academy Press.

Cunradi, C. B., Caetano, R., Clark, C., & Schafer, J. (2000). Neighborhood poverty as a predictor of intimate partner violence among white, black and Hispanic couples in the United States: A multi-level analysis. *Annals of Epidemiology, 10*(5), 297–308.

Daniels, J. W., & Murphy, C. M. (1997). Stages and processes of change in batterers' treatment. *Cognitive Behavior Practice, 4,* 123–145.

Dutton, M. A. (1996). Battered women's strategic responses to violence: The role of context. In J. L. Edleson & Z. C. Eisikovits (Eds.), *Future interventions with battered women and their families.* Thousand Oaks, CA: Sage.

Eby, K., Campbell, J. C., & Sullivan, C. M. (1995). Health effects of experiences of sexual violence for women with abusive partners. *Health Care for Women International, 16,* 563–576.

Federal Bureau of Investigation. (1996). *Crime in the United States—1996.* Washington, DC: U.S. Government Printing Office.

Feldhaus, K. M., Koziol-McLain, J., Amsbury, H. L., Norton, I. M., Lowenstein, S. R., & Abbott, J. T. (1997). Accuracy of three brief screening questions for detecting partner violence in the emergency department. *JAMA, 277,* 1357–1361.

Fishbein, M., Triandis, H. C., Kanfer, F. H., Becker, M., Middlestadt, S. E., & Eichler, A. (2001). Factors influencing behavior and behavior change. In A. Baum, T. A. Tevenson, & J. E. Singer (Eds.), *Handbook of health psychology.* Mahwah, NJ: Erlbaum.

Fogarty, L. A., Heilig, C. M., Armstrong, K., Cabral, R., Galavotti, C., Gielen, A. C., & Green, B. M. (2001). Long-term effectiveness of a peer-based intervention to promote condom and contraceptive use among HIV-positive and at-risk women. *Public Health Reports, 116*(Suppl. 1), 103–119.

Gelles, R. J., & Cornell, C. P. (1990). *Intimate violence in families* (2nd ed.). Thousand Oaks, CA: Sage.

Gielen, A. C., Fogarty, L., Armstrong, K., Green, B. M., Cabral, R., Milstein, B., Galavotti, C., & Heilig, C. (2001). Promoting condom use with main partners: A behavioral trial for women. *AIDS and Behavior, 5*(3), 193–204.

Gielen, A. C., McDonnell, K. A., O'Campo, P., & Burke, J. G. (2005). Suicide risk and mental health indicators: Do they differ by abuse and HIV status? *Women's Health Issues, 15*(2), 89–95.

Gielen, A. C., O'Campo, P. J., & McDonnell, K. A. (2002). Intimate partner violence, HIV status, and sexual risk reduction. *AIDS and Behavior, 6*(2), 107–116.

Goodman, L., Dutton, M. A., Weinfurt, K., & Cook, S. (2003). The Intimate Partner Violence Strategies Index. *Violence Against Women, 9,* 163–186.

Grimley, D. M., DiClemente, R. J., Prochaska, J. O., & Prochaska, G. W. (1995). Adolescent pregnancy, STD, and HIV: A promising new approach. *Family Life Educator, 13,* 7–15.

Hadley, S. M., Short, L. M., Lezin, N., & Zook, E. (1995). WomanKind: An innovative model of health care response to domestic violence. *Women's Health Issues, 5*(4), 189–198.

Heise, L. L. (1998). Violence against women: An integrated, ecological framework. *Violence Against Women, 4,* 262–290.

Heise, L., Ellsburg, M., & Gottemoeller, M. (1999). *Ending violence against women.* Baltimore, MD: Johns Hopkins University School of Public Health Population Information Program.

Hudson, W. W., & Mcintosh, S. R. (1981). The assessment of spouse abuse: Two quantifiable dimensions. *Journal of Marriage and Family, 43,* 873–885.

Jacobson, N. S., Gottman, J. M., Berns, S., & Shortt, J. W. (1996). Psychological factors in the longitudinal course of battering: When do couples split up? When does abuse decrease? *Violence and Victims, 11,* 371–392.

Janinski, J. L., & Williams, L. M. (1998). *Partner violence: A comprehensive review of twenty years of research.* Thousand Oaks, CA: Sage

Jones, A. S., Gielen, A. C., Campbell, J. C., Schollenberger, J., O'Campo, P., Dienemann, J. A., Kub, J., & Wynn, E. C. (1999). Annual and lifetime prevalence of partner abuse in a sample of female HMO enrollees. *Women's Health Issues, 9*(6), 295–305.

Keefe, F. J., Lefebvre, J. C., Kerns, R. D., Rodenberg, R., Beaupre, P., Prochaska, J., Prochaska, J. O., & Caldwell, D. C. (2000). Understanding the adoption of arthritis self-management: Stages of change profiles among arthritis patients. *Pain, 87,* 303–313.

Kelly, J. A., Murphy, D. A., Washington, C. D., Wilson, T. S., Koob, J. J., Davis, D. R., Ledezma, G., & Davantes, B. (1994). The effects of HIV/AIDS intervention groups for high-risk women in urban health clinics. *American Journal of Public Health, 84,* 1918–1922.

Kessler, R., McGonagle, K., Nelson, C., Hughes, M., Swartz, M., & Blazer, D. (1994). Sex and depression in the national Comorbidity Survey, II. *Journal of Affective Disorders, 30,* 15–26.

Koss, M. P., Ingram, M., & Pepper, S. L. (2000). Male partner violence: Relevance to health care providers. In A. Baum, T. A. Revenson, & J. E. Singer (Eds.), *Handbook of health psychology.* Mahwah, NJ: Erlbaum.

Lauby, J., Semaan, S., Cohen, A., Leviton, L., Gielen, A. C., Pulley, L., Walls, C., & O'Campo, P. (1998). Self-efficacy, decisional balance and stages of change for condom use among women at risk for HIV infection. *Health Education Research, 13*(3), 343–356.

Leserman, J., Drossman, D. A., & Hu, Y. J. (1998). Selected symptoms associated with sexual and physical abuse history among female patients with gastrointestinal disorders. *Psychological Medicine, 28,* 417–425.

McCauley, J., Kern, D. E., Kolodner, K., Dill, L., Schroeder, A. F., DeChang, H. K., Ryden, J., Bass, E. B., & Derogatis, L. R. (1995). The battering syndrome: Prevalence and clinical characteristics of domestic violence in primary care internal medicine practices. *Annals of Internal Medicine, 123,* 737–746.

McDonnell, K. A., Gielen, A. C., & O'Campo, P. (2003). Does HIV status make a difference in the experience of lifetime abuse? Descriptions of lifetime abuse and its context among low income urban women. *Journal of Urban Health, 80,* 494–509.

McDonnell, K. A., Gielen, A. C., O'Campo, P. R., & Burke, J. G. (2005). Abuse, HIV status and health related quality of life among low income women. *Quality of Life Research, 14,* 945–957.

McFarlane, J., & Parker, B. (1994). Preventing abuse during pregnancy: An assessment and intervention protocol. *American Journal of Maternal Child Nursing, 19,* 321–324.

McFarlane, J., Malecha, A., Gist, J., Watson, K., Batten, E., Hall, I., & Smith, S. (2002). An intervention to increase safety behaviors of abused women: Results of a randomized clinical trial. *Nursing Research, 51,* 347–354.

McFarlane, J., Soeken, K., Reel, S., Parker, B., & Silva, C. (1997). Resource use by abused women following an intervention program: Associated severity of abuse and reports of abuse ending. *Public Health Nursing, 14,* 244–250.

McFarlane, J., Soeken, K., & Wiist, W. (2000). An evaluation of interventions to decrease intimate partner violence to pregnant women. *Public Health Nursing, 17,* 443–451.

McLeroy, K. R., Bibeau, D., Steckler, A., & Glanz, K. (1988). An ecological perspective on health promotion programs. *Health Education Quarterly,* 1988, *15,* 351–377.

Milstein, B., Lockaby, T., Fogarty, L., Cohen, A., & Cotton, D. (1998). Process of change in adoption of consistent condom use. *Journal of Health Psychology, 3,* 349–368.

Mitchell, R. E., & Hodson, R. (1983). Coping with domestic violence: Social support and psychological health among battered women. *American Journal of Community Psychology, 11,* 629–654.

Murphy, C. M., & Baxter, V. A. (1997). Motivating batterers to change in the treatment context. *Journal of Interpersonal Violence, 12,* 607–619.

National Committee for Injury Prevention and Control. (1989). *Injury prevention: Meeting the challenge.* New York: Oxford University Press.

O'Campo, P., Burke, J. G., Peak, G., McDonnell, K., & Gielen, A. (2005). Uncovering the neighborhood influences on intimate partner violence using concept mapping. *Journal of Epidemiology and Community Health, 59*(7), 603–608.

O'Campo, P., Fogarty, L., Gielen, A. C., Armstrong, K., Bond, L., Galavotti, C., & Green, B. M. (1999). Distribution along a stages-of-behavioral-change continuum for condom and contraceptive use among women accessed in different settings. *Journal of Community Health, 24,* 61–72.

O'Campo, P., Gielen, A., Faden, R., Xue, N., Kass, N., & Wang, M. C. (1995). Violence by male partners against women during the childbearing year: A contextual analysis. *American Journal of Public Health, 85,* 1092–1097.

O'Campo, P., McDonnell, K. A., Gielen, A. C., Burke, J. G., & Chen, Y. (2002). Surviving physical and sexual abuse: What helps low-income women? *Patient Education and Counseling, 46,* 205–212.

Okun, L. E. (1986). *Women abuse: Facts replacing myths.* Albany, NY: SUNY Press.

Parker, B., McFarlane, J., Soeken, K., Silva, C., & Reel, S. (1999). Testing an intervention to prevent further abuse to pregnant women. *Research in Nursing, 22,* 59–66.

Perz, C. A., DiClemente, C. C., & Carbonari, J. P. (1996). Doing the right thing at the right time? The interaction of stages and processes of change in successful smoking cessation. *Health Psychology, 15*(6), 462–468.

Peterson, R., Saltzman, L. E., Goodwin, M., & Spitz, A. (1997). *Key scientific issues for research on violence occurring around the time of pregnancy.* Atlanta, GA: Centers for Disease Control and Prevention.

Pitzner, J. K., & Drummond, P. D. (1997). The reliability and validity of empirically scaled measures of psychological/verbal/control and physical/sexual abuse: Relationship between current negative mood and a history of abuse independent of other negative life events. *Journal of Psychosomatic Research, 43*(2), 125–142.

Plichta, S. B. (1996). Violence and abuse: Implications for women's health. In M. M. & K. S. Collins (Eds.), *Women's health: The Commonwealth Survey* (pp. 237–272). Baltimore, MD: Johns Hopkins University Press.

Plichta, S. B., & Falik, M. (2001). Prevalence of violence and its implications for women's health. *Women's Health Issues, 11*(3), 244–258.

Polacsek, M., Celentano, D. D., O'Campo, P., & Santelli, J. (1999). Correlates of condom use stage of change: Implications for intervention. *AIDS Education and Prevention, 11*, 38–52.

Prochaska, J. O. (1994). Helping patients at every stage. *Behavioral Approaches to Addictions, 3*, 2–7.

Prochaska, J. O., & DiClemente, C. C. (1982). Transtheoretical therapy: Toward a more integrated model of change. *Psychotherapy: Theory, Research and Practice, 19*, 276–288.

Prochaska, J. O., & DiClemente, C. C. (1983). Stages and processes of self-change of smoking: Toward an integrative model of change. *Journal of Consulting and Clinical Psychology, 51*, 390–395.

Prochaska, J. O., & DiClemente, C. C. (1986). Toward a comprehensive model of change. In R. Miller & N. Heather (Eds.), *Treating addictive behaviors* (pp. 3–27). New York: Plenum.

Prochaska, J. O., DiClemente, C. C., & Norcross, J. C. (1992). In search of how people change: Applications to addictive behaviors. *American Psychologist, 47*(9), 1102–1114.

Prochaska, J. O., Redding, C. A., Harlow, L. L., Rossi, J. S., & Velicer, W. F. (1994). The transtheoretical model of change and HIV prevention: A review. *Health Education Quarterly, 21*, 471–486.

Prochaska, J. O., Velicer, W. F., Rossi, J. S., Goldstein, M. G., Marcus, B. H., Rakowski, W., Fiore, C., Harlow, L. L., Redding, C. A., & Rosebloom, D. (1994). Stages of change and decisional balance for 12 problem behaviors. *Health Psychology, 13*, 39–46.

Rath, G. D., & Jarratt, L. G. (1990). Battered wife syndrome: Overview and presentation in the office setting. *South Dakota Journal of Medicine, 43*, 19–25.

Rhodes, K. V., & Levinson, W. (2003). Interventions for intimate partner violence against women: Clinical applications. *JAMA, 289*, 601–605.

Rossi, S. R., Rossi, J. S., Rossi-DelPrete, L. M., Prochaska, J. O., Banspach, S. W., & Carleton R. A. (1994). A processes of change model for weight control for participants in community-based weight loss programs. *International Journal of the Addiction, 29*(2), 161–177.

Sackett, L. A., & Saunders, D. G. (1999). The impact of different forms of psychological abuse on battered women. *Violence and Victims, 14*(1), 105–117.

Sallis, J. F., & Owen, N. (1997). Ecological models. In K. Glanz, B. K. Rimer & F. M. Lewis (Eds.), *Health behavior and health education: Theory, research and practice* (2nd ed.). San Francisco: Jossey-Bass.

Sallis, J. F., & Owen, N. (2002). Ecological models of health behavior. In K. Glanz, B. K. Rimer, & F. M. Lewis (Eds.), *Health behavior and health education: Theory, research and practice* (3rd ed.). San Francisco: Jossey-Bass.

Shepard, M. F., & Campbell, J. A. (1992). The Abusive Behavior Inventory: A measure of psychological and physical abuse. *Journal of Interpersonal Violence, 7,* 291–305.

Stark, E., & Flitcraft, A. (1996). *Women at risk: Domestic violence and women's health.* Thousand Oaks, CA: Sage.

Stark, E., Flitcraft, A., Zuckerman, D., Grey, A., Robison, J., & Frazier, W. (1981). *Wife abuse in the medical setting: An introduction for health personnel.* Rockville, MD: National Clearinghouse on Domestic Violence.

Stark, E., & Flitcraft, A. H. (1991). Spouse abuse. In M. L. Rosenberg & M. A. Fenley (Eds.), *Violence in America: A public health approach.* New York: Oxford University Press.

Straus, M. A., Hamby, S. L., Boney-McCoy, S., & Sugarman, D. B. (1996). The Revised Conflict Tactics Scales (CTS2). *Journal of Family Issues, 17,* 283–316.

Sullivan, C. M., & Bybee, D. I. (1999). Reducing violence using community-based advocacy for women with abusive partners. *Journal of Consulting and Clinical Psychology, 67,* 43–53.

Thakker, R. R., Gutierrez, P. M., Kuczen, C. L., & McCanne, T. R. (2000). History of physical and/or sexual abuse and current suicidality in college women. *Child Abuse and Neglect, 24*(10), 1345–1354.

Tjaden, P., & Thoennes, N. (1998). *Prevalence, incidence and consequences of violence against women: Findings from the National Violence Against Women Survey.* Washington, DC: National Institute of Justice, and Centers for Disease Control and Prevention.

Tolman, R. M. (1999). The validation of the Psychological Maltreatment of Women Inventory. *Violence and Victims, 14,* 25–37.

Trochim, W. (1989). Concept mapping: Soft science or hard art? *Evaluation and Program Planning, 12,* 87–110.

U.S. Department of Health and Human Services. (2000). *Healthy people 2010.* Washington, DC: U.S. Government Printing Office.

Walker, L. E (1979). *The battered woman.* New York: HarperCollins.

Wathen, C. N., & MacMillan, H. L. (2003). Interventions for violence against women: Scientific review. *JAMA, 289,* 589–600.

Weissman, M., & Kleman, G. (1992). Depression: Current understanding and changing trends. *Annual Review of Public Health, 13,* 319–339.

Wingood, G. M., DiClemente, R. J., & Raj, A. (2000). Adverse consequences of intimate partner abuse among women in non-urban domestic violence shelters. *American Journal of Preventive Medicine, 19*(4), 270–275.

Wise, L. A., Zierler, S., Krieger, N., & Harlow, B. L. (2001, Sept. 15). Adult onset of major depressive disorder in relation to early life violent victimization: A case-control study. *Lancet,* 881–887.

Wyatt, G. E. (1992). The sociocultural context of African American and white American women's rape. *Journal of Social Issues, 48*(1), 77–91.

CHAPTER SIXTEEN

APPLYING BEHAVIORAL THEORY
TO SELF-DIRECTED VIOLENCE

Alex E. Crosby, David W. Coombs, Leigh Willis

Injury from self-directed violence, which includes suicidal behavior, is a major public health problem in the United States (Institute of Medicine, 2002) and throughout the rest of the world (World Health Organization, 1996; Krug, Dahlberg, Mercy, Zwi, & Lozano, 2002). In the United States, suicide has ranked among the twelve leading causes of death since 1975. In 2002, it was the eleventh leading cause of death overall in the United States, responsible for 31,655 deaths (Kochanek, Murphy, Anderson, & Scott, 2004); it was the third leading cause of death among people aged fifteen to twenty-four years; fourth among people aged twenty-five to forty-four years; and eighth among those aged forty-five to sixty-four years (Anderson & Smith, 2005). Although suicide is a problem among youth and young adults, overall rates of death due to suicide continue to be highest among persons aged sixty-five years and older (Stevens et al., 1999).

The number of suicides reflects only a small portion of the impact of suicidal behavior. Many more people are hospitalized due to nonfatal suicidal behavior than are fatally injured, and an even greater number are treated in ambulatory settings or are not treated at all for injuries due to suicidal acts than those who are hospitalized (Rosenberg et al., 1987). The comparative descriptions of suicidal ideation and behavior show some important differences; for example, the rate of suicide in males is higher than that in females, but studies of suicidal thoughts and nonfatal suicidal behavior routinely show females with higher rates (U.S. Public Health Service, 2001). Prior studies have shown a high prevalence of nonfatal suicidal behavior among adults. The National Hospital Ambulatory Medical Care Survey estimated 509,000 visits to U.S. hospital emergency departments for self-directed violence in 2000 (McCaig & Burt, 2004). Other research indicates that over 70 percent of people who engage in suicidal behavior never seek health services (Diekstra, 1982). As a result, prevalence figures based on health records substantially underestimate the societal burden.

Injuries and deaths resulting from self-directed violent behaviors represent a substantial drain on the economic, social, and health resources of the nation. One method of estimating the economic cost of suicide includes using four factors: medical expenses of emergency intervention and nonemergency treatment for suicidality; the lost and reduced productivity of people suffering from suicidality; the lost productivity of the loved ones grieving a suicide; and lost wages of those dying by suicide. One analysis estimated that in 1998 alone, suicide accounted for $11.8 billion of lost productivity. In this same study, the direct (health care services, funerals, autopsies, and police investigations) and indirect costs (lost productivity) for the approximately thirty thousand suicides that occur nationally is $25 billion (Institute of Medicine, 2002). Compounding these costs are the unquantifiable costs of loss of life and the emotional trauma experienced by surviving family, friends, and communities that are affected by each person's fatal or nonfatal suicidal behavior (Crosby & Sacks, 2002).

Despite the widespread impact of self-directed violence in the United States, the problem has frequently been perceived as solely as a problem affecting European American males (Davis, 1979) and the affluent (Earls, Escobar, & Manson, 1990). Among non–European Americans, only the incidence of suicide among Native Americans has been widely noted (U.S. Department of Health and Human Services, 1986).

Epidemiology of Suicidal Behavior

In this section we describe the epidemiology of the problem of self-directed violence. (Unless otherwise noted, the source of all mortality data is the Centers for Disease Control and Prevention's Web-based Injury Statistics Query and Reporting System using population data from the U.S. Bureau of the Census.)

From 1998 to 2002, 151,401 suicides were counted in the United States. In 2002, 31,655 U.S. residents took their own lives, making suicide the eleventh leading cause of death for that year. Between 2001 and 2002, the age-adjusted death rate for fatal self-directed violence increased by 1.9 percent, the second straight year of increase, reversing a downward trend shown from 1998 to 2000. The summary data do not illustrate the variation with which suicide risk and the methods of suicide occur across age, sex, ethnic groups, and geographical regions within the United States.

Years of potential life lost before the age of 75 (YPLL-75), one measure of premature mortality, is another way of defining the burden of a health problem on the population. In terms of YPLL-75, suicide was the fifth leading cause of YPLL for U.S. residents in 2002. It accounted for 919,364 years of potential life lost, which represents approximately 4.6 percent of YPLL-75 for all causes of death and was preceded in rank by the following causes, in order: cancer, heart disease, unintentional injury, and conditions of the perinatal period.

Age- and Sex-Specific Suicide Rates

In 2002, overall patterns, as in previous decades, showed adults aged sixty-five years and older had the highest rates; children had the lowest rates. The highest number of suicides occurred among the age group thirty-five to forty-four years. This pattern differs when suicides are examined by sex. Approximately 80 percent of suicide victims are males, and their rates are 4.4 times greater than those of females. In the United States, the male pattern of age groups with the highest rate and highest number of suicides is similar to the overall pattern. Among females, the highest rate and the highest number of suicides are among those aged forty to forty-nine.

Race/Ethnicity- and Age Group–Specific Suicide Rates

Five major ethnic groups are examined in this study: European American non-Latino, African American non-Latino, Latino, Asian-Pacific Islander, and Native American. The last group includes both American Indians and Alaskan Natives. Examining the patterns of suicide rates by age group along with race/ethnicity demonstrates two general patterns. Among three groups (European American non-Latinos, Latinos, and Asian-Pacific Islanders), the rates are low among children, have a sharp rise during adolescence and young adulthood, remain relatively level for middle-aged adults, and then show the highest rates among those aged sixty-five years and older. In contrast, suicide rates among African American non-Latinos and Native Americans are low among children, but have the highest rates among adolescents and young adults; the rates then decline for middle-aged adults and have relatively low rates among those aged sixty-five and older. In each of the racial and ethnic groups, suicide rates were higher for males than for females.

Method of Suicide

Firearms were the leading method used in suicides in the United States in 2002 and accounted for 54 percent of all suicides. The next most commonly reported methods were suffocation (20.4 percent), poisoning (17.3 percent), falls (2.3 percent), and cutting (1.8 percent). Other, or unspecified, means accounted for 4.1 percent of all suicides in 2002. The methods of suicide in 2002 varied by sex. Among males, firearms accounted for the majority of suicides (59.8 percent), followed by suffocation (21.1 percent), poisoning (12.0 percent), and then other methods. Poisoning was also the principal means of suicide used by females (37.3 percent), followed by firearms (35.5 percent), suffocation (16.6 percent), and other methods. The methods of suicide in 2002 also varied by ethnicity. Firearms were the leading method of suicide among European American non-Latino (56.7 percent), African American non-Latino (56.1 percent), and Latino (43.1 percent). Among Asian/Pacific Islanders and Native Americans, suffocation was the leading method.

Geographical Variation

In 2002, age-adjusted suicide rates varied substantially across states, from 21.0 in Alaska to 5.1 in the District of Columbia. As in previous decades, age-adjusted suicide rates in the northeastern states were generally lower than those in other regions, followed by the Midwest. The states in the South and West regions had the highest rates. When state-specific age-adjusted suicide rates for the United States were ranked by quartiles, the rates from ten of the thirteen western states ranked in the highest quartile.*

Morbidity

Only within the past twenty years have nationally representative statistics been available for suicidal thoughts and behavior among adolescents in the United States. Since 1990, the Youth Risk Behavior Surveillance System (YRBSS), a school-based system, has measured health risk behaviors (including suicidal thoughts and behavior) among high school students using a self-report questionnaire. In the surveys, students answered four questions about seriously considering suicide, making a suicide plan, attempting suicide, and making a medically treated suicide attempt during the twelve months preceding the survey. In 2003, high school students reported the following: seriously considered suicide: males 12.8 percent, females 21.3 percent; made a suicide plan: males 14.1 percent, females 18.9;

---

*Northeast: Connecticut, Maine, Massachusetts, New Hampshire, New Jersey, New York, Pennsylvania, Rhode Island, and Vermont. Midwest: Illinois, Indiana, Iowa, Kansas, Michigan, Minnesota, Missouri, Nebraska, North Dakota, Ohio, South Dakota, and Wisconsin. South: Alabama, Arkansas, Delaware, District of Columbia, Florida, Georgia, Kentucky, Louisiana, Maryland, Mississippi, North Carolina, Oklahoma, South Carolina, Tennessee, Texas, Virginia, and West Virginia. West: Alaska, Arizona, California, Colorado, Hawaii, Idaho, Montana, Nevada, New Mexico, Oregon, Utah, Washington, and Wyoming.

attempted suicide: males 5.4 percent, females 11.5 percent; attempted suicide that required medical attention: males 2.4 percent, females 3.2 percent (Grunbaum et al., 2004). The National Electronic Injury Surveillance System developed by the Consumer Product Safety Commission was adapted in July 2000 to include all types and external causes of nonfatal injuries treated in a nationally representative sample of U.S. hospital emergency departments. During 2003, an estimated 411,128 persons were treated in the United States for nonfatal self-inflicted injuries (rate: 141.4 per 100,000 population). Among females, 232,439 were seen for these injuries (rate: 161.3); among males, 178,568 were seen (rate: 121.8). Overall, self-inflicted injury rates were highest among adolescents and young adults. Most (90 percent) self-inflicted injuries were the result of poisoning or being cut or pierced with a sharp instrument.

Prevention and Theories Applied to Suicidal Behavior

While several studies (Krug et al., 2002; U.S. Public Health Service, 2001) have documented that many people around the globe are indirectly and directly affected by suicidal behavior, two important questions come to mind: "Can we prevent it?" and if so, "How do we prevent it?" Unlike some other fields of injury research presented in this book and other areas of health-related research, the field of suicidal behavior prevention has been stifled by numerous barriers, some unique to the nature of this phenomenon (De Leo, 2002; Institute of Medicine, 2001), including lack of application of existing theories of behavior change and the development of a true behavioral theory. Therefore, the remainder of this chapter is devoted to the following topics: issues and obstacles in suicide prevention research, the state of suicide theory, behavior change theories as they apply to suicide, suicidal behavior prevention programs, and two examples of how theories of behavior change can be used for suicide prevention.

Issues and Obstacles

A literature search on suicidal behavior provides a plethora of studies that identify risk and protective factors; however, a search on suicidal behavior prevention reveals the scarcity of empirically based and tested prevention efforts (Hawton, Arensman, & Townsend, 1998; Institute of Medicine, 2002). Some of the inability to conduct prevention research is due to methodological issues, such as small sample sizes and convenience sampling of psychiatric patients and attempters (De Leo, 2002). Furthermore, a majority of interventions that have been tested are clinical interventions and have limited their strategy to a traditional mental health approach that relies almost exclusively on medical treatment. This traditional approach restricts any multidisciplinary insight that could bolster these efforts. Another key issue is that many suicidal behavior prevention efforts are nested in interventions designed primarily to change behaviors that share similar risk factors, chiefly interpersonal violence; hence, suicidal behavior prevention is often an afterthought and consequently is not rigorously evaluated. Although suicidal behavior research is not perceived as sensational and stirring to the public and politicians as some other violence-related topics and so is often neglected, it is imperative that research regarding suicide prevention be adequately funded in conjunction with other related subjects and as a unique entity. There are many in the public and within the health care industry who are skeptical about the preventability of suicide (Morgan & Evans, 1994; Eagles, Klein, Gray, Dewar, & Alexander, 2003). How much less willing might the public be to commit resources to this area if professionals themselves are unconvinced?

Overall, while there is a great deal of empirical knowledge about factors associated with suicidal behavior, the field needs to move toward importing or constructing theories and then focusing on prevention.

State of Suicide Theory

The paucity of theory and theory building in scientific explanations of suicide has been periodically noted by suicidologists (see, for example, Cornette, Abramson, & Bardone, 2000; Maris, 1981; Rogers, 2001). Cornette et al. (2000) attribute this to the complexity of suicide and its heterogeneity, while Rogers (2001) cites Serlin (1987) that research funded by the National Institute of Mental Health has been mainly pragmatic and technological involving a search for discrete risk and protective factors predictive of suicidal behaviors. The result has been listings of biological and psychosocial correlates of suicide or, as Rogers (2001) noted a disjointed set of relationships observed in empirical studies, and not a synthesized body of knowledge.

Maris, Berman, and Silverman (2000) present twelve such relationships with high levels of research support. These relationships include the following: the positive association between age and the suicide rate is strongest for white males; suicide victims are more socially isolated than those who engage in nonfatal suicidal behavior or die from natural causes; between 7 and 20 percent of all persons suffering from alcoholism will eventually die by suicide; and among patient populations, those with depressive illness have the highest suicide rates, whereas persons with schizophrenia have the greatest absolute prevalence of suicide. It is noteworthy that these empirical findings are generic and thus not meant to predict specific suicides; in any large group of older, isolated, depressed, and alcoholic white males, most will never kill themselves because of other, possibly unknowable, protective factors. In fact, prediction of persons who will exhibit future suicidal behavior has proven to be extremely poor (Goldstein, Black, Nasrallah, & Winokur, 1991). Thus, Rogers (2001) concludes that very little is known about how risk and protective factors work together in leading to a decision to attempt or commit suicide. Yet there are still warning signs that indicate a relatively higher probability or possibility of suicidal thinking or behavior.

With or without theoretical grounding, how useful has this kind of research been in preventing suicidal behavior? Many correlates identified have been incorporated into psychosocial instruments to assess individuals for signs and symptoms such as depression, hopelessness, suicidal thinking, and the potential for suicide. They have also been summarized into simple lists of signs and symptoms for informing and training practitioners, gatekeepers, and anyone else interested in identifying and intervening potentially suicidal persons. Anecdotal evidence has led some to believe that the many assessments and interventions have in fact prevented individuals from killing themselves. This conclusion is suggested by some recent local reductions in suicide rates and U.S. rates for adolescent males (Westray, 2001; Gould, Greenberg, Velting, & Shaffer, 2003). However, definitive proof is lacking. Obviously we can never know how many were intervened with and did not commit suicide because of the intervention. Moreover, while some researchers (Joyce, 2001) attribute the decline to increased use of antidepressants, Rogers (2001) and others (Helgason, Tomasson, & Zoega, 2004) disagree.

The conflicting interpretations raise other questions as well: Are there "theories" of suicide that have been empirically tested and used in suicide prevention? If so, did they help prevent suicide? The answers depend in part on how theory is defined. Dictionary definitions boil down to scientific theory as a set of testable, interrelated, lawlike propositions deduced from axioms or commonly held assumptions that integrate empirically verified observations and can be used to explain patterns of human behavior. With respect to suicidology, Maris et al. (2000) indicate that systematic theory construction would ideally generate hypotheses and research findings that are logically or mathematically deduced from a set of definitions. With this kind of theory, researchers could integrate research results into more general theoretical domains or contexts such as behaviorism, cognitive theory, or learning theory. This version of theory would also involve the integration of its different components into a model for understanding suicidal behavior and force investigators to specify their definitions and assumptions.

Maris et al. (2000) note that by these standards very few formal theories of suicide have been put forth; they present a hypothetical example of systematic theory construction to illustrate what is needed. Their psychosocial model is an interrelated set of five axioms and two assumptions with individual suicide as the main outcome. The first axiom posits that suicide is directly related to hopelessness and depression. The factors in turn are related to external events, such as repeated failure, prolonged negative interactions, chronic isolation, and marital problems, eventually devolving to the fifth axiom positing chronic depression, failure, prolonged negative interactions, and social isolation as directly related to (implicitly dependent on) early trauma in a multiproblem family of origin. These and other correlates of individual suicide are said to be influenced in their effects by male sex, age, and religiosity. The authors also point out that real-life causal networks are exceedingly complex; they involve multiple variables and often have complex interaction. Also predictor variables may affect suicide over time with changes in causal relationships occurring over a lifetime. These are examples— of the problems in theory construction for this injury problem.

Rogers (2001) adds another caveat by suggesting that an individual's current suicidal behavior is usually explained by previous suicide-related behaviors and characteristics such as nonfatal suicidal behavior, depression, and expressions of hopelessness. This results in post-hoc theorizing. As an illustration, Rogers cites Platt's research (1992) in which results were used after the fact to test Bandura's social learning theory (1977). Rogers and Carney (1994) describe an appropriate test of theory as one that begins by specifying a theory and then derives testable hypotheses. Using rigorous scientific methods would allow researchers to link the results back to the theory.

Is there a less rigorous definition or standard for scientific theory that can be used? In fact, less rigorous theoretical explanations abound in the social sciences, including suicidology (see, for example, Lester, 1990). There are microlevel "theories" linking demographic and psychosocial characteristics to individual suicide. Well-known examples are hopelessness and depression theories of suicide developed by Beck (Beck, Kovacs, & Weissman, 1975; Beck, Kovacs, & Weissman, 1975). Also in this category would be the theory of "psychache," offered by Shneidman (1993). There are sociocultural theories that explain suicide rate variations within and between population groups, while others describe sociocultural conditions that motivate individuals to commit suicide. The classic example is the work of Durkheim (1951) in which levels of social isolation and normlessness (anomie) are linked to differential suicide rates in Europe and mediated by socioeconomic conditions.

More recently, Pescosolido and Georgianna (1989) elaborated on Durkheim's work by showing that religious disintegration weakened both social integration and sources of social support. Other examples include Henry and Short's research (1954) into the relationship between the business cycle, socioeconomic conditions, and suicide rates, positing relationships between suicide rates and the degree of status malintegration in a society. They speculated that the poor were protected against suicidal behavior due in part to lower economic expectations and strong relational systems that afforded them the avenue of venting their aggression toward higher classes and not toward themselves. Recent studies (Stack, 2000) have tested and elaborated the theoretical ideas of Durkheim, Henry and Short, and others with respect to relationships between socioeconomic status (SES), economic conditions, and suicide rates. These studies have in some cases (societal economy) verified the earlier theories that the greater the prosperity, the lower the suicide rate but in other cases (SES) rejected those theories.

There is also the interpersonal-psychological theory developed by Joiner (2005). The central theme of this theory is that serious suicidal behavior requires each of three interpersonal-psychological precursors: (1) the acquired capability to enact lethal self-injury, (2) the sense that one is a burden on loved ones, and (3) the sense that one does not belong to or is not connected with a valued group or relationship. If acquired capability for suicide is absent, an individual cannot die by suicide even if she or he wants to; if an individual feels that she or he contributes to loved ones or society (that is, does not feel a burden) or feels a sense of belongingness, the will to live remains intact, and the individual will not die by suicide even if she or he can. Joiner (2005) argues that each of these factors is a necessary but not sufficient antecedent of serious forms of suicidal behavior, especially death due to suicide. He contends that the model is consistent with a diverse array of suicide-related facts and phenomena (for example, gender and age differences in suicide rates and decreased suicide rates during times of national crisis).

It has been documented that psychotherapy focused on negative thoughts about self, others, and the future (cognitive therapy) is the leading treatment for suicidal behavior (Rudd, Joiner, & Rajab, 2001). Rudd et al. (2001) developed and described a particular form of cognitive therapy for suicidal behavior, emphasizing problem solving and emotional control. Therapies like these may work because they are systematically correct and amend patients' views that they are a burden on others and do not belong to valued relationships and groups. Through their emphasis on mindfulness, planning, and emotional and behavioral regulation (Linehan, 1993), they may also inhibit the expression of the acquired capability for lethal self-harm and may discourage involvement in provocative experiences that strengthen this acquired capability. Potential prevention efforts too may be informed by the three components of this model. Efforts that enhance belongingness and efficacy may be protective—for example, pairing a new member of a neighborhood with someone who is knowledgeable and willing to acquaint this person with features of the community. Efforts that unintentionally foster habituation to suicidal stimuli (such as graphic pictures of those who died by suicide) may backfire, and the possibility has been documented that some prevention efforts have apparently promoted rather than decreased suicidal behavior (Lester, 1992).

These "theories" are perhaps more properly called theoretical models. Thus, a recent request for application (RFA) for suicide research (National Institutes of Health, 2003) advised that applicants "carefully consider definitions of suicidality . . . and approaches to measurement . . . and theoretical models of distal and proximate risk and protective factors, and models of behavioral and social change that have implications for reducing suicide risk." Maris et al. (2000) describe causal modeling as a simplification of the processes involved in suicidal outcomes to understand how a network of variables might predict suicide. They present an example of causal modeling comprising five independent variables—sex, age, depression, social isolation, and substance abuse—with suicide as the outcome. However, assuming "complex interactions with feedback," they derive eleven possible relationships among the variables. Thus, we have a model that is at once oversimplified but too complex to verify empirically. In their judgment, "models" like these are not really theories but rather statistical diagrams that may or may not be grounded in a broader theoretical context such as cognitive theory.

A different kind of model applied to suicide prevention is exemplified in Clarke, Frankish, and Green (1997) in which the PRECEDE part of the PRECEDE-PROCEED model was used to identify and compare causes of suicide among indigenous adolescents in Australia, New Zealand, Canada, and the United States. The model provides a framework for planning and implementing health education and promotion programs (See also Chapter Seven, this volume, for a detailed discussion of PRECEDE-PROCEED. The PRECEDE part diagnoses major issues attending a health problem by identifying the victims and potential victims, the scope of the problem, the network of immediate and underlying causes, and the potential obstacles to planning prevention programs. Causal factors are identified and prioritized in diagnostic categories like situational and social, epidemiological, and behavioral and environmental. Factors in the last category are subcategorized as behavioral, cultural, family, and socioeconomic. Then an educational and organizational diagnosis is made that identifies predisposing, reinforcing, and enabling factors for the problem. Examples of these include group attitudes and beliefs about suicide, social support availability or lack of it from peers and professionals, and accessibility of resources such as guns to commit suicide. Finally, an administrative and policy diagnosis is done to determine environmental and cultural obstacles to planning and implementing interventions.

Applying the PRECEDE model allows one to consider numerous risk and protective factors in a population (and their interrelationships) simultaneously. This in turn enables one to identify gaps in information needed, as well as to develop and compare specific ideas about interventions at different levels. In this sense, PRECEDE is more of an organizational and methodological device than a theory.

Given the lack of theory, according to the classic definition, one might reasonably insist, as Rogers (2001) does, that at a minimum, a theory or a theoretical model should (1) interrelate empirically derived correlates into a meaningful and understandable picture of suicidal behavior; (2) point to empirically testable hypotheses that can refine or elaborate the theory; (3) specify conditions for predicting specific hypothetical outcomes, such as variations or changes in suicidal behaviors; and (4) explain research outcomes, that is, why predicted events did or did not occur and how this affects the theoretical context. Theories that do this will foster a greater understanding of suicide and suicidal behaviors and it is hoped will lead to successful prediction and prevention.

We then asked which suicide intervention programs used scientific theory or theoretical models as a basis for planning and with what results. In North America alone, there have been numerous suicide intervention and prevention programs during the past thirty years. We searched the scientific literature for those that published their results. We could not identify any programs that explicitly described a theory or theoretical model on which the program was based. No doubt some used ideas derived from well-known theorists like Durkheim or Bandura, but none explicitly presented a theory or model and showed how the intervention was derived from that theory or model. In this context, it is interesting to observe that Lester (1990, 2000), while lamenting the absence of scientific theory, advocates examination of theories in criminology, deviance, victimology, and even economics for their utility in explaining suicidal behavior.

Suicidal Behavior Prevention Programs

The majority of strategies for preventing suicidal behavior have traditionally focused on high-risk individuals using a clinically based, provider-to-patient model. Another prevention model is classified based on the population group it focused on (Gordon, 1983). This model has been increasingly used for suicidal behavior prevention. However, recent comprehensive reviews of suicidal behavior prevention programs have shown only minimal evidence of that any programs, whether clinically oriented or population-level type, actually have reduced suicidal acts (Hawton et al., 1998; Bing & Harstall, 2004; Institute of Medicine, 2001; Krug et al., 2002).

The population group model focuses attention on how certain populations are chosen and employs the terms *universal, selective,* and *indicated* to categorize the groups that are subjects of the program (Gordon, 1983). Universal strategies address all segments of a population regardless of vulnerability. Selective strategies address sections of the population that are at risk (that is, have a greater probability of developing the problem than normal). Indicated strategies address specific high-risk individuals (those already exhibiting a known risk factor or early signs of the disease or problem).

Universal strategies that include population-based programs may have a greater impact on decreasing mortality over those focused on individuals. They may be able to lower the risk of adverse health outcome for an entire population and potentially prevent many more cases than strategies that target a small number of high-risk persons (Rosenman, 1998). Universal strategies include media campaigns (Shanahan, Elliott, & Dahlgren, 2000; Washington State Department of Health, 1995) that seek to provide information, modify negative social norms, or create an environmental change. These campaigns often address an aspect of suicidal behavior called *contagion*, defined as the process by which one suicide facilitates the occurrence of a subsequent suicide. The pathway of contagion can be direct (imitating someone else's suicidal behavior) or indirect (occurrence of suicides in the community or in the media may produce a familiarity with and acceptance of the idea of suicide) (Gould, Wallenstein, & Davidson, 1989). Other prevention strategies aim to reduce access to means, such as firearms (Loftin, McDowell, Wiersma, & Cottey, 1991; Ludwig & Cook, 2000), self-poisoning (Gunnel et al., 1997; Bowles, 1995), gas (Kreitman, 1976; Marzuk et al., 1992), or high places (Marzuk et al., 1992). Some efforts have lowered access to proximal risk factors for suicidal behavior like alcohol misuse (Birckmayer & Hemenway, 1999). Universal programs also include modification of potentially hazardous media (primarily news) suicide portrayal (Sonneck, Etzersdorfer, & Nagel-Kuess, 1994; Annenberg Public Policy Center et al., 2002). Many school-based programs have used a universal approach with awareness and skills training projects (Centers for Disease Control and Prevention, 1992; White & Jodoin, 1998). These programs are designed to educate the participants about suicide and available resources and teach various skills such as decision making or social skills.

Several types of strategies operating at the selective level have been used for suicidal behavior prevention. Examples include screening programs that identify and assess at-risk groups (Centers for Disease Control and Prevention, 1992). Programs using a gatekeeper training model instruct participants to identify and refer persons at risk for suicidal behavior. Those who are trained can be school staff, community members, or physicians (White & Jodoin, 1998; Rutz, von Knorring, & Walinder, 1989). Another type of selected program offers support and skills training (Eggert, Nicholas, & Owen, 1995). Hot lines and crisis centers may also be categorized as selective. There are few studies that have evaluated these strategies, and those that have reach inconsistent findings (Mishara & Daigle, 2001).

Indicated prevention strategies include clinical or medical interventions (Haynes, 1991; American Academy of Child and Adolescent Psychiatry, 2001), family support training, skill-building support groups for high-risk individuals (Thompson, Eggert, Randell, & Pike, 2001), case management, and referral resources for crisis intervention and treatment (Linehan, 1997). Included in this category are programs that address suicidal behavior prevention among those who are incarcerated (Hayes, 1995).

Several organizations have used integrated approaches. While these are challenging to design, execute, and evaluate, because activities occur on multiple levels of prevention, they may have the best chance of success (Litts, Moe, Roadman, Janke, & Miller, 1999; Serna, May, & Sitaker, 1998).

There are also programs designed to address other health problems that have potential for reducing suicidal behavior. These programs are not suicide specific but may apply to a range of suicide-inclusive factors, for example, factors that may relate to several health issues like early antisocial behavior, substance abuse, or child maltreatment (Durlak & Wells, 1997; National Health and Medical Research Council and Department of Health and Aged Care, 1999). Interventions for suicide-inclusive factors have the promise to bring a wider range of health benefits in that they may reduce more than one adverse outcome.

Behavior Change Theories Applied to Interventions

One of the authors (D.C.) has proposed the transtheoretical model of change (TM) (Prochaska & Velicer, 1997; Prochaska & DiClemente, 1982) as a tool for evaluating (or staging) a potentially suicidal person in terms of how seriously she or he is contemplating suicide and is ready to act (Coombs et al., 2001–2002). The TM's potential value for interventions is in identifying where one is with respect to changing a behavior such as smoking, risky sexual practices, or engaging in self-directed violence. The classic TM also evaluates a smoker (or potentially suicidal person) in terms of psychosocial change processes like self-efficacy and social support that indicate both the person's readiness to change and resources available to stimulate movement from one stage of readiness to another. This information allows an interventionist to tailor a person-specific intervention to help the person move toward the desired new behavior—for example, practicing safer sex or away from suicide. The TM has not been previously applied to suicide prevention. The proposed tool reverses the classic TM, which attempts to stimulate positive behaviors, by, for example, assessing the degree to which a smoker is ready to quit smoking into a form intended to extinguish negative (suicide-related) behaviors. (The TM is described in more detail in Chapter Two, this volume, and an application to intimate partner violence is provided in Chapter Fifteen, this volume.)

Two other possibilities are the transactional model of stress and coping (TMSC) and social marketing (SM). Lazarus and Cohen (1977) developed the TMSC to show how individuals evaluate negative events in terms of the event's impact, perceived severity, and their coping abilities (Wenzel, Glanz, & Lerman, 2002). The TMSC adapts concepts such as perceived severity, personal susceptibility, and self-efficacy from the better-known health belief model. When a major stressor occurs—divorce, loss of work, or death in the family, for example—it is normal to feel overwhelmed by emotions and unable to cope. Transient suicidal thoughts may occur (Hirschfeld & Russell, 1997). Suicidal thoughts may persist and increase in someone who is continually overwhelmed by such thoughts and believes he or she can never cope.

The TMSC describes these processes. A highly stressful event or circumstance initially triggers an evaluation of its importance or strength, referred to as the *primary appraisal*. An individual also considers his or her susceptibility and likely reaction to the event's effects, short and long term, along with the event's severity in terms of emotional distress it can cause. This evaluation can create the perception of an extremely threatening and potentially long-lasting situation, greatly increasing distress. If the evaluation is less negative—effects are perceived as transitory—or the event seems irrelevant, little or no threat is felt (Andreasen, 2001). A *secondary appraisal* of a highly threatening event assesses one's control over its anticipated duration and effects. If one feels unable to cope with the effects and manage emotional reactions, threat feelings increase. Some researchers believe that a person's coping styles are thought to be stable personality traits (Gibbs, 1989); however, Lazarus and Folkman (1984), Andreasen, (2001), and Lazarus (1991) view coping abilities as constantly adapting cognitive and behavioral processes. Strong social support for coping behaviors can significantly increase perceptions of control, thereby reducing feelings of threat (Chang, 1998; Wright & Heppner, 1991).

SM, which is less of a theory of behavior change and more of a strategic planning model useful for behavior change programs, has been used worldwide to promote diverse health behaviors ranging from oral rehydration therapy to condom use for HIV prevention. Because SM uses product marketing techniques to promote behavioral changes (Simons-Morton, Greene & Gottlieb, 1995), it appears appropriate for increasing the acceptability of communicating about a stigmatized topic like suicide. One of the challenges is to communicate that suicidal thoughts are not infrequent but always to be taken seriously without increasing the social acceptability of suicidal behavior itself. The five basic SM concepts (Green & Kreuter, 2005; Simons-Morton, Greene, & Gottlieb, 1995) are consumer orientation, audience segmentation, channel analysis, strategy or overall product planning, and process tracking.

In a recent trial (Hodges et al., 2005) TMSC and SM were used to create suicide information and awareness materials for primary care provider offices. The effort drew on theoretical principles in the TMSC (Wenzel et al., 2002; Simons-Morton et al., 1995) and the SM (Green & Kreuter, 2005; Maibach, Rothschild, & Novelli, 2002; Simons-Morton et al., 1995) to design posters and brochures that would be viewed by patients who are depressed or suicidal or know someone who is, then provide motivation for them to seek help from the health care provider. SM was used to choose color, font styles, photomodels, and written content (Simons-Morton et al., 1995).

Consumer orientation was verified by a critique and subsequent revision of these materials with a convenience sample of the target audience: primary care patients. Audience segmentation was used early to assess the moral values, potential biases, and literacy levels of the primary care patient base. This information was used to develop and revise written content. Channel analysis located sites where patients were likely to notice the materials, such as examination rooms where patients are left alone devoid of other distractions. Strategy was to destigmatize talking about suicide in a clinic setting so at-risk patients were not afraid to seek help. Process tracking involves asking patients about the attention-getting qualities of the materials and acceptability of content and providers if patients exposed to the materials asked questions about suicide or sought help. Process data enable adjustments to the methods and materials if serious problems are discovered early. The TMSC information about coping strategies was adapted to help deal with devastating situations, such as loss of a loved one (Wenzel et al., 2002). The TMSC examines each incident of fatal or nonfatal suicidal behavior as a unique occurrence triggered by life circumstances and events. However, the path from precipitating events or circumstances to suicidal behavior can be described in terms of underlying commonalities.

TMSC concepts suggest how to prevent an extremely distressed and suicidal person from moving toward a suicide attempt or suicide. For example, many such persons have an active social support network, although stigma-related feelings prevent help seeking. The poster and brochure photographs of formally suicidal persons are intended to reduce stigma by indicating that suicidal persons come from many different backgrounds and are much like the readers. Negative life events (personal stressors) are not openly addressed on the poster and brochure. The photos are intended to suggest a favorable outcome. The headline on the material is designed to attract attention: "Which of these people have been suicidal?" The answer at the bottom of the poster or last page of the brochure reveals: "all of them, and two have made suicide attempts." These elements suggest that the models were able to get help, cope, and attain a positive outcome.

Both the SM and TMSC helped in the design of materials with the potential to convince patients that suicidal thoughts can occur to anyone and are manageable, and the clinic is a safe, appropriate place to seek help. Additional resources were presented for patients uncomfortable with discussing suicide concerns face-to-face. Most important, the materials act as a point of decision prompt to cue the patient with suicidal thoughts to seek help, whether from a primary care provider or other sources listed in the materials. The workshop on the Science of Public Messages for Suicide Prevention listed an eight-point research agenda to help develop an evidence-based guide for prevention campaigns. Four were addressed by the poster and brochure: use of positive, health-promoting messages in addition to warning signs; use of theory-based conceptual models; assessment of audience cultural norms in developing format and content; and testing approaches to be used (the best channels for message transmission).

Conclusion

Injury from self-directed violence, which includes suicidal behavior, is a major cause of recorded mortality and morbidity throughout the world. Many experts agree that suicidal behavior is underreported in official data (for example, medical records and death certificates); as a result, prevalence figures based on health records substantially underestimate the societal burden. The measurable human and economic costs of suicide are enormous; compounding these costs are the unquantifiable costs of loss of life and the emotional trauma experienced by surviving family, friends, and communities affected by each person's fatal or nonfatal suicidal behavior.

This discussion of the application of behavioral science theory and methods to suicidal behavior identifies several areas in need of further efforts. First, there is a need for well-conceived theories of suicidal behavior designed according to the classical definition of theory. There is a critical need for theories that examine the dynamic interaction of risk and protective factors (individual, family, peer, community, and societal level) as they influence suicidal behavior. Second, the field needs empirical testing of these theories, including development of measurement tools that are able to assess the relevant components of the theories. An element of the testing should involve longitudinal cohort studies, which may be able to identify the relationship between suicidal behavior-specific factors along with relationship between factors that may be relevant for suicidal behavior, other forms of violence, as well as other adverse outcomes or diseases. Third, the paucity of theory-based prevention programs is striking and needs to be remedied. There is a need for multidisciplinary population-based strategies that have the potential to yield the greatest amount of reduction in injuries and deaths (Rosenman, 1998). Also needed are broader implementation and evaluation of programs that focus on factors that influence multiple adverse behaviors or outcomes, including suicidal behavior measures. Several categories of prevention have shown promise: primary prevention among children and youth (Durlak & Wells, 1997), universal strategies focusing on a low-risk population (Catalano et al., 2004), and comprehensive strategies that use multiple avenues of access to the population (Knox, Litts, Talcott, Catalano-Feig, & Caine, 2003) but require further study or replication. Fourth, the persistent stigma that hinders help seeking for suicide-related problems, along with the perception that suicidal behavior is not preventable in certain populations including some health professionals (Hjelmeland & Knizek, 2004), indicates that awareness of past and current research successes has not been communicated effectively.

References

American Academy of Child and Adolescent Psychiatry. (2001). Summary of the practice parameters for the assessment and treatment of children and adolescents with suicidal behavior. *Journal of American Academy of Child and Adolescent Psychiatry, 40*, 495–499.

Anderson, R. N., & Smith, B. L. (2005). *Deaths: Leading causes for 2002.* Hyattsville, MD: National Center for Health Statistics.

Andreasen, A. R. (Ed.). (2001). *Ethics in social marketing.* Washington, DC: Georgetown University Press.

Annenberg Public Policy Center, Centers for Disease Control and Prevention, National Institute of Mental Health, Office of the Surgeon General, Substance Abuse and Mental Health Administration, American Foundation for Suicide Prevention, & American Association for Suicidology. (2002). Reporting on suicide: Recommendations for the media. *Suicide and Life-Threatening Behavior, 32*, vii-xiii.

Bandura, A. (1977). *Social learning theory.* Upper Saddle River, NJ: Prentice Hall.

Beck, A. T., Kovacs, M., & Garrison, B. (1985). Hopelessness and eventual suicide: A ten-year prospective study of patients hospitalized with suicide ideation. *American Journal of Psychiatry, 142*(5), 559–563.

Beck, A. T., Kovacs, M., & Weissman, A. (1975). Hopelessness and suicidal behavior: An overview. *Journal of the American Medical Association, 234*(11), 1146–1159.

Bing, G., & Harstall, C. (2004, July). For which strategies of suicide prevention is there evidence of effectiveness? *WHO Regional Office for Europe's Health Evidence Network.* http://www.euro.who.int/eprise/main/WHO/Progs/HEN/Syntheses/suicideprev/20040712_2.

Birckmayer, J., & Hemenway, D. (1999). Minimum-age drinking laws and youth suicide, 1970–1990. *American Journal of Public Health, 89*, 1365–1368.

Bowles, J. R. (1995). Suicide in Western Samoa: An example of a suicide prevention program in a developing country. In R.F.W. Diekstra, W. Gulbinat, I. Kienhorst, & D. DeLeo (Eds.), *Preventive strategies on suicide.* Netherlands: Leiden and Brill.

Catalano, R. F., Berglund, M. L., Ryan, J.A.M., Lonczak, H. S., & Hawkins, J. D. (2004). Positive youth development in the United States: Research findings on evaluations of positive youth development programs. *Annals of the American Academy of Political and Social Science, 591,* 98–124.

Centers for Disease Control and Prevention. (1992). *Youth suicide prevention programs: A resource guide.* Atlanta, GA: Centers for Disease Control.

Centers for Disease Control and Prevention. (2004, Oct.). Web-based Injury Statistics Query and Reporting System (WISQARS). http://www.cdc.gov/ncipc/wisqars.

Chambers, D. A., Pearson, J. L., Lubell, K., Brandon, S., O'Brien, K., & Zinn, J. (2005). The science of public messages for suicide prevention: A workshop summary. *Suicide and Life-Threatening Behavior, 35,* 134–145.

Chang, E. C. (1998). Dispositional optimism and primary and secondary appraisal of a stressor: Controlling for confounding influences and relations to coping and psychological and physical adjustment. *Journal of Personality and Social Psychology, 74*(4), 1109–1120.

Clarke, V. A., Frankish, C. J., & Green, L. W. (1997). Understanding suicide among indigenous adolescents: A review using the PRECEDE model. *Injury Prevention, 3*(2), 126–134.

Coombs, D. W., Fish, L., Grimley, D., Chess, E., Ryan, W., Leeper, J. D., Miller, H. L., & Willis, S. (2001–2002) The transtheoretical model of change applied to developing suicidal behavior. *OMEGA: The Journal of Death and Dying, 44,* 345–359.

Cornette, M. H., Abramson, L., & Bardone, A. M. (2000). Toward an integrated theory of suicidal behaviors: Merging the hopelessness, self-discrepancy, and escape theories. In T. Joiner & M. D. Rudd (Eds.), *Suicide science: Expanding the boundaries.* Boston: Kluwer.

Crosby, A. E., & Sacks, J. J. (2002). Exposure to suicide: Incidence and association with suicidal ideation and behavior. *Suicide and Life-Threatening Behavior, 32,* 321–328.

Davis, R. (1979). Black suicide in the seventies: Current trends. *Suicide and Life Threatening Behavior, 9,* 131–140.

De Leo, D. (2002). Why are we not getting any closer to preventing suicide? *British Journal of Psychiatry, 181,* 372–374.

Diekstra, R.F.W. (1982). Epidemiology of attempted suicide in the EEC. In J. Wilmott & J. Mendlewicz (Eds.), *New trends in suicide prevention.* New York: Karger.

Durkheim, E. (1951). *Suicide: A study in sociology.* New York: Free Press. (Originally published in 1897)

Durlak, J. A., & Wells, A. M. (1997). Primary prevention mental health programs for children and adolescents: A meta-analytic review. *American Journal of Community Psychology, 25,* 115–152.

Eagles, J. M., Klein, S., Gray, N. M., Dewar, I. G., Alexander, D. A. (2003). Role of psychiatrists in the prediction and prevention of suicide: A perspective from north-east Scotland. *British Journal of Psychiatry, 178,* 494–496.

Earls, F., Escobar, J. I., & Manson, S. M. (1990). Suicide in minority groups: Epidemiologic and cultural perspectives. In S. J. Blumenthal & D. J. Kupfer (Eds.), *Suicide over the life cycle: Risk factors, assessment, and treatment of suicidal patients.* Washington, DC: American Psychiatric Press.

Eggert, L. L., Nicholas, L. J., & Owen, L. M. (1995). *Reconnecting youth: A peer group approach to building life skills.* Bloomington, IN: National Educational Service.

Gibbs, M. S. (1989). Factors in the victim that mediate between disaster and psychopathology: A review. *Journal of Traumatic Stress, 2,* 489–514.

Goldstein, R. B., Black, D. W., Nasrallah, A., & Winokur, G. (1991). The prediction of suicide: Sensitivity, specificity, and predictive value of a multivariate model applied to suicide among 1906 patients with affective disorders. *Archives of General Psychiatry, 48,* 418–422.

Gordon, R. (1983). An operational classification of disease prevention. *Public Health Reports, 98,* 107–109.

Gould, M. S., Greenberg, T., Velting, D. M., & Shaffer D. (2003). Youth suicide risk and preventive interventions: A review of the past ten years. *Journal of the American Academy of Child and Adolescent Psychiatry, 42,* 386–405.

Gould, M. S., Wallenstein, S., & Davidson, L. (1989). Suicide clusters: A critical review. *Suicide and Life-Threatening Behavior, 19,* 17–29.

Green, L. W., & Kreuter, M. W. (2005). *Health program planning: An educational and ecological approach* (4th ed.). New York: McGraw-Hill.

Grunbaum, J. A., Kann, L., Kinchen, S. A., Ross, J. G., Hawkins, J., Lowry, R., Harris, W. A., McManus, T., Chyen, D., & Collins, J. (2004). Youth risk behavior surveillance—United States, 2003. *Morbidity and Mortality Weekly Report, 53*(SS-2), 1–96.

Gunnel, D., Hawton, K., Murray, V., Garnier, R., Bismuth, C., Fagg, J., & Simkin, S. (1997). Use of paracetamol for suicide and non-fatal poisoning in the UK and France: Are restrictions on availability justified? *Journal of Epidemiology and Community Health, 51,* 175–179.

Hawton, K., Arensman, E., & Townsend, E. (1998). Deliberate self-harm: Systematic review of efficacy of psychosocial and pharmacological treatments in prevention repetition. *British Medical Journal, 317,* 441–447.

Hayes, L. M. (1995). *Prison suicide: An overview and guide to prevention.* Mansfield, MA: National Center on Institutions and Alternatives.

Haynes, M. A. (1991). Suicide prevention: A U.S. perspective. In R. B. Goldbloom & R. S. Lawrence (Eds.), *Preventing disease: Beyond the rhetoric.* New York: Springer-Verlag.

Helgason, T., Tomasson, H., & Zoega, T. (2004). Antidepressants and public health in Iceland. *British Journal of Psychiatry, 184,* 157–162.

Henry, A. F., & Short, J. (1954). *Suicide and homicide.* New York: Free Press.

Hirschfeld, R. M., & Russell, J. M. (1997). Assessment and treatment of suicidal patients. *New England Journal of Medicine, 337,* 910–915.

Hjelmeland, H., & Knizek, B. (2004). The general public's view on suicide and suicide prevention and their perception of participating in a study on attitudes towards suicide. *Archives of Suicide Research, 8,* 345–359.

Hodges, D. K., Coombs, D. W., Rand, E., Fulcher, W., Leeper, J., & Quinnett, P. (2005). *The use of behavioral theory in developing suicide prevention materials.* Unpublished manuscript.

Institute of Medicine. (2002). *Reducing suicide: A national imperative.* Washington, DC: National Academy Press.

Joiner, T. E. (2005). *Why people die by suicide.* Cambridge, MA: Harvard University Press.

Joyce, P. R. (2001). Improvements in the recognition and treatment of depression and decreasing suicide rates. *New Zealand Medical Journal, 114,* 535–536.

Knox, K. L., Litts, D. A., Talcott, G. W., Catalano-Feig, J., & Caine, E. D. (2003). Risk of suicide and related adverse outcomes after exposure to a suicide prevention program in the U.S. Air Force: Cohort study. *British Medical Journal, 327,* 1376–1380.

Kochanek, K. D., Murphy, S. L., Anderson, R. N., & Scott, C. (2004). *Deaths: Final data for 2002.* Hyattsville, MD: National Center for Health Statistics.

Kreitman N. (1976). The coal gas history: United Kingdom suicide rates, 1960–1971. *British Journal of Preventive and Social Medicine, 30,* 86–93.

Krug, E. G., Dahlberg, L. L., Mercy, J. A., Zwi, A., & Lozano, R. (Eds.). (2002). *World report on violence and health.* Geneva: World Health Organization.

Lazarus, R. S. (1991). Cognition and motivation in emotion. *American Psychologist, 46,* 352–367.

Lazarus, R. S., & Cohen, J. B. (1977). Environmental stress. In I. Altman & J. F. Wohlwill (Eds.), *Human behavior and environment* (Vol. 2). New York: Plenum.

Lazarus, R. S., & Folkman, S. (1984). *Stress, appraisal and coping.* New York: Springer.

Lester, D. (1990). *Understanding and preventing suicide: New perspectives.* Springfield, IL: Charles C. Thomas.

Lester, D. (1992). *Why people kill themselves: A 1990s summary of research findings on suicidal behavior* (3rd ed.). Springfield, IL: Charles C. Thomas.

Lester, D. (2000). Decades of suicide research: Wherefrom and whereto? In T. Joiner & M. D. Rudd (Eds.), *Suicide science: Expanding the boundaries.* Norwell, MA: Kluwer.

Linehan, M. M. (1993). *Cognitive-behavioral treatment of borderline personality disorder.* New York: Guilford Press.

Linehan, M. M. (1997). Behavioral treatments of suicidal behaviors: Definitional obfuscation and treatment outcomes. In D. M. Stoff & J. J. Mann (Eds.), *The neurobiology of suicide: From the bench to the clinic.* New York: New York Academy of Sciences.

Litts, D. A., Moe, K., Roadman, C. H., Janke, R., & Miller, J. (1999). Suicide prevention among active duty air force personnel—United States, 1990–1999. *Morbidity and Mortality Weekly Report, 48,* 1053–1057.

Loftin, C., McDowell, D., Wiersma, B., & Cottey, T. J. (1991). Effects of restrictive licensing of handguns on homicide and suicide in the District of Columbia. *New England Journal of Medicine, 325,* 1615–1620.

Ludwig, J., & Cook, P. J. (2000). Homicide and suicide rates associated with implementation of the Brady Handgun Violence Prevention Act. *Journal of the American Medical Association, 284,* 585–591.

Maibach, E. W., Rothschild, M., & Novelli, W. (2002). Social marketing. In K. Glanz, B. Rimer, & F. M. Lewis (Eds.), *Health behavior and health education: Theory, research, and practice* (3rd ed.). San Francisco: Jossey-Bass.

Maris, R. W. (1981). *Pathways to suicide: A survey of self-destructive behaviors.* Baltimore, MD: Johns Hopkins University Press.

Maris, R. W., Berman, A. L., & Silverman, M. M. (2000). *Comprehensive textbook of suicidology.* New York: Guilford Press.

Marzuk, P. M., Leon, A. C., Tariff, K., Morgan, E. B., Stajic, M., & Mann, J. J. (1992). The effect of access to lethal methods of injury on suicide rates. *Archives of General Psychiatry, 49,* 451–158.

McCaig, L. F., & Burt, C. W. (2004). *National hospital ambulatory medical care survey: 2002 emergency department summary.* Hyattsville, MD: National Center for Health Statistics.

Mishara, B., & Daigle, M. (2001). Helplines and crisis intervention services: Challenges for the future. In D. Lester (Ed.), *Suicide prevention resources for the millennium.* Philadelphia: Brunner-Routledge.

Morgan, H. G., & Evans, M. O. (1994). How negative are we to the idea of suicide prevention? *Journal of the Royal Society of Medicine, 87*(10), 622–625.

National Health and Medical Research Council and Department of Health and Aged Care. (1999). *National youth suicide prevention strategy—Setting the evidence-based research agenda for Australia.* Canberra: Department of Health and Aged Care, Commonwealth of Australia.

National Institutes of Health. (2003, Aug. 7). Research on the reduction and prevention of suicidality. PA-03-161. *Federal Register*. Bethesda, MD: Author.

Pescosolido, B. A., & Georgianna, S. (1989). Durkheim, suicide and religion: Toward a network theory of suicide. *American Sociological Review, 54,* 33–48.

Platt, S. (1992). Epidemiology of suicide and parasuicide. *Journal of Psychopharmacology, 6*(Suppl. 2), 291–299.

Prochaska, J. O., & DiClemente, C. C. (1982). Transtheoretical therapy toward a more integrative model of change. *Psychotherapy: Theory, Research and Practice, 19*(3), 276–287.

Prochaska, J. O., & Velicer, W. F. (1997). The transtheoretical model of health behavior change. *American Journal of Health Promotion, 12,* 38–48.

Rogers, J. R. (2001). Theoretical grounding: The "missing link" in suicide research. *Journal of Counseling and Development, 79,* 16–25.

Rogers, J. R., & Carney, J. V. (1994). The theoretical and methodological considerations in assessing the "modeling effect" in parasuicidal behavior: A comment on Platt (1993). *Crisis, 15,* 83–89.

Rosenberg, M. L., Gelles, R. J., Holinger, P. C., Zahn, M. A., Stark, E., Conn, J. M., Fajman, N. N., & Karlson, T. A. (1987). Violence: Homicide, assault and suicide. In R. W. Amler & H. B. Dull (Eds.), *Closing the gap: The burden of unnecessary illness.* New York: Oxford University Press.

Rosenman, S. J. (1998). Preventing suicide: What will work and what will not. *Medical Journal of Australia, 169,* 100–102.

Rudd, M. D., Joiner, T., & Rajab, M. H. (2001). *Treating suicidal behavior: An effective, time-limited approach.* New York: Guilford Press.

Rutz, W., von Knorring, L., & Walinder, J. (1989). Frequency of suicide on Gotland after systematic postgraduate education of general practitioners. *Acta Psychiatrica Scandinavica, 80,* 151–154.

Serlin, R. C. (1987). Hypothesis testing, theory building, and the philosophy of science. *Journal of Counseling Psychology, 34,* 365–371.

Serna, P., May, P., & Sitaker, M. (1998). Suicide prevention evaluation in a Western Athabaskan American Indian Tribe—New Mexico, 1988–1997. *Morbidity and Mortality Weekly Report, 47,* 257–261.

Shanahan, P., Elliott, B., & Dahlgren, N. (2000). *Review of public information campaigns addressing youth risk-taking: A report to the National Youth Affairs Research Scheme.* Sandy Bay, Tasmania: Australian Clearinghouse for Youth Studies.

Shneidman, E. S. (1993). Commentary: Suicide as psychache. *Journal of Nervous and Mental Disease, 181,* 147–149.

Simons-Morton, B. G., Greene, W. H., & Gottlieb, N. H. (1995). *Introduction to health education and health promotion.* Long Grove, IL: Waveland Press.

Sonneck, G., Etzersdorfer, E., & Nagel-Kuess, S. (1994). Imitative suicide on the Viennese subway. *Social Science and Medicine, 38,* 453–457.

Stack, S. (2000). Work and the economy. In R. W. Maris, A. L. Berman, & M. M. Silverman (Eds.), *Comprehensive textbook of sociology.* New York: Guilford Press.

Stevens, J. A., Hasbrouck, L., Durant, T. M., Dellinger, A. M., Batabyal, P. K., Crosby, A. E., Valluru, B. R., Kresnow, M., & Guerrero, J. L. (1999). Surveillance for injuries and violence among older adults. *Morbidity and Mortality Weekly Report, 48,* 27–50.

Thompson, E. A., Eggert, L. L., Randell, B. P., & Pike, K. C. (2001). Evaluation of indicated suicide risk prevention approaches for potential high school dropouts. *American Journal of Public Health, 91,* 742–752.

U.S. Department of Health and Human Services. (1986). *Report of the Secretary's Task Force on Black and Minority Health, Vol. 1: Executive summary.* Washington, DC: U.S. Government Printing Office.

U.S. Public Health Service. (2001). *National strategy for suicide prevention: Goals and objectives for action.* Washington, DC: U.S. Department of Health and Human Services.

Washington State Department of Health. (1995). *Youth suicide prevention plan for Washington State.* Olympia: Washington State Department of Health.

Wenzel, L. B., Glanz, K., & Lerman, C. (2002). Stress, coping and health behavior. In K. Glanz, B. Rimer, & F. Lewis (Eds.), *Health behavior and health education: Theory, research and practice* (3rd ed.). San Francisco: Jossey-Bass.

Westray, H. Jr. (2001, Oct.). *The Maryland suicide prevention model: A caring community saves lives.* Paper presented at the Thirteenth Annual Maryland Youth Suicide Prevention Conference, Baltimore, MD.

White, J., & Jodoin, N. (1998). *"Before-the-fact" interventions: A manual of best practices in youth suicide prevention.* Vancouver: British Columbia Ministry for Children and Families.

World Health Organization. (1996). *Prevention of suicide: Guidelines for the formulation and implementation of national strategies.* New York: United Nations.

Wright, D. M., & Heppner, P. P. (1991). Coping among nonclinical college-age children of alcoholics. *Journal of Counseling Psychology, 38,* 465–472.

CHAPTER SEVENTEEN

YOUTH VIOLENCE PREVENTION

Theory and Practice

Darrell Hudson, Marc A. Zimmerman, Susan Morrel-Samuels

Youth violence is a serious public heath problem. Despite a relative decrease in the incidence of violence among youth compared with the peak rates of the early 1990s, it continues to be a major contributor to the premature mortality and morbidity of adolescents and young adults throughout the United States. The Centers for Disease Control and Prevention (2004a) notes that youth violence includes aggressive behaviors such as verbal abuse, bullying, hitting, slapping, or fighting that do not generally result in serious injury or death but do have significant consequences on adolescent health nonetheless. Although researchers often conflate violent behavior with verbal abuse, delinquency, and less serious aggressive behavior in different studies, this chapter focuses on violent behavior and attitudes that are associated with physical assault.

According to the Centers for Disease Control and Prevention (CDC), homicide is the second leading cause of death for young people aged ten to twenty-four, across all gender, racial, and ethnic groups. In 2002, the CDC documented 5,219 homicides among youth aged ten to twenty-four and reported an average of over fourteen murders per day. While most epidemiological data focus on homicide, youth violence

This chapter was supported by grants from the Centers for Disease Control and Prevention (R49/CCR518605, U48/CCU515775) to the University of Michigan for Flint's Youth Violence Prevention Center and the Prevention Research Center of Michigan.

accounts for a large proportion of injuries among youth. In 2002, more than 877,000 youths aged ten to twenty-four were injured as a result of assaults (Centers for Disease Control and Prevention, 2004a). Of these injuries, about one in thirteen required hospitalization (Centers for Disease Control and Prevention, 2004b).

Adolescents are most frequently victimized by their peers. According to estimates by the Bureau of Justice Statistics (2002), youth aged twelve to twenty years are offenders in approximately 72 percent of all assaults on others of their age group. According to the Department of Juvenile Justice, youth aged ten to seventeen years have been involved as offenders in approximately 25 percent of serious violent crimes even though they comprise less than 12 percent of the U.S. population.

Youth violence has significant economic implications as well. Violence-related incidents consume about 3 percent of total medical spending each year. The costs of violence, however, are far broader than simple medical expenditures. The World Health Organization (WHO) reports that violence-related expenses account for about 3 percent of the gross national product for the United States (World Health Organization, 2002). Overall, the annual costs of youth violence in the United States have been estimated to be close to $6 billion (Miller, Fisher, & Cohen, 2001). For an individual youth, the costs of incarceration and medical expenses have been reported to range between $1.9 million to $2.6 million (Cohen, 1998). It has been estimated that urban victims of murder under age eighteen incur a societal cost that averages over $4 million in combined medical expenses, lost earnings, and diminished quality of life for survivors (Miller et al., 2001). In addition, the average assault costs over $8,500 for youth below eighteen years of age who reside in urban areas.

Members of racial and ethnic minorities are at even greater risk of being victims or perpetrators of youth violence. Among those ten to twenty-four years old, homicide is the leading cause of death for African Americans. African Americans have homicide victimization rates that are nearly fourteen times higher than their white counterparts (Dalhberg, 1998). Homicide has been identified as the second leading cause of death for Hispanics and the third leading cause of death for Native Americans, Alaskan Natives, and Asian Pacific Islanders. In addition, youth violence disproportionately affects males, who constituted 85 percent of the victims of homicides reported in 2001. Males also witness interpersonal violence more frequently than females do (Centers for Disease Control and Prevention, 2004b).

Although awareness of and concern about youth violence prevention are growing among public health professionals, research on youth violence with a public health perspective is lacking. The CDC's National Center for Injury Prevention and Control (NCIPC), for example, noted in its Injury Research Agenda that youth violence and suicide are vital areas of concern that require public health involvement (National Center for Injury Prevention and Control, 2002). The NCIPC's research agenda outlined the importance of foundational, developmental, and evaluation research that examines the efficacy and effectiveness of proposed interventions and programs, and the dissemination of research to the scientific community and policymakers. Focusing specifically on youth violence, the CDC agenda calls for the dissemination of prevention interventions that have been effective and investigation of ways in which the benefits of programs can be generalized and replicated. Additional research priorities identified by the NCIPC include evaluation of the effectiveness of parenting programs, development and evaluation of strategies to decrease youth access to firearms, identification of modifiable sociocultural and community factors that influence youth violence, and identification of modifiable factors that protect youth from becoming victims or perpetrators of violence.

This chapter briefly highlights some of the etiological research related to youth violence and provides a critical review of several youth violence prevention interventions that have had formal evaluation. We focus on youth violence prevention efforts that were implicitly or explicitly theory based and included some form of process or outcome evaluation.

Social and Behavioral Antecedents

Studies of violent behavior among youth have traced its antecedents to a variety of individual, peer, family, and societal factors. For the purposes of this chapter, we focus on factors that are amenable to behavioral interventions. Among individual risk factors, several researchers have found that early aggressive behavior (Dahlberg, 1998; Guerra, Huesmann, Tolan, & Van Acker, 1995; Huesmann, Eron, Lefkowitz, & Walder, 1984; Herrenkohl et al., 2000) and antisocial behavior in childhood (Capaldi & Patterson, 1993; Loeber et al., 1993; Ellickson & McGuigan, 2000) are predictive of later violent behaviors. In a national study of adolescents, Resnick et al. (1997) found that deviant behavior and poorer school performance were also associated with violent behavior. A literature review by Pepler and Slaby (1994) identified several individual factors that may lead to violent behavior, including limited academic, problem-solving, and negotiation skills.

One source of risk for adolescents is attitudes and beliefs about violent behavior. Youth who believe violence is a viable, effective, and normative means to solve problems are more likely to engage in violent behavior (Jemmott, Jemmott, Hines, & Fong, 2001). Guided by the theory of planned change, prevention efforts often try to modify such attitudes by attempting to influence perceived norms and providing youth with alternate solutions. Jemmott et al. (2001), for example, assessed fighting behavior and attitudes and intentions about fighting among African American and Hispanic middle school students. They found that participants who had more favorable attitudes toward fighting felt that they would be less likely to be able to avoid fighting and were more supportive of fighting as a way to solve problems. Towns (1996) found that elementary school students who were victimized by violence, whose friends or relatives were imprisoned, or who feared retaliation from perpetrators of violence in their community reported more positive attitudes toward violence as an effective way to solve problems. A study by Vernberg, Jacobs, and Hershberger (1999) indicated that both previous victimization and proviolence attitudes were associated with violent behavior.

Patterns of aggressive behavior may emerge during childhood that increase the probability that youth will engage in violent behavior during adolescence (Eron & Huesmann, 1990). Eron and Huesmann point out that social influences from friends (peers), family, and other adults can reinforce these behavioral patterns. The influence of peer groups on aggressive behavior has been widely documented by researchers (Cairns & Cairns, 1991; Hill, Soriano, Chen, & LaFromboise, 1994; Dahlberg, 1998; Zimmerman, Steinman, & Rowe, 1998; Herrenkohl et al., 2000). Aggressive children may be rejected by their more socially competent peers (Cairns & Cairns, 1991), leading them to establish relationships in marginalized groups of individuals who engage in antisocial behavior. Members of these peer groups may reinforce each other's aggressive behavior and limit experiences of prosocial problem-solving methods (Parker & Asher, 1987). Loeber and Stouthamer-Loeber (1998), for example, found that an adolescent's risk for delinquency increases by associating with delinquent peers.

Researchers have found that parent-child conflict, inadequate parental monitoring, and low parental involvement are related to the development of problem behaviors in adolescents (Ary et al., 1999; Dishion, Patterson, & Kavanaugh, 1992; Orpinas, Murray, & Kelder, 1999). Zimmerman, Steinman, and Rowe (1998) found that support from both mothers and fathers helped protect urban African American youth from the risk posed by friends' violent behavior. Osofsky (1999) concluded in a review of the research literature that children who witness domestic violence are at increased risk for future violent behavior and victimization. Herrenkohl et al. (2000) report that favorable parental attitudes toward violence as an effective problem-solving strategy and criminality were also predictive of future violent behavior of their children.

Schools provide a critical context for peer interaction that may increase the risk for youth violent behavior. Astor, Meyer, & Behre (1999) identified loosely monitored territories in and around school that increased risk for violent occurrences, such as parking lots and cafeterias. Ellickson and McGuigan (2000) found that attendance at middle schools with high levels of drug use was predictive of later violent behavior. In some school environments, students may view violent behavior as normative and use violence as a means of gaining social acceptance and status (Fagan & Wilkinson, 1998).

Research also suggests that neighborhoods characterized by poverty, unemployment, drug activity, easy access to firearms, and crowded, deteriorated housing create a context where youth violence is more likely to occur (McLoyd, 1990; Greenberg & Schneider, 1994; Guerra et al., 1995; Wilson, 1987; Dalhberg, 1998; Hammond & Yung, 1991; Prothrow-Stith, 1995). Exposure to violence in the media has also been associated with higher levels of antisocial behavior, more acceptance of violence as a solution to problems, increased hostility, reduced arousal while witnessing violence, and less sympathy for the victims of violence (Paik & Comstock, 1994; Huesmann & Guerra, 1997; Molitor & Hirsch, 1994; Mullin & Linz, 1995).

Individual-Based Interventions

Most violence prevention interventions operate at the individual level, but some programs focus on contextual factors such as socioeconomic conditions, low parental supervision, and inconsistent parental discipline (Commission on the Prevention of Youth Violence, 2000). Interventions that focus on the individual may be classified by their emphasis on primary, secondary, or tertiary prevention (Table 17.1).

Primary Prevention

Primary prevention programs are typically designed for the general population and seek to mitigate potential risks and promote factors that enhance resiliency. Secondary violence prevention efforts focus on individuals who face heightened risk for violence due to characteristics, behaviors, or environmental factors that increase their vulnerability and seek to ameliorate these factors to prevent violent behavior. Tertiary programs address those who have already engaged in violent behavior and focus on preventing future violence. These prevention programs may be delivered in a variety of settings, frequently defined by the population they are intended to reach.

Numerous school-based interventions have been designed to prevent youth violence and other problem behaviors among children and adolescents (Farrell, Meyer, Kung, & Sullivan, 2001; Ngwe, Liu, Flay, Segawa, & Aya, 2004). Schools may be the optimal setting for implementation of primary prevention programs because youth spend many hours each day in school, and peer relationships often influence behavior (Farrell et al., 2001; Conduct Problems Research Group, 1999). In addition, schools provide a convenient setting for interventions because issues such as recruitment, transportation, and facilities to conduct the intervention are more easily

TABLE 17.1. VIOLENCE PREVENTION INTERVENTIONS.

Source	Program Characteristics	Evaluation Design	Sample Characteristics	Theory Applied	Findings
Ngwe, Liu, Flay, Segawa, & Aya (2004).	This study was designed to test the efficacy of the Aban Aya Youth Project. The intervention was geared toward reducing youth violence among African American youth by focusing on mediating factors such as behavioral intentions, attitudes, and peer behaviors. The program had three interventions: two focusing on risk behaviors of youth violence and another focusing on health-enhancing behaviors. All three interventions were multiyear and school based. Each curriculum consisted of twenty-one lessons for fifth graders, eighteen lessons for sixth graders, and sixteen lessons for seventh and eighth graders. All lessons were delivered by a trained health educator.	Baseline and three-year follow-up assessments. Also tested mediating factors across two intervention and control groups.	571 urban African American elementary school males. Groups had about 389 youth in the intervention groups and 182 youth assigned to the control group.	Theory of reasoned action	Differences found among the mediating factors between the treatment and control groups, $p < 0.05$; program effect for violent behaviors as well, $p < 0.05$.
Farrell, Meyer, & White (2001).	Community-based intervention, Responding in Peaceful and Positive Ways (RIPP), which was designed to prevent violence among early adolescents in a school setting. The RIPP program provided a curriculum designed to teach "knowledge, attitudes and skills to promote nonviolence, positive communication and achievement." Interventionists used a problem-solving model, specifically using behavioral repetition and mental rehearsal of the problem-solving model, experiential learning techniques, and didactic learning modalities. The curriculum consisted of twenty-five weekly sessions taught by prevention specialists during the school day.	Pretest-posttest control group design. Sixth-grade classrooms randomly assigned to intervention or control group. School disciplinary reports for violence-related behavior and self-reported violent behaviors were the outcome measures.	Sample was predominantly African American (96 percent) with mean age of 11.7 ± 0.6. Intervention and control groups each had about 300 sixth graders.	Perry and Jessor's health promotion framework (1985). This framework is designed to "decrease health-compromising factors while increasing health-promoting factors in the areas of behavior, intrapersonal characteristics and environmental characteristics."	Control group had 2.2 times greater rates of disciplinary actions and 5 times greater rates of in-school suspensions due to violent behaviors compared to intervention group. Control group participants were 2.5 times more likely to report injury from fighting than the intervention participants.

TABLE 17.1. VIOLENCE PREVENTION INTERVENTIONS, Cont'd.

Source	Program Characteristics	Evaluation Design	Sample Characteristics	Theory Applied	Findings
Komro et al. (2004).	The program consisted of the ten-session middle school D.A.R.E. curriculum or D.A.R.E. Plus curriculum, which used the ten-session middle school D.A.R.E. curriculum in addition to school, family, and neighborhood prevention strategies. There was also a delayed-program control condition. The D.A.R.E.-only condition used the ten-session middle school curriculum. The D.A.R.E. Plus condition used the ten-session middle school D.A.R.E. curriculum in addition to school, family, and neighborhood prevention strategies. The D.A.R.E. Plus program included a four-session peer-led classroom program, postcards with preventive messages sent home to participants' parents, student-planned after-school activities, and neighborhood teams that worked to create safer school and neighborhood environments.	Evaluation designed to assess the effectiveness of the D.A.R.E. and D.A.R.E. Plus compared to a delayed program control condition. Outcome measures included expectations and beliefs youth had about participation in violence and violent behavior.	Sample consisted of twenty-four predominantly white middle schools in urban, suburban, and rural schools from the Minneapolis/St. Paul metropolitan area. The 4,976 youth in the study were mostly white (79.2 percent) and equally represented males and females.	Social cognitive theory	Males in the D.A.R.E. Plus group reported less physically violent behavior than the males in the control group ($p = 0.03$). Males in the D.A.R.E. Plus group had lower expectations for violence than the D.A.R.E.-only group and control group ($p = 0.02$ and $p = 0.01$, respectively). Males in the D.A.R.E. Plus group also reported more reasons not to be violent than the control group ($p = 0.04$). No differences for females for the other violence-related behavioral outcomes across all three conditions.
Ialongo et al. (1999).	This condition focused on helping to improve teachers' behavioral management in the classroom. The Family-School Partnership focused on enhancing parent-teacher communication and child behavior management strategies.	The Classroom-Centered intervention was designed to provide academic skills and improve academic performance by focusing on language arts and mathematics skills. The evaluation included pre- and postassessments of children's behavior and academic skills.	678 first-grade students and their families at nine urban schools participated. 86.8 percent were African American and 53.2 percent were male. 62.3 percent of the students in the sample received free lunch at school.	Intervention was driven by the life course/social field theory (Kellam, Branch, Agrawal, & Ensminger, 1975; Kellam & Rebok, 1992). This theory asserts that people are presented with social tasks during each stage of life, and the successful completion of these tasks is positively related to their psychological well-being.	The Classroom Centered condition was most effective for achievement and classroom behavior. This condition was also the most effective intervention for males in the sample for aggressive behavior when compared with the control group ($p = 0.02$); teachers reported fewer problems for males in the Classroom Centered group for first ($p = .03$) and second grades ($p = 0.001$). Among

Study	Description	Methods	Sample	Theory	Results
					females, teachers reported fewer problems for the Classroom Centered condition than the control group for grades 1 ($p = .01$) and 2 ($p = 0.0001$). The Family-School Partnership was successful in engaging parents, but parents of low-achieving students participated least.
Webber-Stratton (1998).	Parenting program designed for low-income mothers of children enrolled in several Head Start centers. The PARTNERS experimental intervention component provided a supplement to Head Start programs by including eight to nine weekly sessions designed to increase parental involvement, strengthen parenting competence, enhance child social competence, and build home-school connections in a group format. Specific aspects of the intervention were designed to focus on parent and teacher training. Both aspects were designed to increase involvement in the classroom and at home.	Families from nine Head Start centers were randomly assigned to intervention and control groups. Outcome measures included parent and teacher assessment of children's behaviors, conduct problems, and social competence at school and at home. Parental involvement was also assessed.	345 families were assigned to the intervention group and 167 families to the control group. Children in the sample had a baseline age of 4.7 years, and their mothers were 29.4 years old. 95 percent of children resided with their biological mother, of whom 55 percent were single mothers. The average yearly income was reported at about $10,000. The sample was predominantly white and 53 percent male.	The PARTNERS intervention was driven by developmental theory that focused on multiple risk factors within the family, child, and school settings and how these factors interact to influence the development of conduct problems in young children.	Parental competence was improved in both short-term (three months postintervention) and long-term (one year postintervention) assessments among mothers in the intervention group compared to control group mothers. Parents in the intervention group reported more consistent discipline styles than control group mothers ($p < 0.001$) and greater reduction in physically and verbally negative discipline ($p < 0.001$) than parents in the control group. Teachers reported that mothers in the intervention group had increased involvement in the education of their children compared to the control group mothers ($p < 0.01$). Children of mothers in the intervention

TABLE 17.1. VIOLENCE PREVENTION INTERVENTIONS, Cont'd.

Source	Program Characteristics	Evaluation Design	Sample Characteristics	Theory Applied	Findings
Webber-Stratton (1998), *Continued*					program had fewer conduct problems ($p < 0.05$) and decreased deviant and noncompliant behavior ($p < 0.001$) than those of the control group. At follow-up (twelve to eighteen months postintervention), intervention effects remained for parents' discipline strategies ($p < 0.001$) and most child behavior variables ($p < 0.05$).
Irvine, Biglan, Smolkowski, Metzler, & Ary (1999).	The intervention was composed of twelve weekly sessions designed for groups of parents with middle school children with mild to moderate behavior problems. The classes focused on improving parents' ability to provide positive reinforcement, parent-child communication, and monitoring.	Children were identified and referred by schools or social service agency staff on the basis of twelve child risk behaviors. Families were randomly assigned to an immediate treatment group or a wait-list control group. Parents' and children's behavior were measured using self-report measures. Outcomes were measured immediately after the program and three months, six months, twelve months, and eighteen months postintervention.	The intervention included 303 primarily white mothers with children whose average age was 12.2 years. 61 percent of the children were male.	No specific theory is mentioned. Authors state that the program is rooted in evidence about the role of coercive family interactions in the development of youth problem behaviors.	The ATP evaluation indicated that program parents reported fewer incidences of harsh behavior and overreaction than wait-list parents. More improvement in the behavioral measures for the program group children immediately following the intervention compared to the wait-listed comparison group.

| Zun, Downey, & Rosen (2004). | Interventionists assigned youth who had been injured due to interpersonal violence to a social service agency and health care services to provide the youth with case management for a six-month period. Youth were recruited while they visited a level 1 trauma center emergency room in an urban area. Youth were randomly assigned to a control group or intervention group. The intervention group received individual counseling as well as access to services such as programs in personal development and education. | Participants were randomly assigned to the treatment ($N = 96$) or control group ($N = 92$). The evaluation included posttest assessments at six- and twelve-month intervals and included measures of violence, values, delinquency, peer influences, and future expectations. | Youth aged ten to twenty-four who were patients in hospital emergency rooms who were victims of violence. The majority of the sample was male (82.5 percent) and African American (65.4 percent). | Health belief model | Authors found no difference in attitudes about violence among treatment group participants compared to the control group. |

addressed (Commission on Violence and Youth, 1993). School-based interventions are also advantageous because they can focus on high-risk youth or provide a more universal intervention to which all students are exposed (Ialongo et al., 1999; Farrell et al., 2001). Schools can provide a setting for special programming for at-risk youth whom they identify using their own data (for example, school performance or behavior problems). Alternatively, schoolwide programs can reach all youth regardless of individual characteristics because most schools have attendance requirements for youth up to age sixteen.

Ngwe et al. (2004) report on the Aban Aya Youth Project (AAYP), a longitudinal efficacy trial designed to reduce risk-taking behavior among urban African American youth that included two experimental conditions and a control group. The program was implemented in grades 5 to 8 among twelve randomly assigned elementary schools. Overall, 571 fourteen-year-old African American males participated in the AAYP study. The youth were followed over a four-year period and completed various self-report measures related to attitudes about violence, participation in violent behavior, behavioral intentions related to violence, and perceptions of friends' behavior and friends' encouragement to engage in problem behaviors. Both males and females participated in the program; however, the authors included only males in this analysis. One experimental condition, the school-community program, included a social development curriculum that focused on risk behaviors for violence, substance use, and unsafe sexual behaviors; a parent support group to promote child-parent communication; schoolwide support groups to integrate intervention skills into the school environment; and a community program to establish relationships among parents, schools, and local businesses. Another experimental condition included only the social development curriculum, but not the support and linkages to the community. The social development curriculum included individual skill building for problem solving, interpersonal relations, and critical thinking. The control group focused on encouraging overall health-enhancing behaviors like physical activity, nutrition, and oral health. Ngwe et al. (2004) found that the school-community intervention was more effective than either the social development group alone or the control group in reducing an increase of violent behaviors.

Although an underlying theory is not explicitly described by Ngwe et al., their intervention did focus on components of the theory of reasoned action as evidenced by attention on perceived norms and attitudes. The longitudinal design and use of two experimental conditions and a control group are especially strong aspects of the study design. This intervention is promising because it addressed factors that may mediate the relationship between risks and violent behavior such as perceived norms and attitudes toward violence.

Another school-based intervention, the Responding in Peaceful and Positive Ways (RIPP) program, was designed to prevent violence among sixth graders (Farrell et al., 2001). Schools were randomly assigned to the RIPP intervention or a control group. The RIPP intervention focuses on social-cognitive problem-solving and violence prevention skills, such as avoiding violent situations. The intervention also included a peer mediation component that was available to all students to help with conflict resolution. Twenty-five weekly prevention sessions were led by three prevention specialists who were African American, corresponding to the ethnicity of the majority of participants in the intervention group. The fidelity of the intervention was documented using checklists for all the planned procedures and tasks completed by research assistants. Farrell et al. (2001) found that the control group was 2.2 times more likely to receive disciplinary actions and 5.0 times more likely to receive in-school suspensions due to violent behaviors than intervention group participants at the first posttest, but these differences did not persist at the twelve-month follow-up. They also found that youth in the intervention condition were 2.5 times less likely to report injuries due to fighting and used the school peer mediation program more often than youth in the control group. Notably, Farrell et al. (2001) found that the program was most effective for students who reported higher rates of aggressive behavior prior to entry into the program. This is particularly interesting because the program was designed to be a universal intervention. Their evaluation suggests that school-based violence prevention programs that focus on higher-risk participants may be especially effective.

The Minnesota Drug Abuse Resistance Education (D.A.R.E.) Plus Project also included two violence prevention conditions and a comparison group (Komro et al., 2004). The evaluation of this program was designed to assess the effectiveness of the D.A.R.E. and D.A.R.E. Plus interventions on expectations and beliefs youth had about participation in violence. While the program has been widely implemented across the country, prior evaluations of the D.A.R.E. program have indicated no effects on drug use prevention (Lynam et al., 1999). Although researchers have criticized the D.A.R.E. program due to the lack of a theoretical framework, Komro et al. state that the notion of reciprocal determinism (that is, person-environment-behavior) in social learning theory (Bandura, 1986; Flay & Petraitis, 1994; Komro et al., 1999) and Perry's conceptual model of adolescent health promotion (Perry, 1999) were used in this project.

The D.A.R.E.-only condition used the ten-session middle school D.A.R.E. curriculum. The D.A.R.E Plus condition used the ten-session middle school D.A.R.E. curriculum in addition to school, family, and neighborhood prevention strategies. The D.A.R.E. Plus program included a four-session peer-led classroom program, postcards with preventive messages sent home to participants' parents, student-planned after-school activities, and neighborhood teams that worked to create safer school and neighborhood environments. This program took place in twenty-four middle schools in urban, suburban, and rural locations in the Minneapolis–St. Paul metropolitan area. The 4,976 youth in the study were mostly white (79.2 percent), and males and females were equally represented.

Outcome measures were administered to the study participants at baseline (in fall 1999), as well as two follow-up measurements. One follow-up occurred at the end of the seventh-grade school year (spring 2000), and another measure was collected at the completion of the eighth grade (spring 2001). Evaluation scales included measures of physical and verbal violence, as well as weapon carrying and victimization items. Komro et al. found that males included in the D.A.R.E. Plus group reported less physical and verbal violent behavior than the males in the control group. The males in the D.A.R.E. Plus group reported marginally lower physical violent behavior compared to males in the D.A.R.E.-only group, but males in the D.A.R.E. Plus group reported lower expectations for violence than the D.A.R.E.-only and control groups. Males in the D.A.R.E. Plus group also reported more reasons not to be violent than both the D.A.R.E.-only and control groups. Komro et al. (2004) found that females in the D.A.R.E. Plus group had lower rates of victimization than the D.A.R.E.-only group, but they found no differences across groups for females for any other outcome measure. These results suggest that violence prevention efforts that take a comprehensive approach that includes family, school, and community components may be especially useful. The ineffectiveness of this prevention program among females, however, suggests that females may be motivated to engage in violent behavior by different factors from their male counterparts.

Ialongo et al. (1999) describe another multifaceted approach to school-based violence prevention. They evaluated two interventions designed for first graders enrolled in Baltimore schools. The intervention was driven by the life course–social field theory that posits that successful performance with social task demands early in life may increase the likelihood of success with demands later in life. Three first-grade classrooms in the nine elementary schools were randomly assigned to one of three conditions: classroom centered, family-school partnership, and control. The classroom-centered intervention was designed to provide academic skills and improve academic performance by focusing on language arts and mathematics skills. This condition also focused on helping improve behavioral management among teachers and provided incentives to maintain students' involvement in the intervention. The family-school partnership focused on enhancing parent-teacher communication and child behavior management strategies. This aspect of the program provided a comprehensive approach, with communication training for parents and teachers, home-school communication and learning activities, and a series of workshops for parents to improve their parenting skills. Students in the control group received the standard school setting. The evaluation process included pre- and postassessments of children's behavior and academic skills.

Ialongo et al. (1999) found that the classroom-centered condition was most effective for student achievement and classroom behavior. This condition was most effective for the males for aggressive behavior when compared with the control group. Teachers also reported fewer problems for males in this condition. Among females, teachers reported fewer behavior problems for youth in the classroom-centered condition compared to the control group. The family-school partnership was successful in engaging parents in the program but did not produce the expected effects on youth behavior. This study was informative because it explicitly outlined the theory used; applied a comprehensive, universal approach; and included pre- and postintervention assessments. The intervention also used three different comparison groups with two experimental conditions. Another strength of this program is that it focused on first graders and may be one of a few primary prevention interventions for this age group. This study also provides evidence that association between poor achievement in early academic settings and later aggression-related problems may be modifiable by interventions that focus on behavioral and curricular components as well as improving off-task and inattentive behaviors.

Consistent with other findings, this intervention was most effective for males, providing further evidence for the need to develop effective programs for females. Parent-focused interventions are designed to strengthen parenting skills, involvement, and monitoring to protect youth from engaging in violent behaviors. Researchers have found that parent-child conflict, inadequate parental monitoring, and low parental involvement are related to the development of problem behaviors in adolescents (Ary et al., 1999; Dishion et al., 1992). Zimmerman, Steinman, and Rowe (1998) found that support from both mothers and fathers helped protect urban African American youth from the risk posed by friends' violent behavior. Taylor and Biglan (1998) review empirically based, behavioral family interventions designed to reduce delinquent behavior among children and adolescents. They state that family behavioral interventions grew out of analyses of the theoretical notion that parents reinforce children's behavior through contingencies such as giving praise, offering privileges, and showing adequate attention to disciplinary issues. Taylor and Biglan mention that family-based interventions have been found to be effective for a broad range of behavioral problems among various settings and populations. Successful family-based interventions typically focus on skill-building programs for parents designed to improve parental practices. These interventions are designed to help parents establish social norms and environments that discourage delinquent, aggressive, and violent behavior.

As with interventions geared specifically toward individual youth, primary prevention programs that focus on families are frequently offered in educational settings. Webber-Stratton (1998) evaluated the effectiveness of a parenting program designed for low-income mothers of children enrolled in several Head Start centers. The PARTNERS experimental intervention component provided a supplement to Head Start programs by including eight or nine weekly sessions designed to increase parental involvement, strengthen parenting competence, enhance child social competence, and build home-school connections in a group format. Specific aspects of the intervention were designed to focus on parent and teacher training to increase involvement in the classroom and at home. The PARTNERS intervention was driven by developmental theory that focused on multiple risk factors within the family and school settings and how these factors interact to influence the development of conduct problems in young children. Parents enrolled in the control condition took part in the regular center-based Head Start program. Most participants were white (63 percent).

Results indicated that measures of parental competence were improved in both short-term (three months postintervention) and long-term (twelve months postintervention) assessments among mothers in the intervention group as compared to control group mothers. Specifically, parents in the intervention group reported more consistent discipline styles than control group parents. They also reported fewer physically and verbally negative discipline techniques compared to the control group. Teachers reported that mothers in the intervention group increased their involvement in the education of their children compared to the control group mothers. Most notably, however, children of mothers in the intervention program had fewer conduct problems and decreased deviant and noncompliant behavior than their counterparts in the control group. The intervention effects remained for parents' discipline strategies and most child behavior variables at the twelve-month assessment. The short- and long-term effects of this intervention add to the evidence that programs that focus on improving the parenting skills of parents of young children may be particularly beneficial strategies for primary prevention. This program provides another example of a primary prevention school-based program that emphasizes collaboration between parents and teachers and is designed to strengthen children's personal assets (skills) and external resources (parental competence).

The family may also be the focus of secondary prevention efforts. The Adolescent Transition Program (ATP) was designed for parents whose children are at risk for substance use, academic failure, and antisocial behavior (Irvine et al., 1999). Although no specific theory is mentioned, the program is rooted in evidence about the role of coercive family interactions in the development of youth problem behaviors. Families in eight small Oregon communities were randomly assigned to an immediate treatment group or a wait-list control group. The intervention was composed of twelve weekly sessions designed for groups of parents with middle school children with mild to moderate behavior problems. The classes focused on improving parents' ability to provide positive reinforcement, parent-child communication, and monitoring (problem solving and consistent, fair discipline). Children were identified and referred by schools or social service agency staff on the basis of twelve child risk behaviors. The intervention encompassed 303 primarily white mothers with children whose average age was twelve years. The ATP evaluation indicated that program parents reported fewer incidences of harsh behavior and overreaction than wait-list parents. Irvine et al. (1999) also found greater improvement in the behavioral measures of the program group children immediately following the intervention compared to the wait-listed comparison group. Unfortunately, they were unable to document persistent behavioral changes in comparison with the control group. Furthermore, reductions in behavioral problems were not replicated in the wait-list control group.

Another school-based effort that appears to hold promise is the Multisite Violence Prevention Project (Multisite Violence Prevention Project, 2004), designed to address aggressive and violent behaviors among middle school students in North Carolina, Georgia, Illinois, and Virginia. This school-based project uses an ecological model as the guiding theoretical framework in an effort to influence individual-, familial-, school-, and community-related factors associated with youth violence. The intervention will focus on sixth-grade students and will incorporate a universal approach called the Guiding Responsibility and Expectations for Adolescents for Today and Tomorrow (GREAT) program. This program has two components: one that focuses on students and another that focuses on teachers. In the student component, prosocial norms and behaviors are developed by strengthening social, emotional, and cognitive skills for managing conflicts. The teacher component is designed to encourage sixth-grade teachers to prevent aggression by maintaining classrooms that foster respect and reinforce problem-solving skills. Evaluation data are not available at this time, but the evaluation design includes assessment of program effectiveness for reducing violent behavior and assessment of program process, fidelity, and dosage.

Secondary and Tertiary Prevention

Secondary and tertiary violence prevention programs may be delivered in settings where those who are at elevated risk, or have already experienced violence, are likely to receive other services. Because many individuals who are victims or perpetrators of youth violence often come through the doors of hospitals and juvenile courts, several interventions have focused on these settings (Jones-Brown & Weston-Henriques, 1997; Scott, Taylor, Plotkin, Tepas, & Fryberg, 2002). These adolescents are vulnerable and may be at critical teachable moments in their lives when a doctor or law enforcement officer may help alter the trajectory of youth who have been involved with violence. Some individually directed prevention programs have attempted to change behavior through programs that increase knowledge, social skills, and problem-solving ability among violent offenders while they are incarcerated.

Jones-Brown and Weston-Henriques (1997) describe a program—Communities Organized to Regain Their Environment (CORE)—with an eight-month curriculum for incarcerated youth aged fifteen to eighteen. Participants were granted early release from correctional facilities and supportive after-care in exchange for completing the program. Youth were matched with mentors recruited from nearby communities and matched by youths' ethnicity, sex, socioeconomic background, and vocational interests. Jones-Brown and Weston-Henriques identify specific strengths of the program, such as providing positive male role models for youth who also provide informational and tangible support, such as transportation. Their findings suggest that providing appropriate mentors appears to be an effective strategy to prevent future violent behavior among at-risk, minority youth, but most of the findings presented were anecdotal. Jones-Brown and Weston-Henriques also report lessons learned from their program that include the importance of an effective recruiting and systematic training for mentors.

Zun et al. (2004) evaluated a program designed for patients ten to twenty-four years old in hospital emergency rooms who were victims of violence. Participants were randomly assigned to the treatment ($N = 96$) or control group ($N = 92$). Case managers provided access to primary and preventive health care and social services, individualized case management plans, and anger management training. Control group participants were provided only a list of available services. No specific theory is described that guided the study. In addition, although the evaluation includes posttest assessments at six- and twelve-month intervals and included measures of violence, delinquency, values, peer influences, and future expectations, results have not yet been reported.

Flint's Youth Violence Prevention Center (YVPC) includes a brief intervention that also focuses on youth presenting in the emergency room (ER; http://www.saferflintteens.com). This intervention focuses on youth who are patients in an urban hospital setting and refers them to an interactive computer Web site for follow-up at home or in other locations with computer access. These interactive modules encourage youth to avoid using violence in anger-invoking situations and provide additional online violence prevention resources for youth and parents. Social learning theory and the aggression replacement training (ART) model drive this intervention. The ART model is based on the assumption that youth are deficient in prosocial behaviors, including negotiating differences and responding effectively to teasing and anger (Goldstein, Glick, & Gibbs, 1998). Descriptive results from the pilot study indicate that of 115 twelve to seventeen year olds completing an initial survey in the ER, 86 percent reported engaging in physical violence: 58 percent hit someone, 33 percent were involved in group fighting, 32 percent reported a conflict involving a weapon, and 21 percent carried a weapon (Cunningham, 2005). One month after their ER visit, 24 percent of teens logged on to the Web site without any remuneration. Frequency of Internet use was the only baseline characteristic that significantly predicted visiting the Web site. Analyses of follow-up interviews with the study participants are currently being conducted to examine the effects of the intervention.

Youth violence prevention interventions that focus on individual behavior change appear to be most effective when they incorporate specific skill-building activities and include family involvement. Primary prevention programs that are school based and focus on younger children show promise. Many of the programs in this review included mostly white youth and appeared to be most effective for males. Yet, minority youth are at greater risk for violence and victimization, so research on the effectiveness of interventions for minority youth is needed. Similarly, with a growing female involvement in violent behavior, more research that focuses on adolescent females is necessary.

Community-Based Interventions

Few community-based youth violence prevention interventions are reported in the literature, and those described typically do not include pre-post comparison group designs. Merzel and D'Afflitti (2003) note, however, that the few community-based approaches studied have had only limited success. New intervention efforts are seeking to fill this gap in violence prevention research. The Neighborhood Solutions for Neighborhood Problems program provides an example of a community-based approach that incorporates both primary and secondary violence prevention strategies (Randall, Swenson, & Henggeler, 1999). The leaders of this program developed collaborative relationships among an academic research center, a state health department, and community organizations in a high-risk neighborhood. The multidimensional intervention included a systems therapy approach to address clinical concerns; an early warning system in schools to identify and monitor at-risk youth aged four to seventeen years; and recreational, vocational, and after-school activities. Although this intervention design is promising, the evaluation does not include a comparison group, and no explicit theory is described to guide the intervention. Nevertheless, the community-based approach helps to ensure local relevance, cultural sensitivity, and use of community resources.

Youth Empowerment Solutions for Peaceful Communities connects middle school students with neighborhood organizations to design and carry out community improvement projects (Zimmerman, Reischl, & Morrel-Samuels, 2004). The intervention is based on empowerment and ecological theories (Kawachi, Kennedy, & Wilkinson, 1999; Zimmerman, 1995, 2000). It posits that engaging youth and adults in creating environmental changes that promote peaceful neighborhoods will affect the community as a whole, not just those directly participating in the intervention. This project will organize middle school students into teams, led by a youth council. The students conduct a community assessment using observational and photovoice techniques (Wang, 2004). The youth teams then work with neighborhood organizations to develop and carry out community improvement projects such as community gardens, neighborhood cleanups, or public artwork. The youth and neighborhood groups receive technical assistance and material support from local nonprofits. Social marketing is also employed to raise community awareness and investment in the program. The project tracks changes in attitudes and behaviors among the population of two middle schools, injury and crime rates, and residents' fear of crime in their neighborhood in the intervention and comparison neighborhoods.

Community-level violence prevention programs have several notable advantages. First, they address the contexts within which youth violence occurs rather than focusing on deficits among youth growing up in risky environments. Second, community approaches have the potential to engage grassroots organizations and institutions, such as police, courts, and schools, in creating and sustaining community resources that support healthy development for all children and families. Third, community approaches raise the responsibility for youth violence prevention to all residents. It takes a village to raise a child, and it takes the community to ensure they grow up in a safe environment. Fourth, interventions designed at the community level inevitably require involvement of local organizations and residents that can help make the intervention more relevant and appropriate for the youth for whom it is intended. This can help address cultural, gender, age, or socioeconomic issues that may be pertinent for the intervention. Yet community-level interventions pose challenges for researchers because it is difficult to assess programs effects. Community interventions are complex and typically involve measuring multiple variables in natural settings that are affected by many factors outside the control of investigators.

Conclusions

Despite the attention that youth violence has received, the effect it has on adolescent health generally, and its disproportionate effect on males and members of racial and ethnic minorities, few interventions addressing prevention of youth violence have been theory driven, empirically tested, and critically evaluated. In addition, most of the programs that have been evaluated have included predominantly white youth. Few interventions designed to be culturally sensitive or tailored have been developed or evaluated for their effectiveness (Wright & Zimmerman, in press). Interestingly, Wright and Zimmerman note that programs that do focus attention on specific racial and ethnic minority groups (mostly African Americans) do not specifically identify ways in which they have culturally tailored their interventions. It can be challenging to consider the many and complex contexts in which youth live, but it may be necessary to tailor interventions relevant to and consistent with the values, norms, and social contexts of the audience for the intervention (Wright & Zimmerman, in press).

The NCIPC has identified best practices of youth violence prevention (Thornton, Craft, Dahlberg, Lynch, & Baer, 2002). This best practices book offers several suggestions for matching strategy to the context. Schools, for example, are a critical setting for teaching social problem-solving skills because this approach is consistent with the academic learning environment. Best practices also include the involvement of parents and other members of the community because they must share in the responsibility for making communities safe for adolescent development. The best practices noted in the book also suggest that using a universal approach designed for all students within a specific school may be useful to help change social norms and attitudes about youth violence.

Nation et al. (2003) identified nine critical characteristics for prevention programs that focus on problem behaviors among adolescents. They reviewed research and programs that focused on adolescent substance abuse, risky sexual behavior, school failure, and juvenile delinquency. Three of the most important characteristics they identified were application of theory, sociocultural relevance, and effectiveness evaluation. They also noted that the most effective interventions included programs that were comprehensive, used various teaching methods, provided adequate dosage, provided opportunities for positive relationships, were appropriately timed, and used well-trained staff members.

Yet as our review suggests, researchers have typically focused on identifying individual risk factors for youth violence and developing interventions to address them, and most of the rigorously evaluated primary prevention efforts concentrate on individual-level change. Individual-level interventions typically stress building peer mediation, problem solving, anger management, and other interpersonal skills. Secondary and tertiary prevention efforts also address primarily individual-level change, but direct attention to youth who are at heightened risk or have already perpetrated violence or been victims. Secondary prevention may take place in hospital ERs or among youth in alternative educational settings, who may have experienced violence as perpetrators or victims. Tertiary prevention efforts generally focus on adjudicated or incarcerated youth to help rehabilitate them into less violent lives once they return to their communities. These interventions are often designed to address the individual and may neglect important family, school, and community influences on youth violence.

Researchers are beginning to recognize the need to look beyond the individual in designing violence prevention programs. This may be in part due to the increasing interest in adolescent resiliency (Fergus & Zimmerman, 2005) and the assets and resources in youths' lives that help them overcome risks they face for negative outcomes such as violent behavior. A resiliency approach may change our attention from risk reduction to enhancing positive factors found to help youth overcome the risks. This shift in focus may transform youth violence prevention from a deficit individual blame orientation to a more ecologically driven, strengths-based process that involves multiple sectors of communities. Families, schools, and community organizations need to be involved to develop the supportive and peaceful environments youth require for healthy development. Nevertheless, the complexity and unpredictability of community settings create great challenges in demonstrating causal relationships between a specific intervention and observed outcomes. Yet ecological and injury control theories suggest that the most effective prevention strategies are those that address multiple levels and settings to change the environmental contexts for individual behaviors (Kawachi et al., 1999; Cohen et al., 2003). It is vital that researchers and practitioners work together to develop programs that address the multiple causal pathways for youth violence; include individual, family, and community-based strategies; and are tailored to the populations they are intended to benefit.

References

Ary, D. V., Metzler, C. W., Noell, J. W., Duncan, T. E., Biglan, A., & Smolkowski, K. (1999). Development of adolescent problem behavior. *Journal of Abnormal Child Psychology, 12,* 141–150.

Astor, R. A., Meyer, H. A., & Behre, W. J. (1999). Unowned places and times: Maps and interviews about violence in high schools. *American Educational Research Journal, 36,* 3–42.

Bandura, A. (1986). *Social foundations for thought and action: A social cognitive theory.* Upper Saddle River, NJ: Prentice-Hall.

Bureau of Justice Statistics. (2002). *Criminal victimization in the United States, statistical tables.* Retrieved Dec. 2004 from http://www.ojp.usdoj.gov/bjs/abstract/cvusst.htm.

Cairns, R. B., & Cairns, B. D. (1991). The sociogenesis of aggressive and antisocial behaviors. In J. McCord (Ed.), *Facts, frameworks, and forecasts.* New Brunswick, NJ: Transaction Publishers.

Capaldi, D. M., & Patterson, G. R. (1993). *The violent adolescent male: Specialist or generalist?* Paper presented at the biennial meeting of the Society for Research in Child Development, New Orleans, LA.

Centers for Disease Control and Prevention. (2004a). Web-based Injury Statistics Query and Reporting System (WISQARS). National Center for Injury Prevention and Control, Centers for Disease Control and Prevention. www.cdc.gov/ncipc/wisqars. February 18. 2004.

Centers for Disease Control and Prevention. (2004b). *Youth violence: Fact sheet.* Retrieved Dec. 2004 from http://www.cdc.gov/ncipc/factsheets/yvfacts.htm.

Cohen, L., Miller, T., Sheppard, M., Gordon, E., Ganz, T., & Atnafou, R. (2003). Bridging the gap: Bringing together intentional and unintentional injury prevention efforts to improve health and well-being. *Journal of Safety Research, 34,* 473–483.

Cohen, M. A. (1998). The monetary value of saving a high-risk youth. *Journal of Quantitative Criminology, 14,* 5–33.

Commission on the Prevention of Youth Violence. (2000). *Youth and violence: Medicine, nursing, and public health connecting the dots to prevent violence.* Retrieved Sept. 13, 2004, from http://www.ama-assn.org/violence.

Commission on Violence and Youth. (1993). *Violence and youth: Psychology's response.* Washington, DC: American Psychological Association.

Conduct Problems Research Group. (1999). Initial impact of the fast track prevention trial for conduct problems: The high risk sample. *Journal of Consulting and Clinical Psychology, 67*(5), 631–647.

Cunningham, R. (2005). *Inventory of outcomes: NCIPC-funded youth violence research.* Unpublished manuscript.

Dahlberg, L. L. (1998). Youth violence in the United States: Major trends, risk factors and prevention approaches. *American Journal of Preventive Medicine, 14,* 259–272.

Dishion, T., Patterson, G. R., & Kavanaugh, K. (1992). An experimental test of the coercion model: Linking theory measurement and intervention. In J. McCord & R. E. Tremblay (Eds.), *Preventing antisocial behavior: Interventions from birth through adolescence* (pp. 253–282). New York: Guilford Press.

Ellickson, P. L., & McGuigan, K. A. (2000). Early predictors of adolescent violence. *American Journal of Public Health, 90*(4), 566–572.

Eron, L. D., & Huesmann, L. R. (1990). The stability of aggressive behavior—even unto the third generation. In M. Lewis & S. M. Miller (Eds.), *Handbook of developmental psychology* (pp. 147–156). New York: Plenum Press.

Fagan, J., & Wilkinson, D. L. (1998). Social contexts and functions of adolescent violence. In D. S. Elliott, B. A. Hamburg, & K. R. Williams (Eds.), *Violence in American schools: A new perspective* (pp. 55–93). Cambridge: Cambridge University Press.

Farrell, A. D., Meyer, A. L., Kung, E. M., & Sullivan, T. N. (2001). Development and evaluation of school-based violence prevention programs. *Journal of Clinical Child Psychology, 30*(2), 207–220.

Farrell, A. D., Meyer, A. L., & White, K. S. (2001). Evaluation of responding in peaceful and positive ways (RIPP): A school based prevention program for reducing violence among urban adolescents. *Journal of Clinical Child Psychology, 30*(4), 451–463.

Fergus, S., & Zimmerman, M. A. (2005). Adolescent resilience: A framework for understanding healthy development in the face of risk. *Annual Review of Public Health, 26,* 399–419.

Flay, B. R., & Petraitis, J. (1994). The theory of triadic influence: A new theory of health behavior with implications for preventive interventions. *Advances in Medical Sociology, 4,* 19–44.

Goldstein, A. P., Glick, B., & Gibbs, J. C. (1998). *Aggression replacement training: A comprehensive intervention for aggressive youth.* Champaign, IL: Research Press.

Greenberg, M., & Schneider, D. (1994). Violence in American cities: Young black males is the answer, but what was the question? *Social Science and Medicine, 39*(2), 179–187.

Guerra, N. G., Huesmann, L. R., Tolan, P. H., & Van Acker, R. (1995). Stressful events and individual beliefs as correlates of economic disadvantage and aggression: Implications for preventive interventions among inner-city children. *Journal of Consulting and Clinical Psychology, 63*, 518–528.

Hammond, W. R., & Yung, B. R. (1991). Preventing violence in at-risk African American youth. *Journal of Health Care for the Poor Underserved, 2*(3), 359–373.

Hansen, W. B., & McNeal, R. B. (1997). How DARE works: An examination of program effects on mediating variables. *Health Education and Behavior, 24*(2), 165–176.

Herrenkohl, T., Maguin, E., Hill, K., Hawkins, J., Abbott, R., & Catalano, R. (2000). Developmental risk factors for youth violence. *Journal of Adolescent Health, 26*, 176–186.

Hill, H. M., Soriano, F. I., Chen, S. A., & LaFromboise, T. D. (1994). Sociocultural factors in the etiology and prevention of violence among ethnic youth. In L. D. Eron, J. H. Gentry, & P. Schlegel (Eds.), *Reason to hope: A psychosocial perspective on violence and youth* (pp. 59–97). Washington, DC: American Psychological Association.

Huesmann, L., Eron, L., Lefkowitz, M., & Walder, L. (1984). Stability of aggression over time and generations. *Developmental Psychology, 20*, 1120–1134.

Huesmann, L. R., & Guerra, N. G. (1997). Children's normative beliefs about aggression and aggressive behavior. *Journal of Personality & Social Psychology, 72*(2), 408–419.

Ialongo, N. S., Werthamer, L., Kellam, S. G., Brown, C. H., Wang, S., & Lin, Y. (1999). Proximal impact of two first-grade preventive interventions on the early risk behaviors for later substance abuse, depression, and antisocial behavior. *American Journal of Community Psychology, 27*(5), 599–641.

Irvine, A. B., Biglan, A., Smolkowski, K., Metzler, C. W., & Ary, D. V. (1999). The effectiveness of a parenting skills program for parents of middle school students in small communities. *Journal of Consulting and Clinical Psychology, 67*(6), 811–825.

Jemmott, J. B., Jemmott, L. S., Hines, P. M., & Fong, G. T. (2001). The theory of planned behavior as a model of intentions for fighting among African American and Latino adolescents. *Maternal and Child Health Journal, 5*(4), 253–263.

Jones-Brown, D. D., & Weston-Henriques, Z. (1997). The promise and pitfalls of mentoring as a juvenile justice strategy. *Social Justice, 24*, 253–263.

Kawachi, I., Kennedy, B. P., & Wilkinson, R. G. (1999). Crime: Social disorganization and relative deprivation. *Social Science and Medicine, 48*, 719–731.

Kellam, S. G., Branch, J. D., Agrawal, K. C., & Ensminger, M. E. (1975). *Mental health and going to school: The Woodlawn program of assessment, early intervention, and evaluation.* Chicago: University of Chicago Press.

Kellam, S. G., & Rebok, G. W. (1992). Building developmental and etiological theory through epidemiologically based preventive intervention trials. In J. McCord & R. E. Tremblay (Eds.), *Preventing antisocial behavior: Interventions from birth to adolescence* (pp. 162–195). New York: Guilford.

Komro, K. A., Hu, F. B., & Flay, B. R. (1999). A public health perspective on urban children and youth. In O. Reyes, H. J. Walberg, & R. P. Weissberg (Eds.), *Interdisciplinary perspectives on children and youth.* Thousand Oaks, CA: Sage.

Komro, K. A., Perry, C. L., Veblen-Mortenson, S., Stigler, M. H., Bosma, L. M., Munson, K. A., & Farbakhsh, K. (2004). Violence-related outcomes of the D.A.R.E. Plus project. *Health Education and Behavior 31*(3), 335–354.

Loeber, R., Wung, P., Keenan, K., Giroux, B., Stouthamer-Loeber, M., Van Kammen, W. B., & Maughan, B. (1993). Developmental pathways in disruptive childhood behavior. *Development and Psychopathology, 5*, 103–133.

Loeber, R., & Stouthamer-Loeber, M. (1998). Development of juvenile aggression and violence. Some common misconceptions and controversies. *American Psychologist, 53*(2), 242–259.

Lynam, D. R., Milich, R., Zimmerman, R., Novak, S. P., Logan, T. K., Martin, C., Leukefeld, C., & Clayton, R. (1999). Project DARE: No effects at 10-year follow up. *Journal of Consulting and Clinical Psychology, 67*(4), 590–593.

McLoyd, V. C. (1990). The impact of economic hardship on black families and children: Psychological distress, parenting, and socioemotional development. *Child Development, 61*(2), 311–346.

Merzel, C., & D'Afflitti, J. (2003). Reconsidering community-based health promotion: Promise, performance, and potential. *American Journal of Public Health, 93*(4), 529–533.

Miller, T. R., Fisher, D. A., & Cohen, M. A. (2001). Costs of juvenile violence: Policy implications. *Pediatrics, 107*(1), e3.

Molitor, F., & Hirsch, K. W. (1994). Children's toleration of real-life aggression after exposure to media violence: A replication of the Drabman and Thomas studies. *Child Study Journal, 24*, 191–207.

Multisite Violence Prevention Project. (2004). The multisite violence prevention project: Background and overview. *American Journal of Preventive Medicine, 2*(1), 3–11.

Mullin, C. R., & Linz, D. (1995). Desensitization and resensitization to violence against women: Effects of exposure to sexually violent films on judgments of domestic violence victims. *Journal of Personality and Social Psychology, 69*(3), 449–459.

National Center for Injury Prevention and Control. (2002). *CDC injury research agenda.* Atlanta, GA: Centers for Disease Control and Prevention.

Nation, M., Crusto, C., Wandersman, A., Kumpfer, K. L., Seybolt, D., Morrissey-Kane, E., & Davino, K. (2003). What works in prevention: Principles of effective prevention programs. *American Psychologist, 58*(6/7), 449–456.

Ngwe, J. E., Liu, L. C., Flay, B. R., Segawa, E., & Aya, A. (2004). Violence prevention among African American adolescent males. *American Journal of Health Behavior, 28*(Suppl. 1), 824–837.

Orpinas, P., Murray, N., & Kelder, S. (1999). Parental influences on students' aggressive behaviors and weapon carrying. *Health Education and Behavior, 26*(6), 774–787.

Osofsky, J. D. (1999). The impact of violence on children. *Future of Children, 9*(3), 33–49.

Paik, H., & Comstock, G. (1994). The effects of television violence on anti-social behavior. A meta-analysis. *Communication Research, 21*, 516–546.

Parker, J. G., & Asher, S. R. (1987). Peer relations and later personal adjustment: Are low-accepted children at risk? *Psychological Bulletin, 102*(3), 357–389.

Pepler, D. J., & Slaby, R. G. (1994). Theoretical and developmental perspectives on youth and violence. In L. D. Eron, J. H. Gentry, & P. Schlegel (Eds.), *Reason to hope: A psychosocial perspective on violence and youth* (pp. 27–58). Washington, DC: American Psychological Association.

Perry, C. L. (1999). *Creating health behavior change: How to develop community-wide programs for youth.* Thousand Oaks, CA: Sage.

Perry, C. L., & Jessor, R. (1985). The concept of health promotion and the prevention of adolescent drug abuse. *Health Education Quarterly, 12*(2), 169–184.

Prothrow-Stith, D. B. (1995). The epidemic of youth violence in America: Using public health prevention strategies to prevent violence. *Journal of Health Care for the Poor and Underserved, 6*(2), 95–101.

Randall, J., Swenson, C. C., & Henggeler, S. W. (1999). Neighborhood solutions for neighborhood problems: An empirically based violence prevention collaboration. *Health Education and Behavior, 26*(6), 806–820.

Resnick, M. D., Bearman, P. S., Blum, R. W., Bauman, K. E., Harris, K. M., & Jones, J. (1997). Protecting adolescents from harm: Findings from the National Longitudinal Study on Adolescent Health. *JAMA, 278*, 823–832.

Scott, K. K., Taylor, P. M., Plotkin, A. J., Tepas, J. J., & Fryberg, E. (2002). Turning point: Rethinking violence—Evaluation of program efficacy in reducing adolescent violent crime recidivism. *Journal of Trauma, Injury, Infection and Critical Care, 53*, 21–27.

Taylor, T. K., & Biglan, A. (1998). Behavioral parenting skills programs: A review of the literature for clinicians. *Clinical Child and Family Psychology Review, 1*, 41–60.

Thornton, T. N., Craft, C. A., Dahlberg, L. L., Lynch, B. S., & Baer, K. (2002). *Best practices of youth violence prevention: A sourcebook for community action* (rev. ed.). Atlanta, GA: Centers for Disease Control and Prevention. National Center for Injury Prevention and Control.

Towns, D. P. (1996). "Rewind the world!": An ethnographic study of inner-city African American children's perceptions of violence. *Journal of Negro Education, 65*, 375–389.

Vernberg, E. M., Jacobs, A. K., & Hershberger, S. L. (1999). Peer victimization and attitudes about violence during early adolescence. *Journal of Clinical Child Psychology, 28*(3), 386–395.

Wang, C. C. (2004). Using photovoice as a participatory assessment and issue selection tool. In M. Minkler & N. Wallerstein (Eds.), *Community-based participatory research for health*. San Francisco: Jossey-Bass.

Webber-Stratton, C. (1998). Preventing conduct problems in Head Start children: Strengthening parenting competencies. *Journal of Consulting and Clinical Psychology 66*(5), 715–730.

Wilson, W. J. (1987). *The truly disadvantaged*. Chicago: University of Chicago Press.

Wright, J. C., & Zimmerman, M. A. (in press). Culturally sensitive interventions to prevent youth violence. In N. Guerra & E. Smith (Eds.), *Ethnicity, culture, and youth violence prevention*. Washington, DC: American Psychological Association Press.

World Health Organization. (2002). *World report on violence and health: Summary*. Geneva, Switzerland: Author.

Zimmerman, M. A. (1995). Psychological empowerment: Issues and illustrations. *American Journal of Community Psychology, 23*, 581–599.

Zimmerman, M. A. (2000). Empowerment theory: Psychological, organizational and community levels of analysis. In J. Rappaport & E. Seidman (Eds.), *Handbook of community psychology* (pp. 43–63). New York: Plenum Press.

Zimmerman, M. A., Reischl, T., & Morrel-Samuels, S. (2004). *Youth empowerment solutions for peaceful communities*. Unpublished proposal to the Centers for Disease Control and Prevention.

Zimmerman, M. A., Steinman, K. J., & Rowe, K. J. (1998). Violence among urban African American adolescents: The protective effects of parental support. In X. B. Arriaga & S. Oskamp (Eds.), *Addressing community problems: Psychological research and interventions* (pp. 78–103). Thousand Oaks: Sage.

Zun, L. S., Downey, L., & Rosen, J. (2004). An emergency department–based program to change attitudes of youth toward violence. *Journal of Emergency Medicine, 26*(2), 247–251.

PART FOUR

CROSS-CUTTING ISSUES

CHAPTER EIGHTEEN

SUPERVISION AS A BEHAVIORAL APPROACH TO REDUCING CHILD-INJURY RISK

Barbara A. Morrongiello, Jennifer Lasenby

I n Canada and the United States, as in most other industrialized countries, unintentional injuries are the leading cause of death for children beyond one year
of age (Canadian Institute of Child Health, 2000; Rodriguez, 1990). For example, in the United States, the number of unintentional injury deaths to children
is greater than the next nine causes of death combined (Centers for Disease Control and National Center for Injury Prevention and Control, 2000). Unintentional
injuries are also a leading cause of hospitalization among children (National Center for Health Statistics, 1997). Not surprisingly, because of the scope of this health
issue, there have been numerous calls for research to identify factors that contribute to injury risk during childhood so that more effective prevention programming can be developed (Finney et al., 1993; Miller, Romano, & Spicer, 2000;
Roberts & Brooks, 1987).

One factor that is receiving increasing attention is the role of caregiver supervision in child-injury risk (Gitanjali et al., 2004; Morrongiello, 2005). Surprisingly,
young children most often experience injuries at home when they are presumably being supervised by a caregiver (Rivara, 1995; Shannon, Brashaw, Lewis, &
Feldman, 1992). In fact, some estimates indicate that 90 percent of injuries to
young children occur in or around their home (National Safety Council, 1991;
Rivara, Calonge, & Thompson, 1989). Despite the obvious importance that supervision plays in understanding child-injury risk, there is relatively little empirical research on this risk management strategy. Most research on caregivers'

management of injury risk to children has focused on their use of home safety devices to prevent children from accessing hazards (Gallagher, Hunter, & Guyer, 1985; Gielen, Wilson, Faden, Wissow, & Harvilchuck, 1995; Greaves, Glik, Kronenfeld, & Jackson, 1994; Kelly, Sein, & McCarthy, 1987; Mock et al., 2002; Paul, Sanson-Fisher, Redman, & Carter, 1994; Santer & Stocking, 1991; Woolf, Lewander, Filippone, & Lovejoy, 1987). Hence, as will become evident in this chapter, we have relatively limited knowledge of supervision as a behavioral approach to reducing child-injury risk (see Morrongiello, 2005, for an extensive review).

Despite how often supervision is mentioned as a contributing factor for injury in the literature, few have even attempted to formally define the term (Gitanjali et al., 2004; Morrongiello, 2005; Morrongiello, Ondejko, & Littlejohn, 2004a). Based on the studies in which the term has been used, a reasonable definition would seem to be that *supervision* refers to behaviors that indicate attention (watching, listening) and level of proximity (touching, within reach, beyond reach), with these behaviors judged over time to index the extent of continuity (constant, intermittent, or not at all).

This chapter discusses evidence that bears on the question of how supervision influences children's injury risk, reviews two behavioral programs that have sought to change caregiver supervision (one targeting daycare workers and the other targeting parents), and concludes with suggestions for future research.

Indirect Evidence of a Link Between Supervision and Child-Injury Risk

There is considerable indirect evidence to suggest that supervision influences children's risk of injury. For example, a child's risk of injury increases substantially when the child lives with a single caregiver (Rivara & Mueller, 1987), in a home with multiple siblings (Nathens, Neff, Goss, Maier, & Rivara, 2000; Scholer, Mitchel, & Ray, 1997), or with a substance-abusing caregiver (Westfelt, 1982), which are all characteristics that can compromise a caregiver's capacity to attend closely to a child's activities.

Lapses in caregiver attention have been implicated in a variety of types of children's injuries, including pedestrian injuries (Maleck, Guyer, & Lescohier, 1990; Rivara, Bergman, & Drake, 1989; Wills et al., 1997a, 1997b), drowning (Feldman, Monastersky, & Feldman, 1993; Landen, Bauer, & Kohn, 2003), poisoning (Beautrais, Fergusson, & Shannon, 1982; Brayden, MacLean, Bonfiglio, & Altemeier, 1993; Ozanne-Smith, Day, Parsons, Tibballs, & Dobbin, 2001), choking on small toys (Pollack-Nelson & Drago, 2002), dog bites (Brogan, Bratton, Dowd, & Hegenbarth, 1995), playground injuries (Buck, 1988), injuries that can result from handling of hazardous substances in grocery stores (Harrell & Reid, 1990), injuries that can result from exposure to household safety hazards (Glik, Greaves, Kronenfeld, & Jackson, 1993), injuries on escalators (Platt, Fine, & Foltin, 1997), and fall-related injuries (Alwash & McCarthy, 1987; Harrell, 2003; Board of Trustees, 1991). Of course, one limitation of these studies is that supervision was never directly assessed. Rather, most investigators simply considered the circumstances of the injury and concluded that supervision must have been inadequate and a contributor to children's risk of injury.

Studies that directly assess supervision and relate this to childhood injury risk are rare. For example, Morrongiello and Dawber (1998) studied mothers and their toddlers (two to three and a half years of age) using a contrived-hazards method that involved creating in the laboratory a naturally appearing situation with potential injury-risk hazards (that is, hazards that appear real but have been modified to eliminate injury risk) and then monitoring how caregivers and their children behaved in this seemingly natural injury risk environment.

Results revealed that mothers were predominantly reactive supervisors (they responded once their child approached a hazard) rather than anticipatory supervisors (intervening in anticipation of the child's approaching a hazard). Moreover, as can be seen in Figure 18.1, boys were more likely than girls to behave in ways that elevated injury risk (see also Coppens & Gentry, 1991; Ginsburg & Miller, 1982; Rosen & Peterson, 1990). Boys approached more hazards to look at than girls did and were more likely than girls to immediately touch and retrieve hazardous items. Moreover, boys required more frequent intervention by caregivers and different types of supervision strategies than girls did. Verbal redirection strategies (for example, "Move away from there") were effective for daughters but not sons, resulting in the need for mothers to use more physical redirection strategies (for example, taking the boy's hand and moving him away) for sons than daughters. Thus, boys required both more frequent and more effortful supervision strategies by parents than girls to ensure their safety in hazardous situations. One implication of these findings for intervention is that programs to increase supervision may have to consider the sex of the child to be supervised in defining what constitutes an increase in supervision sufficient to ensure the child's safety in risk environments. The evidence to date suggests that boys require closer supervision than girls to ensure their safety in the same environments.

More recently, questionnaire indexes of supervision have been used to examine relations between general styles of supervision and children's history of injuries. Morrongiello and Hogg (2004) had mothers complete a Beliefs About Supervision questionnaire in which they were presented common situations in which a young child might be playing (for example, in their bedroom) and asked

FIGURE 18.1. AVERAGE NUMBER OF BEHAVIORS SHOWN BY BOYS AND GIRLS AS A FUNCTION OF TYPE OF INJURY HAZARD IN THE CONTRIVED-HAZARDS SETTING.

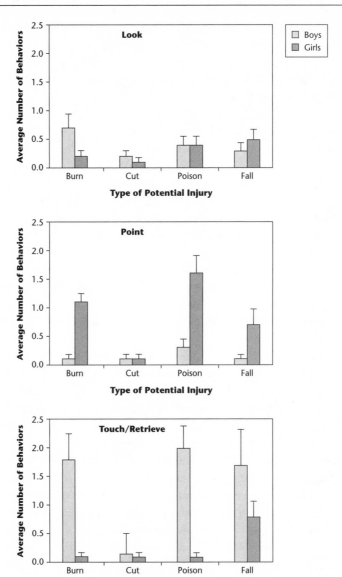

Standard error bars are also indicated.

Source: Morrongiello and Dawber (1998). Reproduced with permission from Oxford University Press.

to indicate the youngest age at which they believe a child could be allowed to be in that situation without constant supervision and the frequency (in minutes) with which they would then check on a child in that situation. Results with mothers of children six to ten years revealed two distinct patterns or styles of supervision, and relating these to children's injury history scores revealed one supervision style was a risk factor and the other was a protective factor for injury.

Among Frequent Monitors, caregivers cite younger ages at which children can be without constant supervision and they manage injury risk by checking on them frequently. Mothers who endorsed this style of supervision had children with a history of more frequent injuries. In contrast, among Infrequent Monitors, caregivers would not leave children alone without constant supervision until at older ages and they would then check on them infrequently on the assumption that the child was now old enough to manage risk himself or herself. Mothers having this style of supervision had children with a history of fewer injuries. Similar results linking these two styles of supervision to children's injury histories also have been found for children two to two and a half years of age (Morrongiello et al., 2004a). From an intervention perspective, the fact that one can discern two distinct styles of supervision and one of these elevates children's risk of injury more than the other suggests that targeting parents with a high-risk supervisory style may be especially effective to maximize having an impact to reduce the frequency of children's injuries.

The Parent Supervision Attributes Profile Questionnaire (PSAPQ; Morrongiello & House, 2004) comprises four subscales (Morrongiello & Corbett, in press) that measure underlying attributes and beliefs that give rise to supervision decisions: protectiveness, tolerance for risk taking, beliefs about children's need for supervision, and a belief that fate controls a child's health status. From an intervention perspective, this may prove to be an especially fruitful approach for effecting changes in supervisory behaviors because targeting the underlying bases for supervision decisions is likely to be critical to effect changes in these behaviors. Initial tests to establish the validity of this measure and its relevance to understanding child-injury risk have yielded quite promising results. Scores on the PSAPQ positively related to actual observed supervisory behaviors on playgrounds, thereby confirming the construct validity of the measure. In addition, scores on the PSAPQ related to children's injury history scores, confirming the predictive validity of the measure. In addition, a recent study of parents' home supervision reveals relations between scores on the PSAPQ and actual supervisory behaviors, as well as child injury history scores (Morrongiello, Corbett, McCourt, & Johnston, in press a, in press b). Hence, the PSAPQ has proven valid for indexing supervision in at least two settings in which children spend a great deal of time. Ongoing research, using a case-control design (cases are children seeking medical treatment for injury; controls are age and sex matched children who are seeking medical treatment for non-injury events), is expected to help in the formulation of cutoff scores to differentiate high-risk from low-risk supervisor scores on the PSAPQ (Morrongiello & Brison, in progress). From a practical point of view, the PSAPQ may prove useful for the identification of high-risk parent supervisors who merit intervention.

A recent study has examined sibling supervision and related this to children's history of home injuries (Morrongiello & MacIssac, 2005). Although sibling supervision is commonplace, there has been virtually no research on this phenomenon. Interviews about daily schedules and the amount of time older siblings looked after younger ones were conducted with mothers having a younger child (eighteen to thirty-six months of age) and an older child ($M = 72$ months, $SD = 24$ months). Results revealed that of the time both children and a parent were home together, the older sibling was the primary supervisor of the younger one about 11 percent of the time. Relating sibling supervision times with injury history scores for the younger child revealed that children with a history of more frequent injuries were more often supervised by an older sibling than children with a history of fewer injuries. Interestingly, younger siblings were rated by parents as being significantly more likely to comply with the parents' commands and requests about safety than with those of their older siblings. Hence, the means by which supervision relates to injury risk in sibling supervision pairs may have more to do with the level of noncompliance shown by the younger sibling than with the quality of supervision that is provided by the older sibling. Previous research also has highlighted the important contribution to injury risk of children's compliance with requests about safety during the preschool years (Morrongiello, Midgett, & Shields, 2001). These types of findings suggest that supervision may interact with child attributes to determine injury risk, which is a possibility that is receiving increasing attention in the literature (see Morrongiello, 2005; Schwebel & Barton, 2005, for further discussion) and certainly merits further study.

In summary, several lines of evidence link supervision to children's history of injuries, providing indirect support for the premise that supervision is a key determinant of child-injury risk. For purposes of planning interventions, the results indicate that boys and girls have different needs for supervision to ensure their safety and that certain patterns of supervision are more likely to elevate child-injury risk than others. There is also evidence that older siblings routinely supervise younger ones and this is associated with increased injury risk, although this association may relate more to noncompliance by the supervisee than to the patterns of supervision shown by older siblings. To advance our understanding of supervision, we need prospective studies that relate actual patterns of supervision to immediate injury. We also need studies that address the issue of how common these patterns of supervision are for children. For example, if a pattern of supervision occurs infrequently and is highly associated with injury, then it is highly significant for understanding injury risk. However, if this pattern regularly occurs at non-injury times, then other factors (for example, child behavioral attributes or level of environmental risk) must be interacting with this pattern of supervision to create risk of injury at some times and not others. As revealed in the next section, only a few studies addressing these issues have been completed.

Direct Evidence Linking Supervision with Child Injury

The most compelling evidence that supervision influences children's risk of injury comes from a recently completed prospective study in which mothers completed injury recording diaries and telephone interviews over the course of twelve weeks, providing self-reports about children's home injuries and diary records of caregiver supervision (Morrongiello et al., 2004a, 2004b). These data were then used to identify determinants of in-home injuries (such as falls, cuts, or burns) experienced by toddlers and to develop a taxonomy of supervision that differentially related to injury risk among two- to three-year-old children.

As shown in Figure 18.2, the findings confirm that different patterns of supervisory behaviors can be discerned and that these are associated with different levels of risk of home injury for young children. Moreover, the taxonomy revealed that distinct patterns of supervision were differentially associated with injuries for boys and girls. Boys essentially required constant supervision to manage injury risk, whereas for girls, intermittently checking on the child was sufficient to manage injury risk. Hence, these findings were consistent with those reported based on a contrived-hazards methodology that revealed that boys required more frequent and more effortful supervision strategies than girls to manage their risk of injury when hazards were present (see Figure 18.2).

Moreover, parents' perceptions of injury risk varied as a function of room in the home, and this had implications for how long they would leave their child alone in each room (see Figure 18.3). In the top panel of Figure 18.3 mothers' ratings of perceived injury risk (range is 1–6) is shown and in the bottom panel the longest time mothers left their children alone (in minutes) is shown as a function of room in the home. Standard error bars are also indicated. Ratings of risk were negatively related to time the child was left alone for high-risk rooms. For both the kitchen and the bathroom, which were perceived as high-risk environments for their children, parents allowed their child less time alone ($r = -.31$ and $-.41$, respectively, $p < .05$). Most important, the time children were left unsupervised related directly to injury rates: there was a positive relation between time-left-alone scores and the frequency of children's injuries in the kitchen and bathroom environments ($r = .41$ and $.35$, respectively; $p < .05$). Hence, in high-risk environments, closer supervision by

FIGURE 18.2. PROPORTION OF INJURIES OCCURRING TO
BOYS AND GIRLS AS A FUNCTION OF LEVEL OF SUPERVISION.

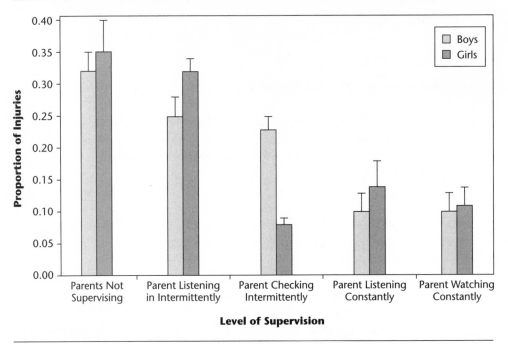

Note: standard error bars are also indicated. Boys, *N* = total injuries; girls = *N* = 137 injuries.

Source: Morrongiello et al. (2004b). By permission of Oxford University Press.

parents was associated with a reduced risk of injury for children, and leaving children unsupervised was associated with increased injury risk.

Just how often are young children typically left unsupervised when at home with a parent? In order to obtain base rate information about supervision, Morrongiello and her colleagues recently completed a study in which mothers of children two through five years of age tracked level and type of supervision from the time the child awoke until the time the child went to bed for ten randomly selected days within a few-week period, including several weekdays and several weekend samples (Morrongiello, Corbett, McCourt, & Johnston, in press a, in press b). A variety of reliability checks were built into the study design and indicated good reliability in maternal reporting about supervision.

Results revealed that the children were awake approximately 6.50 hours per day, with some level of supervision occurring 96 percent of the time and the mother acting as the primary supervisor 78 percent of the time. Hence, children

FIGURE 18.3. DATA DEMONSTRATING RELATIONS BETWEEN PARENTAL PERCEPTIONS OF INJURY RISK AND SUPERVISION.

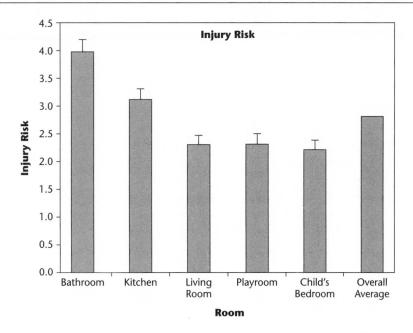

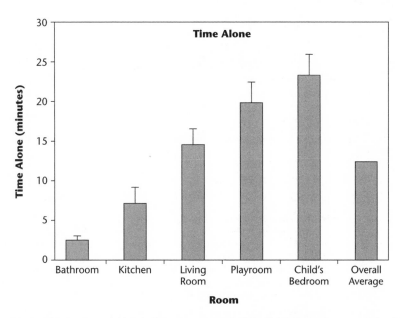

Source: Morrongiello et al. (2004b). By permission of Oxford University Press.

were routinely left completely unsupervised about 4 percent of the time when at home. Nonetheless, as found in previous work (see Figure 18.2) and shown in Table 18.1, level of supervision varied considerably across different circumstances and was poorer when the child was out of view than in view of the supervisor. Moreover, children were often out of view of supervisors (approximately 20 percent of the entries). Hence, on a typical day, children were routinely out of view and receiving only intermittent supervision from caregivers at home (for example, intermittent listening in on the child, going to check on the child periodically).

Supervision scores related to several injury history scores. As shown in Table 18.2, the more the child was in view of the supervisor, the fewer minor injuries (they required only minor parental attention, if anything), non-minor injuries (they were moderate to severe injuries that required treatment of some type), and medical-attended injuries the child experienced. The poorer the level of supervision provided when the child was in view, the greater was the history of medical-attended injuries. Poor supervision when the child was out of view was associated with a history of more minor injuries. Not surprisingly, the more time the child was completely unsupervised, the more minor and non-minor injuries were reported for the child.

In summary, when taken together, the results from these two studies suggest that although young children are not often left completely unsupervised, they are commonly out of view and supervised from a distance. Moreover, several distinct patterns of supervision are evident and occur often, with some patterns elevating

TABLE 18.1. AVERAGE SUPERVISION SCORE UNDER DIFFERENT CIRCUMSTANCES.

Circumstance	Supervision Score
Child in view of supervisor	8.43 (0.34)
Child and supervisor doing something together	9.00 (0)
Independent activities	7.09 (0.85)
Child out of view of supervisor	5.25 (1.71)
Child is alone	4.79 (1.83)
Child is with other children	5.17 (1.78)

Note: 1 = unsupervised; 2 = going to check on child only when parent hears something to indicate this is needed; 3 = checking every 10 minutes or longer; 4 = checking every 8–9 minutes; 5 = checking every 6–7 minutes; 6 = checking every 4–5 minutes; 7 = checking every 2–3 minutes; 8 = listening in constantly but child is not in constant view; 9 = child is in view and constantly supervised. Standard deviations are in parentheses.

Source: Morrongiello et al. (in press a). By permission of Oxford University Press.

TABLE 18.2. CORRELATIONS SHOWING THE RELATION OF MATERNAL HOME SUPERVISION TO CHILDREN'S INJURY HISTORY SCORES.

	Injury Risk Measure from the IHQ[b]		
Supervision[a]	Minor	N-Minor	Medical
IV	−.25*	−.40**	−.24*
S-IV	−.06	−.12	−.26*
S-OV	−.19*	−.04	−.15
OS	−.25*	−.07	−.12
NS	.27*	.21*	.03

[a]IV = proportion of time when the mother has the child in view; S-IV = supervision score when child is in view of the mother; S-OV = supervision score when child is out of view of the mother; OS = overall supervision score (collapsed over all entries); NS = proportion of time when mother is responsible for the child but is not supervising at all.

[b]IHQ = Injury History Questionnaire; Minor = summary score for minor injuries since birth that mother has treated; N-Minor = summary score for non-minor injuries since birth; Medical = summary score for injuries since birth that were treated by a doctor or dentist.

*$p < .05$. **$p < .01$.

Source: Morrongiello et al. (in press b). By permission of Oxford University Press.

risk of injury more than others (see Figure 18.1). Hence, several aspects of these data provide evidence of a direct link between caregiver supervision and child-injury risk.

For purposes of intervention, the taxonomy of supervision developed based on parental reports provides useful information about which patterns of supervision elevate the risk of home injury. Moreover, the taxonomy reveals which supervisory patterns differentially elevate injury risk for boys as compared to girls (see Figure 18.2). Thus, for interventions to be effective in reducing injury risk, one may need to obtain greater increases in supervision by caregivers of sons than daughters.

Behavioral Programs to Increase Supervision

The paucity of data addressing the question of how supervision influences children's risk of injury has made it difficult to determine what the nature and scope of interventions would have to be in order to increase supervision behaviors. In fact, we could identify only two completed interventions on this issue. Of the two programs found, one focuses on parents and the other on daycare providers.

Focusing on parents, Brown, Roberts, and Boles (2005) sought to increase parents' perceptions of children's supervision needs and parents' actual home safety practices; no direct measures of actual supervision were taken, so the study can address only the issue of changing parents' perceptions of what constitutes adequate supervision. The intervention sought to effect changes in these areas by targeting parents' perceptions of their child's risk of injury in the home (that is, perceived vulnerability).

Parents of children four to seven years of age participated in the study and were randomly assigned to one of three conditions: (1) a simulated hazard condition (SHC) in which their child was videorecorded during an unsupervised free play time, resulting in a video record of their child interacting with zero to six available contrived hazards in the lab setting (pill dispenser, cigarette lighter, hunting knife, soldering iron, spray cleaner, BB gun), and these videotapes were then shared with the parent to provide clear evidence of their child's vulnerability for injury when left unsupervised; (2) a video control condition (VCC) in which the parent saw a video of a five year old of the same sex as his or her own child interacting with three hazard-room items (pills, lighter, gun); and (3) a control condition (CC) in which the parent viewed a child development videotape. Prior to participating in the video conditions, a home visit was conducted to complete a standardized home hazard checklist (Home Assessment Prevention Inventory, HAPI-R; Mandel, Bigelow, & Lutzker, 1998); this formed the parents' home safety–practices score. Mothers also were presented four vignettes describing hazardous home situations and were asked to rate the acceptability of five possible parent supervision behaviors; this formed the parents' perceptions of child supervision needs score. Mothers also completed a measure of perceived vulnerability for their child experiencing injury, and this was repeated after viewing the videotape in order to determine if any of the interventions significantly influenced perceived vulnerability.

Results revealed no effects on perceived vulnerability ratings. Hence, none of the video interventions successfully increased parents' perceptions of their child's vulnerability for injury. Nonetheless, there were some significant changes in parents' ratings of appropriate levels of supervision and home hazard scores. Following exposure to the videotape in the SHC, parents' ratings of acceptable supervision in the vignettes task were more conservative, indicating an increase in endorsement of closer supervision practices; these effects were obtained for SHC in comparison to the control group, with scores for the VC falling in between these extremes and not differing significantly from either. Parents in the SHC group also had significantly fewer home hazards on the HAPI-R two weeks after exposure to the intervention. Hence, this intervention seemed to motivate parents subsequently to reduce hazards in the home. Whether this motivation to act also translated into greater actual supervision of their children at home, however, cannot be determined because no measures of supervision were taken. Thus, it remains to be determined if one can effect increases in supervision without evoking increases in perceptions of children's vulnerability for injury. Results of a recent study in our lab are relevant to this point.

Morrongiello and Kiriakou (2004) examined the factors that motivated parents to engage in home safety practices for preventing six types of common injuries to children: burns, poisoning, drowning, cuts, strangulation/suffocation/choking, and falls. They found that parents' home safety practices were motivated by different factors depending on the type of potential injury. Parental beliefs about child vulnerability had greater influences on practices to prevent severe injuries (drowning, poisoning) than for predicting practices to prevent other types of injuries (falls). Thus, depending on the type of injury one seeks to prevent, different factors will need to be targeted to evoke changes in parents' supervision practices. In Brown et al.'s study (2005), therefore, a focus on parents' perceptions of child injury vulnerability may have been more appropriate for some injury hazards than others, resulting in nonsignificant changes when they collapsed across all types of injury. Thus, it may be premature to conclude from their findings that changes in perceptions of injury vulnerability are not essential for an intervention to be successful (that is, to evoke increases in supervision or reductions in hazards in the home).

With regard to methodology, the findings of Brown et al. (2005) suggest that a video-based intervention may have merit as an approach to evoke changes in supervision. However, further research is needed to fully explore how to maximize the effectiveness of this approach. It may be more effective, for example, to limit the focus to hazards actually present in a parent's home. For example, seeing one's child interact with a gun may evoke fear, but it may be unlikely to elicit changes in supervision if the parent knows that there are no guns at home (in other words, the, child's actual vulnerability to injury from guns is negligible). It is possible too that exposing parents to fear-evoking video images, such as their child interacting with serious hazards that do not apply to their home, may actually have a counterintuitive negative effect on supervision. Rather than leading to closer supervision, there may be relief that this is not an issue they have to worry about, leading parents to focus more on how their home is different from those of other families in which children are at far greater risk of injury ("other parents, such as those with guns in the home, need to supervise more closely, but I don't have to because the hazard does not apply to my home").

In summary, though this initial study cannot address the question of whether supervision actually increased following exposure to the intervention, there was evidence that the intervention promoted action by parents to reduce environmental hazards in the home. These actions did not appear to be driven by increased perceptions of vulnerability, though further research is needed to explore more fully how perceived vulnerability relates to parental safety behaviors and if these relations vary with injury type (Morrongiello & Kiriakou, 2004). Another setting in which supervision influences child injury rates is in daycare centers. It has been estimated that 65 percent of children in the United States who are three through five years of age spend their weekdays in child care settings (Cohen, 2001). Supervision, particularly during free play periods on school playgrounds, can be a daunting task but is essential to ensuring that children engage in safe play. In fact, playground equipment is the leading cause of injury in school and child care settings, with over 70 percent of child care centers annually reporting at least one playground injury requiring professional medical treatment (Alkon et al., 2004; Gratz, 2004; Mack, Hudson, & Thompson, 1999). Hence, improving supervision during playground play may substantially reduce children's risk of injury at schools and daycare centers.

Focusing on daycare providers, Schwebel and his colleagues (Schwebel, Summerlin, Bounds, & Morrongiello, in press) recently evaluated a program to reduce children's risk of injury on playgrounds by rewarding children for safe play and having teachers provide these rewards, thereby improving supervision and monitoring by the teachers. Initial testing of this Stamp-in-Safety Program with teachers of children aged four to six years yielded promising results.

For the intervention, teachers were told to give each child at least one stamp during the forty-five-minute playground session and to give stamps at a constant and regular pace throughout the session. Hence, the anticipated effect was that teacher supervision would be improved as a consequence of their need to distribute stamps to the children during free play. Measures of children's and teachers' behaviors were evaluated on the playground before, during, and after the intervention, as well as during a six-month postintervention assessment. During each of the data collection phases, coders recorded six playground behaviors: teachers talking to other adults, teachers warning children about dangerous activity, teachers explaining to children why an activity was dangerous, teachers redirecting children away from dangerous activities, teachers' locations on the playground (they tended to stay in the core area and showed little change in this during the entire study), and children's unintentional injuries (there was only one reported during the entire study).

Applied behavior analysis techniques were used to plot behavior change, with inferential statistics applied to identify changes that were statistically significant. Redirections and explanations showed similar patterns and therefore were collapsed to create a single category of positive teacher verbalizations about child safety.

Figure 18.4 illustrates trends in both the warnings and the redirections and explanations variables. As shown, warnings about dangerous behavior were most

FIGURE 18.4. TEACHERS' WARNINGS, REDIRECTIONS, AND EXPLANATIONS ABOUT DANGEROUS PLAYGROUND ACTIVITY.

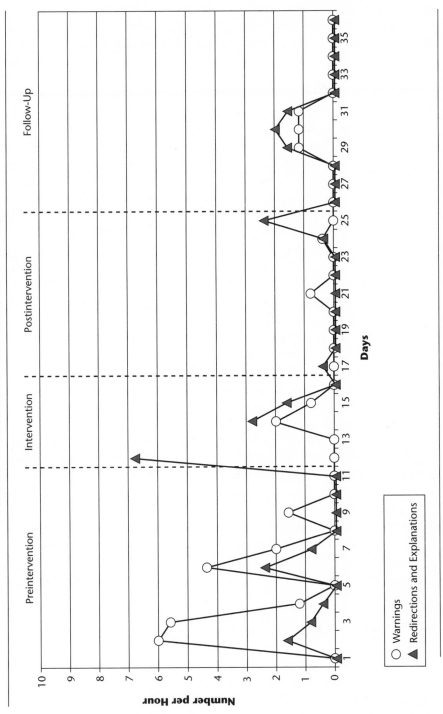

Source: Schwebel et al. (in press). Reproduced with permission.

common before the intervention, decreased during the intervention as children learned how to behave more safely on the playground, and decreased to a statistically significant degree immediately postintervention. Although the rate of warnings increased somewhat six months later during the follow-up assessment, they remained statistically lower than the preintervention rate.

Explanations showed a slightly different pattern. During the intervention, when teachers were actively educating the children about safe play, explanations were significantly elevated. The rate decreased from intervention to postintervention, although not to a statistically significant extent, and returned back to preintervention levels by the six-month follow-up assessment. Redirections showed a pattern similar to explanations, but differences were not statistically significant.

Figure 18.5 illustrates the amount of time teachers talked among themselves. As shown, the number of times teachers were seen talking to adults dropped a statistically significant degree from preintervention to intervention, and then increased somewhat, although not to a statistically significant degree, during postintervention assessments. Hence, the intervention resulted in a decrease in adult directed talking and an increase in supervisory behaviors shown by teachers on playgrounds.

In summary, a number of measures indicated improved supervision and monitoring of the children by their teachers as a result of this behavioral intervention. Teachers' explanations about playground dangers and redirections to safer behavior peaked during the intervention, when they were increasing their supervision and training children about safe behavior. Teachers also spent less time talking to other adults during and after the intervention compared to before the intervention. There was evidence that the intervention improved the frequency of children's safe play behaviors. Specifically, teachers needed to give warnings to children about dangerous behavior most frequently prior to the intervention, but this declined during and after the intervention, which is what one would expect if children showed decreased risky behaviors and increased safe play in response to reinforcement for safe play behaviors. It is interesting to note that, although supervision behaviors changed, teachers viewed the program as one aimed at increasing children's safe playground play rather than one targeting supervision. Whether this type of *indirect* approach to effecting change would also work to improve parents' supervision of children at home remains to be determined but it merits consideration.

Directions for Future Research

Many research questions remain to be addressed, particularly if we wish to develop interventions to effect changes in supervision in order to reduce children's risk of injury. Several suggestions are provided below.

FIGURE 18.5. TEACHERS TALKING TO OTHER ADULTS WHEN ON THE PLAYGROUND.

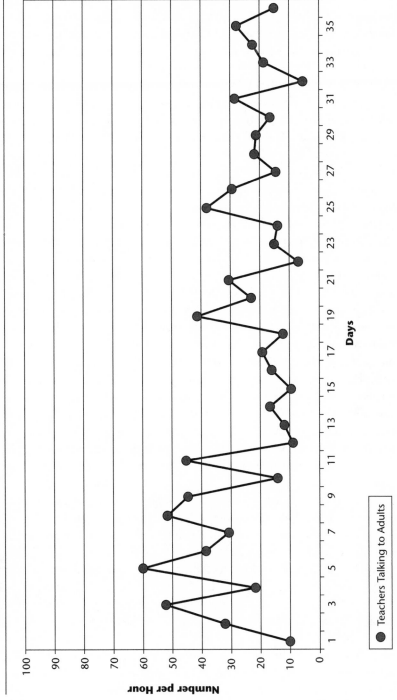

● Teachers Talking to Adults

Source: Schwebel et al. (in press). Reproduced with permission.

First, we know virtually nothing about the extent to which children's risk of injury varies with supervisor. A study examining adults' reactions to young children in hypothetical situations found women more likely than men to intervene under certain conditions (Fagot, Kronsberg, & MacGregor, 1985). Similarly, a study of parental beliefs about the benefits to children of experiencing minor injuries revealed that fathers endorsed stronger beliefs than mothers that children learn from injury experiences and "toughen up" from such experiences (Lewis, DiLillo, & Peterson, 2004). Prior research with school-age children indicates that children assume fathers will supervise less closely and be more tolerant of risk activities than mothers (Morrongiello & Bradley, 1997). Whether these perceptions by children are valid and result in children experiencing more injuries with father than mother supervisors would certainly be important to know for purposes of efficiency in targeting interventions. Similarly, although evidence suggests young children may be at greater risk of injury when supervised by an older child, there is little definitively known about how such effects are realized. Would babysitting training make a difference, or is the issue related more to how the younger child reacts to the babysitter than with how the babysitter actually supervises?

Second, it would be useful to know what factors naturally occur and effect changes in caregivers' patterns of supervision. For example, do caregivers alter their patterns of supervision as children develop or in response to children's injuries or near misses? Prior research with school-age children suggests that parents do not alter safety practices in response to children's injuries (Peterson, Bartelstone, Kern, & Gillies, 1995). However, these findings may not apply for younger children or for supervision. Identifying those naturally occurring triggering events that evoke changes in supervision may provide insights into factors to target in interventions that aim to alter patterns of supervision.

Third, identifying caregiver personality attributes that relate to supervision may assist in the identification of high-risk caregivers for purposes of early intervention (for example, during pregnancy) to prevent child injury. For example, recent research by Morrongiello and her colleagues has revealed certain personality attributes, which are stable and easily measured, that are highly correlated with supervision behaviors. Specifically, conscientiousness was found to relate positively to supervision (Morrongiello et al., 2004a) and neuroticism to correlate negatively with supervision (Morrongiello, Corbett, McCourt, & Johnston, in press b) of young children. There may be additional attributes that are important to supervision and may contribute to identifying high-risk caregivers.

Fourth, research is needed to identify the determinants of supervision decisions that are amenable to change and to identify the best means by which to effect change in these determinants. For example, prior research indicates that the factors that predict parents' safety practices vary with type of injury (Morrongiello

& Kiriakou, 2004). Hence, perceptions of vulnerability play a greater role in predicting practices to prevent poisoning and drowning than falls. These findings can provide a basis for interventionists to determine what factors to target to evoke greater supervision in particular injury risk situations (for example, those that can lead to drowning). There is some evidence already that supervision decisions are based on caregivers' perceptions of their child's vulnerability for injury. For example, mothers show closer supervision of children in rooms they consider to be high-risk environments (see Figure 18.3). Hence, targeting perceptions of vulnerability may lead to greater supervision. The study by Brown et al. (2005) found increases in safety-promoting environmental modifications following an intervention that did not affect perceptions of vulnerability. However, they did not measure caregiver supervision. Thus, the study does not address the issue of whether evoking changes in a caregiver's perceptions of their child's injury vulnerability will lead to improved supervision.

Fifth, further research is needed to determine how supervision is related to childhood pedestrian injuries, a leading cause of death and serious injury for children five to nine years of age (Roberts, 1995). Wazana, Krueger, Raina, and Chambers (1997) found that children who had been injured as pedestrians had parents who were 2.6 times less likely to provide good supervision and that they discontinued the supervision of their child two years sooner than parents of children who had not suffered pedestrian injuries. Similarly, Roberts (1995) found that risk to children who were accompanied by an adult was half that of children who were not supervised. Although these findings highlight the role of supervision in understanding children's risk of pedestrian injury, little is known about what factors influence parents' decisions about what level of supervision their child needs to ensure safety when crossing streets. For example, evidence indicates that parents tend to overestimate their children's road-crossing abilities, particularly five- to six-year-old children, which is within the age range that is at the greatest risk for pedestrian injuries (Dunne, Asher, & Rivara, 1992). It would be informative to examine the relation between parents' estimations of children's abilities and their supervision of children's street crossing (for example, whether poorer supervision is predicted by high estimations of children's abilities). As well, it would be useful to determine if parents interpret the presence of peers as increasing or decreasing children's risk of pedestrian injury. Prior research suggests that peers increase risk (Wills et al., 1997a). If parents assume, however, that peer presence reduces risk (for example, more children to look for traffic), they may misjudge children's abilities as a group to cross safely, resulting in the provision of inadequate supervision. Research indicates too that children have a tendency to run ahead or fall behind adults as they cross the street, adults often set bad examples by crossing the street inappropriately, and when crossing with adults, children are often passive and are not encouraged to practice their safety skills (van der Molen, van den Herik, & van der Klaauw, 1983). Thus, these findings suggest that supervision may interact with other factors (such as how children behave) in determining injury risk, particularly in pedestrian contexts.

Along these same lines, we would argue that the greatest need for research is to explore how supervision interacts with child attributes and level of environmental risk to elevate injury risk (see Morrongiello, 2005, for further discussion). The general assumption in the child injury literature is that supervision has a direct impact on child-injury risk (a unidirectional model of caregiver-to-child influence). There is accumulating evidence, however, that the relation between supervision and child-injury risk derives from a transactional process, that is, the extent to which supervision plays a risk or protective factor depends on child attributes × caregiver supervision × level of environmental risk (Morrongiello et al., 2004a, 2004b). Hence, one must also consider mediating or moderating relations in specifying how supervision influences child-injury risk (Schwebel & Barton, 2005). It may be, for example, that supervisory patterns that serve a protective function in one setting are a risk factor for injury in another setting due to differences in a child's behavior or level of environmental risk across settings. Thus, it may prove to be the case that interventions need to be highly specific and narrowly focused to be effective in targeting supervision (that is, targeting supervision in a specific environment or with respect to a certain type of injury in that environment).

References

Alkon, A., Genevro, J. L., Tschann, J. M., Kaiser, P., Ragland, D. R., & Boyce, W. T. (2004). The epidemiology of injuries in four child care centers. *Archives of Pediatric and Adolescent Medicine, 153,* 1248–1254.

Alwash, R., & McCarthy, M. (1987). How do child accidents happen? *Health Education Journal, 46,* 169–171.

Beautrais, A. L., Fergusson, D. M., & Shannon, F. T. (1982). Childhood accidents in a New Zealand birth cohort. *Australian Paediatric Journal, 18,* 238–242.

Board of Trustees. American Medical Association. (1991). Use of infant walkers. *American Journal of Diseases of Children, 145,* 933–934.

Brayden, R. M., MacLean, W. E., Jr., Bonfiglio, J. F., & Altemeier, W. (1993). Behavioral antecedents of pediatric poisonings. *Clinical Pediatrics, 32,* 30–35.

Brogan, T. V., Bratton, S. L., Dowd, M. D., & Hegenbarth, M. A. (1995). Severe dog bites in children. *Pediatrics, 96,* 947–950.

Brown, K., Roberts, M. C., & Boles, R. E. (2005). Effects of parental viewing of children's risk behavior on home safety practices. *Journal of Pediatric Psychology, 30*(7), 571–580.

Buck, D. J. (1988). Safe on playgrounds? The nature and causes of children's playground accidents and opportunities for prevention. *Public Health, 102,* 603–611.

Canadian Institute of Child Health. (2000). *The health of Canada's children: A CCIH profile* (3rd ed.). Ottawa: Canadian Institute of Child Health.

Centers for Disease Control and National Center for Injury Prevention and Control. (2000). *Ten leading causes of death by age group: 1996.* Atlanta, GA: CDC.

Cohen, S. S. (2001). *Championing child care.* New York: Columbia University Press.

Coppens, N. M., & Gentry, L. K. (1991). Video analysis of playground injury-risk situations. *Research in Nursing and Health, 14,* 129–136.

Dunne, R. G., Asher, K. N., & Rivara, F. P. (1992). Behavior and parental expectations of child pedestrians. *Pediatrics, 89*(3), 486–490.

Fagot, B. I., Kronsberg, S., & MacGregor, D. (1985). Adult responses to young children in risky situations. *Merrill Palmer Quarterly, 31,* 385–395.

Feldman, K. W., Monastersky, C., & Feldman, G. K. (1993). When is childhood drowning neglect? *Child Abuse and Neglect, 17,* 329–336.

Finney, J. W., Christophersen, E. R., Friman, P. C., Kalnins, I. V., Maddux, J. E., Peterson, L., Roberts, M., & Wolraich, M. (1993). Society of Pediatric Psychology Task Force Report: Pediatric psychology and injury control. *Journal of Pediatric Psychology, 18,* 499–526.

Gallagher, S. S., Hunter, P., & Guyer, B. (1985). A home injury prevention program for children. *Pediatric Clinics of North America, 32,* 95–112.

Gielen, A. C., Wilson, M. E., Faden, R. R., Wissow, L., & Harvilchuck, J. D. (1995). In-home injury prevention practices for infants and toddlers: The role of parental beliefs, barriers, and housing quality. *Health Education Quarterly, 22,* 85–95.

Ginsburg, H. J., & Miller, S. M. (1982). Sex differences in children's risk-taking behavior. *Child Development, 53,* 426–428.

Gitanjali, S., Brenner, R., Morrongiello, B. A., Haynie, D., Rivera, M., & Cheng, T. (2004). The role of supervision in child-injury risk: Definition, conceptual, and measurement issues. *Injury Control and Safety Promotion, 11,* 17–22.

Glik, D. C., Greaves, P. E., Kronenfeld, J. J., & Jackson, K. L. (1993). Safety hazards in households with young children. *Journal of Pediatric Psychology, 18,* 115–131.

Gratz, R. R. (2004). Unintentional injury in early childhood group settings. *Children's Health Care, 21,* 239–249.

Greaves, P., Glik, D. C., Kronenfeld, J. J., & Jackson, K. (1994). Determinants of controllable in-home child safety hazards. *Health Education Research, 9,* 307–315.

Harrell, W. A. (2003). Effect of two warning signs on adult supervision and risky activities by children in grocery shopping carts. *Psychological Reports, 92,* 889–898.

Harrell, W. A., & Reid, E. E. (1990). Safety of children in grocery stores: The impact of cartseat use in shopping carts and parental monitoring. *Accident Analysis and Prevention, 22,* 531–542.

Kelly, B., Sein, C., & McCarthy, P. L. (1987). Safety education in a pediatric primary care setting. *Pediatrics, 79,* 818–824.

Landen, M. G., Bauer, U., & Kohn, M. (2003). Inadequate supervision as a cause of injury deaths among young children in Alaska and Louisiana. *Pediatrics, 111,* 328–331.

Lewis, T., DiLillo, D., & Peterson, L. (2004). Parental beliefs regarding developmental benefits of childhood injuries. *American Journal of Health Behavior, 28*(Suppl. 1), S61–S68.

Mack, M. G., Hudson, S. D., & Thompson, D. (1999). Playground safety in the United States, 1998–1999. *Morbidity and Mortality Weekly Report, 48,* 329–332.

Maleck, M., Guyer, B., & Lescohier, I. (1990). The epidemiology and prevention of child pedestrian injury. *Accident: Analysis and Prevention, 22,* 301–313.

Mandel, U., Bigelow, K. M., & Lutzker, J. R. (1998). Using video to reduce home safety hazards with parents reported for child abuse and neglect. *Journal Family Violence, 13*, 147–162.

Miller, T. R., Romano, E. O., & Spicer, R. S. (2000). The cost of childhood unintentional injuries and the value of prevention. *Future of Children, 10*, 137–163.

Mock, C., Arreola, R. C., Trevino, P. R., Almazan, S.V., Enrique, Z. J., Gonzalez, S. R., Simpson, K., & Torre, M. (2002). Childhood injury prevention practices by parents in Mexico. *Injury Prevention, 8*, 303–330.

Morrongiello, B. A. (2005). The role of supervision in child-injury risk: Assumptions, issues, findings, and future directions. *Journal of Pediatric Psychology, 30*, 536–552.

Morrongiello, B. A., & Bradley, M. D. (1997). Sibling power: Influence of older siblings' persuasive appeals on younger siblings' judgments about risk taking behaviors. *Injury Prevention, 3*, 23–28.

Morrongiello, B. A., & Brison, R. *A case-control study to examine the role of supervision in child-injury risk.* Unpublished manuscript.

Morrongiello, B. A., & Corbett, M. (in press). *Parents' supervision of pre-schoolers in the home: The validity of questionnaire measures of supervision. Injury Prevention.*

Morrongiello, B. A., Corbett, M., McCourt, M., & Johnston, N. (in press a). Unintentional injuries in young children: I. The nature and scope of caregiver supervision of children at home. *Journal of Pediatric Psychology.*

Morrongiello, B. A., Corbett, M., McCourt, M., & Johnston, N. (in press b). Unintentional injuries in young children: II. The contribution of caregiver supervision, child attributes, and parent attributes. *Journal of Pediatric Psychology.*

Morrongiello, B. A., & Dawber, T. (1998). Toddlers' and mothers' behaviors in an injury-risk situation: Implications for sex differences in childhood injuries. *Journal of Applied Developmental Psychology, 19*, 625–639.

Morrongiello, B. A., & Hogg, K. (2004). Mothers' reactions to children misbehaving in ways that can lead to injury: Implications for gender differences in children's risk taking and injuries. *Sex Roles, 50*, 103–118.

Morrongiello, B. A., & House, K. (2004). Measuring parent attributes and supervision behaviors relevant to child injury risk: Examining the usefulness of questionnaire measures. *Injury Prevention, 10*, 114–118.

Morrongiello, B. A., & Kiriakou, S. (2004). Mothers' home-safety practices for preventing six types of childhood injuries: What do they do, and why? *Journal of Pediatric Psychology, 29*, 285–297.

Morrongiello, B. A., & MacIssac, T. *Children supervising children: When, where, why, and with what outcomes?* Unpublished manuscript.

Morrongiello, B. A., Midgett, C., & Shields, R. (2001). Don't run with scissors: Young children's knowledge of home safety rules. *Journal of Pediatric Psychology, 26*, 105–115.

Morrongiello, B. A., Ondejko, L., & Littlejohn, A. (2004a). Understanding toddlers' in-home injuries: I. Context, correlates, and determinants. *Journal of Pediatric Psychology, 29*, 415–431.

Morrongiello, B. A., Ondejko, L., & Littlejohn, A. (2004b). Understanding toddlers' in-home injuries: II. Examining parental strategies, and their efficacy, for managing child injury risk. *Journal of Pediatric Psychology, 29*, 433–446.

Nathens, A. B., Neff, M. J., Goss, C. H., Maier, R. V., & Rivara, F. P. (2000). Effect of an older sibling and birth interval on the risk of childhood injury. *Injury Prevention, 6*, 219–222.

National Center for Health Statistics. (1997). *Health, United States, 1996–1997, and injury chartbook.* Hyattsville, MD: Author.

National Safety Council. (1991). *Accident facts.* Chicago: Author.

Ozanne-Smith, J., Day, L., Parsons, B., Tibballs, J., & Dobbin, M. (2001). Childhood poisoning: Access and prevention. *Journal of Paediatrics and Child Health, 37,* 262–265.

Paul, C., Sanson-Fisher, R., Redman, S., & Carter, S. (1994). Preventing accidental injury to young children in the home using volunteers. *Health Promotion International, 9,* 241–249.

Peterson, L., Bartelstone, J., Kern, T., & Gillies, R. (1995). Parents' socialization of children's injury prevention: Description and some initial parameters. *Child Development, 66,* 224–235.

Platt, S. L., Fine, J. S., & Foltin, G. L. (1997). Escalator-related injuries in children. *Pediatrics, 100,* e2.

Pollack-Nelson, C., & Drago, D. A. (2002). Supervision of children aged two through six years. *Injury Control and Safety Promotion, 9,* 121–126.

Rivara, F. P. (1995). Developmental and behavioral issues in childhood injury prevention. *Journal of Developmental and Behavioural Pediatrics, 16,* 362–370.

Rivara, F. P., Bergman, A. B., & Drake, C. (1989). Parental attitudes and practices toward children as pedestrians. *Pediatrics, 84,* 1017–1021.

Rivara, F. P., Calonge, N., & Thompson, R. S. (1989). Population-based study of unintentional injury incidence and impact during childhood. *American Journal of Public Health, 79,* 990–994.

Rivara, F. P., & Mueller, B. A. (1987). The epidemiology and causes of childhood injuries. *Journal of Social Issues, 43,* 13–31.

Roberts, M. (1995). *Handbook of pediatric psychology.* New York: Guilford Press.

Roberts, M., & Brooks, P. (1987). Children's injuries: Issues in prevention and public policy. *Journal of Social Issues, 43,* 105–118.

Rodriguez, J. G. (1990). Childhood injuries in the United States: A priority issue. *American Journal of Diseases of Children, 144,* 625–626.

Rosen, B. N., & Peterson, L. (1990). Gender differences in children's outdoor play injuries: A review and an integration. *Clinical Psychology Review, 10,* 187–205.

Santer, L. J., & Stocking, C. B. (1991). Safety practices and living conditions of low-income urban families. *Pediatrics, 88,* 1112–1118.

Scholer, S. J., Mitchel, E. F., Jr., & Ray, W. A. (1997). Predictors of injury mortality in early childhood. *Pediatrics, 100,* 342–347.

Schwebel, D., & Barton, B. (2005). Contributions of multiple risk factors for child injury. *Journal of Pediatric Psychology, 30,* 553–561.

Schwebel, D. C., Summerlin, A. L., Bounds, M. L., & Morrongiello, B. A. (in press). The Stamp-in Safety Program: A behavioural intervention to reduce behaviors that can lead to unintentional playground injury in a preschool setting. *Journal of Pediatric Psychology.*

Shannon, A., Brashaw, B., Lewis, J., & Feldman, W. (1992). Nonfatal childhood injuries: A survey at the Children's Hospital of Eastern Ontario. *Canadian Medical Association Journal, 146,* 361–365.

van der Molen, H. H., van den Herik, J., & van der Klaauw, C. (1983). Pedestrian behaviour of children and accompanying parents during school journeys: An evaluation of a training programme. *British Journal of Educational Psychology, 53,* 152–168.

Wazana, A., Krueger, P., Raina, P., & Chambers, L. (1997). A review of risk factors for child pedestrian injuries: Are they modifiable? *Injury Prevention, 3,* 295–304.

Westfelt, J. (1982). Environmental factors in childhood accidents. *Acta Pediatrica Scandinavica 291*(Suppl.), 1–75.

Wills, K. E., Christoffel, K. K., Lavigne, J. V., Tanz, R. R., Schofer, J. L., & Donovan, M. (1997a). Patterns and correlates of supervision in child pedestrian injury. The Kids 'N' Cars Research Team. *Journal of Pediatric Psychology, 22*, 89–104.

Wills, K. E., Tanz, R. R., Christoffel, K., Schofer, J. L., Lavigne, J. V., & Donovan, M. (1997b). Supervision in childhood injury cases: A reliable taxonomy. *Accident Analysis and Prevention, 29*, 133–137.

Woolf, A., Lewander, W., Filippone, G., & Lovejoy, F. (1987). Prevention of childhood poisoning: Efficacy of an educational program carried out in an emergency clinic. *Pediatrics, 80*, 359–363.

CHAPTER NINETEEN

REDUCING POSTTRAUMATIC STRESS AFTER INDIVIDUAL AND MASS TRAUMA

Courtney Landau Fleisher, Nancy Kassam-Adams

Shannon Brown and her mom had already spent two nights at the Red Cross shelter. The hurricane winds were beginning to die down enough that officials believed it was safe for families to investigate the damage to their homes. Shannon did not want to see her home. The last couple of nights she barely got any sleep, as she kept imagining the roof of the school gym being ripped off by the howling winds and carrying her away. She would go over to the awards showcase when people around her started talking about the storm. Ms. Brown noticed that her daughter was not acting like herself, but she was also preoccupied with trying to arrange for her son, Jermane, to get home as he had been away when the storm hit. Ms. Brown was also trying to reach other members of the family, both local and those who lived far away. She hoped Shannon's behavior would return to normal when she was able to be away from all the commotion of the shelter.

The damage to the house was substantial, and it was going to require several days of work before they'd be able to stay at home. Jermane returned, and Shannon was happy to see someone who had not been around during the hurricane. Although she could tell it was difficult for Shannon to be at their house, Ms. Brown would not allow her to wander too far, particularly due to the danger of the debris in the neighborhood. To keep her occupied, Shannon's mother tried to start her on a safe clean-up job, but Shannon became very upset and couldn't engage in it. Ms. Brown was overwhelmed by trying to manage her daughter's distress as well as the clean-up responsibilities necessary for the family to return to a safe and comfortable home.

Mrs. Lee had been riding bikes with her two sons, Jeffrey and Shane, on a Sunday, following last in line so that she could keep an eye on her children as they rode together. Coming up from behind them, a car hit Mrs. Lee's bike, flipped her, knocked her unconscious, and left the scene of the collision. Jeffrey, the older son, had Shane stay with their mother while Jeffrey rode into town to get help. The ambulance arrived fifteen minutes later to find Shane crying while trying to get his mother to regain consciousness. Mr. Lee and Jeffrey arrived shortly after. As the emergency medical services (EMS) transported Mrs. Lee to the hospital, Mr. Lee and the two boys followed in the family car. By the time they had arrived at the hospital, Mrs. Lee had regained consciousness. Her fractures were addressed in the emergency department, and she was admitted to the hospital overnight for testing and observation.

Three weeks after the bike collision, the Lee family is struggling to return their lives to normal. Jeffrey and his parents share great anger toward the driver of the car, not only for causing the collision but for leaving the scene and putting Jeffrey and Shane in a very difficult situation. Shane has been largely quiet regarding his feelings about the collision. However, he and Mr. Lee have each found themselves anxious when the family has to be apart, which has made getting out of the house for school and work somewhat difficult. Shane told his father that he has a hard time getting out of his head the image of his mom lying unconscious on the pavement, an image his father replays in his head at times too. Shane's teacher reports that Shane has been more on edge and that he yelled at a friend in class when a borrowed pencil was returned broken. The family notices the struggle they have been having, and the Lees have decided to seek professional help for their family in coping.

As these cases illustrate, individuals and families exposed to frightening or potentially life-threatening experiences may have acute or prolonged traumatic stress reactions that have an impact on broad areas of functioning. Although most people are resilient and do well, a significant minority of children and adults exposed to traumatic events develop persistent, distressing sequelae. The importance of attending to traumatic stress reactions is underscored by their potential impact on recovery of physical health and functioning.

These cases highlight how individuals and families like the Browns and Lees display acute behavioral and emotional reactions. As is evidenced in the Lee family, reactions can occur even when a person was not witness to the trauma. The avoiding Shannon did by leaving the conversation when the storm came up, the reexperiencing Shane and his dad suffered when the images of mom lying on the ground kept replaying in their minds even after she was recovered and at home, and the increased arousal Shane displayed when he overreacted to the broken pencil at school are all posttraumatic stress symptoms (PTSS). Most individuals experience some of these types of symptoms in the days and weeks following a traumatic event. For some, these symptoms are intense and persist for many weeks to months. If the symptoms are severe enough, continue beyond a month, and interfere with important areas of the person's life, the diagnosis of posttraumatic stress disorder (PTSD) is considered.

In this chapter, we explore PTSS/PTSD as a way of understanding individuals' reactions to traumatic events, discover how frequently such reactions occur and how often they occur at a disorder level, and learn what makes these reactions happen. In addition, we focus on what behavioral scientists and other professionals can and cannot do to address PTSS and PTSD after a potentially traumatic event and how to assess the presence of PTSS/PTSD in trauma-exposed populations. The chapter concludes with a discussion about directions for future research.

Traumatic Stressors and Sequelae of Exposure

Posttraumatic stress disorder was initially described in populations of combat veterans. Over time, the range of events considered to be traumatic stressors has expanded, and PTSD is now recognized after an array of traumatic events. According to the current definition of PTSD in the *Diagnostic and Statistical Manual of Mental Disorders* (the DSM-IV-TR; American Psychiatric Association, 2004), to be considered a traumatic stressor, an event must involve actual or threatened death, serious injury, or a threat to the physical integrity of oneself or others, and instill a sense of fear, hopelessness, or horror in the individual. Traumatic events may strike large groups of people at once (mass trauma), such as natural and man-made disasters and terrorism, or individuals or smaller groups of people (individual trauma), as is the case for rape and sexual assault, childhood abuse, injury, and serious illness (Norris et al., 2002). Traumatic stress reactions have been investigated in a wide range of injury populations, including individuals experiencing gunshot wounds (Gill, 2002), assaults or domestic violence (Kilpatrick et al., 2003; Resnick, Acierno, Holmes, Dammeyer, & Kilpatrick, 2000; Roy-Byrne et al., 2004), motor vehicle crashes (Stallard, Velleman, & Baldwin, 1998; Winston, et al., 2002; Zink & McCain, 2003), pedestrian or bicycle injuries (Daviss et al., 2000; Winston et al., 2002), falls (Daviss et al., 2000), burns (Baur, Hardy, & Van Dorsten, 1998; Saxe et al., 2001; Van Loey, Maas, Faber, & Taal, 2003), sports-related injuries (Daviss et al., 2000; Stallard et al., 1998), and injuries sustained in the course of disasters or terrorist incidents (Briere & Elliott, 2000; Norris, Perilla, Riad, Kaniasty, & Lavizzo, 1999).

Regardless of the type of precipitating traumatic event (mass or individual), most individuals directly involved experience a disruption in their behavior and emotions following the event. Reactions generally fall into the areas of reexperiencing the event, emotional numbing or avoiding stimuli related to the trauma, and increased arousal. Individuals exposed to traumatic events may experience distressing dreams, memories, feelings, and behaviors that are associated with the traumatic experience. To cope with the overwhelming emotions stirred up by the recurring memories of the trauma, exposed individuals may attempt to avoid thoughts and reminders of the event. They may attempt to turn off their feelings, thus leading to emotional numbness, social isolation, and appearing emotionally flat. In addition, exposed individuals tend to lose their sense of security, anticipate further danger, and can become hypervigilant and easily startled.

Generally, exposed individuals report at least one of these responses, but they tend to be short-lived, dissipating within days or a couple of weeks. These transient reactions fall within a posttraumatic stress framework, but the intensity and duration of the symptoms do not reach disorder status. *PTSS* is a term that has been used to describe the subclinical symptom presentation of traumatic stress reactions in individuals exposed to traumatic stressors. A subset of those exposed to traumatic stressors develops sufficient symptoms and impairment to be diagnosed with PTSD. These individuals continue to display the behavioral and emotional reactions for at least one month, and these responses interfere with important areas of functioning in their lives.

The emotional distress of experiencing PTSS/PTSD reactions can itself be disabling, but the symptoms and behaviors associated with traumatic stress reactions may also interfere with recovery of physical, social, and occupational functioning after a trauma. For example, Richmond (1997) found that traumatic stress was a key predictor of disability following traumatic injury. In addition, traumatic stress has been linked to poorer health outcomes in a variety of trauma-exposed populations (Schnurr, 1996).

Incidence of PTSS and PTSD

PTSD is a relatively common mental health disorder. Epidemiological surveys indicate that in the general adult population, about 8 percent, or one in twelve persons, have met diagnostic criteria for PTSD at some point in their lifetime (Breslau, 2001; Kessler, Sonnega, Bromet, Hughes, & Nelson, 1995). Lifetime PTSD prevalence is higher among women (10 percent) than among men (5 percent), and this difference persists even when controlling for type of trauma (Kessler et al., 1995; Schnurr, Friedman, & Bernardy, 2002). For children and adolescents, the epidemiological evidence is more limited, but large community surveys have estimated similar lifetime PTSD prevalence (about 7 percent) in younger populations

(Giaconia et al., 1995). Prevalence of diagnostic PTSD may not reflect the full extent of population impact of traumatic stress symptoms. The proportion of individuals experiencing PTSS or "partial PTSD" (clinically significant levels of PTSS that do not meet full criteria for a PTSD diagnosis) appears to equal or exceed the number with diagnostic PTSD (Stein, Walker, Hazen, & Forde, 1997).

The importance of attending to PTSD prevention and treatment is underscored by the broad impact that PTSD appears to have on health outcomes, health care use, and occupational functioning (Kessler, 2000; Schnurr, 1996; Walker et al., 2003). PTSS and partial PTSD have also been demonstrated to have a substantial impact on functioning (Marshall et al., 2001; Stein et al., 1997). The effects of exposure to trauma may be long-lasting, with PTSD symptoms persisting for many years (Briere & Elliott, 2000).

Differing types of potentially traumatic events vary in the degree and impact of associated traumatic stress that is observed among exposed individuals. Among mass trauma events, those involving mass violence appear to result in higher posttraumatic stress impact for exposed individuals, in comparison with natural or technological disasters (Norris et al., 2002). Among individual traumatic events, those that involve assaultive violence are associated with the greatest risk for traumatic stress reactions, with rape as the event most likely to lead to PTSD (Kessler et al., 1995). Because of the sheer frequency of their occurrence, traffic crashes, such as the one experienced by the Lee family, also stand out as one of the most common precipitants of PTSD in the general population. Norris (1992) estimated that motor vehicle crashes alone result in PTSD in 28 per 1,000 adults in the United States at some point in their lifetime. In children, between 13 and 45 percent of those experiencing traumatic injury go on to develop significant PTSD symptoms (Aaron, Zaglul, & Emery, 1999; Daviss et al., 2000; Kassam-Adams & Winston, 2004; Stallard et al., 1998). Among populations specifically experiencing injury, human agency is a risk factor for greater traumatic stress reactions. No studies have directly compared traumatic stress reactions after intentional and unintentional injury; however, reports have generally yielded findings that traumatic events of a more interpersonal nature, such as victims of physical or sexual assault, experience greater adverse psychological impact than those that do not have that component (Foa, Ehlers, Clark, Tolin, & Orsillo, 1999; Kessler et al., 1995; Norris et al., 2002).

A common public perception is that high-profile mass tragedies like the attacks of September 11, 2001, the Asian tsunami on December 26, 2004, and hurricanes Katrina and Rita in August and September of 2005, respectively, yield particularly high rates of PTSD, but the evidence only partially supports this perception. Following the 9/11 terrorist attacks, initial rates of PTSD in the New York metropolitan area and among those directly exposed to the Pentagon attack in Washington,

D.C., were higher than preexisting community samples, but increased PTSD symptoms were not observed across the rest of the country (Galea et al., 2002; Greiger, Fullerton, & Ursano, 2003; Schlenger et al., 2002). Approximately 60 percent of the New York and Washington, D.C., parents surveyed reported having at least one child upset by the aftermath of September 11 (Schlenger et al., 2002). Psychosocial reactions other than PTSD (depression, general clinical distress) were not more prevalent than community samples (Greiger et al., 2003; Schlenger et al., 2002). Several studies found that individuals experiencing acute reactions of greater intensity were more likely to develop PTSD two to six months later (Grieger et al., 2003; Galea et al., 2002; Simeon, Greenberg, Knutelska, Schmeidler, & Hollander, 2003). By six months after the event, PTSD rates had declined to those expected in existing community samples (Galea et al., 2003). Differences in Manhattanites' use of mental health services before versus after the disaster were not substantial, but individuals panic-stricken during the attack, those with previous stressors, women, and individuals younger than sixty-five years of age experienced an increase in use (Boscarino, Galea, Ahern, Resnick, & Vlahov, 2002).

Public attention is often drawn to high-profile events that capture media attention because of their sudden occurrence, horror, or large numbers of individuals affected. In discerning where public health efforts at prevention or treatment of PTSD should be directed, it may be useful to think of a typology of potentially traumatic events:

> *High profile–low frequency* events that affect large numbers of people simultaneously, such as natural disasters and terrorist attacks
>
> *High profile–high severity* events, especially those that involve assaultive violence, that may have broader public impact even when the number of those directly exposed is relatively small, such as sniper attacks and school shootings
>
> *Low profile–high frequency* events that primarily affect individuals or families one at a time, such as community violence or traffic crashes

Each of these types of events brings a different set of challenges and opportunities for designing, evaluating, and implementing effective PTSD prevention and intervention efforts.

Etiology of Traumatic Stress Reactions

Quantifying the impact of trauma by event types is not enough to explain the range of individual responses to potentially traumatic events. Aspects of the individual's particular experience of a disaster, such as injury, property loss, and fear of death, are much better predictors of psychological outcome than are broad disaster types (Briere & Elliott, 2000). Similarly, the literature on injury and traumatic stress has consistently found that subjective experience of the injury event and its aftermath is a much better predictor of traumatic stress reactions than objective measures of injury severity.

Much traumatic stress research has focused on identifying the risk or resilience factors (both individual and contextual) that affect adaptation and recovery in trauma-exposed individuals. Recent quantitative reviews of the literature have identified key factors that affect adaptation after individual and mass trauma, with largely congruent results. Key risk factors for worse mental health outcomes among adult and child disaster survivors include individual factors such as more severe exposure to the event (injury, life threat, loss), female gender, ethnic minority status, lower socioeconomic status (SES), prior psychiatric history, and less relevant coping experience, as well as contextual factors such as family distress, interpersonal conflict or lack of supportive home atmosphere, living in a disrupted or traumatized community context, and weak or deteriorating social resources (Norris et al., 2002). Among adults exposed to a wide variety of types of trauma, risk factors for the occurrence of PTSD include trauma severity, lack of social support, greater posttrauma life stress, female gender, lower SES, less education, psychiatric history, and history of prior trauma (Brewin, Andrews, & Valentine, 2000). There has not been a similar quantitative review focused on children and adolescents exposed to a full range of (nondisaster) traumatic events; however, the research literature suggests that a similar set of risk and resilience factors is salient for youth and that parent and family responses have a particularly large impact on child recovery from trauma (Foy, Madvig, Pynoos, & Camilleri, 1994).

In addition to identifying and quantifying risk factors for the development of PTSD, researchers and clinicians have attempted to explain the underlying psychological and physiological mechanisms that lead to persistent reexperiencing, avoidance, and arousal symptoms in some individuals exposed to traumatic events. Ideally, prevention and treatment for posttraumatic stress will be grounded in a solid theoretical and empirical understanding of these mechanisms. A thorough review of these models is beyond the scope of this chapter, but excellent reviews of cognitive, developmental, social learning, and other models for understanding etiology of PTSD are available (Meiser-Stedman, 2002; Pynoos, Steinberg, & Piacentini, 1999).

Intervening to Reduce or Prevent PTSS Postinjury

On an individual level, the response of victims following a mass trauma event and that of victims of lower-profile but more common individual traumatic events is much the same. Specific considerations must be taken into account when trauma affects large numbers of people at the same time. In particular, the traumatic event may have a devastating impact on the community, which may affect continued trauma exposure, available resources to assist victims, and resulting social support for the victims. While studies have not specifically investigated the general consequences for peripherally involved communities after mass trauma events, comparing cities across the nation following the terrorist attacks of September 11, geographical proximity to the World Trade Centers at the time of the event predicted PTSD (Schlenger et al., 2002). Following both mass and individual trauma, many victims are distressed; demonstrate avoidance, reexperiencing, and hyperarousal behaviors; and may benefit from early preventive intervention. Many of the potential methods for early intervention and prevention are the same regardless of the type of trauma experienced. We will focus on the example of injury because it is a common type of individual trauma, because injury or threat of injury is a core element of mass trauma, and because it is illustrative of many of the opportunities for intervening to reduce or prevent PTSS. Following the injury example, we will touch on special issues to address following mass trauma.

Events such as traumatic injury provide a relatively unique opportunity for intervention because medical professionals are frequently involved with victims almost immediately after the event. Following traumatic injury, there are several potential entry points for intervention to modify the ensuing PTSS, and some of these interventions are already part of health care practice, though they may not have been framed as PTSS interventions. The case of the Lee family can help illustrate entry points for assessment and intervention.

Although Mrs. Lee was unconscious when the EMS arrived, these first responders could have intervened to mitigate Shane's PTSS by reducing his exposure to further traumatic images. EMS workers often prevent witnesses from further exposure by moving them away from where professionals are working on the injured individual. The EMS worker could have further served as a grounding influence for Mr. Lee by reminding him to use natural coping strategies, such as staying with his sons and calling a trusted friend or neighbor to meet them at the hospital. There is no evidence that there is one set of optimal coping responses effective for all individuals in the aftermath of a traumatic event; however, coping strategies such as social withdrawal or increased use of alcohol or other substances appear to be maladaptive (Vlahov et al., 2002). Best practice suggestions (Litz, Gray, Bryant, & Adler, 2001) include encouraging the use of existing social supports and the provision of psychological first aid (Terrorism and Disaster Branch, National Child Traumatic Stress Network [NCTSN] and National Center for PTSD [NCPTSD], 2005), such as encouraging survivors to eat regularly and return to a normal sleep schedule as much as possible.

Assessment and intervention in the emergency room (ER) offers another opportunity for medical professional involvement to reduce or prevent PTSS. Identifying and addressing a patient's risk for future psychological sequelae during an ER visit for traumatic injury presents many challenges. Chief among these are time limitations, and the difficulty of differentiating normal reactions to trauma from distress reactions that presage continuing problems. The majority of injured individuals will experience some PTSS, but only a portion of these will develop PTSD or other adverse sequelae. Therefore, looking at the more immediate needs of patients, trauma-informed health care professionals should be able to provide basic interventions to patients that will minimize the potential for ongoing trauma and maximize continuity of care. In the case of the Lee family, with Mrs. Lee awake and alert, trauma-informed health care professionals could have made efforts to limit the traumatic aspects of the medical care provided. Explaining medical procedures while they are being performed and allowing family members to be present (when the situation is unlikely to subject them to further traumatic exposure) may be calming and soothing to both the patient and their family.

Conducting a brief formal assessment in the acute care setting is another manner in which professionals can intervene to address PTSS. The Screening Tool for Early Predictors of PTSD (STEPP) has been developed to screen for risk factors for development of PTSD in injured children and their parents. The STEPP can guide clinicians in making evidence-based decisions for allocating scarce mental health resources for traumatic stress (Winston, Kassam-Adams, Garcia-España, Ittenbach, & Cnaan, 2003). While the STEPP may help identify those in need of targeted clinical intervention, the use of resources to provide universal intervention to assist most people who experience some level of distress is also warranted.

For individuals who remain in the hospital, health care professionals should be aware that traumatic stress reactions may interfere with the health and functioning of the patient and may have implications for poorer medical outcomes. Following exposure to traumatic events, patients may be more anxious about medical procedures. Efforts to allow the patient as much control in the situation as possible will facilitate treatment and potentially limit further traumatic exposure. Providing basic education to patients and families about traumatic stress and the potential for reactions to arise when reminders occur, and encouraging the use of established methods of coping, may be simple and effective ways to mitigate the interference that traumatic stress reactions could otherwise have on the patient's health and functioning. For those exhibiting signs of severe distress, initiation of a mental health consultation to provide assistance in coping and teaching specific strategies such as relaxation breathing may be the best interventions.

Following acute treatment in the ER or an inpatient hospital stay, patients are often discharged with instructions to follow up with their primary care provider (PCP). Anticipatory guidance about common traumatic stress symptoms following injury is an intervention that can be incorporated into the standard discharge instructions. Patient information sheets describing PTSS and some ways of coping, as well as a statement about traumatic stress in the medical discharge summary, may be salient reminders for patients and families (Robertson, Klein, Bullen, & Alexander, 2002). Checking in with the family a few weeks after discharge about behavioral and emotional adjustment emphasizes the importance of a good emotional as well as physical recovery. Providing information about local programs or agencies qualified to treat PTSS for those experiencing continued distress yields an additional point for intervention.

Zatzick and colleagues (2004) developed and studied a stepped, collaborative care model for intervening with adult patients following motor vehicle crash and assault injuries. Using a multidisciplinary team based in a trauma center, the authors found that relative to those receiving usual care, fewer patients receiving the collaborative care intervention met criteria for PTSD over time. As a method of intervention, the collaborative care approach depended heavily on specialized mental health professionals. Initially case managers conducted bedside visits. Case managers facilitated entry into the intervention and had contact with patients for assessments. At three months postinjury, care was stepped up for those who were diagnosed with PTSD. As treatment progressed, case managers became less involved with the patient, and the psychologist and psychiatrist executed most of the intervention. This model is an example of extending and expanding a more conventional, clinical intervention to address the needs of acutely injured patients while they are still in the medical setting and continuing to support their connection to care over the course of several months. The collaborative care model places more of the responsibility for continuity of care on the multidisciplinary team of professionals rather than solely on the recently injured patient.

A stepped intervention that employs some of the intervention points described earlier is currently being piloted at the Children's Hospital of Philadelphia to address PTSS following pediatric injury. This manualized approach is evidence-based and focuses on early parent-child interactions. An initial round of screening is performed with child patients and their parents presenting in the ER with all types of unintentional injury, and an informational handout on coping after an injury is provided to the families. Those whose screening scores indicate greater risk for persistent traumatic stress receive brief anticipatory guidance along with the handout and are contacted again in two weeks to assess how the parent and child are coping. Those who report continued distress at follow-up are invited to participate in a one-session preventive intervention geared at increasing parent accuracy in assessing the child's needs, increasing appropriate communication between parent and child, and helping parents provide optimal coping assistance to children. Take-home materials and a follow-up telephone contact help to extend the impact of this single session. This approach is consistent with National Institute of Mental

Health models for best practice in preventive care in matching the degree and type of intervention provided to the individual's level of risk: universal interventions are provided to all individuals exposed to a potentially traumatic event, selected interventions target individuals with identified risk factors who need further assessment or intervention, and indicated treatment is offered to individuals with clear distress or psychopathology (National Institute of Mental Health, 1998).

Improving communication between health care providers along the continuum of postinjury care may provide opportunities for enhancing secondary prevention of persistent PTSS. For example, this type of systems intervention might address the continuity of care through transfer of information from acute to outpatient settings. With appropriate patient permissions, PCPs can be made aware of their patient's acute treatment for traumatic injury and be requested to attend to potential PTSS during the next visit. This may occur through inclusion of traumatic stress information in the surgeon's discharge letter to the patient's PCP or using automated alerts built into electronic medical record systems that alert PCPs when a patient has been treated for an injury. An automated alert system that provides sample assessment questions and assists PCPs in offering anticipatory guidance and information to parents of newly injured children has recently been developed by our team at the Children's Hospital of Philadelphia. PCPs have the opportunity to follow patients over time and may be optimally placed to monitor the patient's reactions after an acute traumatic event such as injury. Persistent and complicated concerns that arise may be referred to the traditional mental health system for intervention.

Outside the medical system, community institutions such as schools and workplaces can help monitor recovery. Communication to the school or work environment from the hospital (with appropriate permission from patients) or from the patient's family can facilitate recovery of the patient or family member. Once released from the hospital, injured patients must reintegrate into their daily lives and routines. This time period represents another intervention point for professionals. As was evidenced in the case example, this transition caused challenges for the Lee family. Shane demonstrated some reexperiencing symptoms and increased irritability, as evidenced by his outburst at school. Informing Shane's teacher and the school nurse or school counselor about Shane's family's experience may help them help him get back into his normal routines at school and provide the extra support he may need during the aftermath of the biking incident. The transition back to school is an excellent opportunity for intervention to promote a healthy recovery. Providing school professionals with empirically based methods of assisting children following such an event can help achieve this goal.

Sometimes children at school are aware of the injury or may have even seen the event take place. Friends and classmates may begin to question whether they will be safe from such an incident or have other reactions to the event. Providing information about common reactions to traumatic injury and instilling the expectation that reactions will go away over time can be an intervention to help schoolmates process the event and move forward with their everyday activities. Such information could be provided in a group format by a school professional like the school nurse or counselor.

Just as reentry into school can be difficult but helpful for a child, returning to work can help an adult recover from a traumatic injury event. Returning to work provides an opportunity for life to return to normal as much as possible after the event. Hospital personnel may partner with the work setting to help anticipate accommodations the individual may need when resuming work responsibilities. Encouraging individuals to share the experience with trusted others at work could yield additional support for any stress at work. Similarly, when individuals can alert a supervisor from the beginning, it may facilitate requests for absence if follow-up appointments are needed to ensure proper healing. These strategies may ease the transition back to work and the return to regular activities, which promotes healing.

Broad-Scale Debriefing Following Mass Trauma Events

Widespread exposure through the news media to mass trauma events evokes in many an emotional response and a desire to reach out to the community. This was exemplified after September 11 when individuals from across the country converged on New York City to offer their services. A popular type of early intervention has been to provide psychological debriefing for those exposed to mass trauma. In some communities, the Brown family and others at the shelter after the hurricane might have been offered the most frequently used and recognized method of debriefing, critical incident stress debriefing (CISD). In this intervention, the goals would have been for Shannon and her mother to learn about stress reactions and adaptive coping, about normal reactions to trauma, for them to process their emotions and share about the event in the group, and, if warranted, possibly to take advantage of further intervention. CISD has also often been offered by agencies and organizations to emergency services providers and first responders as a mandatory session within days of a traumatic event (Mitchell & Everly, 1995). The potential benefit of this approach is that it provides information about reactions to trauma and adaptive ways of coping in a systematic fashion to a large number of people.

While this approach would appear to meet the need to help victims exposed to traumatic events, caution is warranted. The effectiveness of the approach has not been supported by the available empirical evidence (Rose & Bisson, 1998;

Rose, Bisson, & Wessely, 2001), and some evidence suggests it may actually exacerbate subsequent PTSS (Bisson, Jenkins, Alexander, & Bannister, 1997). Further research using more rigorous methodology is needed to identify components of the approach that are useful in modulating the short- and long-term consequences of exposure to trauma for individuals and organizations (Litz et al., 2001).

What alternatives are available for individuals like Shannon, her mother, and others who experienced the hurricane? Within the past several years, researchers have begun to rigorously examine early interventions (for adults) designed to prevent posttraumatic psychological sequelae. This literature suggests the promise of some effective, targeted early interventions (Rauch, Hembree, & Foa, 2001; Rose et al., 2001). To our knowledge, no published study has examined the effectiveness of early interventions for children to prevent later posttraumatic distress. From the adult literature, promising approaches include psychoeducation that promotes natural processes of coping and social support (Litz et al., 2001; Rauch et al., 2001), education about and suggestions for coping with specific reactions such as hyperarousal (Litz et al., 2001; Resnick et al., 2000), and interventions that increase social support and reduce maladaptive coping strategies (Litz et al., 2001; Norris, Byrne, Diaz, & Kaniasty, 2001). The cutting edge of current research and practice in early intervention after a trauma is systematic examination of which interventions work, for whom, during which time period after the trauma, and in which service delivery context (Litz et al., 2001). The adult literature strongly supports the notion of screening trauma-exposed individuals to target interventions to those at most risk rather than universal application of preventive interventions (Litz et al., 2001). Discussion of treatments for PTSD is beyond the scope of this chapter, but interested readers are referred to Foa, Keane, and Friedman (2000) for a comprehensive compendium reviewing many treatment models.

Screening Individuals at Risk for PTSS/PTSD

Many assessment tools are available to identify PTSS and to diagnose PTSD. The most accurate way to ascertain a diagnosis of PTSD is through the use of a structured interview, in which a trained clinician asks a set of standardized questions and, based on the responses, determines whether the individual should be diagnosed with PTSD. Examples of well-validated structured interviews are the Diagnostic Interview for Children and Adolescents (DICA; Welner, Reich, Herjanic, Jung, & Amado, 1987), the Clinician Administered PTSD Scale (CAPS; Blake et al., 1995) and the CAPS for Children and Adolescents (CAPS-CA; Newman & Ribbe, 1996), and the Structured Interview for Disorders of Extreme Stress (SIDES; Pelcovitz et al., 1997). Assessment with such measures requires the time of a specially trained mental health professional. Given that the majority of trauma-exposed individuals ultimately adjust successfully and the scarcity of mental health resources, the use of structured or semistructured interviews to yield a PTSD diagnosis is unlikely to occur outside of specialized mental health service systems and would be an inefficient use of resources if applied to all exposed individuals.

The use of self-report questionnaires to identify those with PTSD symptoms is an economical alternative to conducting thorough evaluations on all trauma-exposed individuals. Questionnaires can be administered by individuals without specialized mental health training, though their interpretation should be guided by a mental health professional. Examples of psychometrically sound self-report measures of PTSS include the UCLA Post-Traumatic Stress Disorder Reaction Index (PTSD-RI; Steinberg, Brymer, Decker, & Pynoos, 2004), the Impact of Events Scale–Revised (IES-R; Weiss & Marmar, 1997), the PTSD Symptom Scale–Self-Report (PSS-SR; Wohlfarth, Van den Brink, Winkel, & Ter Smitten, 2003), the Posttraumatic Diagnostic Scale (PTDS; Foa, Cashman, Jaycox, & Perry, 1997), the Child PTSD Symptom Scale (CPSS; Foa, Johnson, Feeny, & Treadwell, 2001), the PTSD Checklist (PCL; Ruggiero, Del Ben, Scott, & Rabalais, 2003), and the Acute Stress Checklist for Children (ASC-KIDS; Kassam-Adams, in press).

A less formal approach to screening involves inquiring about the individual's experience of the incident and resources for coping with the event in the course of conversation. A recently developed protocol for emergency and acute care health professionals emphasizes ways of integrating professional response to traumatic stress into the course of care with the *D-E-F* mnemonic: *D*istress, *E*motional support, and *F*amily (National Child Traumatic Stress Network, 2004). At the scene or in the aftermath of a traumatic event, first responders such as police officers, emergency medical technicians (EMTs), rescue workers, and health care professionals must focus their attention on the most basic responsibilities (the *A-B-Cs; a*irway, *b*reath sounds, and *c*irculation) of their job: ensuring the safety of the scene and attending to the physical well-being of the victim. When the *A-B-Cs* are accomplished, these professionals can focus on the *D-E-F* to promote the victim's psychosocial recovery: attending to the individual's distress, ensuring the individual has adequate emotional support, and providing support for the family (Exhibit 19.1).

Preventive intervention messages following this type of assessment have as a primary goal educating the individual and family about the common range of reactions following an event. It can be helpful to reassure the individual that feeling upset or frightened for a while, thinking about the incident when not wanting to, or feeling jumpy are common reactions in the first few days and weeks following a traumatic event. It is useful to plan for ways they can help themselves and ensure that social support is present during the recovery process. When reactions are

EXHIBIT 19.1. INFORMAL ASSESSMENT QUESTIONS TO GAUGE PTSS AND PSYCHOSOCIAL NEEDS IN THE AFTERMATH OF A TRAUMATIC EVENT.

1. Ask about the meaning and impact of the experience for the individual:
   - "What was it like for you when [*fill in incident here*] happened?"

   Listen for:
   - Whether the individual describes feeling terrified or horrified by what occurred.

2. Assess general coping:
   - "How are you doing since the experience?"

   Listen for:
   - Whether the individual has a plan to deal with upsetting emotions and whether she is able to invoke her plan.

3. Help contextualize the individual's experience and assess coping resources:
   - "Most people feel upset or jumpy after a scary event like you experienced. What are some ways you have to soothe yourself or help yourself feel better?"

   Listen for:
   - Healthy methods like taking a bath or talking with friends as opposed to maladaptive methods like extreme social withdrawal or increased use of alcohol or drugs.

4. Assess social support:
   - "Who do you have to talk to about what happened?"

   Listen for:
   - An indication that the individual has at least one person to talk to.

severe, are significantly interfering with the individual's functioning, and do not appear amenable to the intervention described, a referral to a mental health professional or agency that treats individuals with PTSD is prudent. Therefore, access to good mental health resources is necessary for those conducting screening in the aftermath of trauma.

There are several benefits to having professionals who are not mental health specialists, such as police officers, EMTs, nurses, or rescue workers, conduct screenings. First, having these other professionals conduct screening can help to destigmatize the reactions of the potentially traumatized individual. When seen as part of routine treatment following a traumatic experience, the victim may not view the inquiry in a threatening manner. Second, the use of non–mental health professionals to conduct the screenings allows mental health professionals to focus efforts on treatment of those experiencing the greatest need. Third, many first-responder professionals are genuinely concerned with the impact of events on those they see and welcome training in incorporating responses to trauma victims if these responses are easily integrated into current practice and do not increase time demands. A challenge in light of scarce mental health resources is to identify the referral and consultation resources that would allow these professionals a sense of closure knowing that those in need can get help.

Screening by first-responder professionals following a trauma may be an efficient way to identify those in need of further services, but many individuals are exposed to trauma that goes undetected by professionals or agencies. Individuals exposed to domestic violence when the police were not called, those witnessing neighborhood violence, or those experiencing a very scary injury that did not need medical intervention may not come to the attention of professionals who could intervene. Most of these individuals will experience some distress, but they will return to baseline functioning over time. Those who do not, however, are a difficult group to reach to ensure proper assessment and intervention. As with many other public health concerns, one place to access many of these individuals is in primary care doctors' offices.

PCPs have increasingly incorporated screening for health concerns, such as levels of lead in the blood, child abuse and neglect, domestic violence, drug and alcohol abuse, and even depression in adult populations, during primary care visits. This venue has become a useful outlet for addressing such concerns because of the frequency with which individuals visit their PCP and because of the safety of discussing these issues with a respected professional with whom the individual has an established relationship. Primary care can also be a good setting for assessment of exposure to traumatic experiences and traumatic stress reactions. In the context of an established relationship between patient and PCP, the assessment can be conducted with a few brief questions, and when a referral is necessary, the PCP, often the gatekeeper to mental health treatment, can provide it. One important hurdle is that the amount of information the PCP must cover before addressing mental health concerns often exceeds the time available in scheduled visits.

The issue of traumatic stress reactions in primary care settings has received some attention in the literature. Incidence of full or partial PTSD in the primary care setting suggests that attention to this mental health concern is warranted. In adults, between 11.8 and 31.0 percent of primary care patients were found to have PTSD (Lang, Laffaye, Satz, Dresselhaus, & Stein, 2003; Stein, McQuaid, Pedrelli, Lenox, & McCahill, 2000), and 23 percent of children in a pediatric ambulatory clinic were identified as having PTSD (Cohen & Mannarino, 2003). An alternative to using the PCP's clinical time to conduct a screen for traumatic exposure and traumatic stress responses has examined the use of self-report scales. Two such self-report scales, the PTSD Checklist and the Beck Anxiety Inventory–Primary Care, have been used and positively evaluated as screeners for detecting PTSD in primary care settings (Lang et al., 2003; Mori et al., 2003; Stein et al., 2000). Their relatively brief format, requiring about five to seven minutes of the patient's time, and the efficiency with which they can be scored and evaluated with respect to the traumatic stress reactions of the patient make these self-report screeners viable as a means to evaluate PTSD in primary care. Further evaluation of the feasibility of assessing trauma exposure and traumatic stress reactions in primary care is necessary, and particular attention should be focused on developing the most efficient methods to assess the problem. As more efficient assessment methods become available, primary care screening for PTSD, like other public health concerns, can become a reality.

Conclusion and Future Research

The behavioral and emotional reactions of individuals exposed to frightening and extremely distressing events can be understood as traumatic stress reactions following a traumatic event. These reactions are common, occurring in most exposed individuals, but they often resolve over time. The prevalence and impact of PTSS and PTSD following traumatic exposure highlight the broad scope and intense nature of this issue. Given the high percentage of individuals experiencing lifetime incidence of exposure to traumatic events and the preponderance of individuals who suffer at least temporary distress following exposure, PTSS and PTSD are public health concerns.

Research and clinical findings have highlighted the initial adverse effect of traumatic events, including reexperiencing of the event and general hypervigilance occurring in trauma-exposed individuals. As noted, most initial distress resolves with time, but a significant minority of individuals will endure persistent, and perhaps chronic, symptoms associated with the traumatic experience. Behavioral scientists have become increasingly involved in research on preventing potentially traumatic events ranging from HIV infection to intentional and unintentional injury (Snider & Satcher, 1997), and translating these findings into public health initiatives aimed at preventing exposure to these events (Gielen & Sleet, 2004). Empirically-supported treatments are available to intervene with individuals diagnosed with PTSD. However, the nature of PTSS and PTSD, and the symptoms that follow exposure to a traumatic event, make secondary preventive intervention an important goal in reducing adverse reactions to trauma.

In this chapter, we have highlighted the role behavioral scientists have played in developing screening techniques to identify exposed individuals at risk for developing PTSS/PTSD (Blake et al., 1995; Foa et al., 2001; Steinberg et al., 2004; Welner, Reich, Herjanic, Jung, & Amado, 1987; Winston et al., 2003) to improve the efficiency of secondary preventive intervention. An important contribution of behavioral science is ensuring that screening techniques take into account the logistical and other challenges faced by those attempting to implement screening. Thus, we have highlighted nontraditional approaches that may be used to address traumatic stress reactions, including intervention by first responders and medical professionals (National Child Traumatic Stress Network, 2004). These innovations are empirically grounded, but they require additional research to validate their efficacy.

Uniform intervention in the form of psychological debriefing with all trauma-exposed individuals has not proven itself effective in reducing traumatic stress reactions. However, elements of debriefing approaches may have effective components that can be adapted for modified approaches to secondary prevention. Research that investigates individual aspects of psychological debriefing to determine whether there are positive, active ingredients to the intervention can facilitate development of more effective early interventions. Also in their secondary prevention role, behavioral scientists have developed promising targeted early interventions (Rauch et al., 2001; Rose et al., 2001): psychoeducation strategies promoting the natural processes of coping and social support and reducing maladaptive coping strategies (Litz et al., 2001; Norris et al., 2001; Rauch et al., 2001) and anticipatory guidance around specific reactions (Litz et al., 2001; Resnick et al., 2000).

To identify those in greatest need of intervention, development and identification of brief screening instruments, with strong predictive validity, which can be used by non–mental health specialists, will be an important contribution to the field. This may take the form of self-report instruments or identifying key questions that can help professionals determine which individuals are at greatest risk of developing PTSD and, thus, most in need of intervention.

In addition to screening for risk, development and assessment of interventions immediately posttrauma is an important research goal for traumatic stress studies. We have highlighted opportunities that exist for intervention, particularly in the medical system, that involve modification to existing methods of treatment that theoretically can serve to mitigate traumatic stress reactions. However, to assess their effectiveness, interventions need to be systematically examined to determine which interventions work, for whom, at what point in time, and administered in which service delivery context. Traditional interventions continue to be developed to address PTSD, but the effectiveness of the unique opportunity to intervene soon after trauma exposure is important to harness because of the proximity of treating professionals around the time of exposure. It is important not to waste these valuable resources.

There are many research opportunities for assessment and early intervention for posttraumatic stress reactions. The interdisciplinary nature of intervention surrounding trauma exposure creates exciting new approaches to combine injury prevention and mental health skills to address this mental health concern. With the large percentage of individuals exposed to traumatic experiences, development of effective assessment and intervention tools can have a wide-reaching impact on injury prevention and public health.

References

Aaron, J., Zaglul, H., & Emery, R. E. (1999). Posttraumatic stress in children following acute physical injury. *Journal of Pediatric Psychology, 24*(4), 335–343.

American Psychiatric Association. (2004). *Diagnostic and Statistical Manual of Mental Disorders, 4th edition, Text Revision (DSM-IV-TR)*. Washington, DC: Author.

Baur, K. M., Hardy, P. E., & Van Dorsten, B. (1998). Posttraumatic stress disorder in burn populations: A critical review of the literature. *Journal of Burn Care and Rehabilitation, 19*(3), 230–240.

Bisson, J. I., Jenkins, P. L., Alexander, J., & Bannister, C. (1997). Randomised controlled trial of psychological debriefing for victims of acute burn trauma. *British Journal of Psychiatry, 171*, 78–81.

Blake, D. D., Weathers, F. W., Nagy, L. M., Kaloupek, D. G., Gusman, F. D., Charney, D. S., & Keane, T. M. (1995). The development of a clinician-administered PTSD scale. *Journal of Trauma, 8*(1), 75–90.

Boscarino, J. A., Galea, S., Ahern, J., Resnick, H., & Vlahov, D. (2002). Utilization of mental health services following the September 11th terrorist attacks in Manhattan, New York City. *International Journal of Emergency Mental Health, 4*, 143–155.

Breslau, N. (2001). The epidemiology of posttraumatic stress disorder: What is the extent of the problem? *Journal of Clinical Psychiatry, 62*(Suppl. 17), 16–22.

Brewin, C. R., Andrews, B., & Valentine, J. D. (2000). Meta-analysis of risk factors for posttraumatic stress disorder in trauma-exposed adults. *Journal of Clinical and Consulting Psychology, 68*(5), 748–766.

Briere, J., & Elliott, D. (2000). Prevalence, characteristics, and long-term sequelae of natural disaster exposure in the general population. *Journal of Traumatic Stress, 13*(4), 661–680.

Cohen, J. A., & Mannarino, A. P. (2003). *Posttraumatic stress in primary care*. Paper presented at the Society for Developmental and Behavioral Pediatrics, Pittsburgh, PA.

Daviss, W., Racusin, R., Fleischer, A., Mooney, D., Ford, J., & McHugo, G. (2000). Acute stress disorder symptomatology during hospitalization for pediatric injury. *Journal of the American Academy of Child and Adolescent Psychiatry, 39*(5), 569–575.

Foa, E. B., Cashman, L., Jaycox, L., & Perry, K. (1997). The validation of a self-report measure of posttraumatic stress disorder: The Posttraumatic Diagnostic Scale. *Psychological Assessment, 9*(4), 445–451.

Foa, E., Ehlers, A., Clark, D., Tolin, D., & Orsillo, S. (1999). The posttraumatic cognitions inventory (PTCI): Development and validation. *Psychological Assessment, 11*(3), 303–314.

Foa, E., Johnson, K., Feeny, N., & Treadwell, K. (2001). The Child PTSD Symptom Scale: A preliminary examination of its psychometric properties. *Journal of Clinical Child Psychology, 30*(3), 376–384.

Foa, E., Keane, T., & Friedman, M. (Eds.). (2000). *Effective treatments for PTSD: Practice guidelines from the International Society for Traumatic Stress Studies.* New York: Guilford Press.

Foy, D., Madvig, B., Pynoos, R., & Camilleri, A. (1994). Etiologic factors in the development of posttraumatic stress disorder in children and adolescents. *Journal of School Psychology, 34*(2), 133–145.

Galea, S., Ahern, J., Resnick, H., Kilpatrick, D., Bucuvalas, M., Gold, J., & Vlahov, D. (2002). Psychological sequelae of the September 11 terrorist attacks in New York City. *New England Journal of Medicine, 346*, 982–987.

Gielen, A. C., & Sleet, D. (2003). Application of behavior-change theories and methods to injury prevention. *Epidemiologic Reviews, 25*, 65–76.

Giaconia, R., Reinherz, H., Silverman, A., Pakiz, B., Frost, A., & Cohen, E. (1995). Traumas and posttraumatic stress disorder in a community population of older adolescents. *Journal of American Child and Adolescent Psychiatry, 34*(10), 1369–1380.

Gill, A.S.C. (2002). Risk factors for pediatric posttraumatic stress disorder after traumatic injury. *Archives of Psychiatric Nursing, 16*(4), 168–175.

Grieger, T. A., Fullerton, C. S., & Ursano, R. J. (2003). Posttraumatic stress disorder, alcohol use, and perceived safety after the terrorist attack on the Pentagon. *Psychiatric Services, 54*, 1380–1382.

Kassam-Adams, N. (in press). The acute stress checklist for children (ASC-Kids): Development of a child self-report measure. *Journal of Traumatic Stress.*

Kassam-Adams, N., & Winston, F. K. (2004). Predicting child PTSD: The relationship between ASD and PTSD in injured children. *Journal of the American Academy of Child and Adolescent Psychiatry, 43*(4), 403–411.

Kessler, R. C. (2000). Posttraumatic stress disorder: The burden to the individual and to society. *Journal of Clinical Psychiatry, 61*, 4–12.

Kessler, R. C., Sonnega, A., Bromet, E., Hughes, M., & Nelson, C. B. (1995). Posttraumatic stress disorder in national comorbidity survey. *Archives of General Psychiatry, 52*(12), 1048–1060.

Kilpatrick, D. G., Ruggiero, K. J., Acierno, R., Saunders, B. E., Resnick, H. S., & Best, C. L. (2003). Violence and risk of PTSD, major depression, substance abuse/dependence, and comorbidity: Results from the National Survey of Adolescents. *Journal of Consulting and Clinical Psychology, 71*(4), 692–700.

Lang, A. J., Laffaye, C., Satz, L. E., Dresselhaus, T. R., & Stein, M. B. (2003). Sensitivity and specificity of the PTSD checklist in detecting PTSD in female veterans in primary care. *Journal of Traumatic Stress, 16*(3), 257–264.

Litz, B., Gray, M., Bryant, R., & Adler, A. (2001). Early intervention for trauma: Current status and future directions. *Clinical Psychology: Science and Practice, 9*, 112–134.

Marshall, R., Olfson, M., Hellman, F., Blanco, C., Guardino, M., & Struening, E. (2001). Comorbidity, impairment, and suicidality in subthreshhold PTSD. *American Journal of Psychiatry, 158*, 1467–1473.

Meiser-Stedman, R. (2002). Towards a cognitive-behavioral model of PTSD in children and adolescents. *Clinical Child and Family Psychology, 5*(4), 217–232.

Mitchell, J. T., & Everly, G. S. (1995). *Critical incident stress debriefing: An operations manual for the prevention of traumatic stress among emergency services and disaster workers.* Ellicott City, MD: Chevron.

Mori, D. L., Lambert, J. F., Niles, B. L., Orlander, J. D., Grace, M., & LoCastro, J. S. (2003). The BAI-PC as a screen for anxiety, depression, and PTSD in primary care. *Journal of Clinical Psychology in Medical Settings, 10*(3), 187–192.

National Child Traumatic Stress Network. (2004). *Pediatric medical traumatic stress toolkit.* Retrieved Oct. 23, 2005, from http://www.nctsn.org/nccts/nav.do?pid=hom_main.

National Institute of Mental Health. (1998). *Priorities for prevention research at NIMH.* Bethesda, MD: Author.

Newman, E., & Ribbe, D. (1996). Psychometric review of the clinician-administered PTSD Scale for Children. In B. Stamm (Ed.), *Measurement of stress, trauma and adaptation.* Lutherville, MD: Sidran Press.

Norris, F. (1992). Epidemiology of trauma: Frequency and impact of different potentially traumatic events on different demographic groups. *Journal of Consulting and Clinical Psychology, 60*(3), 409–418.

Norris, F., Byrne, C., Diaz, E., & Kaniasty, K. (2001). *Psychosocial resources in the aftermath of natural and human-caused disasters: A review of the empirical literature, with implications for intervention.* White River Junction, VT: National Center for Post-Traumatic Stress Disorder.

Norris, F. H., Friedman, M. J., Watson, P. J., Byrne, C. M., Diaz, E., & Kaniasty, K. (2002). Sixty thousand disaster victims speak: Part I. An empirical review of the empirical literature, 1981–2001. *Psychiatry, 65*(3), 207–239.

Norris, F. H., Perilla, J. L., Riad, J. K., Kaniasty, K. Z., & Lavizzo, E. A. (1999). Stability and change in stress, resources, and psychological distress following natural disaster: Findings from Hurricane Andrew. *Anxiety, Stress, and Coping, 12*(4), 363–396.

Pelcovitz, D., van der Kolk, B., Roth, S., Mandel, F., Kaplan, S., & Resick, P. (1997). Development of a criteria set and a structured interview for disorders of extreme stress (SIDES). *Journal of Traumatic Stress, 10*(1), 3–16.

Pynoos, R. S., Steinberg, A. M., & Piacentini, J. C. (1999). A developmental psychopathology model of childhood traumatic stress and intersection with anxiety disorders. *Biological Psychiatry, 46*(11), 1542–1554.

Rauch, S., Hembree, E., & Foa, E. (2001). Acute psychosocial preventive interventions for posttraumatic stress disorder. *Advances in Mind-Body Medicine, 17*(3), 187–190.

Resnick, H., Acierno, R., Holmes, M., Dammeyer, M., & Kilpatrick, D. (2000). Emergency evaluation and intervention with female victims of rape and other violence. *Journal of Clinical Psychology, 56*, 1317–1333.

Richmond, T. S. (1997). An explanatory model of variables influencing postinjury disability. *Nursing Research, 46*(5), 262–269.

Robertson, C., Klein, S., Bullen, H., & Alexander, D. A. (2002). An evaluation of patient satisfaction with an information leaflet for trauma survivors. *Journal of Traumatic Stress, 15*(4), 329–332.

Rose, S., & Bisson, J. (1998). Brief early psychological interventions following trauma: A systematic review of the literature. *Journal of Traumatic Stress, 11*(4), 697–710.

Rose, S., Bisson, J., & Wessely, S. (2001). *Psychological debriefing for preventing post traumatic stress disorder (PTSD).* Oxford: Update Software.

Roy-Byrne, P. P., Russo, J. E., Michelson, E., Zatzick, D. F., Pitman, R. K., & Berliner, L. (2004). Risk factors and outcome in ambulatory assault victims presenting to the acute emergency department setting: Implications for secondary prevention studies in PTSD. *Depression and Anxiety, 19,* 77–84.

Ruggiero, K. J., Del Ben, K., Scott, J. R., & Rabalais, A. E. (2003). Psychometric properties of the PTSD Checklist–Civilian Version. *Journal of Traumatic Stress, 16*(5), 495–502.

Saxe, G. N., Stoddard, F. J., Courtney, D., Cunningham, K., Chawla, N., Sheridan, R. L., King, D. W., & King, L. A. (2001). Relationship between acute morphine and the course of PTSD in children with burns. *Journal of the American Academy of Child and Adolescent Psychiatry, 40*(8), 915–921.

Schlenger, W. E., Caddell, J. M., Ebert, L., Jordan, B. K., Rourke, K. M., Wilson, D., Thalji, L., Dennis, J. M., Fairbank, J. A., & Kulka, R. A. (2002). Psychological reactions to terrorist attacks: Findings from the National Study of Americans' Reactions to September 11. *Journal of American Medical Association, 288,* 581–588.

Schnurr, P. (1996). Trauma, PTSD, and physical health. *PTSD Research Quarterly of the National Center for PTSD, 7*(3), 1–6.

Schnurr, P. P., Friedman, M. J., & Bernardy, N. C. (2002). Research on posttraumatic stress disorder: Epidemiology, pathophysiology, and assessment. *Journal of Clinical Psychology, 58*(8), 877–889.

Simeon, D., Greenberg, J., Knutelska, M., Schmeidler, J., & Hollander, E. (2003). Peritraumatic reactions associated with the World Trade Center disaster. *American Journal of Psychiatry, 160,* 1702–1705.

Snider, D. E., & Satcher, D. (1997). Behavioral and social sciences at the Centers for Disease Control and Prevention. *American Psychologist, 52*(2), 140–142.

Stallard, P., Velleman, R., & Baldwin, S. (1998). Prospective study of post-traumatic stress disorder in children involved in road traffic accidents. *British Medical Journal, 317,* 1619–1623.

Stein, M. B., McQuaid, J. R., Pedrelli, P., Lenox, R., & McCahill, M. E. (2000). Posttraumatic stress disorder in the primary care medical setting. *General Hospital Psychiatry, 22,* 261–269.

Stein, M., Walker, J., Hazen, A., & Forde, D. (1997). Full and partial posttraumatic stress disorder: Findings from a community survey. *American Journal of Psychiatry, 154*(8), 1114–1119.

Steinberg, A., Brymer, M., Decker, K., & Pynoos, R. (2004). The University of California at Los Angeles post-traumatic stress disorder reaction index. *Current Psychiatry Reports, 6*(2), 96–100.

Terrorism and Disaster Branch, National Child Traumatic Stress Network and National Center for PTSD. (2005). *Psychological first aid field operations guide.* Retrieved Oct. 23, 2005, from http://www.nctsn.org/nccts/nav.do?pid=hom_main.

Van Loey, N.E.E., Maas, C.J.M., Faber, A. W., & Taal, L. A. (2003). Predictors of chronic posttraumatic stress symptoms following burn injury: Results of a longitudinal study. *Journal of Traumatic Stress, 16*(4), 361–369.

Vlahov, D., Galea, S., Resnick, H. S., Ahern, J., Boscarino, J. A., Bucuvalas, M. J., Gold, J., & Kilpatrick, D. G. (2002). Increased use of cigarettes, alcohol, and marijuana among Manhattan, New York, residents after the September 11th terrorist attacks. *American Journal of Epidemiology, 155*(11), 988–996.

Walker, E., Katon, W., Russo, J., Ciechanowski, P., Newman, E., & Wagner, A. (2003). Health care costs associated with posttraumatic stress disorder symptoms in women. *Archives of General Psychiatry, 60,* 369–374.

Weiss, D. S., & Marmar, C. R. (1997). The Impact of Events Scale–Revised. In J. P. Wilson & T. M. Keane (Eds.), *Assessing psychological trauma and PTSD* (pp. 399–411). New York: Guilford Press.

Welner, Z., Reich, W., Herjanic, B., Jung, K. G., & Amado, H. (1987). Reliability, validity, and parent-child agreement studies of the Diagnostic Interview for Children and Adolescents (DICA). *Journal of the American Academy of Child & Adolescent Psychiatry, 26*(5), 649–653.

Winston, F., Kassam-Adams, N., Garcia-España, J. F., Ittenbach, R., & Cnaan, A. (2003). Screening for risk of persistent posttraumatic stress in injured children and their parents. *JAMA, 290,* 643–649.

Winston, F. K., Kassam-Adams, N., Vivarelli-O'Neill, C., Ford, J. D., Newman, E., Baxt, C., Stafford, P., & Cnaan, A. (2002). Acute stress disorder symptoms in children and their parents after pediatric traffic injury. *Pediatrics, 109*(6), e90.

Wohlfarth, T. D., Van den Brink, W., Winkel, F. W., & Ter Smitten, M. (2003). Screening for posttraumatic stress disorder: An evaluation of two self-report scales among crime victims. *Psychological Assessment, 15*(1), 101–109.

Zatzick, D., Roy-Byrne, P., Russo, J., Rivara, F., Droesch, R., Wagner, A., Dunn, C., Jurkovich, G., Uehara, E., & Katon, W. (2004). A randomized effectiveness trial of stepped collaborative care for acutely injured trauma survivors. *Archives of General Psychiatry, 61*(5), 498–506.

Zink, K. A., & McCain, G. C. (2003). Post-traumatic stress disorder in children and adolescents with motor vehicle–related injuries. *Journal for Specialists in Pediatric Nursing, 8*(3), 99–106.

CHAPTER TWENTY

LAW, BEHAVIOR, AND INJURY PREVENTION

Frederic E. Shaw, Christopher P. Ogolla

Since the 1970s, injury experts have recognized the importance of law as a critical element in behavior change, and innovations in injury law have brought many successes. Laws requiring automobile occupants to wear safety belts have dramatically reduced the risk of serious injury and death in crashes. Laws requiring helmet use have reduced traumatic brain injuries. Pool fencing laws have prevented toddlers from drowning. Laws that extend the licensing age for teen drivers have reduced automobile-related injuries. Indeed, the word *injury* itself comes from the Latin *in-juris*, which literally means "not law" or "not right."

Burris (1999) has identified the four roles of law in society: (1) governing and protecting the possession and transfer of wealth and goods, (2) endowing (or failing to endow) individuals with rights that equip them to avoid disease (and injury), (3) providing settings (legislatures, bureaucracies, courts) and a vocabulary for debating important social issues, and (4) regulating the meaning of identities and behaviors, categorizing some as favored and others as disfavored. Law intertwines with injury prevention in each of these roles.

Law does not function in isolation from other modalities or strategies for behavioral change. Indeed, the successes attributable to law are in part related to the fact that law has an educational and promotional component. Law is an effective complement to other behavior change efforts, such as education and persuasion.

In this chapter, we examine the basis of the law of injury prevention and how law can change the behaviors and actions of individuals, corporations, and populations. We then comment on the main wellspring of law, the legislatures, and how lawmakers are influenced to create new laws that affect injury-related behaviors.

Law and the U.S. Legal System

Laws are the rules by which members of society have agreed to live as part of a social contract. The philosopher Thomas Hobbes envisioned a lawless world as an unnerving place: "no letters; no society; and which is worst of all, continual fear, and danger of violent death; and the life of man, solitary, poor, nasty, brutish, and short" (Hobbes, 1986). To avoid this fate, we agree collectively to obey the commands of legitimate democratic government. In return, we gain the protection and comforts of living in civil society (Mill, 1860).

For public health, this rationale for law is crystallized in the landmark U.S. Supreme Court case, *Jacobson* v. *Massachusetts* (1905). The case arose when, during a smallpox outbreak in 1902, a local preacher in Cambridge, Massachusetts, refused on principle to submit to mandatory vaccination. He was tried, convicted, and fined five dollars. Rather than pay the fine, he appealed his conviction through the state courts to the U.S. Supreme Court.

In the *Jacobson* opinion, the Supreme Court denied Jacobson's appeal and set out a principle that underlies nearly all of public health law (citing *Crowley* v. *Christensen*, 1890, pp. 26–27): "The possession and enjoyment of all rights are subject to such reasonable conditions as may be deemed by the governing authority of the country essential to the safety, health, peace, good order and morals of the community. Even liberty itself, the greatest of all rights, is not an unrestricted license to act according to one's own will."

Laws are usually written in terms of duties and rights. The most fundamental rights in U.S. law are defined by the U.S. Constitution and the state constitutions. Rights can also be granted by federal, state, or local lawmaking bodies in treaties, statutes, regulations, or ordinances. And they can be viewed in a moral, legal, or economic and utilitarian context (Holmes, 1897).

Underlying the law is the concept of justice, which implies noninterference, moral rightness, equality, and the idea that no person should be placed at a disadvantage except for fault and according to established procedure. The concept of justice comes to American law through the Declaration of Independence, which states that "all men are created equal; that they are endowed by their Creator with certain unalienable rights," and "among these are life, liberty, and the pursuit of happiness."

At the top of the legal hierarchy is the Constitution, the supreme law of the land. All legal powers flow from this single document. Other subordinate sources

of law are treaties and federal statutes adopted by Congress, administrative regulations made by federal agencies under a delegation of authority from Congress,
presidential executive orders, state constitutions, state statutes passed by state legislatures, and state administrative regulations adopted by state executive agencies.
Underlying nearly all American law is the common law, a system of judge-made
law inherited from Great Britain and interpreted by courts for hundreds of years.

Judicial courts of appeal also make law in the sense that they settle disputes
and, in doing so, create precedents that must be followed by lower courts under
the legal principle of *stare decisis* (Latin, "to stand by the decision"). This principle
creates stability in the law because judges within a jurisdiction, whether state or
federal, are obliged to follow precedents established by their own appellate courts.
For example, if a state supreme court upheld an act by the legislature requiring
motorcyclists to wear helmets, all lower courts in the state would be bound by this
decision.

The Constitution and Federalism

The U.S. Constitution is the highest law of the nation, and no statute (a written
law passed by Congress or a state legislature), treaty, ordinance (a local written law),
regulation (an administrative rule with the force of law adopted by a federal or state
agency), or judicial ruling may stand if it contravenes the Constitution. The Constitution sets out the structure of the U.S. government and defines the roles of the
federal government, the states, and the various political entities within them.

A theme within the Constitution is division of power. The constitutional
drafters wished to create a central government of limited, enumerated powers
and reserve the balance of powers to the states. Article I, section 1 of the Constitution endows Congress not with *all* legislative power but with "the legislative powers herein granted." Thus, in the U.S. political system, the federal government has
only the powers specifically listed in the Constitution, such as the power to lay and
collect taxes, borrow money, and regulate commerce with foreign nations and
among the states. Powers not mentioned in the Constitution remain with the states
(although the so-called elastic clause in Article I, section 8 gives Congress the
power to "make all laws which shall be necessary and proper" for carrying out
the powers and purposes of the Constitution). One power retained by the states
is the police power, the general power of the states to keep order and protect the
health and safety of their own populations. The majority of public health powers are a subset of the police power. The police power of the states is strong and
broad—strong because it is only rarely limited by the courts (see *Queenside Hills Co.
v. Saxl*, 1946) and broad because it is absolute, so long as it does not violate the
federal Constitution.

Federalism refers to the sharing of power between the states and the federal government. Under our constitutional scheme, the states' sovereignty preceded, and was not disturbed by, the establishment of the federal government. When the Constitution was ratified, the states ceded specific powers to the federal government. The sovereignty of the states was later guaranteed by the ratification of the Tenth Amendment, which states, "The powers not delegated to the United States by the Constitution, nor prohibited by it to the States, are reserved to the States respectively, or to the people."

Although the states have control over the majority of public health matters within their borders through their police power, the federal government has exerted strong influence over public health since the early years of the Republic (Parmet, 2002), mainly by using two of its enumerated powers: the power to regulate interstate commerce and the spending power (Art. I, sec. 8). Courts have interpreted the interstate commerce power broadly, and this interpretation has allowed the federal government to expand its authority. Congress's spending power allows the federal government to place conditions on monetary grants to the states in order to promote actions it wishes the states to take. It is a powerful lever, because few states are in a position to refuse federal largess. In daily practice, the division of public health powers between the federal government and the states is a cooperative and pragmatic one, with the federal government mainly concerned with external and interstate threats and the states concerned mainly with threats inside their own borders.

Individual Rights

As noted previously about the *Jacobson* case, public health practice often involves a legal tension between the liberty of individual persons and the duty of the state to protect the whole population. In the United States, individual rights are protected by the Bill of Rights, which are the first ten amendments to the Constitution, ratified in 1791. Of the amendments, the First, Second, Fourth, Fifth, Tenth, plus a later amendment, the Fourteenth dovetail with public health.

The Fifth and Fourteenth Amendments guarantee that the government (whether federal or state) cannot deprive persons of "life, liberty, or property, without due process of law." At its essence, this means that the government cannot deprive persons of these possessions in an arbitrary or capricious way. Due process is a constant concern in public health practice, and especially in injury control, because promoting injury prevention behaviors (such as requiring safety belt use) often involves interfering with the liberty of individual persons.

Courts divide the right of due process into two categories: procedural and substantive due process. *Procedural due process* means that the government may not

deprive a person of life, liberty, or property without going through a fair proce-
dure, including at a minimum, notice, a hearing, and an impartial decision maker.
Substantive due process goes beyond procedure to the rationale for the deprivation.
It means that the government must have a justification for interference.

Liberty is the interest most often implicated in public health law. The
Supreme Court has defined liberty to be more than just physical freedom; it includes among others such basic rights as the right to contract, engage in an oc-
cupation, acquire useful knowledge, marry, establish a home, and raise children
(*Meyer* v. *State of Nebraska*, 1923). The oft-debated right to privacy, typified by cases
such as *Griswold* v. *Connecticut* and *Roe* v. *Wade*, originates in substantive due process.

The Regulatory State

Congress or state legislatures can create laws directly by passing statutes or indirectly through statutory delegations to administrative agencies. The second
method, and the body of law that surrounds it, is called *administrative law*. Because
the majority of public health law is embodied in delegations of authority to executive agencies, it is often considered a branch of administrative law.

In injury prevention, the creation of administrative rules is sometimes preferred over the creation of statutes. Rule making is viewed as preferable to legislation for addressing complex structural or behavioral standards because
legislatures are not well suited to developing detailed technical rules, such as specifications for the construction of residential swimming pool fences. Sometimes the
regulatory route is preferred because it is seen as less susceptible to influence or
pressure from special interest groups. Legislatures sometimes delegate rule making to administrative agencies when they wish the final decisions to be insulated
from political criticism (Mendeloff, 1988).

A century ago, legislatures would be more likely to address social problems
by direct action—through the adoption of statutes. However, as society and government have become larger and more complex, legislatures have increasingly
delegated public health actions to administrative agencies. Thus, over time, law
has become less statutory and more regulatory (Breyer & Stewart, 1992). This is
especially true in injury law, as manifested by rules for consumer safety and auto
safety, which set legal standards for how products or cars are built or perform.

After regulations have been adopted, they may be challenged in court by parties who are aggrieved by them, and courts may invalidate regulations if they
violate constitutional standards or statutory requirements. For example, under
the federal Administrative Procedure Act, first adopted in 1946, which controls
some federal rule making, a reviewing court must set aside any agency action that
is "arbitrary, capricious, an abuse of discretion, or otherwise not in accordance

with law"; "contrary to constitutional right, power, privilege, or immunity"; or "in excess of statutory jurisdiction, authority, or limitations, or short of statutory right" (Administrative Procedure Act, §706, 2005). In practice, courts seldom hold that public health regulations are unconstitutional. As Richards and Rathbun (1998) have observed, courts show great deference to public health agencies, in large part because courts do not have the expertise to make decisions on highly technical matters.

Role of Law in Injury Prevention

Law can affect the occurrence of injuries in three basic ways: (1) changing the social meaning of risks and injuries and the laws that help prevent them, (2) changing the physical and social environment, and (3) changing individual behavior—by commanding persons to either refrain from taking certain risky actions or to undertake preventive actions. The third is the most difficult because it relies on changing the everyday behaviors of people.

Humans have great difficulty judging risk. The average person depends on his or her common experience, interpreted through a set of shaky heuristics, to judge risks, and these are notoriously inaccurate (Tversky & Kahneman, 1974). Consider the risk of death in a motor vehicle crash. The annual risk that a U.S. resident will die in a car crash is on the order of 1 in 19,000 (National Safety Council, 2005), a level low enough that the majority of persons may not perceive enough danger to take preventive actions voluntarily. Thus, many people would not wear auto safety belts if their only motivation to do so were based on their everyday perception of risk. (See Chapter Five, this volume.)

Law can provide a substitute set of motivations. Under a legal requirement to wear safety belts, the basis of motivation is shifted away from the perception of the risk of injury to the perception of the risk of being caught and punished, or perhaps more precisely, the risk of rebuke. By using law, injury prevention behavior is facilitated not just because the risk of being caught is often perceived to be higher than the risk of being injured but also because the law creates a common social expectation of obedience.

Law can play a role in each of William Haddon's list of ten strategies for injury prevention (Table 20.1). Legal interventions can also be introduced in each phase of Haddon's three phases of injury control: preevent, event, and postevent (Institute of Medicine, 1985). Legal interventions can play an important role in motivating behavior using both active strategies (placing children in the back seat every time they ride in a vehicle) and passive strategies (installing four-sided fences around residential swimming pools).

TABLE 20.1. HADDON'S TEN STRATEGIES TO INTERFERE WITH THE ENERGY TRANSFER/INJURY PROCESS AND EXAMPLES OF LEGAL INTERVENTIONS.

Haddon Strategy	Example of Strategy	Example of a Legal Tactic	Type of Law
1. Prevent the creation of the hazard	Stop producing poisons	Hold manufacturers legally liable for damages caused by defective products	Litigation
2. Reduce the amount of the hazard	Package toxic drugs in smaller, safer amounts	Require manufacturers to reduce amount of toxic drugs per package	Legislation or regulation
3. Prevent the release of a hazard that already exists	Make bathtubs less slippery	Require or create incentives for tub makers to change tub surfaces	Legislation
4. Modify the rate or spatial distribution of the hazard	Require automobile air bags	Adopt federal requirements for air bags	Regulation
5. Separate, in time or space, the hazard from that which is to be protected	Use sidewalks to separate pedestrians from automobiles	Require or create incentives for developers to install sidewalks in new subdivisions	Legislation
6. Separate the hazard from people by a material barrier	Insulate electrical cords	Hold manufacturers legally liable for damages caused by defective electrical cords	Litigation
7. Modify relevant basic qualities of the hazard	Make crib slat spacings too narrow to strangle a child	Ban sale of cribs with wide slat spacings	Regulation
8. Make people more resistant to damage from the hazard	Improve the host's physical condition through appropriate nutrition and exercise programs	Require education about nutrition and exercise in schools	Legislation or regulation
9. Begin to counter the damages already done by the hazard	Provide emergency medical care	Require all telephone companies to make 911 the emergency call number	Legislation (federal) and regulation
10. Stabilize, repair, and rehabilitate	Provide acute care and rehabilitative facilities	Provide Medicaid and Medicare coverage for advanced fracture treatment methods	Regulation (state and federal)

Source: Adapted from *Protecting the Public: Legal Issues in Injury Prevention* by Tom Christoffel and Stephen Teret, copyright Oxford University Press, Inc. 1991. Used by permission of Oxford University Press, Inc.

Changing Social Meaning

One way that law works is by regulating the meaning of identities and behaviors, categorizing some as favored and others as disfavored (Lessig, 1995). By doing this, law defines the social meaning of both preventive actions and risk-taking behaviors. This can have an important impact on how the law is perceived and used and on its efficacy and effectiveness in changing behavior.

Governments often use the social meaning of law to advance their ends. Lessig (1995) recalls how the Soviet Russian government used social meanings in the 1960s to change the use of motorcycle helmets (Lessig, 1995). In the 1950s, the Soviet government reacted against motorcycle helmets and vilified riders who wore them because the helmets were manufactured in the West. However, in the 1960s, when Soviet Russian factories began to manufacture motorcycle helmets, the government's policy goals changed. At that point, the government sought to tarnish only those who wore imported helmets.

Bonnie (1986) has emphasized that legal controls can influence behavior by "symbolizing and expressing the official government view of the behavior" and generating "derivative effects" on behavior patterns by influencing attitudes and beliefs (Bonnie, 1986, p. 143). He wrote, "Expressions of the law, over time, may affect attitudes about right or wrong and about desirable and undesirable conduct and ultimately—in this indirect way—may influence behavior" (p. 183). People obey the law because they fear detection and punishment, but also because they see law as a pronouncement of new or changed social norms to which they wish to conform.

However, the declarative effects of law do not always produce the desired behaviors. As Bonnie has observed, when no consensus exists on which behavior is acceptable, the government's announcement of its preference might actually lead to more of the disapproved behavior among alienated and disaffected groups. This reverse effect has played a major role in the repeal of motorcycle helmet law in the United States (Wasserstrom, 2001) (Figure 20.1). Lessig refers to this as the "Orwell effect," when the mere knowledge that a behavioral preference comes from the government produces reverse behavior. To guard against this, governments sometimes try to minimize their own visibility as they attempt to change social meaning, hoping that by doing so, they can avoid reaction.

Changing the Physical Environment

While many writers characterize the general approach to injury prevention as the three E's of education (linked to behavior change), environment (product modification), and enforcement (laws, statutes, or regulations), in the practical world all three are interrelated (Sleet & Gielen, 1998; Gilchrist, Saluka, & Marshall, 2006).

FIGURE 20.1. UNIVERSAL HELMET LAW STATES, UNITED STATES, 1965–2004.

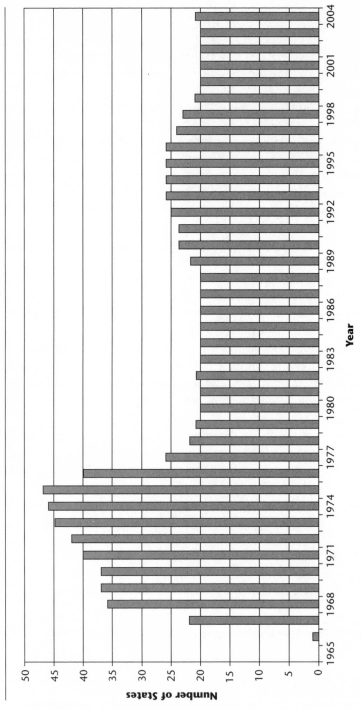

Source: Ulmer and Preusser (2003, Oct.).

Injury prevention depends on reducing environmental threats, changing products to make them safer, and changing individual and population behaviors to reduce risks (Sleet, Liller, White, & Hopkins, 2004). Law plays a part in each of these strategies. Taking an ecological approach in injury prevention recognizes that all three strategies are important, and each builds on the strength of the others (see Chapter Six, this volume; Gielen & Sleet, 2003).

Christoffel and Gallagher (1999) list four approaches to injury prevention that modify the physical environment: (1) minimizing or eliminating the need for the potential hazard, (2) designing safer physical surroundings, (3) designing safer consumer products, and (4) redesigning operating protocols and practices. As the authors state, these measures are not dependent on actions by individuals.

Minimizing or eliminating the need for potential hazards through law is difficult. This approach often requires sweeping societal changes that are costly and must compete with other societal priorities. Using mass transit systems to reduce commuter traffic, for example, might be effective in reducing motor vehicle crashes, but such systems must compete for resources with road construction, health care, and other government services (Christoffel & Gallagher, 1999).

Designing safer consumer products comes about largely because of law. Schieber, Gilchrist, and Sleet illustrate this in their discussion of the enduring struggle for sleepwear flammability regulations (Schieber, Gilchrist, & Sleet, 2000). They describe how the regulations exemplify (1) the benefits of regulating commonly used products; (2) the difficulty with keeping pace with changes in family customs, fashions, and changes in industry; (3) the interplay among government agencies, technical experts, industry, and advocacy groups; and (4) the public's frequent confusion with highly technical matters. They observe, "This issue illustrates how well-intended and effective safety regulations can have difficulty keeping up with changes in fashion and industry, and how changes in regulations can confuse the public and create conflict" (p. 122).

Law is used often to stimulate engineering changes that result in a redesign of products or how they are used (see Chapter Twenty-One, this volume). The regulation of hot tap water temperature is an example. Each year, thousands of children are scalded by overheated tap water. In the past, the thermostat dial setting of hot water heaters was preset at the factory to 140 or 150 degrees, a temperature that can cause burns. One solution was to have the manufacturers reduce the factory setting to 120 degrees (Schieber et al., 2000), and new laws requiring this have been adopted in some jurisdictions (Katcher, 1992). Another example involves burns in children from disposable cigarette lighters. More than two hundred deaths per year, for the past fifteen years, have been related to children igniting disposable cigarette lighters. In 1994, the CPSC mandated that lighter manufacturers develop and install child-resistant features on every lighter sold.

Since the rule took effect in 1994, deaths related to these devices have been reduced by 58 percent (Smith, Green, & Singh, 2002).

Changing Individual Behavior

Law is the traditional way in which governments seek to protect the public good by changing the behavior of individuals. Laws can change social meaning, as described previously, but they also can shape individual behavior through behavior modification or deterrence. But the existence of law is no guarantee of individual behavior change. The public may be unaware of a law, or enforcement of a law may be inadequate or imperceptible. Sometimes the public is aware of a law but does not perceive any benefit from it. In other cases, the public evades or ignores laws because it perceives the law to be rarely enforced or sanctions to be minimal or tolerable. The 55 mile per hour speed limit is such an example. Some laws fail completely, such as the Eighteenth Amendment to the U.S. Constitution (1919), which prohibited "the manufacture, sale, or transportation of intoxicating liquors" in the United States and had to be repealed after just fourteen years.

Despite these limitations, laws and regulations are among the most effective mechanisms for inducing individuals and populations to adopt safer behaviors, provided the laws are carefully crafted and the public is prepared, through education, to accept them as meaningful and helpful to the public good. Laws often will not be effective, however, if they are seen as draconian, burdensome, or an excessive infringement on personal liberty.

Governments have the authority to coerce people to do what is safe for others, and even for themselves. Individuals obey coercive laws on psychological grounds (conditioning based on reward and punishment), economic grounds (rational wealth maximizing), or social grounds (obedience to social customs and mores, status, and peer pressure). Coercive laws accomplish their behavior change goals through incapacitation (removing the person's ability to disobey repeatedly) or deterrence. Deterrence can be specific, meaning that the law punishes to prevent repeat offenses after the first one, or general, whereby the punishment of offenders acts as a lesson to those who have not yet offended (Robertson, 1998).

Coercive laws can be framed positively or negatively. As positive laws, they command certain behaviors, such as stopping at a red light, wearing seat belts, or using hard hats at construction sites. As negative laws, they forbid certain behaviors, such as drunk driving, discarding a refrigerator with the door still attached, or selling food or drink containing wood alcohol. The majority are framed as the latter—as prohibitions—with attached punishments for violation.

The majority of laws aimed at individual behavior change for injury prevention are enacted by the states or localities and are rooted in the states' police power.

For example, in 1981, Christoffel and Teret (1993) conducted an inventory of Massachusetts statutes aimed at preventing unintentional childhood injuries. The inventory identified 124 statutes, of which the majority dealt with motor vehicles, fire, and poison injuries. Some of the statutes were broad or programmatic; others were extremely narrow. They covered such subjects as specifications and rules for pedestrians crossing roadways; safety equipment on school buses; requirements for fire drills in schools, hospitals, and nursing homes; the design of lawnmowers and child car seats; and a ban on eyeglasses with flammable frames. All were aimed at improving the health of the citizenry by reducing the incidence and severity of injuries, and the inventory showed the large quantity, ubiquity, and far-reaching scope of state injury laws.

Studies of the effectiveness of laws aimed at individual behavior have yielded a few general themes. First, as early as 1985, the injury prevention profession had already recognized that "individual behavior change to prevent injuries has been more successful when the behavior was easily observable and required by law" (Institute of Medicine, 1985). The wearing of motorcycle helmets, for example, is easily observable by enforcement officers, and the presence of laws raises the use of helmets from approximately 50 to 100 percent. Second, for some behaviors, the level of enforcement roughly predicts the effectiveness of laws. For example, in one rural Georgia town, when police began confiscating bicycles of any child not wearing a helmet, helmet use increased dramatically (Gilchrist, Scheiber, Leadbetter, & Davidson, 2000). Third, the decrease in injuries caused by behavior laws may not necessarily be as much as expected, because people who are at greatest risk for injuries are also the least likely to obey the laws (Institute of Medicine, 1985).

Robertson (1983) has suggested a number of factors that increase compliance with the law. One is that laws are more likely to be obeyed if a high probability exists for detection and conviction. Robertson has suggested that to obtain an effect that is more than temporary, the detection and conviction rate of a law should be more than 30 percent of the violators. He has also suggested that laws work best when few exceptions exist, conviction occurs soon after detection, and conviction results in a relatively severe punishment. All of these comport with classical behavior change theory and technology (Skinner, 1958). Sleet and Gielen (1998) have suggested that in order for law to work as a force to reduce injury, the law must first be known, it must be understood and interpreted to apply to the individual, resources must be available to comply with the law, and the perceived benefit of the law must outweigh the perceived burden.

Some authors have proposed that some injury prevention mandates may actually cause an increase in risk taking, resulting in a nullification of the preventive effects of the law. For example, when drivers perceive that cars are built safer or that bicycling is safer while wearing a helmet, they might respond by taking more chances, such as speeding in a car or bicycling in a more reckless way. This is called risk compensation or risk homeostasis. Experts differ on the extent to which risk compensation actually occurs (Hedlund, 2000).

Deterrence Through Civil Liability

A tort (from the Latin *tortus,* meaning twist) is a "civil wrong, other than a breach of contract, for which the court will provide a remedy in the form of an action for damages" (Keeton, 1984, p. 2). Generally, a tort interferes with the interests of others and is based on conduct that is socially unreasonable. Torts are important in injury prevention because, although the principal purpose of tort law is to compensate wronged parties, it also has the potential to deter injurious behaviors. For example, tort law can change the behaviors of individuals and thereby reduce the risk of injury to others. It can also affect the actions of manufacturers and dealers and thereby reduce the risk of using products. Deterrence through torts is especially important when legislatures and safety agencies choose not to regulate in a particular area of injury (Christoffel & Gallagher, 1999).

The most important type of tort lawsuit for injury prevention is product liability. Whereas the majority of tort suits are based on a theory of negligence, modern product liability actions are usually based on the existence of a defect in a product and consequent harm to a user, without regard to the fault or negligence of the manufacturer (this is called *strict liability*). The plaintiff must prove, by a preponderance of the evidence (more than 50 percent), that the product was defective in manufacture or design, that it was the cause of the plaintiff's injuries, and that the defect existed when it left the hands of the defendant.

Product liability cases have heightened manufacturers' awareness of the importance of safety in their products (Christoffel & Teret 1993), especially in automobile manufacturing. In *Larsen* v. *General Motors* (1968), the court recognized that automobiles should provide safe transportation or as safe as is reasonably possible. This widened the liability of manufacturers and opened the door for a series of product liability lawsuits that has advanced motor vehicle safety. Product liability lawsuits have advanced safety in motor vehicle equipment (air bags, child car seats, lap safety belts) and in other products (such as hot water vaporizers, explosives, farm machinery, and firearms).

Manufacturers can try to escape liability for defective products by arguing that the plaintiffs contributed to their own injuries through their own negligence (contributory negligence). For example, when a plaintiff sues a ladder manufacturer claiming that the ladder was defective and caused his injuries, if the plaintiff had inspected the ladder and discovered the defect but chose to use the ladder anyway, the manufacturer may try to escape liability or reduce the size of the verdict. Defendants can also claim that the plaintiff assumed certain risks in using the product or that the plaintiff used the product improperly.

Tort law is not a perfect social policy instrument (Christoffel & Teret, 1993), and its deterrent effect is often anemic or muted. Insurance policies can buffer manufacturers against large verdicts, at least temporarily. Huge attorney fees and prolonged litigation can dilute the deterrent effect. Legislatures can reverse court-established liability policies.

Deterrence Through Criminal Sanctions

When persons violate laws or regulations, they can be subject to criminal or administrative penalties. To be punished with a criminal penalty, in general, a person must do something voluntarily that is contrary to law. To merely think of violating a law or to violate the law involuntarily (such as during an epileptic seizure) generally is not sufficient to constitute a criminal act. Because violations of criminal law can result in the most severe punishments meted out by society, the standard of proof used for criminal conviction, "beyond a reasonable doubt," is higher than the one used in civil proceedings. In addition, the criminal law contains constitutional protections to prevent government overreaching and punishing the innocent.

Criminal laws serve three basic functions: (1) incapacitating persons who commit crimes by separating them from society; (2) inflicting punishment on persons who are guilty, on the basis of the moral proposition that wrongdoing deserves punishment; and (3) deterring criminal conduct (Feinberg & Gross, 1986). The power of deterrence varies substantially from law to law and depends on circumstances. Criminal laws often have their greatest deterrent effect on persons who are the least likely to commit crimes—those who have conventional values or strong social ties (Shepherd, 2001).

The traditional connection between criminal law and injury prevention is in intentional injury. Criminal laws (with both their social meaning and deterrent functions) are one of society's main ways of deterring intentional harm to others. However, criminal law is also used to deter harmful conduct that causes unintentional injuries, as with criminal penalties for those who fail to install window guards on all upper-story residences occupied by children (Lazzarini, Scott, & Buehler, 2003).

Criminal laws have been effective in preventing certain types of injuries, such as injuries caused by drunk driving. However, because of their potential to threaten or infringe on human rights, criminal laws are used carefully and "only in the context of a sound legal and ethical framework that safeguards the rights of citizens, families, and detainees" (Shepherd, 2001, p. 1719).

Classic examples of using criminal sanctions to reduce injuries are the different laws regarding drinking alcohol and driving. In the United States, all states have lowered the blood alcohol concentration necessary to constitute "under the influence" to 0.08 grams per deciliter, and epidemiological evidence demonstrates that this reduces alcohol-related fatal crashes 4 to 15 percent (Shults et al., 2001). All states have also increased the minimum legal drinking age to twenty-one years, and this has reduced fatal crashes by 7 to 30 percent (Shults et al., 2001).

Potential Impediments to Using Law to Change Behavior

Although laws are undeniably useful in changing behavior to prevent injuries, individual laws can be challenged as illegal or ineffective. The principal way in which laws are challenged is through a claim that the law contravenes the federal or state constitutions. These challenges are difficult because of the states' broad police power, the courts' strong deference to public health authorities, and the relatively low standard of justification (usually mere rationality) that the state must meet to defend a law successfully.

Illegality

Since enactment of the first injury laws of the previous century, defendants or other aggrieved parties, such as corporations affected by product safety laws, have challenged these laws in court. For example, at the federal level, corporations have challenged regulations on motor vehicles and consumer products on the basis of claims of faulty rule-making procedure, improper legal standards, and excesses of federal authority. At the state level, persons who have been charged with violations of safety laws have contested them on a variety of constitutional or other grounds.

Challenges to Federal Power

Early cases challenging federal authority over safety laws argued that the federal government had exceeded its authority under the Commerce Clause. As in other areas of law in which the Commerce Clause was implicated, few of these cases were successful. Over decades, the courts have gradually expanded their view of Congress's authority to regulate interstate commerce, and, notwithstanding a few cases that seemed to reverse earlier trends (e.g., *United States* v. *Lopez,* 1995), the authority is now so broad that successful challenges remain unusual.

The spending power is the other main source of federal authority in injury prevention. This authority too has been challenged but has been upheld by the federal courts. A landmark case was *South Dakota* v. *Dole* (1987), in which the state of South Dakota challenged a federal statute permitting reductions in highway grants if the state had a minimum drinking age of under twenty-one years. The U.S. Supreme Court upheld the statute and ruled that it was a valid use of the spending power. In doing so, however, the Court cautioned that the spending power is not unlimited. Restrictions on state grants must be in pursuit of the general welfare, must be unambiguous, and probably must be related to the federal interest in particular national projects or programs.

Challenges to State Power

Because the bulk of injury prevention law resides in the states, the majority of challenges to such laws occur in state courts. Usually such claims involve violations of the Fourteenth Amendment right to due process, the Fourth Amendment right to be free of unreasonable searches and seizures, and occasionally the First Amendment right to free speech. Challenges to state public health laws are not often successful.

Courts have upheld states' power to conduct inspections and confiscation of private property (even without compensation in the case of nuisances), regulate the manufacture of products and the delivery of services, control hazards, coerce the behavior of persons, and generally regulate activities associated with public health. The courts are required to balance the public health interests of the state against the rights of individuals, but they give wide latitude to the wisdom of legislatures. As one court wrote, "It is not for the courts to determine which scientific view is correct in ruling upon whether the police power has been properly exercised. 'The judicial function is exhausted with the discovery that the relation between means and end is not wholly vain and fanciful, an illusory pretense . . .'" (*Chiropractic Ass'n of N.Y., Inc.* v. *Hilleboe,* 1962).

The Iowa case of *State* v. *Hartog* (1989) is often cited as a classical judicial explanation of the police power. The defendant, John Hartog, received a citation for failing to use his automobile safety belt, as required by Iowa law. He was found guilty and appealed his conviction on grounds that the Iowa safety belt law was unconstitutional because it violated his Fourteenth Amendment right to privacy and was beyond the state's police power. In disagreeing with Hartog, the court explained that the state's exercise of police power is valid as long as a "reasonable relation to the public welfare" exists. Furthermore, the court said, the state was justified in using the public costs associated with car crashes as a rationale for the safety belt law. Because the costs of car crash injuries are shared by all of society, Hartog was not entitled to decide for himself whether to wear a safety belt.

In deciding whether a "reasonable relation to the public welfare" exists, courts look at two factors: (1) the importance of the state interest and (2) the closeness of the connection between the interest and the requirements of the statute (Christoffel & Teret, 1993). In cases where a fundamental right is affected (for example, those involving liberty, personal autonomy, or privacy, including rights to procreate, marry, or live together as families), or where discrimination against a class of persons might be involved, courts may examine state laws using a higher level of scrutiny than "reasonable relation."

Another constitutional right, the Fourth Amendment right to be free of unreasonable searches and seizures, has been implicated in the use of sobriety check points to detect alcohol-impaired drivers. In *Michigan Department of State Police* v. *Sitz* (1990), the U.S. Supreme Court upheld the checkpoints, citing the magnitude of the drunk driving problem and the relatively small intrusion on motorists, who were being stopped only for about twenty-five seconds each.

Ineffectiveness of Law

The presence of a law does not guarantee the behavior changes needed to prevent injuries. In the legal sphere, the question of effectiveness is important because under the due process principles set out in *Jacobson* and other cases, the government could not adopt intrusive laws that were irrational by way of utter ineffectiveness. Effectiveness also has important economic connotations. Governments sometimes disfavor laws for which the societal cost is greater than the benefit. This does not mean that every law must be demonstrably cost-beneficial. Sometimes, noneconomic values trump economic ones.

Some authors have argued that all new injury prevention laws should be evaluated routinely to avert adverse effects and inefficiency (Schieber et al., 2000). The evaluation of laws is difficult work, however. Effectiveness studies require not just expertise from the field of epidemiology, but also from medicine, health services research, policy, and law. For many laws, obtaining the data needed to study effectiveness is difficult (Institute of Medicine, 1985). Methodological problems also hamper these studies, as with the difficulty in parsing the effect of law amid effects from other factors (Acton, 1998; Robinson, 1998). Such groups as the Task Force on Community Preventive Services (http://www.thecommunityguide.org) and the Cochrane Collaboration (http://www.cochrane.org) have systematically evaluated existing studies on the effectiveness of injury prevention laws. The Task Force, for example, found strong evidence that sobriety checkpoints are effective in reducing alcohol-impaired driving (Centers for Disease Control and Prevention, 2001; Shults et al., 2001) but insufficient evidence to conclude whether firearms laws are effective in reducing firearm-related injuries (Hahn et al., 2005).

Although the measurement of the effectiveness of laws is no easy task, it is usually better to know the effectiveness of a particular law than not to know. A few blatantly ineffective laws can breed cynicism among lawmakers and the public about the effectiveness of all laws aimed at injury-preventing behaviors. Ineffective laws also may drain scarce enforcement or advocacy resources away from more fruitful pursuits. Ideally, the evaluation of laws should be planned at the time the laws are adopted, with careful attention to methodology.

Legislation and Injury Prevention

In democratic societies such as the United States, legislation is the ultimate source of all statutory and regulatory law. Legislation is based in the political process, which includes such activities as researching and developing injury legislation, informing and persuading legislators of the benefits of injury prevention, and supporting political candidates and coalitions that advocate for prevention laws. Injury prevention advocates have scored many legislative successes; improvement in automobile design and equipment and drunk driving laws are just two examples. However, advocates have also been disappointed in some areas of legislation—the repeals of state motorcycle helmet laws, for example.

Some of the disappointments have been caused by a mismatch of countervailing political forces. Public health professionals who work in government are generally prohibited from political advocacy or lobbying. Advocates in the private not-for-profit sector sometimes have a lower ability to influence the legislative process than private commercial interests, in part because they have fewer prerogatives and resources. Other disappointments have occurred because the prevention community sometimes has been unable to appreciate the culture in which the legislative process takes place (Weisbuch, 1987).

The Divergent Cultures of Public Health and Legislatures

Many public health professionals are accustomed to a rational course of preventive public health action—from medical reports to epidemiologic findings to analysis, and finally to well-considered policy. This, however, is not always the course of legislation, which has been characterized not by rationality but by intuition (Sederburg, 1992). To be successful in the legislative process, injury prevention advocates should understand the culture of legislators and the ways in which their culture differs from public health (Brownson & Petitti, 1998). One key difference is the role played by science. In public health, science usually drives social action, and programs must be underpinned by credible scientific data. In lawmaking, however, science is just one of many ingredients. Legislators must consider not just science but all of society's preferences.

Public health advocates and elected lawmakers attain success in different ways (Goodman, Loue, & Shaw, 2005). Public health advocates attain success ultimately by reducing the incidence of public health problems over the long term. Elected lawmakers attain success mainly by fulfilling the expectations of social groups, usually over a relatively short period of time. Legislators respect disease reduction as a societal goal, but they must also ensure that the goal is understood and recognized by the social groups whose expectations the legislators must fulfill. Elected lawmakers usually do not have the luxury of taking positions that violate the expectations of their supporting social groups (Heifetz & Sinder, 1988).

The world of the public health professional, especially epidemiologists, is one of scientific complexity and nuance. For them, scientific truths usually must be qualified and carefully couched so they do not exceed the strength of the data on which they are based. In the elected lawmaker's world, however, nuance often must be sacrificed. To achieve success, elected legislators must often convey truths in vivid, highly simplified, powerful symbols such as colorful political speeches and campaign advertisements (Heymann, 1988).

Epidemiological evidence is the bedrock of public health advocacy, but it is not always primary in political decision making. For example, this evidence has the disadvantage of being complex and often counterintuitive. Most legislators have limited training in science and are not equipped to understand epidemiological or statistical data. However, some legislators (virtually all members of Congress and some state legislators) have staff assistants or trusted advisers who are able to translate and interpret scientific information into terms the legislator can understand.

Public health advocates sometimes use economic analyses to buttress arguments in favor of prevention legislation. These analyses provide a useful scale of where society can get the most return for fiscal investments. In the legislative arena, however, these analyses sometimes are less persuasive than expected. Most legislators (especially those that do not serve on appropriations committees) are not in a position to reallocate resources from less cost-effective social programs into more cost-effective ones. In addition, economic analyses are often trumped by political considerations. Even so, economic analysis has a valuable place in reassuring legislators that the costs of injury prevention legislation are within the bounds of reasonableness.

Factors in the Legislative Process

The best way to understand legislators is to understand their constituents. Legislators must not only be aware of their constituents' perceptions, but must also seize opportunities to influence them. Hedrick Smith (1988) has likened the process by which members of Congress stay in office as a perpetual motion machine, an un-broken succession of elections. Although Smith was writing about Congress, to a lesser degree the same observation applies to state legislators. Jacobson (2004) has observed two important recent trends in the congressional "electoral logic." Both have strong implications for injury prevention advocacy. The first is particularism: "members' notorious affection for policies that produce particularized benefits" (Jacobson, 2004, p. 223). Members have strong incentives to vote for programs, benefits, and tax breaks that are narrowly targeted. The second trend is Congress's increasing desire to serve the "vocal, organized, and active" and pay less atten-tion to persons and groups that are politically inattentive or atomized (Jacobson, 2004, p. 223).

Methods for Legislative Success

Injury prevention advocates sometimes complain about their inability to get leg-islation passed more readily, pointing out perceived obstructions by automobile companies, firearms manufacturers and gun owner groups, children's pajamas makers, other commercial players, and lobbyists. Advocates express frustration with legislators who do not support injury prevention legislation despite strongly favorable scientific evidence. While complaints and frustration are understand-able, injury legislation often has failed because injury prevention advocates have not been willing or able to engage in practical politics to the extent that their ri-vals do. The remainder of this chapter lists some potential methods for attaining greater legislative success:

• *Seek cogency and intramural consensus.* Linder (1987) has described how legisla-tive efforts in injury prevention can be thwarted by a lack of cogency or intramural consensus. Cogency means building arguments that will motivate policymakers and justify legislation. A lack of consensus in injury policy can nurture resistance among opponents. On the practical level, legislators hesitate to back injury legis-lation if they sense that prevention experts do not agree on its merits.

• *Seek maximum immersion in the legislative culture.* Immersion in the legislative process can produce a deep understanding of legislative and political dynamics, including financing and the crucial role of constituencies. Advocates should focus primarily on the practical everyday tug-and-pull of legislation, not just on aca-demics and political science (Matthews, 1988), and legislation and politics at the local level, because local politics drives all state and national political decision making.

• *Know lawmakers and staff personally.* Legislators give greater attention and cre-dence to advocates whom they know personally and trust. Advocates should develop strong personal relationships with legislators well before they need to lobby them on specific issues. Advocates should also recognize the crucial role of legislative staff. Because of the breadth and complexity of the political environment in Congress and state capitols, legislators rely heavily on staff members who develop specialized knowledge of legislative issues.

- *Learn to communicate in legislators' language.* Effective communication with legislators requires, above all, a sense of the political context in which the communication is taking place and sensitivity for the prerogatives and priorities of legislators. Brownson and Malone (2002) have developed a list of ten underlying qualitative factors and approaches for effectively communicating with elected officials. For example, advocates must develop a keen knowledge of the opposition to the issue for which they are advocating and be forthright about their own personal positions. Brevity is crucial. The communication techniques that work well in academic or government injury prevention practice might not work when communicating with legislators.

- *Find insider champions.* Champions inside the political process can play a decisive role in the adoption of injury legislation (Chorba & Vinicor, 1990; Teret, Alexander, & Bailey, 1990). Conversely, one well-placed opponent can scuttle legislation with ease and spoil an intensive advocacy effort (Weisbuch, 1987). Injury prevention advocates should search for insider champions who have the trust of key legislators. Advocates should cultivate legislators who are willing to act as long-term champions for injury legislation in Congress and state legislatures.

- *Use the power of the story.* In politics, human stories are often more powerful than policy analyses and epidemiological studies. Stories place complex policy issues in the context and vernacular of daily life, give them an emotional component, and allow everyday people to see how issues apply to their own lives. Because legislators are sensitive to their constituents, they respect powerful stories that can impress their constituents. Human stories are also often very attractive to the press. McLoughlin and Fennell (2000) have described the effective use of survivor advocacy in favor of legislation for routine installation of interior trunk releases to prevent entrapment in car trunks.

- *Avoid excessively paternalistic legislation that will trigger social backlash.* The reversal of dozens of state motorcycle helmet requirements since 1976, and the inability of public health advocates to reinstate them, is an example of a regulatory backlash by consumers who view these laws as excessively paternalistic. Vogel (1991) has examined four examples of successful grassroots consumer opposition to government health and safety regulations, including seat belt ignition interlocks and motorcycle helmet laws. The risk of consumer backlash is highest for legislation that (1) has a high visibility to consumers, (2) has high saliency, (3) intrudes on the daily lives of citizens, (4) interferes with freedom of choice in matters where consumers believe they are in a better position to judge their self-interest than the government, and (5) upsets large numbers of voters.

• *Envision changes in law as opportunities to alter social meaning.* Lessig (1995) has discussed two techniques that can be used to alter the social meaning of behaviors: tying and ambiguation. In tying, "the social architect attempts to transform the social meaning of one act by tying it to, or associating it with, another social meaning that conforms to the meaning that the architect wishes the managed act to have" (p. 1009). In ambiguation, "the architect tries to give the particular act, the meaning of which is to be regulated, a second meaning as well, one that acts to undermine the negative effects of the first" (p. 1010). Some of the historic success of Mothers Against Drunk Driving was its ability to change, or ambiguate, the social meaning of alcohol-impaired driving. Changes in social meaning can be used to reduce other injury-prone behaviors.

• *Conduct more research on the natural history of legislation.* A neglected area of research in public health law is the life cycle of legislation. Little is known about how public health policies translate into legislation and what factors predict legislative success. This would be a fruitful subject of collaboration among epidemiologists, political scientists, and researchers from other disciplines (for example, anthropologists, social psychologists, and sociologists). Robertson (1998) has cited the need for such research by asking, "What are the origin and sustenance of the lobbying in opposition to laws that reduce injury?" (Robertson, 1998, pp. 145–146).

Conclusions

Perhaps more than any other discipline in public health, injury prevention relies on law for behavior change. The future of injury law in the United States depends to some extent on the general environment for legislative and judicial change. Recent repeals and failures to reinstate state motorcycle helmet laws suggest that legislation restricting some types of personal liberties might not be as acceptable as it was in the past. However, legislatures have shown no appetite for reversing key injury prevention laws (for example, automobile safety belt requirements and drunk driving laws). In the latter case, laws that reduce drinking and driving have actually been strengthened worldwide (Howat, Sleet, Elder, & Maycock, 2004; Peden et al., 2004). At one level, the future of injury legislation will depend on how willing and able prevention advocates are to intertwine themselves with the workings of the legislative process and learn from the methods used by other effective interest groups.

Efforts to reduce injury-producing behaviors will continue to rely on the application of sound behavior change principles—-those based on incentives, rewards, and punishments. To attain even greater successes, advocates will need to take an ecological approach and seek to change behavior by modifying products, environments, and individual behaviors. As it has been in the past, law will be an effective partner in such efforts.

References

Acton, C. (1998). Helmet laws and health. *Injury Prevention, 4,* 171–172.

Administrative Procedure Act. (2005). 5 USCS § 706.

Bonnie, R. J. (1986). The efficacy of law as a paternalistic instrument. In R. A. Dienstbier & G. B. Melton (Eds.), *The law as a behavioral instrument.* Lincoln: University of Nebraska Press.

Breyer, S., & Stewart, R. (1992). *Administrative law and regulatory policy* (3rd ed.). Boston: Little, Brown.

Brownson, R. C., & Malone, B. R. (2002). Communicating public health information to policy makers. In D. E. Nelson, R. C. Brownson, P. L. Remington, & C. Parvanta, (Eds.), *Communicating public health information effectively: A guide for practitioners.* Washington: American Public Health Association.

Brownson, R. C., & Petitti, D. B. (Eds.). (1998). *Applied epidemiology: Theory to practice* (2nd ed.). New York: Oxford University Press.

Burris, S. (1999). Law as a structural factor in the spread of communicable diseases. *Houston Law Review, 36,* 1755–1786.

Centers for Disease Control and Prevention. (2001). Motor-vehicle occupant injury: Strategies for increasing use of child safety seats, increasing use of safety belts, and reducing alcohol-impaired driving. A report on recommendations of the Task Force on Community Preventive Services. *Morbidity and Mortality Weekly Report, 50*(RR-7), 1–13.

Chiropractic Ass'n of N.Y., Inc. v. Hilleboe. (1962). 12 N.Y.2d 109.

Chorba, T., & Vinicor, F. (1990). Enactment of mandatory seatbelt-use legislation: An analysis of the political process in North Carolina. *North Carolina Medical Journal, 51,* 599–607.

Christoffel, T., & Gallagher, S. S. (1999). *Injury prevention and public health.* Gaithersburg, MD: Aspen.

Christoffel, T., & Teret, S. (1993). *Protecting the public: Legal issues in injury prevention.* New York: Oxford University Press.

Elder, R. W., Shults, R. A., Sleet, D. A., Nichols, J. L., Thompson, R. S., Rajab, W., & Task Force on Community Preventive Services. (2004). Effectiveness of mass media campaigns for reducing drinking and driving and alcohol-involved crashes: A systematic review. *American Journal of Preventive Medicine, 27*(1), 57–65.

Feinberg, J., & Gross, H. (1986). *Punishment: Part 5. Philosophy of law* (3rd ed.). Belmont, CA: Wadsworth.

Gielen, A. C., & Sleet, D. (2003). Behavioral approaches to injury prevention. *Epidemiologic Reviews, 25,* 65–67.

Gilchrist, J., Saluka, G., & Marshall, S. (2006). Sport and recreation-related injuries. In L. Doll, J. Mercy, S. Bonzo, & D. Sleet (Eds.), *Handbook of injury and violence prevention.* New York: Springer.

Gilchrist, J., Scheiber, R. A., Leadbetter, S., & Davidson, S. C. (2000, July). Police enforcement as a part of a comprehensive bicycle helmet program. *Pediatrics, 1 Pt.*(1), 6–9.

Goodman, R. A., Loue, S., & Shaw, F. E. (2005). Law and epidemiology. In R. Brownson & D. Petiti (Eds.). *Applied epidemiology* (2nd ed.). New York: Oxford University Press.

Griswold v. *Connecticut* (1965). 381 U.S. 479.

Hahn, R. A., Bilukha, O., Crosby, A., Fullilove, M. T., Liberman, A., Moscicki, E., Snyder, S., Tuma, F., Briss, P. A., & Task Force on Community Preventive Services. (2005). Firearms laws and the reduction of violence: A systematic review. *American Journal of Preventive Medicine, 28*(Suppl. 1), 40–71.

Hedlund, J. (2000). Risky business: Safety regulations, risk compensation, and individual behavior. *Injury Prevention, 6,* 82–90.

Heifetz, R. A., & Sinder, R. M. (1988). Political leadership: Managing the public's problem solving. In R. B. Reich (Ed.), *The power of public ideas.* Cambridge, MA: Harvard University Press.

Heymann, P. B. (1988). How government expresses public ideas. In R. B. Reich (Ed.), *The power of public ideas.* Cambridge, MA: Harvard University Press.

Hobbes, T. (1986). *The Leviathan.* Retrieved Nov. 2, 2005, from http://oregonstate.edu/instruct/phl302/texts/hobbes/leviathan-contents.html. (Originally published in 1660)

Holmes, O. W., Jr. (1897). Path of the law. *Harvard Law Review, 10,* 457, 457–478.

Howat, P., Sleet, D. A., Elder, R., & Maycock, B. (2004). Preventing alcohol-related traffic injury: A health promotion approach. *Traffic Injury Prevention, 5*(3), 208–219.

Institute of Medicine. (1985). *Injury in America.* Washington, DC: National Academy Press.

Jacobson, G. C. (2004). *The politics of congressional campaigns.* New York: Pearson-Longman.

Jacobson v. *Massachusetts.* (1905). 197 U.S. 11.

Katcher, M. (1992). Efforts to prevent burns from hot tap water. In A. B. Bergman (Ed.), *Political approaches to injury control at the state level.* Seattle: University of Washington Press.

Keeton, W. P. (Ed.). (1984). *Prosser and Keeton on the law of torts* (5th ed.). St Paul, MN: West.

Larsen v. *General Motors Corp.* (1968). 391 F.2d 495.

Lazzarini, Z., Scott, S., & Buehler, J. W. (2003). Criminal law and public health practice. In R. A. Goodman, M. A. Rothstein, R. E. Hoffman, W. Lopez, & G. W. Matthews (Eds.), *Law in public health practice.* New York: Oxford University Press.

Lessig, L. (1995). The regulation of social meaning. *University of Chicago Law Review, 62,* 943–1045.

Linder, S. H. (1987). On cogency, professional bias, and public policy: An assessment of four views of the injury problem. *Milbank Quarterly, 65,* 276–301.

Matthews, C. (1988). *Hardball: How politics is played told by one who knows the game.* New York: HarperCollins.

McLoughlin, E., & Fennell, J. (2000). The power of survivor advocacy: Making car trunks escapable. *Injury Prevention, 6,* 167–170.

Mendeloff, J. M. (1988). *The dilemma of toxic substance regulation: How overregulation causes underregulation at OSHA.* Cambridge MA: MIT Press.

Meyer v. *State of Nebraska.* (1923). 262 U.S. 390.

Michigan Department of State Police v. *Sitz.* (1990). 496 U.S. 444.

Mill, J. S. (1860). *On liberty.* Harvard Classics, Volume 25. PF Collier & Son.

National Safety Council. (2005). *What are the odds of dying?* Retrieved May 2005 from http://www.nsc.org/lrs/statinfo/odds.htm.

Parmet, W. E. (2002). After September 11: Rethinking public health federalism. *Journal of Law, Medicine and Ethics, 30,* 201–209.

Peden, M., Scurfield, R., Sleet, D. A., Mohan, D., Hyder, A. A., Jarawan, E., & Mathers, C. (Eds.). (2004). *World report on road traffic injury prevention.* Geneva, Switzerland: World Health Organization.

Queenside Hills Co. v. *Saxl.* (1946). 328 U.S. 80.

Richards, E. P., & Rathbun, K. C. (1998). Public health law. In R. B. Wallace (Ed.), *Public health and preventive medicine* (14th ed.). Stamford CT: Appleton & Lange.

Robertson, L. S. (1983). *Injuries: Causes, control strategies, and public policy.* Lanham, MD: Lexington Books.

Robertson, L. S. (1998). *Injury epidemiology: Research and control strategies.* New York: Oxford University Press.

Robinson, D. (1998). Helmet laws and health. *Injury Prevention, 4,* 170–172.

Roe v. *Wade.* (1973). 410 U.S. 113.

Schieber, R. A., Gilchrist, J., & Sleet, D. A. (2000). Legislative and regulatory strategies to reduce childhood unintentional injuries. *Future of Children, 10,* 111–136.

Sederburg, W. (1992). Perspectives of the legislator: Allocating resources. *Morbidity and Mortality Weekly Report, 41*(Suppl.), 37–48.

Shepherd, J. P. (2001). Criminal deterrence as a public health strategy. *Lancet, 358,* 1717–1722.

Shults, R. A., Elder, R. W., Sleet, D. A., Nichols, J. L., Alao, M. O., Carande-Kulis, V. G., Zaza, S., Sosin, D. M., & Thompson, R. S. (2001). Task Force on Community Preventive Services. Reviews of evidence regarding interventions to reduce alcohol-impaired driving. *American Journal of Preventive Medicine, 21*(4S), 66–88.

Skinner, B. F. (1953). *Science and human behavior.* New York: Macmillan.

Sleet, D., & Gielen, A. (1998). Injury prevention. In S. Gorin & J. Arnold (Eds.), *Health promotion handbook* (pp. 247–275). St. Louis: Mosby.

Sleet, D., Liller, K., White, D., & Hopkins, K. (2004). Injuries, injury prevention and public health. *American Journal of Health Behavior, 28*(Suppl. 1), S6–S12.

Smith, H. (1988). *The power game: How Washington works.* New York: Random House.

Smith, L. E., Green, M. A., & Singh, H. A. (2002). Study of the effectiveness of the US safety standard for child resistant cigarette lighters. *Injury Prevention, 8,* 192–196.

South Dakota v. *Dole.* (1987). 483 U.S. 203.

State v. *Hartog.* (1989). 440 N.W.2d 852.

Teret, S., Alexander, G., & Bailey, L. (1990). The passage of Maryland's gun law: Data and advocacy for injury prevention. *Journal of Public Health Policy, 11*(1), 26–38.

Tversky, A., & Kahneman, D. (1974). Judgment under uncertainty: Heuristics and biases. *Science, 185,* 1124–1131.

Ulmer, R. F., & Preusser, D. F. (2003, Oct.). *Evaluation of the repeal of motorcycle helmet laws in Kentucky and Louisiana.* Washington, DC: U.S. Department of Transportation, National Highway Traffic Safety Administration. Retrieved June 21, 2005, from http://www.nhtsa.dot.gov/people/injury/pedbimot/motorcycle/kentuky-la03/TOC.html.

United States v. *Lopez.* (1995). 514 U.S. 549.

Vogel, D. (1991). When consumers oppose consumer protection: The politics of regulatory backlash. *Journal of Public Policy, 10,* 449–470.

Wasserstrom, A. S. (2001). Validity of traffic regulations requiring motorcyclists to wear helmets or other protective headgear. 72 *American Law Reports* 5th 607.

Weisbuch, J. B. (1987). The prevention of injury from motorcycle use: Epidemiologic success, legislative failure. *Accident Analysis and Prevention, 19,* 21–28.

CHAPTER TWENTY-ONE

HUMAN FACTORS IN PRODUCT AND ENVIRONMENTAL DESIGN FOR INJURY CONTROL

Bryan E. Porter, James P. Bliss

This chapter's focus is the role of human factors for preventing injuries. We introduce readers who may not be familiar with human factors to general concepts within the field, issues for engineers to consider when designing machines for safe human use, reasons that humans misuse or fail to use engineering innovations for safety, and recommendations for increasing safe product use. We discuss lessons learned from human factors approaches to safety and suggest future areas of study.

The System Concept Within Human Factors Engineering

Historically, safety has been a driving impetus within the field of human factors engineering. A primary disciplinary goal of human factors engineering is to apply knowledge about human capabilities and limitations to the design of technology and equipment. By doing so, designers of complex tasks and equipment may create safer and more user-friendly systems. Popular examples of the successful application of human factors principles to technology design include the center

---

Both authors contributed equally to this chapter.

high-mounted stop light (CHMSL) on automobiles (Digges, Nicholson, & Rouse, 1985), the redesign of nuclear power plants following the Three-Mile Island nuclear power incident (Maddox & Muto, 1999), and the design of alarms and warnings to facilitate rapid perception and reaction to dangers (Stanton & Edworthy, 1999).

A cornerstone principle that defines the field of human factors engineering is that humans and technology, together with the surrounding environment, form a system. Proctor and Van Zandt (1994) noted that the combined performance of the system depends on the smooth and consistent functioning of each of its three components. If the human operator, technology, or environment is unreliable, unstable, or flawed, system performance (and likely operator safety) may be in jeopardy.

Sanders and McCormick (1993) pointed out that systems are complex entities, marked by several defining features. The structure of systems may be serial or parallel. Serial systems are marked by sequential components, each accomplishing a unique function. Parallel systems feature redundancy, so that if one component fails, a backup is available. Such redundancy is a critical requirement for systems where safety is at risk. For example, medical monitoring and administration equipment generally includes redundant subsystems to ensure that critical functions are accomplished in a timely and reliable manner. The process of adding equipment to ensure redundancy is known as probabilistic fault tolerance and is part of a larger program of detailed hazard analysis (Goetsch, 2005).

Engineering efforts to improve safety can have ramifications for humans, technology, and the environment. Therefore, it is important that designers of technical safety solutions consider each factor. However, humans, technology, and environments are not always stable, which complicates this process. Physical equipment and technology may fail due to faulty design, age, or deterioration. Environments may improve or degrade over time, and human behavior is prone to distraction, stress, workload, fatigue, or other factors affecting performance (for example, use of drugs and alcohol and experience with a given task). The human component of the system involves perhaps the greatest source of variability.

Researchers have documented predictable performance decrements associated with various cognitive and physical states. For example, human performance is best when arousal is at a moderate level but degrades if arousal is too low or high (Yerkes & Dodson, 1908). Models of attention suggest task performance will suffer if a person must attend to many tasks at one time; however, the degradation can be reduced with practice (Schneider & Shiffrin, 1977). A related influence is task workload. Human performance worsens under conditions of physical and cognitive demands (Lysaght et al., 1989). Examples of physical conditions creating demand are driving and talking on a cell phone, driving with a stick shift (manual transmission), or flying an aircraft manually (without autopilot) while adjusting headphones. Cognitive examples creating demand involve any situation with multiple things to attend to or process such as remembering navigation directions while driving a car and talking to a passenger or talking to a colleague at work about one problem while thinking about the solution to other problems. Fatigue also causes variability in cognitive processing, as well as in the speed and accuracy of physical actions and reactions. In fact, cognitive deficits usually occur before any physical deficits are observed (Haslam, 1985). The variability associated with acquisition of task skill (learning curves) has been known in psychology for many years as have methods for modifying learning acquisition (Reynolds, 1952). Cognitive and physical states have a strong influence on the likelihood of injury.

In addition to these individual factors, interactive influences on system operations can be enormous. For example, a parent cooking dinner may be distracted by competing demands (an individual factor). His or her fatigue may then be exacerbated because of increased time pressure (such as a spouse arriving home late from work). Unfortunately, such individual and interactive influences have implications for safety and make the design of injury-proof environments difficult.

Because human performance is exceedingly complex and variable, considerable effort has been devoted to understanding and predicting human reliability. For example, Swain (1964) developed the Technique for Human Error Rate Prediction at Sandia Laboratories in the 1950s as a way to quantify and track human error during the assembly of nuclear warheads. It features a fairly simplistic approach to quantify errors of commission and omission but breaks down as task performance details and environments become more complex. A more recent technique, the Systematic Human Error Reduction and Prediction Approach (Embrey, 1986), involves creating task and error taxonomies as steps toward quantifying and predicting the errors associated with each.

Safety Engineering Priority Hierarchies

The variability associated with hardware and with the human performer has made the task of designing for safety challenging. The most appropriate ways to ensure safety often fall along a continuum from the most proactive to the least proactive. The National Safety Council (NSC) along with the Occupational Safety and Health Administration (OSHA) and the National Institute for Occupational Safety and Health (NIOSH) at the Centers for Disease Control and Prevention (CDC) have a mandate from the federal government to protect citizens and minimize injury and exposure to unhealthy environments. To accomplish this mission, the NSC has developed a four-stage Safety Engineering Priority Hierarchy that has been widely adopted by society at large, and specifically by American industries.

Design for Minimum Risk

The most effective strategy is to design for minimum risk, which suggests that effective equipment or environmental design can prevent injuries. Including a fuel cutoff switch on automobiles to stop fuel flow in the event of a crash is an example. Such automated devices are particularly effective because they are built into the system. Not all activities can benefit from such approaches. For example, underwater diving, bungee jumping, and motorcycle riding are all inherently risky activities that may not be amenable to designing for minimal risk. Participants, therefore, are encouraged to wear protective equipment or alter the task, which may incidentally reduce enjoyment.

Safety Devices or Safeguards

In industry, the practice of incorporating safety devices or safeguards is common and often required. OSHA has specified regulations for a variety of machines, including abrasive wheel machinery, forging machines, and woodworking machines (CFR 1910, subpart O). There are many possible strategies for safeguards on machinery, including placing physical barriers at the point of operation or incorporating photoelectric or radio-controlled sensors to prevent machine operation. Generally the NSC has established several criteria for safeguards: they should prevent contact between humans and equipment, be secure and durable, protect people or machines from falling objects, create no new hazards or interference, and allow safe maintenance.

Safeguards provide a critical function, particularly in situations where operators might not be vigilant about safety. Having a passive safeguard system may free the worker to focus on other aspects of the task. A natural precursor to implementing safeguards is risk assessment, where task experts judge which normal activities might constitute a threat to workers.

Warning Devices

In some situations, it is difficult or impossible to design the task more safely or implement safeguards. For example, in certain sports activities, personal risk is assumed to be a by-product of participation. In these situations the use of safety warnings that cue people to impending dangers may be the easiest safety strategy, but may not be the most effective. The use of warning devices includes fixed warning labels, or transient alarm signals that appeal to one or more senses. In some ways, the use of warnings represents the easiest way to implement a safety strategy. However, the assumption that people will heed warnings is suspect. The research literature is replete with anecdotes demonstrating nonadherence to warnings and alarms (Bliss, Deaton, & Gilson, 1995; Breznitz, 1984; Rodriguez, 1991).

Several empirical studies show that distrust of alarms is a problem in aviation (Bliss, 2003), mining (Mallett, Vaught, & Brnich, 1993), ship handling (Kerstholt, Passenier, Houttuin, & Schuffel, 1996), medicine (Bitan, Meyer, Shinar, & Zmora, 2004), and automobile driving (Nohre, MacKinnon, & Sadalla, 1998). In most cases, frequent false alarms engender distrust, and therefore complacency.

Other evidence suggests alarms engender complacency because of learned irrelevance, which occurs when a person is continually exposed to the alarm stimulus, such as an emergency fire exit sign, but rarely if ever has had occasion to use the exit in an emergency. For example, McClintock, Shields, Reinhart-Rutland, and Leslie (2001) found that people recognize emergency exit signage and associate it with safety, but do not notice the signage when they are involved in everyday activities. Such emergency exit signage is overabundant in the environment, with few actual emergency events to trigger the use of the emergency exit. Such signs become familiar without cause for action, and the odds of being underused increase when an actual emergency requiring evaluation occurs. One technique to improve these signs' effectiveness and counter learned irrelevance in the United Kingdom is to use blue flashing lights in an emergency, allowing people to form an association between emergencies and exit locations. People are conditioned to notice and respond to blue flashing lights such as those used by ambulances.

Training Programs

The last recommendation by the NSC to increase safety in those instances where people must interact with unsafe equipment or situations is to develop and implement training programs. Research concerning ways to ensure mastery, transfer, and retention of learned information abounds (Adams, 1987; Holding, 1965). However, training as a sole strategy for improving safety has several potential disadvantages. If training materials do not approximate the actual task, the training benefit may not generalize. Also, unlike safeguarding or improving task design, training must be periodically repeated, particularly for people who may not experience hazards frequently. Examples of such tasks may include operating underwater diving equipment or performing maintenance on military vehicles. Such repeated training may be quite costly. Perhaps the biggest disadvantage of training as a safety intervention is that it does not necessarily lead to safer behavior. Trainees may not learn important information or be able to apply the learning to the task, and the learning may not transfer to new or changed task requirements.

Human-Technology Considerations and Injury Prevention

A primary goal of the discipline of human factors engineering is to design or re-design tasks and environments to enhance the safety of participants or opera-tors. Succeeding in this goal requires an appreciation of the limits of all aspects of systems: human behavior, machines, and environments. Meister (1989) pre-sented several aspects of the traditional engineering design process. Specifically, he noted that engineers tend to reuse design approaches that have worked be-fore, they generally rely on their own intuition, they tend to first focus on hard-ware and software constraints, and they typically do not have a good working knowledge of behavioral theories or tendencies. Human factors practitioners strive to compensate for these tendencies by emphasizing user behaviors within the context of an operational system. Human factors input generally occurs within six stages of system design (Bailey, 1982): determining system objectives, defining the system, creating the basic design, designing the human interface, in-corporating aids and facilitators, and conducting tests and evaluations of the completed design.

Within each stage, there are activities that must be performed to ensure safety. In the first two stages, the focus is primarily on the tasks and the flow of infor-mation across system components. The smooth flow of such information is cru-cial, for example, if human operators will be reading displays and activating controls, as in the case of manufacturing operations or in driving. In the design stage, it is important to consider the allocation of responsibilities between the human and the technology. One important aspect of function allocation is an ac-knowledgment of the capabilities and limitations of humans with regard to per-formance and safety. If a primary function of the system will be to transfer hot material to a cooling area, safety considerations would necessitate a mechanical component rather than a human handling the transport.

The fourth stage has particular implications for safety because of the focus on the human-technology interface. Specifically, the design and function of dis-plays, controls, consoles, and work spaces strongly determine the risk assumed by task operators. It is for this reason that most human factors practitioners include risk assessment as an integral part of the interface design stage. Goetsch (2005) noted that risk assessment should seek to specify the severity of potential injuries, frequency of exposure to hazards, possibility of avoiding hazards that occur, and likelihood of injuries if safety control systems fail.

The last two stages that Bailey (1982) discussed are often considered ancillary to the functionality of the system or environment. Unfortunately, because designers often neglect these stages, some systems undergo human factors modification only after someone has been hurt or killed.

An overriding challenge for designers is to predict and understand the user population. For example, users of traffic signals will include all people who drive automobiles, as well as pedestrians. Designing to accommodate such diversity is not trivial and designers have taken one of several approaches: designing for extreme individuals, designing for the average individual, or designing for an adjustable range (Sanders & McCormick, 1993). These design choices are evident in many of the safety devices that exist today. All building occupants should be able to open fire safety doors that automatically shut when fire alarms sound, but designs chosen for safety doors may fail to accommodate many users, such as children, the elderly, and the disabled. Automobile seats are designed to be adjustable; however, the failure of many drivers to adjust them properly before driving reduces the effectiveness of these design features. Designers must be aware of environmental influences on performance. In many cases, the safety of users may be threatened because they must operate in a hot, cold, noxious, poorly lit, noisy, or otherwise stress-filled environment. In addition to the obvious physical challenges, researchers such as Hockey (1986) have documented specific cognitive deficits associated with these stressors. Specifically, Ramsey and Kwon (1988) documented heat-related cognitive deficits for complex cognition, and Ramsey, Burford, Beshir, and Jensen (1983) noted that unsafe behaviors increased as the ambient temperature rose above 73 degrees or fell below 63 degrees Fahrenheit. Noisy environments will typically not hinder cognitive processing unless the tasks performed are highly demanding (Eschenbrenner, 1971). However, poor lighting has long been acknowledged as a detriment to performance (Proctor & Van Zandt, 1994). Because of findings such as these, the European Union has identified stress as an occupational risk, and courts in the United Kingdom have identified excessive stress levels as a workplace risk. Furthermore, OSHA has stipulated limits for specific environmental influences such as noise.

The complexity of human behavior in various environments presents designers of safety interventions with a daunting task. To ensure the effectiveness of such interventions, designers must be able to predict the behavioral tendencies of users.

Perceptual and Cognitive Considerations for Injury Prevention

To further understand injury prevention through human factors, cognitive considerations beginning with perception of physical stimuli must be discussed. Perceptual processes are susceptible to variations in environmental stimuli and are particularly important for reacting to threats. Few people would doubt the importance of vision for driving, for example (see Cavallo, Mestre, & Berthelon, 1997, for visual factors related to time-to-collision judgments). After vision, people probably rely most on auditory perception. As an example, heavy machine operators can damage their hearing, but the equipment (headgear) to protect their hearing can obstruct auditory cues important for avoiding danger.

Touch also plays an important role. Historically, driving a car at high speeds would cause the steering wheel to vibrate. Modern passenger vehicles now feature ultrasmooth rides, minimizing vibrations created by vehicle-road surface interactions, reducing vibrotactile cues regarding speed, and perhaps increasing how much control drivers feel while speeding (Summala, 2005). Prolonged vibrotactile stimulation from using construction equipment may increase whole-body and segmental vibration, leading to musculoskeletal disorders (Kittusamy & Buchholz, 2004).

Vestibular cues affect balance; compromised balance may lead to injury. Construction workers, painters, and firefighters working on ladders may be at greater risk of falling when they have colds. Machine operators with inner ear disturbances may also be at risk, particularly if operating the technology requires keen balance. Colds, illnesses, and medications affect olfactory perception also. This is particularly insidious in environments where fire is a risk, because of human reliance on olfaction to detect smoke.

Cognitive factors play a significant role in how engineering strategies affect injury prevention. Human operators must decide whether the hazard to be avoided is worth the cost and effort of deploying the technology (for example, by purchasing a smoke alarm, using a safety belt, or wearing protective eye gear). Operators' decision-making strategies are important to understand and manipulate to increase the use of engineering strategies.

Many in public health assume that decision makers will choose interventions and policies based on fact and logic. It seems obvious, for example, that walking or running on icy streets increases the risk of falling. Yet people do this all the time. It is also clear that safety belt use decreases the odds of dying in a motor vehicle crash (Evans, 2004). Furthermore, public safety campaigns and laws exist to compel safety belt use. Yet 20 percent of U.S. front-seat occupants do not wear safety belts consistently or at all; more than half of rear occupants do not (Glassbrenner, 2005).

Rational decision-making (or rational choice) models, a part of classical decision theory (Sternberg, 2003), assume people are sensitive to their options, are fully informed of the consequences of these options (odds of outcome), and are fully rational in choosing the option that yields maximal benefit and lowest cost. However, human behavior is not always rational. Instead, people often rely on decision-making strategies involving heuristics and biases (Sternberg, 2003). Heuristics are mental shortcuts used to make decisions without the benefit of evaluating all relevant information.

A poignant example of one such heuristic may affect the decision to wear a vehicle safety belt. A significant minority of people do not wear safety belts, choosing instead to believe that (for example) safety belts reduce chances to survive rather than increase them. Similarly, people may relate personal anecdotes about surviving car crashes because they were thrown from the vehicle. The rational belief is that wearing safety belts is more effective than not wearing them in most crash situations, because flying through windshields and hitting the pavement cannot statistically improve one's chances of avoiding injury and death (Evans, 2004). Yet people persist in thinking that they will be safer when unbuckled.

Kahneman and Tversky (1972) explain this quandary by suggesting that people often employ a representativeness heuristic. Sternberg (2003) provides a cogent explanation of this heuristic. People believe events are more likely when they seem to represent the population of possibilities and appear randomly generated. If events do not register with anecdotal evidence, which is typically based on a small sample of data, people judge them to be less likely. Humans often do not accurately judge the base rates of those events occurring within the population, judging instead that personal experience fairly represents the majority's reality.

A second heuristic is the availability heuristic (Tversky & Kahneman, 1973). It is harder to imagine someone injured from not wearing eye protection when hammering a nail or drilling something into a wall than it is to imagine someone dying from a terrorist attack. A person's assessment of how likely an event is to occur is influenced by how available that event is within his or her memory, and current memories of terrorist victims are more likely.

Another cognitive construct is fear perception, or the belief that a risk is meaningful and real. The study of fear perception is relevant to understanding how people make risky decisions, or even to realize that a decision must be made to avoid risk. Within injury control, there are examples of manipulating risk perception, for example, regarding child safety seats. Child safety seats (and booster seats) are engineered technologies to help children survive crashes and avoid injury. Safety seats have shown their effectiveness for protecting children (Dellinger, Sleet, Shults, & Rinehart, 2006). Will and Geller (2004) focused on increasing perception among caregivers that their child safety seats needed to be checked for installation and use errors. Their review of the issues surrounding parental fear perception indicated that many such caregivers believed they had successfully installed and used seats correctly, even though misuse rates have been estimated to be higher than 70 percent (Decina & Lococo, 2003). Engineering improvements for the driving environment—like child seats—may not generate proper behaviors to use the technology correctly because people simply do not perceive the risk inherent for non-use or incorrect use.

Will (2005) discussed how to better design and implement fear appeals to increase correct use of child safety seats. Her work can apply to a wide range of injury control initiatives. Her main target is to correct the "immunity fallacy" that caregivers have, or the belief that they are not susceptible to the negative consequences that occur when child safety seats are misused or not used. Based on her review of risk communication, she advocated that media messages targeting caregivers should use crash footage to demonstrate the power of crash forces and depict injuries from such crashes to caregivers. Such shock may be necessary to motivate caregivers to pay attention to messages regarding the use of child safety seats. However, Will also pointed out that effective fear appeals must do more than shock people; they must provide needed information and resources to alleviate the fear and prevent the danger. It is not enough to scare people; fear alone will not motivate change (and may activate a "defense mechanism" in the target audience; Sanders & McCormick, 1993, p. 679). Fear plus an action plan to avoid the danger is more effective (Girasek, 2006).

The Influence of Task Workload

People often use cognitive shortcuts or heuristics when they face stressful or difficult tasks. For that reason, it is important to consider the influence of task workload on safety interventions. Engineers should consider the physical requirements of using engineering innovations to prevent injury. There are numerous physiological elements to address when designing products to reduce injury, not the least of which is how the innovation itself may strain or stress humans' ability to use it. Sanders and McCormick (1993) discussed various such physiological measures, including muscle physiology, respiratory and cardiovascular responses, and the strain on these systems, when humans complete various tasks. Reducing injury likelihood requires ensuring the strain does not exceed certain risk limits associated with a task.

Engineers should be aware of how physiological workload is a function of task progression. One clear example involves the issue of aviation safety. Pilots have varying physical requirements to complete their flight duties. Physically (and mentally) their workload is highest during takeoff and landing, when they are monitoring flight information and controlling the plane's moment-to-moment positioning. Therefore, the landing gear lever should be where the pilot can get to it, but not so available that the pilot activates it accidentally. In vehicles, drivers should be able to comfortably reach the accelerator and brake pedals and be able to sit upright sufficiently to see over the dashboard. Sanders and McCormick

(1993) provided several examples of workplace design (seats, work-surface heights, and computer screen angles) that demonstrate how the physical loads to do tasks affect both performance and injury potential.

Cognitive or mental workload is equally critical. Many of the influences that jeopardize safety involve limits of information processing by the brain. Researchers have shown that humans performing complex tasks in high-workload conditions will develop a sort of tunnel vision, whereby peripheral stimuli are screened out (Easterbrook, 1959). Conversely, research also suggests that if humans are underloaded, they will suffer performance degradation in cognitive information encoding (Smallwood, Obonsawin, & Reid, 2003). One consequence of task underload appears to be daydreaming, which has been connected with injury-producing events.

Mental workload is also affected by cognitive resources and task demand (Wickens & Hollands, 2000). As tasks become more difficult and as humans are required to perform more behaviors simultaneously, performance may decrease because of additional cognitive and physical workloads (Wickens & Hollands, 2000). However, not all workload is detrimental. Charlton (2002) reviewed evidence suggesting performance is worsened when the task is so difficult that it exceeds resources, but he also found that easy tasks may be performed better when workload is increased. Wickens and Hollands (2000) suggested that training may increase workload management. Indeed, experts compared to novices are better able to manage high workload levels.

Workload effects on safety can be readily seen in the driving environment. Summala (2005) noted that workload increases or decreases as a function of time constraints and complexity of tasks while in a dynamic environment, such as a moving car at a given speed. Specifically, he suggested that drivers feeling time pressure to complete tasks will either slow their speed to reduce workload or continue and face load problems (increasing risk). Drivers with plenty of time and low workload, in contrast, may perform other tasks or become bored, both leading to increased risk. Summala also discussed the role of motivation, given that driving a car at high speeds is pleasurable for many people. This motive and others may affect the adoption of risk while driving.

The Influence of Situation Awareness

Situation awareness (SA) is another important determinant of safety behaviors. SA is the act of perceiving elements in one's environment, including their temporal and spatial attributes, their significance, and what will happen to these attributes in the immediate and more distant future (Endsley, 1988). Embedded within this definition are three levels of situation awareness. Level 1 SA refers to the act of perceiving the status, attributes, and dynamics of environmental features. For example, a person who is riding a motorcycle on a mountain highway needs to perceive the presence and changing status of upcoming curves, moisture on the highway, and prevailing wind. Level 2 SA refers to the act of comprehending the meaning of the features perceived as a part of level 1 SA. If the motorcycle rider crosses a threshold to a different style of asphalt, he or she would need to process this information in the light of (for example) the motorcycle's capabilities, his or her riding skills, and the ambient weather conditions. An important part of level 2 SA is the processing of features relevant to current and future goals.

The third level of SA is particularly relevant for safety-related actions. Task performers must have the ability to determine what will happen to features of their environment as they continue to interact with them. For example, a motorcycle rider who realizes that the motorcycle is running low on gas must make a decision about when to stop to fill up. Elements of the situation that will influence the decision include the projected rate of fuel use, knowledge of existing fuel stations, and size of the motorcycle's fuel tank. Level 3 SA is implicated within some of the most popular accident models, such as James Reason's "Swiss cheese model" (Reason, 2000). This model asserts that accidents happen because of a progressive chain of relatively innocuous events. Each event may be visualized as a hole within a single piece of cheese. Though individually these holes do not pose serious threats to safety, if they happen to occur together, an accident will result. Level 3 SA is necessary for people to anticipate the holes aligning.

Many other variables influence situation awareness and safety. Some of the more important ones are tolerance of risk, time pressure, and existing task parameters and goals. These additional variables are easily illustrated by considering other safety examples, such as using cellular telephones while driving, driving too fast along a highway, failing to use protective sports equipment, or removing batteries from household smoke alarms.

The Influence of Automation

Converting manual tasks to automated ones has had an important impact on cognitive and physical workload. Manufacturing jobs rely on machines, the cars we drive have many built-in automatic processes to help us reduce load (for example, adjustable seats and collapsible steering wheels to reduce crash load). However, relegating cognitive functions to machines has a mixed effect on perceived workload—sometimes decreasing it, other times increasing it (Parasuraman & Riley, 1997). Parasuraman and Riley reviewed evidence suggesting that workers choose automation to help relieve workload. Other evidence, such as in aviation studies, suggests that automation can increase workload. For example, we have noted that take-offs and landings have higher physiological loads than cruise flying. Automation processes in the cockpit require mental workload to use properly. Just as important, the decision to use the automation often requires cognitive effort and workload. If the benefits of automation are not apparent and the amount of effort required to determine the benefit is too high, a person may decide not to use the technology (Kirlik, 1993), may avoid using it, or may override it.

Overreliance on automation can create additional injury risk. For example, people may allow the automative processes to run unabated, without critical evaluation or monitoring. Parasuraman and Riley (1997) reviewed cases in which pilots used autopilot technology even when it resulted in performance decrements. Other evidence in their review demonstrates seasoned pilots often fail to monitor the automation, instead placing "excessive trust" in the system (p. 239). Another example of complacency is the misplaced reliance on airbags over seat belts even though the policies requiring air bags are not as cost-effective for saving lives as the simple manual technology (Elvik & Vaa, 2004; Evans, 2004; Sleet & Kallberg, 1991).

Automation can sometimes improve performance. To use engineering innovations, humans must trust those systems to perform well. The decision not to use safety belts because one believes they reduce chances to survive in certain crashes is an example of such distrust. In the case of airbag technology, it proved to be more harmful than helpful to small children in the front seat. Our heuristics may certainly guide what automation we choose to trust and therefore use.

Trust in automation is affected by the perception of system reliability (see Parasuraman & Riley, 1997). Airplane pilots sometimes prefer to take manual control of the aircraft because they do not trust the automated speed control or autopilot functions in inclement weather conditions. Similarly, advanced users of personal computers may prefer to use programs that are less automated because they want greater control over program functions. Drivers may opt for less automation than more to retain some control over vehicle maneuverability, even if the automated solution appears superior.

Lessons Learned from Human Factors Research for Injury Control

Some lessons from applying human factors research to injury control include the following:

- Humans and technology, together with the surrounding environment, form a system. To reduce injury, task and equipment designers must focus on each of these elements and how they work individually and together.

- Even given the importance of focusing on the system, it is generally easier and more effective to modify equipment and technology than it is to train individuals to engage in safe behaviors. Therefore, if designers can modify a technology or environment to reduce opportunities for risk, injuries may be reduced.
- The complexity of human behavior makes it difficult to design systems according to a one-size-fits-all philosophy. Decisions regarding cutoffs (for example, with height, weight, and mental workload capability) may not easily or effectively apply to a majority of the target population.
- Heuristics and biases affect perceptions of whether a technology will or will not reduce injury and whether people will adopt and embrace the technology as helpful in avoiding risk. Researchers should consider how fear appeals may alter reliance on heuristics and biases.
- To be effective, human factors approaches to reducing injury should account for cognitive and physical workload. In addition to training for workload management, engineers should manipulate workload levels to enhance performance.
- Humans look to their environments for information about what is going to happen (situation awareness). Automation can help prepare them, but it must be reliable, trustworthy, and cost-effective.
- Technology and engineering interventions are not the panacea for injury prevention without consideration of other techniques, but they are important for any comprehensive injury prevention model. There is a continuing opportunity to design effective automation to assist with safety enhancements if researchers understand human-technology interactions and the behavioral and cognitive factors influencing automation use.

Future Research Needs

There are at least two areas for future research that deserve mentioning. First, human factors researchers should be mindful of behavioral adaptation to technology. Human behavior adapts to the environment, and experiences help to shape and change perceptions of risk and acceptance of workload. For example, there have been numerous discussions and debates within traffic psychology about whether and how drivers adapt to vehicle design and roadway environment changes, with conclusions that such technological changes do not always lead to expected injury reductions (see Summala, 2002). By manipulating and adapting workload variables and understanding how to prevent cognitive deficits, automation complacency, and learned irrelevance, behavior researchers will have the opportunity to improve adaptation.

Second, much of human factors research for injury control has focused on transportation and occupational issues. These are two of the most relevant areas where technology and automation make significant impacts on safety. However, there are other areas of injury control that may benefit from human factors research. One is medical injury control involving surgeries and hospital care (Bogner, 1994). Another involves injury control in environments with little technology or no automation, such as on playgrounds and in sports and recreation. In these examples, the use of evidence-based design criteria is highly relevant (Ratte, Morrison, Lerner, Denham, & Johnson, 1990).

Conclusions

The science of human factors has a legitimate place alongside other approaches to reduce injury. Risk-taking behavior is the result of many variables that interact to create contingencies for particular behaviors (Mattaini, 1996). Human factors and engineering initiatives help build these contingent relationships with other predictors of the behavior. Focusing on how human behavior interacts with technology represents a critical area of future study for injury control.

Finally, in an effort to emphasize the role that human factors play in injury prevention, we offer the following wisdom, adapted from and inspired by Shneiderman (1998):

- "Know thy user" to incorporate appropriate safety interventions for his or her needs.
- "Know thy task" to understand how it will affect user trust, workload, and situational awareness.
- "Know thy environment" to appreciate how other factors such as stress, heat, cold, and noise will interact with the human operator to influence safety.

References

Adams, J. A. (1987). Historical review and appraisal of research on the learning, retention and transfer of human motor skills. *Psychological Bulletin, 101*, 41–74.

Bailey, R. (1982). *Human performance engineering.* Upper Saddle River, NJ: Prentice Hall.

Bitan, Y., Meyer, J., Shinar, D., & Zmora, E. (2004). Nurses' reactions to alarms in a neonatal intensive care unit. *Cognition, Technology and Work, 6*, 239–246.

Bliss, J. P. (2003). An investigation of alarm related incidents in aviation. *International Journal of Aviation Psychology, 13*(3), 249–268.

Bliss, J. P., Deaton, J. J., & Gilson, R. D. (1995). Alarm response behavior under conditions of varying alarm reliability. *Ergonomics, 38*(11), 2300–2312.

Bogner, M. S. (Ed.). (1994). *Human error in medicine.* Mahwah, NJ: Erlbaum.

Breznitz, S. (1984). *Cry wolf: The psychology of false alarms.* Mahwah, NJ: Erlbaum.

Cavallo, V., Mestre, D., & Berthelon, C. (1997). Time to collision judgments: Visual and spatio-temporal factors. In T. Rothengatter & E. C. Vaya (Eds.), *Traffic and transport psychology theory and application* (pp. 97–111). New York: Pergamon Press.

Charlton, S. G. (2002). Measurement of cognitive state in test and evaluation. In S. G. Charlton & T. G. O'Brien (Eds.), *Handbook of human factors testing and evaluation* (2nd ed., pp. 97–126). Mahwah, NJ: Erlbaum.

Decina, L. E., & Lococo, K. H. (2003). *Misuse of child restraints.* Washington, DC: National Highway Traffic Safety Administration. DOT HS 809671.

Dellinger, A., Sleet, D. A., Shults, R., & Rinehart, C. (2006). Motor vehicle injury prevention. In L. Doll, S. Bonzo, J. Mercy, & D. A. Sleet (Eds.), *Handbook of injury and violence prevention.* New York: Springer.

Digges, K., Nicholson, R., & Rouse, E. (1985). *The technical basis for the center high mounted stoplamp.* Warrandale, PA: SAE. Report #851240.

Easterbrook, J. A. (1959). The effect of emotion on cue utilization and the organization of behavior. *Psychological Review, 66,* 183–201.

Elvik, R., & Vaa, T. (2004). *The handbook of road safety measures.* Amsterdam: Elsevier.

Embrey, D. E. (1986). *SHERPA: A systematic human error reduction and prediction approach.* Paper presented at the International Meeting on Advances in Nuclear Power Systems, Knoxville, TN.

Endsley, M. (1988). Design and evaluation for situation awareness enhancement. In *Proceedings of the Human Factors Society 32nd Annual Meeting* (pp. 97–101). Santa Monica, CA: Human Factors Society.

Eschenbrenner, A. J., Jr. (1971). Effects of intermittent noise on the performance of a complex psychomotor task. *Human Factors, 13,* 59–63.

Evans, L. (2004). *Traffic safety.* Bloomfield Hills, MI: Science Serving Society.

Girasek, D. (2006). Communications and risk perception. In A. Gielen, D. A. Sleet, & R. DiClemente (Eds.), *Injury and violence prevention: Behavioral science theories, methods, and applications.* San Francisco: Jossey-Bass.

Glassbrenner, D. (2005). *Safety belt use in 2004-demographic results. Traffic safety facts: Research note.* Washington, DC: National Highway Traffic Safety Administration. DOT HS 809848.

Goetsch, D. L. (2005). *Occupational safety and health* (5th ed.). Upper Saddle River, NJ: Prentice Hall.

Haslam, D. R. (1985). Sustained operations and military performance. *Behavior Research Methods, Instruments, and Computers, 17,* 9–95.

Hockey, G.R.J. (1986). Changes in operational efficiency as a function of environmental stress, fatigue, and circadian rhythms. In K. R. Boff, L. Kaufman, & J. P. Thomas (Eds.), *Handbook of perception and human performance, Vol. 2: Cognitive processes and performance* (pp. 44-1–44-49). Hoboken, NJ: Wiley.

Holding, D. H. (1965). *Principles of training.* London: Pergamon Press.

Kahneman, D., & Tversky, A. (1972). Subjective probability: A judgment of representativeness. *Cognitive Psychology, 3,* 430–454.

Kerstholt, J. H., Passenier, P. O., Houttuin, K., & Schuffel, H. (1996). The effect of a priori probability and complexity on decision making in a supervisory control task. *Human Factors, 38,* 65–78.

Kirlik, A. (1993). Modeling strategic behavior in human-automation interaction: Why an "aid" can (and should) go unused. *Human Factors, 35,* 221–242.

Kittusamy, N. K., & Buchholz, B. (2004). Whole-body vibration and postural stress among operators of construction equipment: A literature review. *Journal of Safety Research, 35,* 255–261.

Lysaght, R. J., Hill, S. G., Dick, A. O., Plamondon, B. D., Linton, P. M., Wierwille, W. W., Zaklad, A. L., Bittner, A. C., Jr., & Wherry, R. J. (1989). *Operator workload: Comprehensive review and evaluation of operator workload methodologies* (Tech. Rep. No. 851). Alexandria, VA: U.S. Army Research Institute for the Behavioral and Social Sciences.

Maddox, M. E., & Muto, W. H. (1999, Apr. 6). Operator Edward Frederick looks back and tells about the systems and training improvements at TMI. *Ergonomics in Design,* 6–12.

Mallett, L. G., Vaught, C., & Brnich, M. J., Jr. (1993). Sociotechnical communication in an underground mine fire: A study of warning messages during an emergency evacuation. *Safety Science, 16,* 709–728.

Mattaini, M. (1996). Public issues, human behavior, and cultural design. In M. A. Mattaini & B. A. Thyer (Eds.), *Finding solutions to social problems: Behavioral strategies for change* (pp. 13–40). Washington, DC: American Psychological Association.

McClintock, T., Shields, T. J., Reinhart-Rutland, A., & Leslie, J. (2001). A behavioral solution to the learned irrelevance of emergency exit signage. In *Human behavior in fire: Understanding human behavior for better fire safety design.* Proceedings of the 2nd International Symposium, Cambridge, Boston. London: Interscience Communications.

Meister, D. (1989). *Conceptual aspects of human factors.* Baltimore, MD: Johns Hopkins University Press.

Nohre, L., MacKinnon, D. P., & Sadalla, E. K. (1998, Oct. 5–9). The effects of warning false alarms on driving speed. In *Proceedings of the 42nd Annual Human Factors and Ergonomics Society Meeting,* Chicago.

Parasuraman, R., & Riley, V. (1997). Humans and automation: Use, misuse, disuse, abuse. *Human Factors, 39,* 230–253.

Proctor, R. W., & Van Zandt, T. (1994). *Human factors in simple and complex systems.* Needham Heights, MA: Allyn & Bacon.

Ramsey, J., Burford, C., Beshir, M., & Jensen, R. (1983). Effects of workplace thermal conditions on safe work behavior. *Journal of Safety Research, 14,* 105–114.

Ramsey, J., & Kwon, Y. (1988). Simplified decision rules for predicting performance loss in the heat. In *Proceedings on Heat Stress Indices.* Luxembourg: Commission of the European Communities.

Ratte, D., Morrison, M., Lerner, N., Denham, S., & Johnson, D. (1990). *Development of human factors criteria for playground equipment safety.* Washington, DC: U.S. Consumer Product Safety Commission. Final Report CPSC-C-88-1231.

Reason, J. T. (2000). Swiss cheese model. In J. Reason, *Managing the risks of organizational accidents.* Burlington, VT: Ashgate.

Reynolds, B. (1952). The effect of learning on the predictability of psychomotor performance. *Journal of Experimental Psychology, 44,* 189–198.

Rodriguez, M. A. (1991). What makes a warning label salient? In *Proceedings of the Human Factors Society 35th Annual Meeting* (pp. 1029–1033). Santa Monica, CA: Human Factors Society.

Sanders, M. S., & McCormick, E. J. (1993). *Human factors in engineering and design* (7th ed.). New York: McGraw-Hill.

Sandman, P. M. (1991). *Risk = Hazard + outrage: A formula for effective risk communication* [Videotape]. (Available from the Environmental Communication Research Program, Cook College, Rutgers University, New Brunswick, NJ 08093.)

Schneider, W., & Shiffrin, R. M. (1977). Controlled and automatic human information processing: I. Detection, search, and attention. *Psychological Review, 84,* 1–66.

Shneiderman, B. (1998). *Designing the user interface: Strategies for effective human-computer interaction.* Reading, MA: Addison-Wesley.

Sleet, D. A., & Kallberg, V. P. (1991). Airbags save lives, but the costs are high. *Nordic Road and Transport Research, 3,* 8–11.

Smallwood, J., Obonsawin, M., & Reid, H. (2003). The effect of block duration and task demands on the experience of task unrelated thought. *Imagination, Cognition and Personality, 22,* 13–31.

Stanton, N. A., & Edworthy, J. (1999). *Human factors in auditory warnings.* Aldershot, England: Ashgate.

Sternberg, R. J. (2003). *Cognitive psychology* (3rd ed.). Belmont, CA: Wadsworth.

Summala, H. (2002). Behavioural adaptation and drivers' task control. In R. Fuller & J. A. Santos (Eds.), *Human factors for highway engineers* (pp. 189–200). New York: Pergamon Press.

Summala, H. (2005). Traffic psychology theories: Towards understanding driving behaviour and safety efforts. In G. Underwood (Ed.), *Traffic and transport psychology: Theory and application* (pp. 383–394). Amsterdam: Elsevier.

Swain, A. D. (1964). *THERP.* (Report No. SC-R-64-1338). Albuquerque, NM: Sandia National Laboratories.

Tversky, A., & Kahneman, D. (1973). Availability: A heuristic for judging frequency and probability. *Cognitive Psychology, 5,* 207–232.

Wickens, C. D., & Hollands, J. G. (2000). *Engineering and human performance* (3rd ed.). Upper Saddle River, NJ: Prentice Hall.

Will, K. E. (2005). Child passenger safety and the immunity fallacy: Why what we're doing isn't working. *Accident Analysis and Prevention, 37,* 947–955.

Will, K. E., & Geller, E. S. (2004). Increasing the safety of children's vehicle travel: From effective risk communication to behavior change. *Journal of Safety Research, 35,* 263–274.

Yerkes, R. M., & Dodson, J. D. (1908). The relation of strength of stimulus to rapidity of habit. *Journal of Comparative Neurological Psychology, 18,* 459–482.

CHAPTER TWENTY-TWO

BEHAVIORAL SCIENCES, INJURY, AND VIOLENCE PREVENTION

Synthesis and Future Directions

Ralph J. DiClemente, Andrea Carlson Gielen, David A. Sleet

The risk of an injury or exposure to violence and its adverse sequelae is one of the most significant and immediate threats to population health and well-being. Injury and violence exact a significant toll on individuals and, ultimately, on society (see Chapter One for a more detailed description of the epidemiology and impact of injury on individuals and society). From an individual perspective, the toll can be measured in terms of morbidity and mortality. Injury-associated morbidity includes pain, suffering, and disability. These adverse sequelae can be acute or chronic, curable or intractable. From an economic and social standpoint, injury and violence continue to exact a significant toll on society, resulting in missed work time, lost productivity, and treatment-associated costs. For these reasons, the prevention of injury and violence must be a public health priority and the behaviors that give rise to injury the subject of careful study.

Recent advances in technology, such as safer vehicles and roadways, smoke alarms and carbon monoxide detectors, bicycle helmets, fire-retardant materials, and poison-prevention packaging, to name but a few, have made important contributions to reducing injury risk. Coinciding with advances in injury protection technology have been changes to legal statutes and laws (see Chapter Twenty). New and stricter laws to discourage driving under the influence of alcohol, the mandatory requirement for using seat belts and child safety seats, reduced speed limits, and stricter building codes that require sprinkler systems have been important in injury prevention. Many of the technological advances have enhanced

485

the likelihood of injury prevention and the prospects for survival for people experiencing an injury. Each of these advances, and others in injury prevention, rely
at least in part on behavior to succeed.

Injury prevention programs that encourage individuals to adopt and maintain injury-preventive behaviors remain an important and practical strategy, regardless of other approaches used to change products and environments. Laws
and technology designed to enhance injury prevention are limited by people's willingness to use technology properly and adhere to laws. It may be useful to look at
models in health promotion that typically implement a variety of strategies simultaneously to maximize the likelihood people will adopt and sustain life-saving
and risk-reducing behaviors.

Programs that enhance people's awareness of the threat posed by injury, increase their perception of personal vulnerability to injury, modify their beliefs, norms,
attitudes, and intentions, and increase the accessibility to and affordability of safety
devices and behavior change resources can decrease the likelihood of injury. While
modifying individuals' injury-related behaviors is admittedly a formidable challenge,
such changes are achievable. Multifaceted, interdisciplinary approaches have succeeded in contributing to substantial changes in injury-related behaviors in the past
two decades through, for example, seat belt use, car seat use, smoke alarm use, poison prevention, violence, and drowning prevention measures. Some well-controlled
intervention trials, such as community mobilizing to reduce alcohol-related trauma
and smoke alarm distribution programs, have yielded promising and effective strategies. Recent advances in the application of health behavior change and communication theory to injury and violence prevention are encouraging signs that carefully
designed and implemented programs can succeed in changing injury prevention behaviors and reducing injury-related morbidity and mortality.

The chapters in this book describe promising advances in the field of injury
and violence prevention with respect to behavior change theory, design, implementation, and evaluation. Intervention approaches are discussed that address an
array of injury risk behaviors, in diverse settings, and with different populations.
This concluding chapter highlights key cross-cutting areas of prevention research
and suggests directions for future behavioral science research in injury and violence prevention.

Injury Prevention Research and
Practice Need to Be Interdisciplinary

The success of prevention efforts is, to a large extent, attributable to the heterogeneity of disciplines that are actively involved in the science of injury prevention.
Because of this diversity, advances in prevention are being made by transcending

disciplinary boundaries in theory, methodology, implementation, and evaluation strategies. The most important advances have been made using transdisciplinary and interdisciplinary approaches that involve not only injury epidemiologists but also social and behavioral science researchers and health promotion practitioners. Examples from the work reviewed in this book include the relationship between human behavior and engineering solutions (Chapter Twenty-One), the use of psychological research in elucidating the role of supervision in preventing injuries (Chapter Eighteen), and the multifaceted, multilevel approaches to reducing drinking and driving crashes (Chapters Ten and Eleven) to name but a few.

The best opportunity to develop a coherent, effective, and interdisciplinary approach to injury prevention research is through the continued integration and collaboration of researchers in the behavioral and social sciences, with public health practitioners, health educators and clinicians, health psychologists, law and policy experts, epidemiologists, engineers, and biostatisticians. Of particular importance is the interaction between researchers and practitioners. As Lawrence Green notes, "if we want more evidence-based practice, we need more practice-based evidence" (2005). The research-practice connection is essential to help find better ways to promote the widespread adoption and use of effective strategies; however, a research analytical framework for studying diffusion, dissemination, and adoption of safety behaviors is absent in the injury prevention literature.

Examples of interdisciplinary collaborations are well represented in the description of home safety interventions in Chapter Thirteen, the work in youth violence presented in Chapter Seventeen, the applications of social cognitive theory in Chapter Three, and some of the examples of community models described in Chapter Four.

There is also growing recognition of and support for those in acute care and rehabilitation to provide behaviorally focused secondary prevention interventions, and trauma centers are increasingly being expected to participate in primary prevention efforts. Collaborations between health services researchers, trauma and rehabilitation care providers, and those trained in the behavioral sciences should increase in the future, leading to rapid advances in secondary prevention strategies. Addressing posttraumatic stress, as described in Chapter Nineteen, is one example of these critically important postevent interventions.

Injury Prevention Behavior Change Interventions Need to Address Multiple Levels of Causality

Historically, the injury epidemic had been largely viewed as an individual-level health phenomenon. This perspective dominated the early days of injury prevention. Subsequently, there was an incremental shift in research focus, from emphasis on the individual to an increased emphasis on the physical environment and how to engineer safety into products and environments (Hale & Glendon, 1987). However, overreliance on passive approaches may result in underreliance on individual responsibility for self-protection. Most recently, there has been a growing recognition of the need for complementary approaches to injury prevention, that is, a comprehensive approach that integrates strategies designed to modify individuals' behavior and their physical environment as part of a multifaceted, coordinated prevention program. Theory development and application is an important cornerstone in this effort to better understand individual factors strategies to motivate individuals to take preventive actions. These are discussed further in Chapter Two.

The public health field generally, and the injury prevention field specifically, have also emphasized the impact of the social environment on safety policies and individuals' behavior. Behavioral scientists, in particular, have realized a host of environmental and structural influences that make a significant contribution to sustaining the injury epidemic (see Chapter Six), but these forces do not operate apart from the actions of individuals.

Researchers and practitioners alike are increasingly acknowledging the importance of social context, that is, the need to understand an individual's behavior within his or her social environment and intervene not only on the individual level but on broader social structural levels. It is clear, for example, that individual-level interventions, while effective at motivating behavior change, may not be sufficient to sustain behavior changes over protracted periods of time, particularly in the face of pervasive countervailing pressures that promote or reinforce risk behavior. Furthermore, addressing behavior change at the individual level lacks sufficient breadth to reach large segments of an at-risk population. Community-level interventions that create and support social norms conducive to injury prevention are needed (Blumenthal & DiClemente, 2004), along with research to document their success. These issues are comprehensively addressed in the discussions of an ecological model (Chapter Six), PRECEDE-PROCEED and the Haddon matrix (Chapter Seven), and community models (Chapter Four).

Interventions targeted at the community level are designed to promote injury-preventive behavior change by providing individuals with information and skills to change behavior through naturally occurring channels of influence in the community and simultaneously to provide a supportive environment that encourages injury-preventive behavior. Changing community norms also reinforces and maintains safety-promoting behaviors. This provides one avenue for ensuring a social context in which individuals will be reminded that the healthier alternative (safer behavior) is preferred in accordance with community standards and norms.

Community-level interventions may have four interrelated outcomes. First, they may promote the adoption of injury-preventive behaviors among persons engaged in risky behaviors. Second, they may help sustain newly acquired injury-preventive behaviors and, it is hoped, solidify these changes so that they are maintained over protracted periods of time. Third, they may serve to amplify individual-level program effects over extended time periods, reducing the potential for relapse to high-risk behaviors. And finally, community-level interventions may foster an atmosphere that discourages the initial adoption of high-risk behaviors. An understanding of these broader, pervasive influences may lead to the development of community-level interventions, initiate policy changes, design institutionally based programs, and promote the development of broader, macrolevel societal changes.

Strategies Are Needed to Improve the Sustainability of Injury Prevention Behavior Change Program Efforts

Another key area in injury prevention research is in the development of strategies to sustain intervention program effects over time. There is ample evidence from health promotion research in other fields that both individual- and community-level interventions can modify injury risk behaviors. However, there are also data suggesting that intervention effects decay over time. In individual-level prevention interventions in other areas of health promotion, one strategy that is frequently used to minimize decay (or attenuation of intervention effects) is to use booster sessions subsequent to delivering the primary "dose" of the intervention. While this has shown efficacy in reconstituting intervention effects in long-term follow-up, it is clearly labor and time intensive, and thus costly.

Alternative approaches are needed and should be explored for specific application in injury prevention. One strategy that holds promise is the use of social marketing or media interventions to enhance health risk communication, motivate adoption of injury-preventive behaviors, reinforce prevention messages, and sustain behavior change (see Chapter Five). An example is the use of media-based interventions or social marketing strategies. As stand-alone interventions or, what is perhaps more effective, in a complementary model in conjunction with other intervention strategies, these health risk communication media-based interventions and social marketing strategies may create a social climate that encourages continued adherence to injury prevention behaviors.

Based on studies of other health behaviors, we believe that mass media, when used appropriately, may help to create an environment conducive to injury prevention. As illustrated in the discussion of health risk communication (Chapter Five), numerous characteristics of injury problems make media appeals to safe behaviors particularly challenging. Nevertheless, it is likely that more sophisticated campaigns that draw heavily on knowledge of the audience and health communication theories could have significant dividends for promoting injury prevention behaviors. Comprehensive injury prevention campaigns that include media have had demonstrable successes, as discussed in several of the chapters in this book.

In particular, mass media can help increase awareness of the injury problem and the benefits of prevention and can create a climate that encourages public or private funding for injury prevention. Thus, the media can be instrumental in creating a social climate that makes a wide spectrum of prevention strategies more acceptable at both the individual and community levels. It is widely recognized that media attention and education around motor vehicle safety issues such as seat belt use, bicycle helmet use, and the hazards of drinking and driving prepared the public for the mandatory legislation that followed, thereby facilitating an understanding and acceptance of new laws. On issues where attempts to pass legislation failed or were overturned (as with motorcycle helmet use), preparation of the public may not have been adequate or persuasive enough (see Chapter Twenty on legislation). While media-based interventions may be effective in preparing the public or stimulating people who are in the contemplation stage (in the stages of change model; Chapter Two), they can be prepared to be informative, entertaining, and personally relevant. In addition, messages about injury disseminated through the mass media may facilitate more open discussion of risk behavior and its adverse consequences. Generating such discussion and framing media messages to focus on needed policy changes is at the root of media advocacy, which has received much attention as a promising approach in public health and may be particularly relevant in injury and violence prevention (Wallack, Dorfman, Jernigan, & Themba, 1993).

Media interventions are not a panacea. It is clear that media-based interventions remain an understudied intervention modality in the United States. Indeed, media may be particularly well suited as part of a complementary prevention strategy in which media messages are timed to overlay an existing individual- or community-level intervention. Whether media campaigns, in isolation or in conjunction with existing injury prevention programs, would enjoy widespread support and success in the United States is arguable. However, media programs, even those that may be less innovative, may still serve to create a social climate conducive to open discussion about the hazards of injury-associated risk behaviors. And as noted above, media messages may reinforce prevention messages for individuals exposed to more intensive interventions. In this way, media campaigns may have a direct impact on individuals' behavior and may indirectly influence behavior by affecting social norms to help sustain newly adopted injury-preventive behaviors or reinforce maintenance of low-risk behaviors in the face of counter-vailing social pressures.

In Search of New and Promising Theoretical Orientations

Theories are developed to predict and explain phenomena. In injury prevention, theories of human behavior are useful in predicting and explaining why people do or do not engage in behaviors that increase their risk for injury. Many theories have been used to guide exploratory research designed to identify the antecedents and determinants of risk behaviors (see Chapters Two through Four for a review of widely applicable individual- and community-level theories). Theory too has played an integral role in guiding the development of programs designed to eliminate or reduce risk behaviors associated with the likelihood of experiencing an injury.

The range of theoretical approaches possible in injury prevention is diverse. Theoretical approaches from a broad spectrum of disciplines have been used to guide observational research into the determinants of injury-related behaviors as well as behavior change interventions designed to reduce injury risk behaviors. A great deal of evidence suggests that theory-based interventions can be effective in promoting injury prevention behaviors. However, many theories related to be-havior, econometrics, environmental psychology, human factors, communications, anthropology, and other aspects of social science remain to be tested in injury prevention.

Testing and refining theory leads to change. As theories become less useful or fail to guide the design and implementation of injury prevention interventions, they should be modified or even discarded in favor of more useful explanatory models. This process of development, elimination, and replacement is incremen-tal and cyclical, allowing new theories to emerge and be synthesized and em-braced. The current theoretical armamentarium has been very useful, particularly the social cognitive theories (see Chapter Three), in furthering our understanding of the interplay of factors that can affect both risk and preventive behavior and how implementation should proceed.

Injury prevention can ultilize new and emerging theoretical models to guide scientific progress and innovative applications or revisions of older models. These new theories and applications should be empirically tested (DiClemente, Crosby, & Kegler, 2002). As in any other science, the field of injury prevention needs to be receptive to innovation and maintain rigorous evaluation standards in the de-velopment of new methods and models.

The Need to Improve Injury Prevention Program Transfer

No injury prevention intervention is perfect. Not every individual exposed to an intervention will adopt the appropriate injury preventive behaviors. Such a goal is unrealistic. Striving for this may even be counterproductive, creating inertia among policy experts, practitioners, and other consumers of prevention research while they search for the "magic bullet" intervention that will protect everyone automatically.

This does not mean that we lower the standard for determining effective injury prevention interventions. Quite the contrary. A failure to adopt and maintain rigorous standards for identifying effective injury prevention interventions is bought at the cost of wasting scarce resources on ineffective programs. It does mean, however, that while the continued efforts of prevention scientists need to be directed at developing more effective injury prevention interventions, existing interventions that have demonstrated programmatic efficacy need to be widely disseminated and adopted by the public.

Ultimately, preventing injury depends not only on the development and evaluation of innovative behavior change approaches, but on how effectively these interventions can be translated and integrated into clinic practice, school curricula, community programs, and other areas. Thus, future research also focuses on identifying mechanisms for the timely translation of effective injury interventions into sustainable community-, clinic-, or school-based programs. Successful translation in injury prevention can benefit from guidelines, theoretical constructs, and approaches already developed in other areas of public health (National Cancer Institute, 2005; Svanstrom, Boleslav, & Grivna, 2004).

While the research output in terms of behavioral approaches to injury prevention has been remarkable (Sleet & Hopkins, 2004), particularly research in the past few years using models or theory-based interventions, the uptake and the integration of this information into ongoing sustainable, programmatic activities have been far less plentiful, even absent. Understanding the barriers that impede the rapid adoption of new injury prevention programs by governmental and community-based organizations is a critical need in the field. As this book points out, we have many interventions known to work, but we have not paid sufficient attention to dissemination. Further study is needed in advancing our understanding of how organizations, including the individual providers within those organizations, are influenced to adopt innovations in injury prevention.

The development of sustainable systems and processes for the efficient transfer of injury prevention programs is contingent on many factors. Foremost is the need for an infrastructure that is responsible for collecting and collating new injury prevention information as well as organizing, managing, and coordinating its active transfer to practitioners and other consumers, including policy analysts, elected officials, health department officials, clinical and social service providers, and prevention program managers in community-based organizations. For efficient program transfer, investing in the development of an infrastructure to design and continually monitor systems and processes needed to promote rapid and widespread use of evidence-based injury prevention strategies is critical. Resources will need to be identified, mobilized, and committed to the ongoing maintenance and support of infrastructure that promotes the rapid dissemination of injury prevention programs.

There is a clear distinction between the passive transfer of injury prevention programs versus the actions required to encourage the uptake and implementation of these programs. To be effective, the transfer of effective strategies to individual and community use is not automatic (Sogolow, Saul, & Sleet, 2006). Rather, it must be an active and purposive application of skills, systems, and resources dedicated to supporting both the transfer and the uptake of new prevention programs. Thus, gaps and inadequacies in the infrastructure responsible for supporting the transfer and uptake of new injury prevention programs will clearly limit how efficiently systems and processes can be designed, implemented, maintained, and evaluated. Without a competent and fully operational infrastructure for dissemination, it is doubtful that the experimental and community research done will translate to have an impact on the injury problem. To support the uptake of effective programs, it will be necessary to invest in training, the provision of relevant materials, and an ongoing program of technical assistance.

The Need to Assess Objective Outcomes in Injury Prevention Research

To a large extent, injury prevention interventions have relied on individuals' self-reported behavior change to assess program efficacy. Typically individuals reported their frequency of a particular injury-associated behavior. In the most rigorous research designs, randomized controlled trials, baseline frequency of risk measures is contrasted with postintervention measures of similar risk behaviors relative to a placebo attention comparison group or control group (see Chapter Nine for a discussion of intervention research methods and evaluation approaches). In essence, these programs provide a measure of programmatic impact (change in injury-associated risk behaviors relative to a referent group). While impact evaluation outcomes are desirable, so too is the need to complement these measures, when feasible, with objective outcomes (that is, actual injuries) for evaluating program efficacy.

Measuring biological end points (injuries), while representing an objective and quantifiable marker, is not always feasible and not always necessary to document the success of an intervention. There are many proxies for injury, including the reduction in injury-related risk behaviors that are predictable precursors to an injury-related event. Observation of changes in these injury-related behaviors is often sufficient to demonstrate the impact of an intervention designed to reduce risk.

Reliance on the actual occurrence of injuries as a measure of program efficacy may not be an appropriate outcome for every study. It is unlikely, for instance, that the incidence of injuries will be changed in a short-term study conducted in a population with little risk behavior or in a community with a low prevalence of a particular injury. Conversely, populations with a high degree of risk behaviors and a high prevalence of a particular injury are ideal for studying the effects of behavioral interventions on injury incidence. Moreover, studies incorporating injury incidence as the primary outcome measure will need to be conducted with samples that are large enough and follow-up that is long enough to provide sufficient statistical power to detect differences in injury incidence. With many injuries a "rare event," efficacy using injury incidence will be increasingly difficult. Future injury prevention intervention studies should incorporate actual injury incidence as an outcome when appropriate and feasible, but also explore the use of intermediate outcomes, such as reductions in injury risk behaviors, improvements in skill, or reductions in exposures.

The Need to Measure Cost-Effectiveness in Injury Prevention Research

The increasing emphasis on cost containment, the emergence of the managed care environment, and the disproportionate increase in the cost of health care versus other expenditures over the past decade have prompted examining cost-effectiveness as one criterion for evaluating health promotion programs. In our current fiscal environment, it becomes imperative that we not only evaluate program efficacy in terms of impact (changes in behavior, attitudes, norms, and knowledge, for example) and outcomes (including changes in morbidity, mortality, and quality of life) but also assess cost-effectiveness. Such information is vitally important to program planners, policymakers, practitioners, and others involved in the design and implementation of health promotion and disease prevention programs.

Arguably, one might question whether injury prevention programs should be held accountable to the standard that a program's economic benefits to society outweigh its financial costs. However, whether one accepts that standard, the application of economic evaluation techniques is as appropriate to injury prevention interventions as to other health programs (Capilouto, 1999). For example, if two injury prevention programs (say, fall prevention among the elderly), using rigorous evaluation methodology, yielded similar impact and outcome evaluations, but one program cost two dollars to avert a fall while the other program cost ten dollars to avert a fall, the cost-effectiveness differential would favor the former program. Indeed, the former program could be markedly expanded to reach many more people and still cost less than the latter program, yielding a substantial population benefit.

Unable to sidestep the issue of cost effectiveness, injury prevention scientists and program planners need to become familiar with the theory and methods used to conduct cost-effectiveness studies (Haddix, Teutsch, Shaffer, & Dunet, 1996; Finkelstein, Corso, & Miller, 2006). This methodology represents an entirely different perspective for many injury researchers and practitioners (Zaza et al., 2001). Most often, injury prevention scientists have had their philosophical, theoretical, and methodological roots in their own discipline, not in economic research. Yet injury prevention specialists will increasingly need to become familiar with cost-effectiveness methods and analysis, establish the cost-effectiveness of these interventions, and implement programs accordingly. This points to the need to conduct interdisciplinary research with colleagues who have expertise in other disciplines.

Need for Structured Reporting of Injury Prevention Interventions

Some journals in the fields of medicine, including the *Journal of the American Medical Association* and the *British Medical Journal,* have adopted structured reporting requirements to enhance study comparability and quality. Working groups have been convened to study and recommend reporting guidelines for biomedical clinical trial research (Begg et al., 1996; Standards of Reporting Clinical Trials Group, 1994). Similarly, reporting guidelines for injury prevention trials would be equally useful.

The growth in injury prevention intervention research has led to new challenges: how to calibrate an intervention's efficacy in relation to other interventions. Variability in the reporting of injury prevention trials severely limits comparability of findings between trials. Moreover, the lack of structured reporting guidelines reduces the level of certainty with which injury interventions could be carefully assessed, weighed against other interventions, and replicated.

Structured reporting is meant to provide other researchers, practitioners, and consumers of injury prevention research with a list of essential elements necessary to adequately describe and, if need be, replicate the study. The purpose is to assist investigators in preparing reports that will facilitate understanding of the study—its rationale, methodology, and statistical analyses—and thus increasing the utility of the findings for practitioners, researchers, and policy experts. A principal advantage of structured reporting is that consumers will have uniform, comparable information to review and evaluate, regardless of variability in investigators' writing styles or reviewers' and journals' policies, which is much needed in making a determination about the validity of the findings and influence decision making about implementation of a particular injury prevention intervention.

The intent of a proposed reporting format is not to discourage investigators from including additional elements in published reports or to discourage investigators in the design and implementation of innovative interventions. Structured reporting does not preclude innovation; it only requires that investigators provide a clear, accurate, and consistent structure for describing the study design, its implementation, specification of the intervention, and data analysis. With the development and evaluation of increasing numbers of injury prevention interventions, structured reporting guidelines will provide a framework that may enhance interpretation of research findings by researchers, practitioners, and policy analysts.

Interactions Between Spheres of Influence: Lessons for the Future

Several converging spheres of influence (among them, law, technology, behavioral science, and economics) will likely result in increased focus on injury prevention research, but some important caveats must be noted if there is truly to be an increase in attention to this area of research. First, injury prevention is a science of diverse disciplines. Much will be gained by embracing the breadth of perspectives from these different disciplines and to engage in transdisciplinary work. However, it is incumbent on injury researchers, behavioral science researchers, and practitioners to work toward convergence of theories and methodologies to improve injury prevention practice. In many ways, injury prevention might be considered an applied science, borrowing from basic methods in other fields, for example, in biomechanics, behavioral and social science, and applying it to injury prevention. Second, not only will the goal of converging the science of injury prevention be advanced by using rigorous, empirically based methodologies, but such methodological rigor will soon be required as managed care organizations and governmental agencies, key resources in health promotion practice (Bronstein, 1999; Capper, 1999), and government funders increasingly require demonstrable evidence of cost-effectiveness of injury prevention programs. It is clear, for example, that the use of theory and methodological rigor is not uniform across different areas of injury research. Indeed, there is marked variability in the use of theory-based interventions and in the use of rigorous randomized controlled trials to assess programmatic efficacy (see Chapter Nine). Third, these increasing requirements to provide documented cost-effectiveness data to support intervention programs will require that injury prevention program planners and interventionists have adequate research training. This will require the training of scientist-practitioners who are capable of both implementing and evaluating injury prevention programs. In fact, academic researchers who are also trained as scientist-practitioners may be best able to appreciate the barriers of service program implementation and best able to advance the field while developing empirically validated programs capable of more broad-scale dissemination than at present.

Conclusions

This volume has outlined the promising developments in theory and design, evaluation, implementation methods, and their application to injury prevention. Examples of different injuries, with varying individual and population risk profiles, and in varying settings with different populations have been highlighted. From this overview, it should be obvious that the field of injury prevention is heterogeneous, multidisciplinary, and rapidly growing. The depth and breadth of research applying social and behavioral sciences to injury prevention is impressive. As new theoretical models and innovative intervention strategies are identified and as societal, health care, and regulatory influences increase their focus on effective prevention strategies, there will be a corresponding increase in the emphasis on the role of the behavioral sciences.

Future injury prevention intervention programs must build on their historical roots. Programs must be developed and evaluated on an ongoing basis to monitor programmatic efficacy—not only by measuring statistically significant changes in theoretically and empirically important mediators and behavioral intentions of injury risk behavior, but more robust indicators as well, such as observed changes in the prelevance of injury risk behaviors and changes in injury itself. Programs must be modified according to evaluation feedback, further refining the intervention and strengthening its potential to effectively promote behavior change. Equally important as program development is a need for effective program translation. Programs that are evaluated and identified as effective should be widely disseminated through diverse channels, and adequate training and program materials should be available to encourage dissemination. Finally, for injury prevention behavioral interventions to progress more rapidly, the development of a comprehensive and coordinated infrastructure to conceptualize, stimulate, and support behavioral science research is necessary. This support needs to involve an array of private and public funding agencies, with careful thought to filling the gaps in behavioral epidemiology, behavioral safety, and other related needs.

Given the human suffering, economic costs, lost productivity, and medical care resources associated with injury, behavioral interventions that demonstrate programmatic efficacy will be an important component in any public health strategy to prevent injury. Furthermore, given the monetary cost of developing and evaluating injury prevention interventions, it is critical that these studies be adequately designed, conducted, analyzed, and reported. While injury prevention programs, adequately funded and innovative in design, offer great potential to effectively reduce risk behaviors and injuries, changes will not happen overnight. Behavior change on a large enough scale will require a comprehensive sustained effort, addressed in an ecological context, and tailored to be relevant and sensitive to the intended population. And, finally, without structured reporting of injury prevention interventions, we run the risk of not identifying potentially effective intervention programs and instead adopting others that may not be effective or have never been empirically demonstrated to be effective.

This is an exciting time to examine injuries from a behavioral perspective. There are new opportunities and new challenges ahead for behavioral scientists to apply their tools, skills, perspectives, and concepts to the public health problem of injuries, but only when they can work side-by-side with public health practitioners and researchers. The application of behavioral and social science theories in injury prevention will help us understand more specifically how behavior and injuries are interlinked. Such information will be valuable in designing injury intervention, prevention, and rehabilitation programs in the future.

References

Begg, C., Cho, M., Eastwood, S., Horton, R., Moher, D., Olkin, I., Pitkin, R., Rennie, D., Schulz, K. F., Simel, D., & Stroup, D. F. (1996). Improving the quality of reporting of randomized controlled trials: The CONSORT statement. *Journal of the American Medical Association, 276,* 637–639.

Blumenthal, D. S., & DiClemente, R. J. (2004). *Community-based health research: Issues and methods.* New York: Springer.

Bronstein, J. M. (1999). The role of health care organizations in health promotion and disease prevention. In J. Raczynski & R. J. DiClemente (Eds.), *Handbook of health promotion and disease prevention* (pp. 607–620). New York: Plenum Press.

Capper, S. (1999). The role of governmental public health agencies. In J. Raczynski & R. J. DiClemente (Eds.), *Handbook of health promotion and disease prevention* (pp. 621–636). New York: Plenum Press.

Capilouto, E. (1999). Determining the cost-effectiveness of health promotion programs. In J. Raczynski & R. J. DiClemente (Eds.), *Handbook of health promotion and disease prevention* (pp. 637–652). New York: Plenum Press

DiClemente, R. J., Crosby, R. A., & Kegler, M. (2002). *Emerging theories in health promotion research and practice: Strategies for enhancing public health.* San Francisco: Jossey-Bass.

Finkelstein, E., Corso, P., & Miller, T. R. (2006). *The Incidence and Economic Burden of Injuries in the U.S., 2000*. New York: Oxford University Press.

Green, L. W. (2005). Retrieved Oct. 30, 2005, from http://lgreen.net/authors/lwgreen.htm.

Haddix, A. C., Teutsch, S. M., Shaffer, P. A., & Dunet, D. O. (1996). *Prevention effectiveness*. New York: Oxford University Press.

Hale, A. R., & Glendon, A. I. (1987). *Individual behavior in the control of danger*. Netherlands: Elsevier.

National Cancer Institute. (2005, June). *President's Cancer Panel: Translating research into cancer care, delivering on the promise*. Bethesda, MD: National Institutes of Health.

Sogolow, E., Saul, J., & Sleet, D. (2006). Toward a dissemination model: Moving science-based injury interventions to practice. In L. Doll, J. Mercy, S. Bonzo, & D. Sleet (Eds.), *Handbook of injury and violence prevention*. New York: Springer.

Sleet, D. A., & Hopkins, K. (Eds.). (2004). *Bibliography on behavioral science research in unintentional injury prevention* [CD-ROM]. Atlanta, GA: Centers for Disease Control and Prevention. www.cdc.gov/pub-res/behavioral.

Standards of Reporting Clinical Trials Group. (1994). A proposal for structured reporting of randomized clinical trials. *Journal of the American Medical Association, 272*, 1926–1931.

Svanstrom, L., Boleslav, J., & Grivna, M. (2004). *Sustainability within safe communities*. Prague: Centrum Urazove Prevence.

Wallack, L., Dorfman, L., Jernigan, D., & Themba, M. (1993). *Media advocacy and public health: Power for prevention*. Thousand Oaks, CA: Sage.

Zaza, S., Carande-Kulis, V. G., Sleet, D. A., Sosin, D., Elder, R., Shults, R., Dinh-Zarr, T., Nichols, J., & Thompson, R. (2001). Methods for conducting systematic reviews of the evidence of effectiveness and economic efficiency of interventions to reduce injuries to motor vehicle occupants. *American Journal of Preventive Medicine, 21*(4s), 23–30.

APPENDIX: FEDERAL INJURY AND VIOLENCE-RELATED DATA SYSTEMS

Joseph L. Annest, David A. Sleet

In recent years, the number and breadth of injury and violence-related databases available to injury prevention researchers and practitioners have grown substantially. Federal agencies, private research organizations, and state and local groups have posted Web sites that contain useful data on unintentional injuries, interpersonal violence, and intentional self-harm. As part of its mission is to reduce morbidity, disability, death, and costs associated with injuries, the National Center for Injury Prevention and Control (NCIPC) at CDC works closely with other federal agencies; national, state, and local organizations; state and local health departments; and academic institutions to provide access to the best available injury-related data. NCIPC also is working to improve the quality and availability of injury data and injury databases. Accurate and comprehensive data are essential for injury research, monitoring trends in injury events, developing and evaluating the effectiveness of injury prevention programs, and providing the basis for decision by policymakers and the public aimed at reducing injuries in America and internationally. CDC is committed to improving injury surveillance and data systems. Part of our efforts, an inventory of federal data systems, was developed to identify current sources of national data on injury mortality, morbidity, and risk factors.

Following is a list of thirty-seven federal data systems that provide injury-related data. In addition, three private injury-related databases are listed where the sponsor maintains the Internet site for public use. Web sites or URLs are provided for each data system where the public can go to get information about the database, survey and surveillance methods, and findings. Data systems are organized by topic. Some data systems are listed more than once depending on their relevance to different topics. This inventory of Web sites is intended to help readers find useful and relevant injury- and violence-related data online. We recognize that Internet Web pages are posted and taken down every day. We do not claim this is a comprehensive list, and we have not evaluated these sites with any standard criteria for usefulness or consumer-friendliness. We have verified that each URL is authentic and linked to the source specified, as of the final publication date of this book. Their listing here implies no endorsement of the data or the sources of the data, except those collected and provided by CDC.

Behavioral Risk Factors and Injury Incidence

Behavioral Risk Factor Survey System (BRFSS), CDC-NCCDPHP, annual survey. http://www.cdc.gov/brfss/

Youth Risk Behavior Survey (YRBS), CDC-NCCDPHP, biennial school-based survey for state/local, occasional national survey. http://www.cdc.gov/nccdphp/dash/yrbs/index.htm

Injury Control and Risk of Injury Survey (ICARIS). National Center for Injury Prevention and Control, CDC, periodic telephone interview survey. No Web site available. Contact Marcie Kresnow at CDC: mkresnow@cdc.gov

National Health Interview Survey (NHIS), CDC-NCHS, annual household survey. http://www.cdc.gov/nchs/nhis.htm

Injury Morbidity Data

National Electronic Injury Surveillance System (NEISS) (CPSC), NEISS All Injury Program (CPSC/CDC-NCIPC), and NEISS-work-related injury (CPSC/CDC-NIOSH)-ongoing. http://www.cpsc.gov/epidemiology/; http://www.cpsc.gov/library/neiss.html; http://www.cdc.gov/ncipc/wisqars; http://www2.cdc.gov/risqs/default.asp (work-related injury)

National Hospital Ambulatory Medical Care Survey (NHAMCS), CDC-NCHS, annual survey. http://www.cdc.gov/nchs/about/major/ahcd/ahcd1.htm

National Ambulatory Medical Care Survey (NAMCS), CDC-NCHS, annual survey. http://www.cdc.gov/nchs/about/major/ahcd/ahcd1.htm

National Hospital Discharge Survey (NHDS), CDC-NCHS, annual survey. http://www.cdc.gov/nchs/about/major/hdasd/nhds.htm

Healthcare Cost and Utilization Project (HCUP), AHRQ. http://www.ahrq.gov/data/hcup/

Indian Health Service-Ambulatory Care and Inpatient Care Systems, IHS, ongoing. http://www.ihs.gov/nonmedicalprograms/ihs%5Fstats/

Injury Deaths and Death Certificates

National Vital Statistics System (NVSS), CDC-NCHS, ongoing. http://www.cdc.gov/nchs/nvss.htm

National Mortality Follow-back Survey-1993 (NMFS93), CDC-NCHS, periodic. http://www.cdc.gov/nchs/about/major/nmfs/nmfs.htm

Automotive Injury Data

Fatality Analysis Reporting System (FARS), NHTSA, motor vehicle traffic crash deaths, ongoing. http://www-fars.nhtsa.dot.gov/

National Automotive Sampling System-General Estimates System (NASS-GES), NHTSA, annual. http://www-nrd.nhtsa.dot.gov/departments/nrd-30/ncsa/ges.html

National Automotive Sampling System-Crashworthiness Data System (NASS-CDS), NHTSA, annual. http://www-nrd.nhtsa.dot.gov/departments/nrd-30/ncsa/cds.html

NHTSA Special Crash Investigation (SCI), NHTSA, (includes air-bag related injuries), ongoing. http://www-nrd.nhtsa.dot.gov/departments/nrd-30/ncsa/sci.html

Air Bag Fatality Summary Report and Tables. Cases shown as having a case status of "Available" can be found at: http://www-nass.nhtsa.dot.gov/BIN/logon.exe/airmislogon

Automotive Behavioral Injury Data

National Occupant Protection Use Survey (NOPUS), NHTSA, periodic. http://www-nrd.nhtsa.dot.gov/departments/nrd-01/summaries/4313ga.html

Motor Vehicle Occupant Safety Survey, NHTSA, biennial. http://www.nhtsa.dot.gov/people/injury/research/occu_protection.html

National Survey of Drinking and Driving Attitudes and Behaviors, NHTSA, periodic. http://www.nhtsa.dot.gov/people/injury/research/alcohol_impaired.html

Occupational Injury Data

National Traumatic Occupational Fatality Surveillance System (NTOF), CDC-NIOSH, ongoing. http://www.cdc.gov/niosh/injury

National Electronic Injury Surveillance System—Work RISQ—Nonfatal work-related injuries. http://www2.cdc.gov/risqs/default.asp

Census of Fatal Occupational Injuries (CFOI), BLS, ongoing. http://www.bls.gov/iif/oshfat1.htm

Survey of Occupational Injuries and Illnesses (SOII), BLS, annual survey. http://www.bls.gov/iif/home.htm

Census of Agriculture (COA), DOC, periodic. http://www.nass.usda.gov/census. Note: Although available reports do not provide injury statistics, the 1992 Census of Agriculture did ask questions about the number of work-related injuries. More recent COAs do not ask about injury.

Violent Death Data

National Incident Based Reporting System (NIBRS), FBI, ongoing. http://www.fbi.gov/hq/cjisd/ucr.htm

Law Enforcement Officers Killed and Assaulted (LEOKA), FBI, ongoing. http://www.fbi.gov/ucr/ucr.htm

National Violent Death Reporting System (CDC-NVDRS), CDC-NCIPC, ongoing. http://www.cdc.gov/ncipc/profiles/nvdrs/facts.htm

Uniform Crime Reports-Supplemental Homicide Reports (UCR-SHR), FBI, ongoing. http://www.fbi.gov/ucr/ucr.htm

Crime and Victimization Data

National Crime Victimization Survey (NCFS), BJS, annual survey. http://www.ojp.usdoj.gov/bjs/cvict.htm

National Child Abuse and Neglect Data System (NCANDS), NCCAN, annual. http://nccanch.acf.hhs.gov/

http://www.hhs.gov/news/press/2003pres/20030401.html

National Incidence Study of Child Abuse and Neglect (NIS), NCCAN, periodic. http://nccanch.acf.hhs.gov/

National Violence Against Women Survey, was conducted only once in 1995–1996 by NIJ and NCIPC. Although there is no Web site, publications from the survey are all available on the Web: http://www.ncjrs.org/pdffiles1/nij/181867.pdf; http://www.ncjrs.org/pdffiles1/nij/183781.pdf; http://www.ncjrs.org/pdffiles/169592.pdf; http://www.ncjrs.org/pdffiles/172837.pdf

Drug Abuse Data

Drug Abuse Warning Network (DAWN), SAMHSA, ongoing. http://www.dawninfo.samhsa.gov

National Survey on Drug Use and Health, formerly called the National Household Survey on Drug Abuse (NHSDA), SAMHSA, annual. http://www.oas.samhsa.gov/nhsda.htm

Monitoring the Future Survey (MTFS), NIDA, school-based, annual. http://www.nida.nih.gov/DrugPages/mtf.html

Other Injury Data

National Fire Incident Reporting System (NFIRS), FA, ongoing. http://www.usfa.fema.gov/inside-usfa/nfirs.cfm. Enter manually on title line of Web search.

Health Care Finance Administration-5% Sample Standard Analysis File (SAF) and Medicare Provider Analysis and Review (MEDPAR) File, HCFA, ongoing. http://www.cms.hhs.gov/statistics/medpar/default.asp

Private (Nonfederal) Injury-Related Data Systems

Trauma care/poisoning data: National Trauma Data Bank (NTDB)–American College of Surgeons, ongoing. http://www.facs.org/dept/trauma/ntdb.html

Toxic Exposure Surveillance System (TESS)—American Association of Poisoning Control Centers, annual. http://www.aapcc.org/poison1.htm

United States Eye Injury Registry—American Society of Ocular Trauma. http://www.useironline.org

NAME INDEX

SUBJECT INDEX

A

AAYP (Aban Aya Youth Project), 378

ABC model: applied to BBS approach, 304; applied to changing behavior, 33; direct persuasion using, 312–313

ABS (antilock braking systems), 224

Abusive Behavior Inventory, 332

Accident: as banned term by U.S. National Traffic Safety Administration, 88; public's persistent use of term, 85, 88; "Swiss cheese" model of, 478

ADI (administrative driver improvement) program, 222

Administrative diagnosis, 139

Administrative law, 446–447

Administrative Procedure Act (1946), 446–447

Adolescents: CDC on motor vehicle injuries/death among, 56; Checkpoints Program to prevent motor vehicle crashes among, 56–58t, 59; GDL (Graduated driver licensing) policy for dri-

ving, 56; sports/recreational injuries in, 257–269; suicide morbidity of, 349–350; youth violence and, 368–388; YRBS (Youth Risk Behavior Survey) on, 174–175, 182–183*fig. See also* Children

Adoption: of innovation, 71; PAP (precaution adoption process) Model on, 91; PAPM (precaution adoption process model), 21, 29–32, 31*fig*

African Americans: AAYP participation by youth, 378; alcohol-related traffic fatalities and, 237; assessing fighting behavior/attitudes of youth, 371

Age: alcohol-related traffic crashes and, 236; fatal and nonfatal home injuries by, 276t–277t, 278; suicide rates by, 348

Agricultural Extension Services, 70

AID (alcohol-impaired driver): characteristics of, 236–238; impaired driving by, 234; relationship between binge drinking and, 240

Air bags: "excessive trust" in, 479; as passive protection, 5–6, 8

Alaskan Natives, homicide as leading cause of death for, 369

Alcohol-related traffic crashes: characteristics of those involved in, 236–238; interventions to reduce, 238, 240–249. *See also* BAC (blood alcohol concentration)

ALR (administrative license revocation), 220

American Academy of Child and Adolescent Psychiatry, 358

American Academy of Pediatrics, 279, 283

American Association of Poison Control Centers, 281

American Association of Retired Persons, 283

American College of Sports Medicine, 258

American Geriatric Society, 280

American Journal of Preventive Medicine, 197

American Psychological Association (APA), 12, 421